SURGERY
A CLINICAL APPROACH

ASK A | **ACCOMPANIED BY CD-ROM** | **D-ROM**

1

11

102

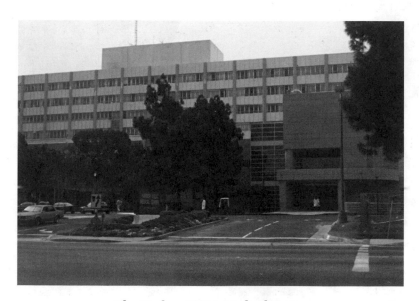

The Harbor-UCLA Medical Center

SURGERY
A CLINICAL APPROACH

EDITED BY

FRED S. BONGARD, M.D.

Associate Professor, Department of Surgery, University of California, Los Angeles, UCLA School of Medicine, Los Angeles, California; Chief, Division of Trauma and Critical Care, Director of Surgical Education, Department of Surgery, Harbor-UCLA Medical Center, Torrance, California

MICHAEL J. STAMOS, M.D.

Associate Professor, Department of Surgery, University of California, Los Angeles, UCLA School of Medicine, Los Angeles, California; Chief, Section of Colon and Rectal Surgery, Department of Surgery, Harbor-UCLA Medical Center, Torrance, California

EDWARD PASSARO, JR., M.D.

Professor, Department of Surgery, University of California, Los Angeles, UCLA School of Medicine; Chief, Surgical Service, Department of Surgery, West Los Angeles Veterans Affairs Medical Center, Los Angeles, California

Illustrations by William Tocci, M.S.

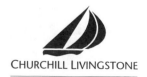

CHURCHILL LIVINGSTONE

New York, Edinburgh, London, Madrid, Melbourne, San Francisco, Tokyo

Library of Congress Cataloging-in-Publication Data

Surgery : a clinical approach / edited by Fred S. Bongard, Michael J.
Stamos, Edward Passaro, Jr. ; illustrated by William Tocci.
    p.   cm.
  Includes bibliographical references and index.
  ISBN 0-443-08994-9 (alk. paper)
  1. Surgery.   I. Stamos, Michael J. II. Passaro, Edward.
  [DNLM: 1. Surgery, Operative. WO 500 S9612 1997]
  RD31.S9114   1997
  617—dc20
  DNLM/DLC
  for Library of Congress   96-41027
                                       CIP

Distributed in the United Kingdom by Churchill Livingstone, Robert Steven-
son House, 1–3 Baxter's Place, Leith Walk, Edinburgh EH1 3AF, and by associated companies, branches, and representatives throughout the world.

Medical knowledge is constantly changing. As new information becomes
available, changes in treatment, procedures, equipment and the use of drugs
become necessary. The editors/authors/contributors and the publishers have,
as far as it is possible, taken care to ensure that the information given in this
text is accurate and up to date. However, readers are strongly advised to confirm that the information, especially with regard to drug usage, complies with
the latest legislation and standards of practice.

The Publishers have made every effort to trace the copyright holders for bor-
rowed material. If they have inadvertently overlooked any, they will be
pleased to make the necessary arrangements at the first opportunity.

Acquisitions Editor: *Marc Strauss*
Production Editor: *Bridgett L. Dickinson*
Production Supervisor: *Laura Mosberg Cohen*
Desktop Publishing Coordinator: *Barbara Ulbrich*
Cover Design: *Jeannette Jacobs*

Printed in the United States of America

First published in 1997   7 6 5 4 3 2 1

CONTRIBUTORS

FRITZ BAUMGARTNER, M.D.

Assistant Professor, Department of Surgery, University of California, Los Angeles, UCLA School of Medicine, Los Angeles, California; Chief, Division of Cardiothoracic Surgery, Department of Surgery, Harbor-UCLA Medical Center, Torrance, California

MARVIN BERGSNEIDER, M.D.

Assistant Professor, Department of Surgery, University of California, Los Angeles, UCLA School of Medicine, Los Angeles, California; Division of Neurosurgery, Department of Surgery, Harbor-UCLA Medical Center, Torrance, California

FRED S. BONGARD, M.D.

Associate Professor, Department of Surgery, University of California, Los Angeles, UCLA School of Medicine, Los Angeles, California; Chief, Division of Trauma and Critical Care, Director of Surgical Education, Department of Surgery, Harbor-UCLA Medical Center, Torrance, California

RINALDO CANALIS, M.D.

Professor, Department of Surgery, University of California, Los Angeles, UCLA School of Medicine, Los Angeles, California; Chief, Division of Head and Neck Surgery, Department of Surgery, Harbor-UCLA Medical Center, Torrance, California

CHRISTIAN DE VIRGILIO, M.D.

Assistant Professor, Department of Surgery, University of California, Los Angeles, UCLA School of Medicine, Los Angeles, California; Division of Vascular Surgery, Department of Surgery, Harbor-UCLA Medical Center, Torrance, California

CARLOS E. DONAYRE, M.D.

Assistant Professor, Department of Surgery, University of California, Los Angeles, UCLA School of Medicine, Los Angeles, California; Division of Vascular Surgery, Department of Surgery, Harbor-UCLA Medical Center, Torrance, California

PAVEL DULGEUROV, M.D.

Assistant Professor of Medicine, Department of Otolaryngology, University of Geneva School of Medicine; Staff Physician, Department of Otolaryngology, University of Geneva Medical Center, Geneva, Switzerland

GERHARD J. FUCHS, M.D.

Associate Clinical Professor, Department of Surgery, University of California, Los Angeles, UCLA School of Medicine, Los Angeles, California

CLAUDINE GYSIN, M.D.

Fellow in Residence, Department of Otolaryngology, University of Geneva School of Medicine, Geneva, Switzerland

CHARLES N. HEADRICK, M.D.

Assistant Clinical Professor, Department of Surgery, University of California, Los Angeles, UCLA School of Medicine, Los Angeles, California; Division of Colon and Rectal Surgery, Department of Surgery, Harbor-UCLA Medical Center, Torrance, California

DAVID K. IMAGAWA, M.D.

Assistant Professor, Department of Surgery, University of California, Irving, College of Medicine, Irving, California; Director UCI/UCLA Liver Transplant Program; Director, UCLA Transplant Laboratory, Los Angeles, California

CYNTHIA M. KELLY, M.D.

Instructor, Department of Surgery, University of California, Los Angeles, UCLA School of Medicine, Los Angeles, California

DANIEL F. KELLY, M.D.

Assistant Professor, Department of Surgery, University of California, Los Angeles, UCLA School of Medicine, Los Angeles, California; Division of Neurosurgery, Department of Surgery, Harbor-UCLA Medical Center, Torrance, California

MILAN KINKHABWALA, M.D.

Assistant Professor, Department of Surgery, Cornell University Medical College; Director, Pancreas Transplant Program, Department of Surgery, New York Hospital-Cornell Medical Center, New York, New York

STANLEY R. KLEIN, M.D.

Associate Professor, Department of Surgery, University of California, Los Angeles, UCLA School of Medicine, Los Angeles, California; Chief, Division of Surgical Oncology, Department of Surgery, Harbor-UCLA Medical Center, Torrance, California

TAI-SHION LEE, M.D.

Professor, Department of Anesthesiology, University of California, Los Angeles, UCLA School of Medicine, Los Angeles, California

MALCOLM LESAVOY, M.D.

Professor, Department of Surgery, University of California, Los Angeles, UCLA School of Medicine, Los Angeles, California; Chief, Division of Plastic and Reconstructive Surgery, Department of Surgery, Harbor-UCLA Medical Center, Torrance, California

MARK S. LITWIN, M.D.

Assistant Professor, Department of Surgery, University of California, Los Angeles, UCLA School of Medicine, Los Angeles, California; Division of Urology, Department of Surgery, Harbor-UCLA Medical Center, Torrance, California

DUNCAN Q. MCBRIDE, M.D.

Associate Professor of Clinical Surgery, Department of Surgery, University of California, Los Angeles, UCLA School of Medicine, Los Angeles, California; Chief, Division of Neurosurgery, Department of Surgery, Harbor-UCLA Medical Center, Torrance, California

THOMAS C. MOORE, M.D.

Professor, Department of Surgery, University of California, Los Angeles, UCLA School of Medicine, Los Angeles, California; Division of Pediatric Surgery, Department of Surgery, Harbor-UCLA Medical Center, Torrance, California

GERALD MOSS, M.D.

Assistant Clinical Professor, Department of Surgery, University of California, Los Angeles, UCLA School of Medicine, Los Angeles, California; Division of Surgical Oncology, Department of Surgery, Harbor-UCLA Medical Center, Torrance, California

SINA NASRI, M.D.

Surgery Fellow, Department of Otolaryngology, Stanford University School of Medicine, Palo Alto, California, and University of California, Los Angeles, UCLA School of Medicine, Los Angeles, California

GIDEON P. NAUDE, M.D.

Clinical Instructor, Department of Surgery, University of California, Los Angeles, UCLA School of Medicine, Los Angeles, California; Division of Trauma and Critical Care, Department of Surgery, Harbor-UCLA Medical Center, Torrance, California

EDWARD PASSARO, JR., M.D.

Professor, Department of Surgery, University of California, Los Angeles, UCLA School of Medicine; Chief, Surgical Service, Department of Surgery, West Los Angeles Veterans Affairs Medical Center, Los Angeles, California

JACOB RAJFER, M.D.

Professor, Department of Surgery, University of California, Los Angeles, UCLA School of Medicine, Los Angeles, California; Chief, Division of Urology, Department of Surgery, Harbor-UCLA Medical Center, Torrance, California

MICHAEL RIDGEWAY, M.D.

Fellow in Surgical Oncology, Department of Surgery, Harbor-UCLA Medical Center, Torrance, California

GENE ROBINSON, M.D.

Division of General Surgery, Department of Surgery, Harbor-UCLA Medical Center, Torrance, California

THOMAS P. SCHMALZRIED, M.D.

Assistant Clinical Professor, Department of Surgery, University of California, Los Angeles, UCLA School of Medicine, Los Angeles, California; Division of Orthopaedic Surgery, Department of Surgery, Harbor-UCLA Medical Center, Torrance, California

MARCO SCOCCIANTI, M.D.

Clinical Instructor, Department of Surgery, University of California, Los Angeles, UCLA School of Medicine, Los Angeles, California; Division of Vascular Surgery, Department of Surgery, Harbor-UCLA Medical Center, Torrance, California

JOEL A. SERCARZ, M.D.

Assistant Professor, Department of Surgery, University of California, Los Angeles, UCLA School of Medicine, Los Angeles, California; Attending Physician, Division of Otolaryngology, Department of Surgery, Harbor-UCLA Medical Center, Torrance, California

R. KENDRICK SLATE, M.D.

Assistant Professor, Department of Surgery, University of California, Los Angeles, UCLA School of Medicine, Los Angeles, California; Division of Plastic and Reconstructive Surgery, Department of Surgery, Harbor-UCLA Medical Center, Torrance, California

BRUCE E. STABILE, M.D.

Professor and Vice-Chairman, Department of Surgery, University of California, Los Angeles, UCLA School of Medicine, Los Angeles, California; Chairman, Department of Surgery, Harbor-UCLA Medical Center, Torrance, California

MICHAEL J. STAMOS, M.D.

Associate Professor, Department of Surgery, University of California, Los Angeles, UCLA School of Medicine, Los Angeles, California; Chief, Division of Colon and Rectal Surgery, Department of Surgery, Harbor-UCLA Medical Center, Torrance, California

HERNAN I. VARGAS, M.D.

Assistant Professor, Department of Surgery, University of California, Los Angeles, UCLA School of Medicine, Los Angeles, California; Division of Surgical Oncology, Department of Surgery, Harbor-UCLA Medical Center, Torrance, California

MARILENE B. WANG, M.D.

Associate Professor-in-Residence, Division of Head and Neck Surgery, Department of Surgery, University of California, Los Angeles, UCLA School of Medicine; Staff Surgeon, ENT Section, Department of Surgery, West Los Angeles Veterans Affairs Medical Center, Los Angeles, California

RODNEY A. WHITE, M.D.

Professor, Department of Surgery, University of California, Los Angeles, UCLA School of Medicine, Los Angeles, California; Chief, Vascular Surgery, Associate Chair, Department of Surgery, Harbor-UCLA Medical Center, Torrance, California

DANIEL ZINAR, M.D.

Associate Professor, Department of Surgery, University of California, Los Angeles, UCLA School of Medicine, Los Angeles, California; Chief, Division of Orthopaedic Surgery, Department of Surgery, Harbor-UCLA Medical Center, Torrance, California

FOREWORD

Surgery: A Clinical Approach represents a unique and very special achievement by the surgical faculty at Harbor-UCLA Medical Center. The idea for the book was spawned by the recognition of an unmet need among today's medical students and house staff. That need relates to the explosion of factual knowledge within the surgical disciplines that all too often leaves the students and residents overwhelmed and bewildered. In response to this conundrum, the editors of this text set out to abstract and codify principles, concepts, and essential surgical knowledge into a form and format that not only should but *could* be assimilated during a brief surgical clerkship. In a unique departure from conventional texts, they have also provided a CD-ROM keyed to the text that is intended to provide the reader with as much relevant data as desired. Thus, *Surgery: A Clinical Approach* has been created specifically to be an introductory text rather than a comprehensive compendium of surgical facts. It has been designed to stress principles and concepts more than the acquisition of data, although the latter has been made readily available. The inclusion of case presentations at the beginning of each chapter is intended to immerse the student immediately into the "real world" of clinical surgery in a way that is stimulating and that facilitates acquisition and integration of the chapter's essential information. It is the wish of the editors and contributors that the book be genuinely fun to read. The addition of "Key Points" highlight boxes, which summarize the most important information, is meant to save the student time and permit rapid and efficient review.

The assembly of this text was, of course, a great amount of work for the authors and a tremendous undertaking on the part of the editors. All who contributed are actively engaged in the education of medical students, residents, and practicing surgeons. More importantly, all are deeply concerned with and committed to teaching and wanted this to be an institutional effort. The character of the book clearly bears the imprint of the faculty's approach to student education. It is our hope that *Surgery: A Clinical Approach* will serve not only to provide clinically useful concepts and information, but also to stimulate the interest and curiosity of all students of surgery.

Bruce E. Stabile, M.D.
Professor and Vice-Chairman
Department of Surgery
University of California, Los Angeles,
UCLA School of Medicine
Los Angeles, California
Chairman
Department of Surgery
Harbor-UCLA Medical Center
Torrence, California

CONTENTS

ABBREVIATIONS

AAA	abdominal aortic aneurysm	**COM**	chronic otitis media
A-aDO$_2$	alveolar-arterial oxygen content gradient	**COPD**	chronic obstructive pulmonary disease
ABI	ankle brachial index	**CPAP**	continuous positive airway pressure
AC	assist control	**CPP**	cerebral perfusion pressure
ACTH	adrenocorticotropic hormone	**CRF**	corticotropin release factor
ADH	antidiuretic hormone	**CsA**	cyclosporine
AFP	α-fetoprotein	**CSF**	cerebrospinal fluid
AHF	antihemophilic factor	**CT**	computed tomography
AIDS	acquired immunodeficiency syndrome	**CVA**	costovertebral angle
ALT	alanine aminotransferase	**CVP**	central venous pressure
AMBU	assisted mechanical breathing unit	**D$_5$W**	5% dextrose in water
ANA	antinuclear antibodies	**DCIS**	ductal carcinoma in situ
AOM	acute otitis media	**DIC**	disseminated intravascular coagulation
APR	abdominal perineal resection	**DIP**	distal interphalangeal
ARDS	adult respiratory distress syndrome	**DNA**	deoxyribonucleic acid
5-ASA	aminosalicylic acid	**DO$_2$**	oxygen delivery
ASD	atrial septal defect	**DVT**	deep venous thrombosis
AST	aspartate aminotransferase	**EBV**	Epstein-Barr virus
ATN	acute tubular necrosis	**ECG**	electrocardiogram
AUA	American Urologic Association	**ECM**	erythema chronicum migrans
(a-v)DO$_2$	arterial-venous oxygen content gradient	**ECMO**	extracorporeal membrane oxygenation
AV	atrioventricular	**EGD**	esophagogastroduodenoscopy
AVM	arteriovenous malformation	**ELISA**	enzyme-linked immunosorbent assay
BCC	basal cell carcinoma	**EMG**	electromyograph
BCG	bacillus Calmette-Guerin	**ERCP**	endoscopic retrograde cholangiopancreatography
ß-hCG	ß-human chorionic gonadotropin	**ESR**	erythrocyte sedimentation rate
BMA	bone marrow aspiration	**ESRD**	end-stage renal disease
BPH	benign prostatic hyperplasia	**ESWL**	extracorporeal shock wave lithotripsy
bpm	beats per minute	**EtOH**	ethanol
CABG	coronary artery bypass graft	**FAP**	familial adenomatous polyposis
CAM	congenital adenomatoid malformation	**FEV$_1$**	forced expiratory volume in 1 second
CaO$_2$	arterial oxygen content	**FFP**	fresh frozen plasma
CAS	carotid artery stenosis	**FNA**	fine needle aspiration
CBC	complete blood count	**FNH**	focal nodular hyperplasia
CEA	carcinoembryonic antigen	**G-CSF**	granulocyte colony-stimulating factor
CHF	congestive heart failure	**GCS**	Glasgow Coma Scale
CIS	carcinoma in situ	**GFR**	glomerular filtration rate
CMV	continuous mandatory ventilation	**GGT**	gamma-glutamyl transpeptidase
CMV	cytomegalovirus	**H$_2$**	histamine-2 (receptor)
CO	cardiac output	**HAT**	hepatic artery thrombosis
CO$_2$	carbon dioxide	**Hb**	hemoglobin

HbSat	hemoglobin saturation	**PE**	pulmonary embolism
Hct	hematocrit	**PGE$_1$**	prostaglandin E$_1$
HgBAic	glycated hemoglobin	**PIP**	proximal interphalangeal
HIDA	dimethyl-iminodiacetic acid	**PMN**	polymorphonuclear neutrophil (leukocyte)
HIV	human immunodeficiency virus	**PO**	oral
HLA	human leukocyte antigen (histocompatibility antigens)	**PO$_2$**	oxygen partial pressure
HNPCC	hereditary nonpolyposis colon cancer	**PPD**	purified protein derivative
HPF	high power field	**PRBC**	packed red blood cell
HR	heart rate	**PSA**	prostate-specific antigen
HTO	high tibial osteotomy	**PT**	prothrombin time
IBD	inflammatory bowel disease	**PTH**	parathyroid hormone; parathormone
ICA	internal carotid artery	**PTT**	partial thromboplastin time
ICP	intracranial pressure	**RA**	test for rheumatoid factors
ICU	intensive care unit	**RBC**	red blood cell
IDA	iminodiacetic acid	**RF**	rheumatoid factor
IL	interleukin	**RIA**	radioimmunoassay
IM	intramuscular	**RIND**	reversible ischemic neurologic deficit
IMA	inferior mesenteric artery	**RNA**	ribonucleic acid
IMV	intermittent mandatory ventilation	**RPLND**	retroperitoneal lymph node dissection
INH	isoniazid	**RQ**	respiratory quotient
IV	intravenous	**SaO$_2$**	arterial oxygen hemoglobin saturation
JNA	juvenile rheumatoid arthritis	**SCC**	squamous cell carcinoma
KOH	potassium hydroxide	**SGOT**	serum glutamic oxaloacetic transaminase
KUB	kidney-ureter-bladder	**SGPT**	serum glutamic pyruvic transaminase
LBO	large bowel obstruction	**SIMV**	synchronized intermittent mandatory ventilation
LCIS	lobular carcinoma in situ	**SLE**	systemic lupus erythematosus
LDH	lactate dehydrogenase	**SMA**	superior mesenteric artery
LES	lower esophageal sphincter	**SOM**	secretory otitis media
LFT	liver function test	**SPEP**	serum protein electrophoresis
MAP	mean arterial pressure	**S$\bar{v}$O$_2$**	mixed venous oxygen hemoglobin saturation
MB	myocardial band	**t-PA**	tissue plasminogen activator
MCP	metacarpophalangeal	**T3**	triiodothyronine
MCV	mean corpuscular volume	**T4**	thyroxine
MEN	multiple endocrine neoplasia	**TB**	tuberculosis
6MP	6-mercaptopurine	**TBSA**	total body surface area
mph	miles per hour	**TCC**	transitional cell carcinoma
MRI	magnetic resonance imaging	**Td**	tetanus toxoid
N$_2$O	nitrous oxide	**TGNM**	cancer classification (tumor grade node metastasis)
NCV	nerve conduction study	**TIA**	transient ischemic attack
NEC	necrotizing enterocolitis	**TIPS**	transjugular intrahepatic portosystemic shunt
NG	nasogastric	**TEA**	transluminal angioplasty
NIH	National Institutes of Health	**TN**	tumor necrosis factor
NL	normal	**TIM**	cancer classification system (tumor node metastasis)
NO	nitric oxide	**TRH**	thyrotropin releasing hormone
NPO	nothing by mouth; nothing per os	**TSP**	thyroid stimulating hormone
NS	normal saline	**TT**	thrombin time
NSAID	nonsteroidal anti-inflammatory drug	**TURP**	transurethral resection of the prostate
OLT	orthotopic liver transplantation	**UGI**	upper gastrointestinal (series)
OM	otitis media	**UTI**	urinary tract infection
OPLL	ossification of the posterior longitudinal ligament	**UPEP**	urine protein electrophoresis
OPO	organ procurement organizations	**US**	ultrasonography
PaO$_2$	arterial oxygen partial pressure	**UUN**	urine urea nitrogen
PCA	patient controlled analgesia	**$\dot{V}$E**	minute volume
PCO$_2$	carbon dioxide partial pressure	**VMA**	vanillylmandelic acid
PCP	phencyclidine	**$\dot{V}$O$_2$**	peripheral consumption of oxygen
PCWP	pulmonary capillary wedge pressure	**VSD**	ventricular septal defect
PDA	patent ductus arteriosus	**WBC**	white blood cell
		WNL	within normal limits

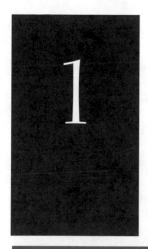

1 ABOUT SURGERY:
A CLINICAL
APPROACH

FRED S. BONGARD

MICHAEL J. STAMOS

EDWARD PASSARO, JR.

*S*urgery: A Clinical Approach was written at the specific request of medical students for a concise but complete textbook of general surgery and the surgical subspecialties that could be read and mastered in limited time. It incorporates a novel approach: a text that is clinically formatted but that stresses principles and concepts, complimented by a CD-ROM. Although several "standard" textbooks are available, they are too complex and lengthy for a clinical clerk to complete during an 8–12 week rotation.

The proliferation of medical knowledge over the past several years has created a compunction among book editors that has compelled them to produce texts of leviathan proportions. This may be well and good for the surgical house officer or the surgical practitioner; however, the mere sight of such books fills medical students with confusion and dread. Further, given the pace of current medical progress, particularly in molecular biology, such tomes are often outdated by the time they are published after 2–3 years of preparation. Without specific guidance, which is seldom available (or desirable), it is difficult to decide what material is useful and relevant and what is superfluous. Our students indicated that a concise work providing pertinent information in a readable and patient-based format would be quite welcome. Realizing that

most students reading this book will not become surgeons, our mission became to produce a book that would provide the student and nonsurgical house officer or practitioner with the information necessary to evaluate and care for patients with surgical disease.

Although intended primarily for the medical student, this book should be useful for surgical residents, as well as other interested physicians. The level of information available extends from the concepts and principles to the latest piece of basic or clinical data available. Formatted this way, the book has the potential to "not get old," as the principles will endure while the factual information is constantly updated through Medline. Theoretically, therefore, the limiting factor to information is the reader's use of the text and CD-ROM, rather than the material itself.

THE AUTHORS

This book was conceived and edited by three general surgeons who teach and practice at hospitals affiliated with the University of California at Los Angeles. All of us meet with medical students at least twice a week and are actively involved in the evaluation and evolution of the surgical curriculum.

The chapter authors are colleagues and associates who also participate regularly in medical education. Many of them lecture and/or take part in student seminars and evaluations. All chapters were written by academic faculty, so that the student can be assured of timeliness and accuracy. We have purposely not invited contributors who are not regularly involved in teaching medical students, to avoid the inclusion of material not essential to a core curriculum. Because of the close working relationship between the editors and authors, we had the unique opportunity to produce a work with a uniform writing and illustration style. Virtually all illustrations were drawn by the same artist according to our specifications, to facilitate interpretation and learning. Every chapter has been thoroughly edited and reviewed to ensure that it conforms with the intended style and content guidelines set forth by the editors.

FORMAT AND ORGANIZATION

Our first and most important step was deciding on a format. At variance with virtually all currently available books, we chose a disease-specific approach. A glance through other books demonstrates that diseases are presented under organ groups. For example, peptic ulcer disease is part of the "Stomach" chapter, while diverticulitis is part of the "Colon and Rectum" chapter. This organization is at variance with the way most clinical clerks learn about disease processes. Ward experiences, and even lectures or problem-based learning sessions, revolve around disease processes. This book has been divided into short chapters that each present one disease, or a few closely related disease processes. This format allows students to gain rapidly the information necessary to evaluate and care for their patients.

After deciding on the overall format, we tackled the chapter design. Each of the three editors wrote a sample chapter in the format he thought most appropriate. We chose three widely disparate topics (acid-base disturbances, colon cancer, and hernias) to allow experimenting with approaches that best lent themselves to different subject areas. Over the course of 12 months, we distributed the chapters to our students and entertained anonymous evaluations. Contrary to some of our expectations as well as current educational dogma, we found that (1) chapter objectives are usually not read, (2) illustrations are

helpful only when integrated into the text, (3) references are ignored unless their importance is explained, and (4) unanswered review questions are generally useless. We also learned that (1) problem-based, patient-oriented, presentation facilitates recall, (2) diagnostic and differential diagnostic data are critically important, (3) outcome and follow-up information is an absolute necessity, (4) brevity is a virtue, and (5) facilities for a quick review (*not* open-ended questions) are helpful. With this in hand, we concentrated our efforts on one sample chapter, producing no less than seven revisions, each one of which was evaluated by our students. In the end, we believe that a useful—and enjoyable—format evolved.

Finally, we revised and honed the Table of Contents. Remembering our mission, we strove to include only that information essential to our audience. The general surgery topics are grouped by system, while other topics are organized by discipline. The topics contained within each subspecialty were chosen by the section editor who practices in that area. Again, only the most important and relevant diseases were included.

CHAPTER ORGANIZATION

We strove to maintain a uniform format between chapters and sections. Wherever possible, chapters are introduced by a brief overview, followed by these six sections:

1. *Case presentations.* The cases were chosen to include relevant historical items as well as physical examination and laboratory findings.

2. *General considerations.* This section contains information on epidemiology, anatomy, physiology, and pathogenesis. We have included timely basic science information only when it contributes to a better understanding of the disease process or its treatment.

3. *Diagnosis.* Physical findings, laboratory and imaging studies, and other diagnostic aids are included here.

4. *Differential diagnosis.* This section was the item most frequently requested by our students. We have included information on why other disease entities should or should not be included in the differential. Because it is often difficult for students to distinguish between diseases, we have paid particular attention to this section.

5. *Treatment.* A narrative of treatment options comprises this section. We have attempted to describe only those treatment regimens that are widely accepted and commonly practiced. When new or controversial regimens are included, specific notation of their place in management is made.

6. *Follow-up.* Because of the temporally limited interaction that students have with their patients, instruction on the na-

ture and extent of postsurgical follow-up is often abridged. Mindful of this shortcoming in the educational process, we designed this section to emphasize disease outcome and follow-up procedures. The frequency and extent of physical and laboratory examinations is stressed so that students and nonsurgical practitioners can plan subsequent care.

Two other features merit discussion. Key phrases within the chapters have been summarized in "Key Points" boxes to emphasize the teaching point. Students report that this helps in the identification of important information, as well as facilitating reviews of the chapter at a later date. As our students have found, this reinforces the material just covered in the chapter and provides a superb mechanism for quick reviews. These sections can also be used when an overview of the disease process is required. Such an outline should prove useful in the few minutes available before or after admitting a patient, to ensure that key areas in the history, physical, and laboratory examinations have been included in the initial evaluation. The highlighted sections should also prove useful when reviewing for ward rounds or examinations. The second notable item is the Suggested Readings section. Included are a few citations of particular importance. Typically, these are re-view articles or discussions of current therapy that are particularly useful to the student. We have purposely omitted basic research studies unless they provide indispensable information. A two- or three-sentence description of the content of each reference is included with the citation. These references should provide ample supplemental information if required or desired. When used as intended, the student should not have to consult Index Medicus unless in-depth or historical information is required.

HOW TO USE THIS BOOK

1. *When preparing for patient management.* Review the introductory comments and cases first. Didactic material throughout the chapter will refer to the cases, in order to reinforce items of particular importance. Then, proceed to the subsequent sections to learn about diagnosis and management.

2. *When reviewing.* Read the "Key Points" boxes for a quick overview of the material. Be sure to review the cases whenever possible, because a great deal of supporting information is contained within them.

HELLO!

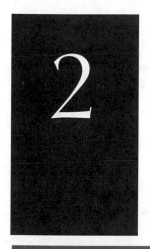

2

FLUIDS,

ELECTROLYTES, AND

ACID-BASE BALANCE

FRED S. BONGARD

Efficient management of fluid and electrolye disorders is an important part of the daily care of inpatients. Unfortunately, the lengthy and esoteric lectures in many books and on rounds make the subject confusing for students. This chapter discusses this vital topic by illustrating the care of two patients and reviews the physiology and mechanics of order writing in fluid and electrolyte/acid-base management.

CASE 1
GASTRIC OUTLET OBSTRUCTION

A 55-year-old male had a long history of peptic ulcer disease. Despite multiple attempts at medical management, he continued to experience epigastric pain and vomiting. On presentation to the emergency room, his abdomen was distended with increased dullness to percussion over the epigastrium. He appeared mildly dehydrated but was not hypotensive and had no orthostatic blood pressure changes. An NG tube returned 1,000 ml of nonbilious material. He was admitted to the hospital and started on an IV infusion of D$_5$W at 150 ml/hr (he weighed 70 kg) with no oral intake.

Over the next several days, the NG tube continued to produce 50 ml/hr of clear nonbilious aspirate. After several days, he began to complain of weakness, generalized fatigue, and constipation. A chemistry panel showed a potassium of 2.8 mEq/L, chloride of 84 mEq/L, and bicarbonate of 31 mEq/L. Potassium replacement was begun with 40 mEq KCl over 6 hours. A repeat electrolyte panel the next day detected a potassium concentra-

tion of 3.0 mEq/L. Blood gas analysis showed a pH of 7.52 and a bicarbonate concentration of 32 mEq/L.

CASE 2
POSTOPERATIVE COMPLICATION

A 52-year-old woman (50 kg) was admitted for elective sigmoid colectomy for diverticular disease. Her operation went well except for unanticipated blood loss of 1 L due to inflammation surrounding her left colon. During the 3-hour operation, she received 5 L of lactated Ringer's solution. The first few days after surgery were uneventful, with the exception of a continued paralytic ileus. She was continued on an IV infusion of D$_5$W with 20 mEq KCl/L. On the fifth day, she began to complain of muscle twitching and anxiety. On the seventh day, she experienced a generalized seizure. During the postictal period she was found to be hypertensive, with marked hyperreflexia. Review of her bedside chart showed that her urine output had been decreasing over the past several days.

5

GENERAL CONSIDERATIONS

Body fluid is found in three spaces: intracellular (42% of total body weight), interstitial (14%), and intravascular (7%). Blood fills the intravascular space and is the portion of the body fluids that clinicians have ready access to. Skeletal muscle makes up most of the intracellular space and is the largest collection of fluids and electrolytes. The interstitial volume is composed of fluid between the other two compartments. Under pathologic conditions, it fills with edema fluid and constitutes part of the *third space*.

Equilibrium between the compartments depends on the relative concentrations of osmotically active particles (osmolals [Osm]) in solution. In clinical usage, the term *tonicity* is interchangeable with *osmolality*. The effective oncotic pressure depends on the number of osmotically active particles that do not pass freely between the semipermeable membranes that separate the compartments. In each compartment, the concentration of particles is normally 285–305 mOsm. An increase in the number of osmolals in one compartment causes a flow of water into that compartment, decreasing its oncotic pressure.

The effect of volume depletion depends on the composition of the fluid lost (Table 2.1). For example, sweat is extremely hypotonic because it contains very little sodium. When a high fever is accompanied by severe sweating, the defect is due primarily to free water loss and results in hypertonic dehydration. This causes fluid to move (translocation) from the interstitial space into the intravascular space, reducing the increased oncotic pressure. Because body secretions are formed by components in the intravascular space, fluid loss due to fistulas, diarrhea, and drains ultimately results in intravascular dehydration. The composition of the fluid lost has a profound effect on the patient's fluid and electrolyte balance. For example, gastric secretions are very high in both chloride and potassium (Table 2.1). Thus, gastric suction leaves the intravascular space low in volume (dehydration), chloride (hypochloremia), and potassium (hypokalemia). When the loss is from the gastrointestinal tract, the resulting hypokalemia may be profound because of the relatively high concentration of potassium in these fluids (Case 1). In an effort to treat the electrolyte imbalance, a sample of the drainage or an aspirate should be sent for chemical analysis when the composition is in doubt.

When considering a patient's fluid requirements, it is useful to think about one's own water intake. The average healthy person consumes about 6 glasses, 8–12 oz each, for a total daily intake of 48–72 oz (1,440–2,160 ml/day). For a 70-kg student, this would be about 20–30 ml/kg/day. Therefore, an adult patient without previous deficits (e.g., vomiting, diarrhea, fistulas) and without ongoing losses (nasogastric [NG] tube loss) the *basal* fluid requirement is 20–30 ml/kg. This varies greatly with a number of factors, such as temperature and the presence of an infection. Smaller patients need less fluid and larger patients need more. A useful rule of thumb for free water requirements is to provide 100 ml/kg/day for the first 10 kg of the patient's weight, 50 ml/kg/day for the next 10 kg, and 20 ml/kg/day for each remaining kilogram. A 70-kg patient requires the following: 10 kg · 100 ml/kg (1 L) + 10 kg · 50 ml/kg (500 ml) + 50 kg · 20 ml/kg (1 L) = 2,500 ml/day of free water. A 23-kg child would need 10 kg · 100 ml/kg (1 L) + 10 kg · 50 ml/kg (500 ml) + 3 kg · 20 ml/kg (60 ml) = 1,560 ml/day of free water. This formula exceeds the normal intake of most healthy people, but with normal renal function the excess is well tolerated and provides a "safety net" to compensate for increased insensible loss of "third spacing" seen with fever or infection. The goal is to maintain adequate intravascular volume to prevent vital organ ischemia.

Fluid and electrolytes are normally lost through three routes: (1) urine output, (2) gastrointestinal loss, and (3) insensible loss. Insensible loss is primarily sweat and respiratory loss that consists primarily of electrolyte free water (sweat has only 35 mEq Na$^+$/L). This constitutes usually only 400 ml/m^2/day, although fever increases insensible loss by 10%/°C. The loss of free water may produce significant hypertonic dehydration, requiring additional free water replacement.

Most (80%) ingested water is absorbed between the distal ileum and the mid-transverse colon. Only 200–400 ml of fluid is ultimately lost in the stool. Surgical patients frequently have increased fluid and electrolyte loss from the gut. Sources include prolonged gastric suction (Case 1), intestinal obstruction, fistulas, and diarrhea. Vomiting.

Urine output varies with a number of factors, including activity level, ambient temperature, and fluid intake. The normal person voids about 4–5 times per day in volumes of 200–250 ml. Following traumatic or surgical stress, increased secretion of aldosterone in response to

TABLE 2.1 *Composition of gastrointestinal secretions*

Type of Secretion	Volume (mL/24 hr)	Na (mEq/L)	K (mEq/L)	Cl (mEq/L)	HCO$_3^-$ (mEq/L)
Saliva	1,000–1,500	5–10	20–30	5–15	25–30
Stomach	1,000–2,000	60–90	10–15	100–130	—
Pancreas	600–800	135–145	5–10	70–90	95–115
Bile	300–600	135–145	5–10	90–110	30–40
Small intestine	2,000–3,000	120–140	5–10	90–120	30–40

decreased intravascular pressure causes a *physiologic* oliguria. Urine excretion may fall as low as 0.5–1.0 ml/kg/hr. This commonly occurs during the immediate postoperative period when acceptable urine output is 0.5–1.0 ml/kg/hr. Under these circumstances, attempts to increase urine output through the use of diuretics are ill advised and may worsen dehydration by leading to loss of both sodium and water. Oliguria is also produced by the action of antidiuretic hormone (ADH), which is secreted in response to increased serum osmolarity resulting from dehydration. Serum osmolality is estimated using the equation

$$\text{Serum osmolality (mOsm)} = 2 \cdot [\text{Na}] + \frac{[\text{glucose}]}{18} + \frac{[\text{BUN}]}{2.8}$$

Normal serum osmolality ranges between 285 and 305 mOsm. Because sodium is the major contributor, increased sodium produces increased osmolality. The hyperglycemia that accompanies diabetes or injudicious use of hyperalimentation may also cause hyperosmolarity. Free water loss causes an increase in the concentration of particles and stimulates the chemoreceptors in the carotid body. These in turn relay information to the hypothalamus, which secretes antidiuretic hormone, promoting the reabsorption of water from the collecting tubules of the kidney to reduce the blood's osmotic pressure.

Basal requirements for electrolytes must also be considered when writing intravenous fluid orders. Normal requirements are 1–1.5 mEq/kg/day for sodium, 0.5–0.75 mEq/kg/day for potassium, and 1–1.5 mEq/kg/day for chloride.

Selection of an intravenous fluid and its rate of infusion is not a daunting task. Although a large number of intravenous fluids are available, only the few used regularly need to be learned (Table 2.2). Most contain a small amount of dextrose (5%, or 50 g/L), to provide limited calories (4 kcal/g dextrose = 200 kcal/L), which prevents protein catabolism.

Dextrose is also added to some solutions (e.g., $D_5 \cdot \frac{1}{2}NS$) to make them isosmotic, to avoid red blood cell (RBC) lysis on infusion. The dextrose quickly crosses cell membranes, where it is used as an energy source, leaving behind only the free water and electrolytes in the intravascular space.

When planning fluid/electrolyte orders, three questions must be answered:

1. What are the patient's existing deficits?
2. What is the basal requirement?
3. What are the ongoing losses? Case 1 will serve as an example.

The 70-kg patient (Case 1) had been vomiting for several days and had 1,000 ml of gastric secretions in his stomach, when an NG tube was placed. These are pre-existing deficits. The degree of dehydration (loss of free water) can be estimated using the *2-4-6 rule*. The patient who is mildly dehydrated (e.g., thirsty, decreased urine output, dry skin, normal blood pressure with minimal orthostatic change) has a fluid deficit of 2% of total body weight. If the dehydration is more pronounced and includes orthostatic blood pressure changes and decreased skin turgor, the free water deficit is approximately 4% of total body weight. When hypotension at rest is present and oliguria is profound, the deficit is 6% of total body weight. In the sample case, the patient appears mildly dehydrated, making his estimated pre-existing loss 2% of his weight, or 1.4 L (1 kg = 1 L). The gastric contents aspirated through the NG tube account for 1.0 L, bringing the pre-existing deficit to 2.4 L.

The electrolyte composition of the fluid lost is important. The patient had been vomiting gastric contents (presumably he had gastric outlet obstruction from peptic ulcer disease), which is close to $D_5 \cdot \frac{1}{2}NS + 20$ KCl in composition (Tables 2.1 and 2.2).

TABLE 2.2 *Composition of intravenous solutions*

Solutions	Glucose (g/L)	Na	Cl	HCO₃	K	Ca	Mg	HPO₄	NH₄
				(mEq/L)					
Extracellular fluid	1,000	140	102	27	4.2	5	3	3	0.3
5% dextrose and water	50	—	—	—	—	—	—	—	—
10% dextrose and water	100	—	—	—	—	—	—	—	—
0.9% sodium chloride (normal saline)	—	154	154	—	—	—	—	—	—
0.45% sodium chloride (half-normal saline)	—	77	77	—	—	—	—	—	—
0.21% sodium chloride (¼ normal saline)	—	34	34	—	—	—	—	—	—
3% sodium chloride (hypertonic saline)	—	513	513	—	—	—	—	—	—
Lactated Ringer's solution	—	130	109	28[a]	4	2.7	—	—	—
0.9% ammonium chloride	—	—	168	—	—	—	—	—	168

[a]Present in solution as lactate, but metabolized to bicarbonate.

Replacement of pre-existing loss is best accomplished over 24 hours, with one-half of the replacement given over the first 8 hours and the remainder over the ensuing 16 hours. This approach should be modified for older patients with the potential for congestive heart failure who cannot tolerate large volume infusions. Conversely, in younger patients who are being prepared for emergency surgery, the deficit can be replaced quickly. In the sample patient, the 2.4-L deficit can be repaired with 150 ml/hr of D_5 + ½NS + 20 mg KCl/L over 8 hours (one-half the estimated loss) followed by 75 ml/hr D_5 + ½NS over the next 16 hours (the second half of the deficit).

Since patients are often not allowed oral intake, both fluid and electrolytes must be provided by the parenteral route. Although formulas can be used to estimate this need, fluid infusion rates and compositions are guided ultimately by urine output and blood chemistry determinations.

For the patient described in Case 1, the calculated maintenance fluid requirement is approximately 2,400 ml/day (100 ml/hr). Since he was not febrile and had no other reason for increased insensible loss (e.g., mechanical ventilation with nonhumidifed gas), there was no need to increase the basal fluid rate. Among the solutions available, D_5W + ½NS + 20 mEq KCl/L will provide the electrolytes required.

Surgical patients frequently have catheters, fistulas, and drains, all of which are sources of ongoing fluid and electrolyte loss. Unless these losses are replaced, dehydration and electrolyte/acid-base imbalances will result. The volume lost can be measured, while the electrolyte composition can be estimated (Table 2.1). If the source of the loss (i.e., a fistula) is unknown, a sample of the effluent should be analyzed for electrolyte composition. Once the electrolyte content is known, an appropriate replacement fluid can be selected.

The patient in Case 1 had an NG tube that continued to produce 50 ml/hr of gastric juice. This can be replaced on a milliliter to milliliter basis with D_5W + ½NS + 20 mEq/L of KCl.

If we combine the three components of pre-existing loss, basal requirement, and ongoing loss, we find that fluid therapy over the first 8 hours should consist of D_5W + ½NS + 20 mEq/L of KCl at 300 ml/hr. For the next 16 hours, it should be reduced to 225 ml/hr. Assuming that the deficit has been replaced, that the patient's urine output is at least 0.5–1.0 ml/kg/hr, and that the output through the NG tube remains relatively constant (at 50 ml/hr), the infusion rate should be further reduced to 150 ml/hr at the end of 24 hours. In the problem described in Case 1, the pre-existing fluid loss, maintenance fluid, and ongoing loss all use the same electrolyte solution. This is often not the case, and either a combination of fluids must be used or a special solution can be prepared by the pharmacy to approximate the patient's needs.

As written, the scenario in Case 1 includes only D_5W, with minimal provisions for replacing electrolyte losses and ongoing requirements. The result was severe dehydration and hyponatremia. Profound derangements of this type can easily be prevented by remembering the three components of fluid therapy. Case 2 is reviewed in detail in Appendix 2.1.

KEY POINTS

• Under pathologic conditions, interstitial space fills with edema fluid and constitutes part of the third space

• Increased number of osmolals in one compartment causes flow of water into that compartment, decreasing oncotic pressure

• Because body secretions are formed by components in the intravascular space, fluid loss due to fistulas, diarrhea, and drains ultimately leads to intravascular dehydration

• Fluid and electrolytes normally lost through three routes: urine output, gastrointestinal loss, and insensible loss

• Decreased intravascular pressure after traumatic or surgical stress leads to increased secretion of aldosterone, causing physiologic oliguria; use of diuretics to increase urine output ill-advised—may worsen dehydration, and loss of sodium and water

• Most intravenous fluids contain small amount of dextrose (5%, or 50 g/L), providing limited calories (4 kcal/g dextrose = 200 kcal/L), preventing protein catabolism (-ve N balance?)

• Dextrose also added to some solutions (e.g., D_5 · ½NS making them isosmotic, to avoid RBC lysis on infusion

• Replacement of pre-existing loss usually accomplished over 24 hours, with one-half of replacement given over first 8 hours, and remainder over next 16 hours

---

FLUIDS AND ELECTROLYTES

Sodium is the principal extracellular cation (Fig. 2.1) and the major contributor to extracellular osmolality. The serum concentration of sodium is not necessarily related to extracellular volume status, although changes in sodium concentration usually produce changes in extracellular fluid volume by shifting free water. Signs and symptoms of hypo- and hypernatremia usually do not occur unless the changes are severe or occur rapidly.

Replacement of electrolyte-rich fluid loss with free water is the most common cause of hyponatremia in surgical patients (Case 2). As the extracellular osmolality falls, free water shifts into the intracellular space, where it may cause nervous system symptoms, including increased tendon reflexes, muscle twitching, convulsions, and hypertension (Case 2). Other findings include excessive salivation, lacrimation, watery diarrhea, and increased intracranial pressure. The symptoms of hyponatremia depend not only on its degree, but also on the speed with which it develops. When hyponatremia occurs rapidly, signs and symptoms appear at a concentration as high as 130 mEq/L. When chronic loss is responsible, findings may not be present until the concentration is as low as 120 mEq/L.

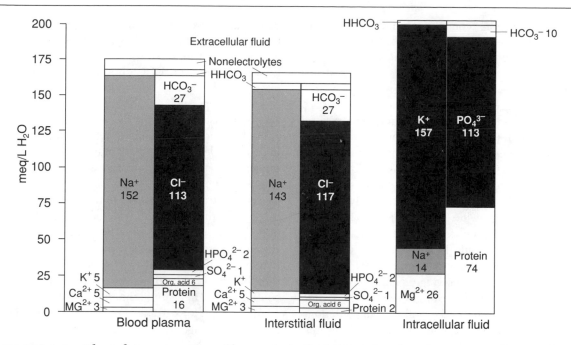

FIGURE 2.1   *Electrolyte composition of human body fluids. Note that the values are in milliequivalents per liter (mEq/L) of water, not of body fluid. (From Leaf A, Newburgh LH: Significance of the Body Fluids in Clinical Medicine. 2nd Ed. Thomas, 1955, with permission.)*

Sodium deficits should be approximated from the serum sodium concentration. Because hyponatremia is frequently caused by excess free water administration, the deficit is often *relative* rather than real. The sodium deficit is calculated as follows:

$$Na \text{ deficit} = (140 \text{ mEq/L} - \text{measured Na}) \cdot (\text{body weight} \cdot 0.6)$$

Because sodium distributes throughout total body water, the quantity (body weight · 0.6) is used. Sodium should be replaced when hyponatremia is profound (<120 mEq/L) or when the loss occurs rapidly and the patient becomes symptomatic. No more than one-half the calculated deficit should be replaced within the first 24 hours. Amyelenosis may result from excessively enthusiastic replacement. Normal saline is used, although hypertonic saline (3% NaCl) may be required in rare circumstances.

Hypernatremia results from the loss of free water in excess of sodium. It causes weakness, restlessness, and delirium. The skin becomes dry and the mucous membranes are sticky. Salivation and tear production are decreased, and an increase in body temperature may also occur. Free water, usually in the form of D_5W, is required and should be administered slowly to prevent a sudden decrease in osmolarity.

Potassium is the principal intracellular cation (Fig. 2.1). Average oral intake of potassium is 50–100 mEq/day, with the majority excreted in the urine. Large amounts of potassium are released from injured and burned tissues, causing hyperkalemia. The symptoms of hyperkalemia are cardiovascular or gastrointestinal and include nausea, vomiting, diarrhea, and constipation. Muscle weakness, loss of deep tendon reflexes, and paralysis occur. Electrocardiographic (ECG) findings include high peaked T waves ("tombstone" T waves), widened QRS complexes, and depressed ST segments. At potassium concentrations greater than 6 mEq/L, T waves may disappear to be followed by diastolic cardiac arrest.

Hyperkalemia should be treated when concentrations exceed 5 mEq/L or when signs or symptoms are present. Management of hyperkalemia revolves primarily around neutralizing the cardiovascular effect of potassium and secondarily on decreasing the actual potassium concentration. Calcium antagonizes the actions of potassium and should be the first drug given. The patient should be given 50–100 ml of calcium chloride by rapid intravenous infusion. Reduction of potassium concentration may be accomplished with the intravenous infusion of glucose and insulin. Potassium enters the cells along with glucose. Although this procedure can rapidly lower the serum potassium, rebound often occurs and potassium levels rise acutely several hours later. The use of ion exchange resins such as polystyrene sulfonate (Kayexalate) are helpful. A slurry of this compound, administered by enema, exchanges sodium for potassium. The exchange resin works slowly and takes several days of repeat administration before potassium levels fall into a normal range. All exogenous sources of potassium should be stopped, and renal function should be checked to ensure that the patient does not have acute renal failure resulting in potassium retention.

Hypokalemia is more common among surgical patients than is hyperkalemia and usually results from insufficient potassium administration in the face of prolonged gastrointestinal loss. Because potassium is exchanged for sodium in the renal tubule, hypovolemia (with production of aldosterone) exaggerates hypokalemia by increasing renal loss. Furthermore, because hydrogen and potassium are in competition for renal reabsorption, alkalosis can also augment renal excretion. Hypokalemia causes decreased contractility of skeletal, smooth, and cardiac muscle. Signs include paralytic ileus, decreased deep tendon reflexes, weakness, and ultimately flaccid paralysis. The ECG exhibits flattening of the T waves, low voltage, depression of ST segments, and appearance of the U wave. Potassium replacement should be instituted for chemical (<3.5 mEq/L) or symptomatic hypokalemia. This is particularly important in patients receiving digitalis because hypokalemia sensitizes the myocardium to the effects of digitalis. In patients who cannot take oral supplementation, intravenous potassium should not be replaced at rates greater than 10–15 mEq/hr. Because potassium is largely an intracellular ion, relatively small decreases in serum potassium reflect large whole body potassium deficiencies. Hence, large quantities of potassium are usually required over several days for adequate replacement of potassium deficiencies. In general, a decrease of 1.0 mEq/L in serum potassium represents a 100–200-mEq whole body defect. When serum potassium is tested shortly after intravenous infusion, a false sense of security is obtained when the concentration has risen. However, as the newly administered potassium equilibrates with the intracellular space, the plasma concentration will drop rapidly. Hence, potassium levels should not be tested until several hours after infusion has been completed.

The whole body content of calcium is 1,000–1,200 g. Dietary intake is approximately 1–3 g, with 200 mg excreted in the urine. Serum calcium is largely under the control of the parathyroid hormone (parathyrine)/calcitonin system. Approximately one-half of the body's calcium is bound to plasma proteins and is un-ionized. A decrease of 1 g/dl of albumin results in a 0.8 mg/dl decrease in the measured total serum calcium concentration. Hence, patients with hypoproteinemia may have a relatively normal calcium concentration in spite of measured hypocalcemia. Most of the remaining calcium is ionized and is responsible for neuromuscular conduction and contraction. The extent of calcium ionization is inversely related to pH. As a result, alkalosis worsens hypocalcemia. The parathyroid glands respond to decreased ionized calcium by secreting parathyrine, which causes increased reabsorption of calcium from the bones, decreased renal excretion of calcium, and increased excretion of phosphate. The signs and symptoms of hypocalcemia usually appear at a serum concentration of 8 mEq/L with normal protein and pH levels. Circumoral paresthesias and tingling in the fingers and toes along with hyperactive deep tendon reflexes are the first signs. Chevostek's and Trousseau's signs, carpopedal spasm, tetany, and convulsions occur with further decreases. The ECG shows prolongation of the QT interval.

Acute hypocalcemia should be treated with an intravenous infusion of either calcium gluconate or calcium chloride. Calcium gluconate contains 93 mg of Ca^{2+} in 10 ml, while calcium chloride contains 273 mg of Ca^{2+} in 10 ml, making calcium chloride the agent of choice. Hypocalcemia may be produced by massive blood transfusions because the citrate preservative in the banked blood chelates calcium. In this case, calcium should be replaced at a dose of 0.2 g of calcium for every 500 ml of blood transfused. A common misconception is that calcium supplementation is required after transfusion for normal hemostasis; however, blood will clot normally with very small calcium concentrations. The supplementation requirement stems from the need for cardiac contractility and excitation-contraction coupling.

Hypercalcemia among surgical patients may stem from hyperparathyroidism, injudicious calcium administration, the milk-alkali syndrome, or the paraneoplastic syndrome. Many tumors are endocrinologically active and produce hormone-like substances such as parathyrine. Symptoms of hypercalcemia include weakness, nausea, vomiting, abdominal complaints, and anorexia. Other findings include back and extremity pain, thirst, polydypsia, polyuria, stupor, and coma. When calcium levels reach 16 mEq/L, immediate treatment should be instituted. The initial management of hypercalcemic crisis is the induction of a saline diuresis. Furosemide causes renal excretion of calcium and lowers the calcium level. Sufficient volumes of saline are required to ensure diuresis and prevent hypovolemia. Other methods to reduce the calcium concentration include phosphate supplementation and the use of corticosteroids and mithramycin. Phosphate supplementation binds calcium and reduces bone reabsorption. It produces metastatic calcium phosphate deposits, which may be deleterious when they form in organs such as the eye or kidney. Corticosteroids decrease the reabsorption of calcium from bone and the intestinal tract and are useful in select patients with systemic diseases such as sarcoidosis, leukemia, or lymphoma. Mithramycin is an antineoplastic drug that decreases osteoclastic activity. Because it may take weeks to act and has several undesirable side effects, it is seldom used.

More than one-half of the body's 2,000-mEq content of magnesium is complexed in bone; the remainder is within the cells. The normal plasma magnesium concentration is 1.5–2.5 mEq/L, constituting a balance between the daily dietary intake of 250 mEq/day and loss in stool. Most body fluids, including many secretions, have a magnesium content of 2–3 mEq/L. Magnesium activates cholinesterase and therefore plays a crucial role in controlling striated muscle activity. Deficits of magnesium lead to uncontrolled myoneural conduction and excessive muscular activity. Magnesium is also an integral part of the phosphorylating enzymes used in carbohydrate metabolism. Hypomagnesemia is common among alcoholics, with gastrointestinal malabsorption syndromes, with chronic diarrhea, after prolonged use of loop diuretics such as furosemide or ethacrynic acid, with pancreatitis or gastrointestinal fistula, and with hypoparathyroidism. Hypomagnesemia produces gross tremors, hyperreflexia, muscle fibrillation, transitory hallucinations, arrhythmias, and Chvostek's and Trousseau's signs (hypomagnesemic tetany). Hypomagnesemia is treated with oral or intravenous magnesium, the latter in the form of magnesium sulfate. Renal function should be assessed before magnesium replacement is given because magnesium accumulates in renal failure. Because 80% of administered magnesium is excreted in the urine, a significant amount must be given to correct even a small deficit. This is best done (in a patient with normal renal function) by giving 20 ml of 20% $MgSO_4$ as an intravenous bolus, followed by 500 ml of 20% $MgSO_4$ every 6 hours (qid) until the concentration normalizes (1 g of magnesium contains 8 mEq of Mg^{2+}). When large doses of magnesium are given, the ECG should be monitored for signs of toxicity (similar to those seen with hyperkalemia) to avert cardiac arrest.

Hypermagnesemia (prolonged levels over 5–6 mEq/L) result in arrhythmia, lethargy, hyporeflexia, and weakness. This occurs most commonly in patients with renal failure or when excessive magnesium replacement has been administered over a long period. Rapid increases in magnesium concentration should be treated by infusion of calcium chloride or calcium gluconate. Hypermagnesemia due to renal failure is best treated by hemodialysis.

Hypophosphatemia is the most common disturbance related to phosphate and is usually secondary to decreased intake among patients receiving total parenteral nutrition (TPN). It may also occur among cirrhotics and in those with either hypo- or hyperparathyroidism. Mild deficits (<3.0 mEq/dl) result in hyperglycemia because intracellular phosphorylation of glucose is required after glucose enters the cell. Hypophosphatemia allows glucose to leak from cells. Moderate nutrition-related deficits occur among alcoholics (<2.0 mEq/dl) and present as weakness, malaise, and chronic debility. Severe deficits (<1.0 mEq/dl) cause decreased energy stores by affecting mitochondrial adenosine triphosphate (ATP) production and by limiting oxygen unloading to the tissue by reducing 2,3-diphosphogluconate (2,3-DPG) concentrations. Hypophosphatemia is treated by administration of either sodium or potassium biphosphate. The patient is given either 1–2 mg/kg PO or isotonic buffered sodium phosphate (200–500 ml tid IV). If phosphate is administered too quickly, it will complex with calcium and produce hypocalcemia, which can lead to hypotension and renal failure.

KEY POINTS

Sodium

- Concentration not necessarily related to extracellular volume status, although changes in sodium concentration usually produce changes in extracellular fluid volume by shifting free water

- Replacement of electrolyte-rich fluid loss with free water most common cause of hyponatremia in surgical patients; symptoms depend not only on degree, but also on speed of development

Potassium

- Potassium is principal intracellular cation

- Symptoms of hyperkalemia are cardiovascular or gastrointestinal (nausea, vomiting, diarrhea, and constipation)

- Hyperkalemia should be treated when concentrations exceed 5 mEq/L or when signs or symptoms present

- Calcium antagonizes actions of potassium; should be first drug given

- Hypokalemia more common among surgical patients; usually results from insufficient potassium administration during prolonged gastrointestinal loss

- Signs include paralytic ileus, decreased deep tendon reflexes, weakness, ultimately flaccid paralysis

- Potassium replacement necessary for chemical (<3.5 mEq/L) or symptomatic hypokalemia, particularly in patients on digitalis, because myocardium sensitized to its effects

- Decreases of 1.0 mEq/L in serum potassium generally represents a 100–200-mEq whole body deficit

Calcium

- Decrease of 1 g/dl albumin results in 0.8-mg/dl decrease in measured total serum calcium concentration

- Signs and symptoms of hypocalcemia usually appear at serum concentration of 8 mEq/L with normal protein and pH levels; first signs are circumoral paresthesias and tingling in fingers and toes, along with hyperactive deep tendon reflexes

- Acute hypocalcemia treated with intravenous infusion of calcium gluconate or calcium chloride

- Symptoms of hypercalcemia include weakness, nausea, vomiting, abdominal complaints, and anorexia

- Initial management of hypercalcemic crisis is induction of saline diuresis

Magnesium

- Most body fluids have magnesium content of 2–3 mEq/L

- Magnesium activates cholinesterase and therefore plays crucial role in controlling striated muscle activity

- Hypomagnesemia produces gross tremors, hyperreflexia, muscle fibrillation, transitory hallucinations, arrhythmias, and Chvostek's and Trousseau's signs

- Hypomagnesemia treated with oral or intravenous magnesium sulfate; with large doses, monitor ECG for toxicity, as in hyperkalemia, to avert cardiac arrest

• Hypermagnesemia (prolonged levels >5–6 mEq/L) result in arrhythmia, lethargy, hyporeflexia, and weakness

Phosphate
• Hypophosphatemia usually secondary to decreased intake among patients receiving total parenteral nutrition

ACID-BASE BALANCE

Acid-base balance depends on the relative concentration of hydrogen ion and its buffer systems. In general, any decrease in bicarbonate (or increase in protons) will result in acidosis, while any increase in bicarbonate (or decrease in protons) will result in alkalosis. Recall that hydrogen ions, bicarbonate, and carbon dioxide are in equilibrium:

$$H^+ + HCO_3^- \leftrightarrow H_2CO_3 \leftrightarrow H_2O + CO_2$$

The increase in proton concentration may occur as a result of the addition of an acid (most metabolic processes produce weak acids) or by an increase in the concentration of carbon dioxide (respiratory failure). Physiologic acids are either volatile or fixed. Fixed acids are those that can only be excreted by the kidneys, while volatile acids (carbon dioxide) are removed by the lungs. A drop in pH because of an increase in fixed acids is termed *metabolic acidosis*; when caused by carbon dioxide accumulation, *respiratory acidosis* has occurred. Decreased hydrogen concentration (increased pH) produces metabolic or respiratory alkalosis.

Changes in the concentration of hydrogen ions are buffered by several systems, including the bicarbonate buffer, protein buffers, and the hemoglobin buffering system. Although changes in the bicarbonate system are the principal early defenses, the protein buffering system is much larger and can absorb greater concentrations of acid than can the bicarbonate system.

The respiratory system responds quickly to the accumulation of metabolic acids. As protons accumulate, they are buffered by the bicarbonate system, producing carbon dioxide and water. An increase of 10 mmHg of carbon dioxide causes a decrease in pH of 0.08. The altered pH stimulates the aortic chemoreceptors, which in turn stimulate the respiratory center to increase the rate and volume of breathing. Such Kussmaul ventilation eliminates carbon dioxide from the blood. This respiratory compensation for metabolic acidosis occurs quickly but is somewhat limited in its ability to offset a large accumulation of acid. Contrary to popular belief, pulmonary retention of carbon dioxide (so-called compensatory respiratory acidosis) does not occur significantly in response to metabolic alkalosis.

The kidney has the greatest capacity to correct disturbances in acid-base balance. It protects against both acidosis and alkalosis by excreting acid during acidosis and al-kali during alkalosis. Renal acidification can lower urine pH to as low as 4.5. This mechanism is so important to homeostasis that virtually all forms of renal insufficiency ultimately result in metabolic acidosis because of the impaired ability to secrete acids.

Common causes of metabolic acidosis among surgical patients include cellular ischemia (hypoxia), diabetic acidosis, ketosis, rhabdomyolysis, and major trauma. Cellular hypoxia, due to shock, cardiac arrest, hypothermia, or heart failure, leads to decreased oxygen delivery for the aerobic metabolism of glucose. This causes lactate to accumulate, producing lactic acidosis. Although relatively uncommon in surgical practice, ingestion of salicylates, paraldehyde, methanol, or acetazolamide (carbonic anhydrase inhibitor) also causes metabolic acidosis. The symptoms of metabolic acidosis include Kussmaul respiration, decreased cardiac output, disorientation, lethargy, and dehydration. When the acidosis is mild (pH >7.2) a rightward shift in the oxyhemoglobin dissociation curve partially compensates for the decreased cardiac output by increasing the unloading of oxygen to the tissues.

To aid in determining the cause of a metabolic acidosis, clinicians frequently divide acidosis into two groups: those with an anion gap and those without. The anion gap is calculated as follows:

$$\text{Anion gap} = 2 \cdot [Na^+] - ([HCO_3^-] + [Cl^-])$$

Because the number of anions and cations must be equal in order to preserve electroneutrality, the total number of cations must equal the total number of measured and "unmeasured" anions. Sodium represents the vast majority of the cations in the extracellular space, while bicarbonate and chloride together constitute most of the anions. However, there is normally a small deficit when the anion concentration is subtracted from the cation concentration. This "gap" is composed of anions not normally measured in routine laboratory determinations. These anions are usually the salts of weak acids, such as lactate, pyruvate, malate, citrate, amino acids, sulfates, and free fatty acids. Under normal conditions, the anion gap is less than 14 mEq/L. Any decrease in the bicarbonate concentration or increase in the number of weak acid salts, or both, will widen the gap and produce an anion gap acidosis. Common causes of high gap acidosis include diabetic ketoacidosis, uremia, aspirin ingestion, lactic acidosis, and infection. Although "nongap" acidosis can occur (from the addition of chloride), it is far less common.

The guiding principle in the treatment of metabolic acidosis (high gap or otherwise) is to identify and correct the underlying process. This may require repair of hypovolemia, drainage of an infection, or improvement of myocardial contractility with the use of an inotropic agent such as dopamine. As this is being done, pharmacologic correction with base may be required if the acidosis has become severe. Sodium bicarbonate is the agent of choice. However, sodium bicarbonate must be used with extreme caution when the patient has an associated respiratory acidosis because neutralization of the excess protons will result in the production of carbon dioxide, which must be excreted by the lungs.

The amount of bicarbonate required can be determined when the base deficit is known. The base deficit is calculated during the automated measurement of blood gases. It represents that portion of the acidosis (or alkalosis) that is due to a metabolic component. Hence, if the pH is 7.2 and the arterial partial pressure of carbon dioxide ($PaCO_2$) is normal (40 mmHg), the acidosis must be of metabolic origin, exclusively, and the base deficit will be elevated (normal = ± 2). On the contrary, if the pH is 7.32 and the $PaCO_2$ is 50, the acidosis is purely of respiratory origin, and the base deficit will be 0. The amount of base required to achieve full correction of the metabolic component of an acidosis is calculated as follows:

mEq base required = 0.4 · base deficit · body weight (kg)

The term 0.4 is used because virtually all of the disturbance occurs in the extracellular space, which is approximately 40% of the total body weight. Hence, if a 70-kg patient with a pH of 7.1 has a base deficit of 15, the required amount of base would be: 15 · (0.4 · 70), or 420 mEq HCO_3^-. Since each ampule of sodium bicarbonate contains 44.6 mEq of base, approximately 9½ ampules of bicarbonate would be needed to reverse the metabolic acidosis completely. Profound disturbances should not be corrected rapidly. Approximately one-half of the calculated requirement should be administered over 8 hours, with the rest given over the ensuing 16 hours. Rapid infusions of bicarbonate can produce profound respiratory acidosis if any element of respiratory failure is present in a spontaneously breathing patient.

Metabolic alkalosis occurs relatively infrequently among surgical patients; however, it may be life-threatening when severe. It consists of the triad of (1) increased pH, (2) increased HCO_3^-, and (3) decreased serum chloride concentration. Because the decline in chloride does not compensate for the rise in bicarbonate, the anion gap increases. Metabolic alkalosis is produced by vomiting, prolonged gastric suction, use of diuretics, and volume depletion (contraction alkalosis). Among critically ill patients, the use of acetate in hyperalimentation solutions is an often unsuspected source.

Prolonged emesis and gastric suction are the two most common causes in surgical patients. Both result in the loss of chloride and protons from the stomach, producing alkalosis and volume contraction. The loss of blood volume causes the secretion of renin and the production of aldosterone, which fosters sodium retention (to compensate for volume loss) and potassium excretion. The decreased

glomerular filtration rate (GFR) (in response to the decreased circulating blood volume) and the lowered potassium "reset" the kidney and allow complete reabsorption of all filtered bicarbonate. A paradoxic aciduria may even occur as the kidneys exchange protons for potassium.

The symptoms and physical findings associated with mild metabolic alkalosis are usually nonspecific and are related to the underlying disorder that caused the alkalosis. Alkalemia acts as a negative inotrope and can cause a decrease in blood pressure beyond that produced by the associated volume depletion. The increased pH also decreases the fraction of ionized serum calcium and reduces the arrhythmia threshold. The leftward shift of the oxyhemoglobin dissociation curve reduces the amount of oxygen unloaded and may contribute to tissue hypoxia.

Metabolic alkalosis should be treated with hydration. Once normal renal function returns, potassium replacement is begun. This therapy increases the GFR and causes the excretion of bicarbonate. In severe cases, or when the alkalosis is not responsive to saline, acetazolamide (carbonic anhydrase inhibitor), arginine hydrochloride, or even 0.1 N HCl may be used. Acetazolamide results in renal loss of bicarbonate, potassium, water, and sodium. The drug typically takes 2–3 days to produce an effect and is normally begun intravenously at a dose of 5 mg/kg once daily.

Respiratory acidosis is present when there is an increased concentration of dissolved carbon dioxide [$PaCO_2$] in the blood. It most commonly occurs in patients with chronic respiratory disease or in those receiving mechanical ventilation with insufficient minute ventilation. Other causes include airway obstruction, respiratory center depression, circulatory collapse, neurogenic disease, and restrictive pulmonary processes. The increased $PaCO_2$ is particularly problematic because dissolved carbon dioxide can quickly cross membranes, such as the blood-brain barrier, to alter metabolic processes. An acute change in $PaCO_2$ produces a change in blood pH within about 10 minutes. Buffering is by the nonbicarbonate system, which has a large capacity; hence, only small changes in pH occur. Once equilibrium is achieved, pH falls by about 0.08 units for every 10-mmHg increase in $PaCO_2$.

The symptoms of respiratory acidosis are nonspecific and are usually related to the underlying cause. In severe cases, fatigue, weakness, and confusion may be present. Physical findings include tremor, asterixis, weakness, incoordination, papilledema, and pyramidal tract findings. Coma may ensue when $PaCO_2$ reaches 70–100 mmHg. Renal compensation causes a metabolic alkalosis by retaining bicarbonate, returning the pH toward normal.

As with all acid-base disturbances, the key to management revolves around identification of the underlying process. For patients with acute or chronic respiratory failure, this may include endotracheal intubation and mechanical ventilation. For those already receiving mechanical ventilation, the increased $PaCO_2$ identifies inadequate alveolar ventilation. This is caused either by improper ventilator settings or by increased physiologic dead space. Minute ventilation is the product of tidal volume and respiratory rate. The typical mechanically ventilated patient requires 10–15 ml/kg of tidal volume at 8–10 breaths/min. Dead space is that proportion of inhaled volume that does not come into contact with exchange surfaces of the lung. Dead space has three components: apparatus, anatomic, and physiologic. Anatomic dead space is that portion of the ventilator volume that remains within the breathing circuit, while anatomic dead space is that fraction that remains within the conducting airways, such as the trachea. Physiologic dead space constitutes the largest and most significant component and is caused by alveoli that have lost either their normal perfusion or their ability to exchange gases. Normal dead space is 30% of tidal volume. This may increase to more than 75% in extremely ill patients. Increased dead space produces a respiratory acidosis by reducing effective ventilation.

Respiratory alkalosis produces an alkalemia with decreased $PaCO_2$ and a normal or decreased bicarbonate concentration. Excitability and excessive mechanical ventilation are the most common causes. In the initial period following injury, the response to pain causes a transient respiratory alkalosis. The normal homeostatic response is excretion of bicarbonate to produce a compensatory metabolic acidosis. In the steady state, the plasma bicarbonate concentration falls by about 0.5 mEq/L for each 1-mmHg decrease in $PaCO_2$. The arterial pH is corrected toward, but does not become, normal.

Symptoms of hyperventilation and severe respiratory alkalosis include hypocalcemic tetany (due to the reduced fraction of ionized calcium), irritability, anxiety, vertigo, and syncope. ECG changes include ST segment or T wave flattening and alterations in the QRS complex.

The key differential diagnosis of primary respiratory alkalosis is from respiratory compensation for underlying metabolic acidosis. Patients with severe underlying infections or diabetic coma often have respiratory compensation for their underlying acidosis.

Because respiratory alkalosis is always caused by hyperventilation, the key to treatment is the demonstration of the underlying disorder. Blood gases will demonstrate whether an associated hypoxia is the cause of hyperventilation. Drug ingestions may also cause central nervous system excitement with hyperventilation. When the patient is receiving mechanical ventilation, a reduction in the minute ventilation or change in the mode setting is usually curative.

KEY POINTS

• Decreased bicarbonate or increased protons results in acidosis; increased bicarbonate or decreased protons results in alkalosis

• A drop in pH because of an increase in fixed acids is metabolic acidosis; when caused by accumulation of carbon dioxide, it is respiratory acidosis; decreased hydrogen concentration (increased pH) is metabolic or respiratory alkalosis

• Increase of 10 mmHg of carbon dioxide causes decrease in pH of 0.8

Metabolic Acidosis
• In metabolic acidosis, lactate accumulation produces lactic acidosis

• Symptoms of metabolic acidosis include Kussmaul respiration, decreased cardiac output, disorientation, lethargy, and dehydration

• Anion gap is composed of anions not normally measured in routine laboratory determinations

• Normal anion gap is less than 14 mEq/L; any decrease in bicarbonate concentration and/or increase in number of weak acid salts widens gap and produces anion gap acidosis

• Guiding principle in treatment of any metabolic acidosis is to identify and correct underlying process

• Base deficit is portion of acidosis or alkalosis due to a metabolic component

• Amount of base required to achieve full correction of metabolic component of acidosis is calculated as mEq base required + 0.4 · base deficit · body weight (kg)

• Rapid infusions of bicarbonate can produce profound respiratory acidosis in presence of respiratory failure in a spontaneously breathing patient

Metabolic Alkalosis
• Decline in chloride does not compensate for rise in bicarbonate, so anion gap always decreases

• Metabolic alkalosis produced by vomiting, prolonged gastric suction, use of diuretics, and volume depletion (contraction alkalosis)

• Prolonged emesis and gastric suction the two most common causes in surgical patients

• Alkalemia acts as a negative inotrope and can cause a decrease in blood pressure beyond that produced by associated volume depletion

Respiratory Acidosis
• Increased $PaCO_2$ particularly problematic because dissolved carbon dioxide can quickly cross membranes, such as blood-brain barrier, to alter metabolic processes

• Once equilibrium achieved, pH falls by about 0.08 units for every 10-mmHg increase in $PaCO_2$

• For patients with acute or chronic respiratory failure, management includes endotracheal intubation and mechanical ventilation

Respiratory Alkalosis
• Respiratory alkalosis produces alkalemia with decreased $PaCO_2$ and normal or decreased bicarbonate concentration;

excitability and excessive mechanical ventilation are most common causes

• Symptoms of hyperventilation and severe respiratory alkalosis include hypocalcemic tetany (due to reduced fraction of ionized calcium), irritability, anxiety, vertigo, and syncope

• Key differential diagnosis of primary respiratory alkalosis is from respiratory compensation for underlying metabolic acidosis

SUGGESTED READINGS

Bongard FS, Sue DY: Fluid, electrolytes, and acid base. In Bongard FS, Sue DY (eds): Current Critical Care Diagnosis and Treatment. Appleton & Lange, E. Norwalk, CT, 1994.

A good chapter with ample detail on fluid and electrolyte disturbances. Contains many of the charts and nomograms that appear in Cogan (see below).

Cogan MG: Fluid and Electrolytes: Physiology and Pathophysiology. Appleton & Lange, E. Norwalk, CT, 1991

A monograph that includes detailed physiologic descriptions of acid-base disorders. It should be used as a reference when detailed information about complex acid-base disorders is needed. It contains several nomograms and charts that may be helpful in diagnosing these disorders.

QUESTIONS

1. *Hypernatremia?*

   A. Always occurs in the presence of volume contraction.

   B. Should be treated whenever present.

   C. Usually occurs in the face of metabolic alakalosis.

   D. Causes an increase in the serum osmolality.

2. *Potassium?*

   A. Is largely an extracellular cation.

   B. Is increased in patients with metabolic alkalosis.

   C. Can be replaced rapidly in deficiency states.

   D. Produces U waves on the ECG in decreased concentration.

3. *Metabolic alkalosis?*

   A. Increases the delivery of oxygen to the tissues.

   B. Increases the fraction of ionized calcium.

   C. Commonly occurs following prolonged gastric suction.

   D. Is not related to the concentration of potassium.

4. *Increased physiologic dead space?*

   A. Produces a metabolic alkalosis.

   B. Produces a respiratory alkalosis.

   C. May require an increased minute ventilation to treat.

   D. Is associated with diuretic use.

(See p. 603 for answers.)

MANAGEMENT

OF CASE 2

Case 2 illustrates the inadvertent creation of hyponatremia, the most common postoperative fluid and electrolyte disturbance. This was caused by the use of a solution containing only D_5W + 20 mEq KCl/L, instead of a more physiologic solution (e.g., D_5W + ½NS + 20 KCl) for maintenance.

The patient's operation took 5 hours, during which time she lost 1 L of blood. Evaporation (insensible) from the peritoneal and visceral surfaces is a major cause of fluid loss during laparotomy. Normally, this loss is replaced by the anesthesiologist with either saline or lactated Ringer's solution at 10 ml/kg/hr. Although this may seem like a large volume, evaporative loss can be considerable. Blood loss during surgery is replaced either with blood (depending on how much is lost and on any pre-existing conditions such as ischemic cardiac disease) or with balanced salt solution (normal saline or lactated Ringer's) in a ratio of 3 ml crystalloid (crystalloid is a term applied to any solution that does not contain high-molecular-weight molecules such as albumin) for each milliliter of blood lost. Colloids, which do contain high molecular weight species, can be used in smaller volumes. Colloid solutions are expensive and offer no real advantages. The 3:1 ratio is required, as most of the replacement solution quickly leaves the intravascular space to enter the interstitium. Using these guidelines, the patient should have received:

Maintenance (open abdomen):

10 ml/kg/hr · 5 hr · 50 kg	2,500 ml
1,000 ml blood loss · 3 ml replacement/ml blood lost	3,000 ml
Expected intraoperative replacement	5,500 ml

From this calculation, we can see that the 5 L of lactated Ringer's solution received in the operating room was appropriate.

To write the postoperative fluid orders, we need to consider three factors: (1) pre-existing loss, (2) maintenance requirements, and (3) ongoing loss.

1. Pre-existing loss

   Our calculation indicates that she may have received about 500 ml too little during surgery. If we follow the rule about the time required for replacement, one-half (250 ml) should be given over the first 8 hours (about 30 ml/hr), with the remainder given over the next 16 hours (250 ml/16 hr = 15 ml/hr). These are relatively small volumes and, since we are primarily concerned about the free water lost from evaporation, we can use the maintenance fluid chosen to replace this loss rather than use a separate solution.

2. Maintenance Requirement

   This can be calculated simply using our estimate for fluid requirement in a 50-kg patient.

100 ml/kg for the first 10 kg	1,000 ml
50 ml/kg for the next 10 kg	500 ml
20 ml/kg for each remaining kg	600 ml
Total 24-hr requirement	2,100 ml (or 90 ml/hr)

3. Ongoing loss

Although this patient does not have any drains in place, we know that a paralytic ileus will form (following manipulation of the bowel) and that fluid will leak into the bowel lumen. This "third spacing" can constitute considerable loss and must be accounted for. Table 2.1 indicates that the volume (primarily small bowel) can be as much as 2,000–3,000 ml/24 hr with a composition similar to that of lactated Ringer's or ½NS + 20 mEq KCl, to which bicarbonate has been added to account for the extra sodium and bicarbonate present. We will estimate the loss at 1,200 ml/day (since we are not draining the entire small bowel, it seems reasonable to begin with a smaller volume), which would require 50 ml/hr.

Adding the requirements:

Pre-existing loss (using lactated Ringer's solution)	30 ml/hr (8 hr)
Maintenance	90 ml/hr
Ongoing loss (using lactated Ringer's solution)	50 ml/hr
Total fluid requirement	170 ml/hr (8 hr)

Because lactated Ringer's solution will serve to replace both the pre-existing and the ongoing losses, we should consider its use for the maintenance fluid as well. It is somewhat higher in sodium that $D_5 \cdot$ ½NS, but its use for 24 hours (during which time the pre-existing loss is replaced) will result in only a relatively small excess of sodium, after which time we can change to a more dilute sodium solution. Therefore, our initial fluid order would be D_5 lactated Ringer's solution at 170 ml/hr for 8 hours, followed by D_5 lacted Ringer's solution at 155 ml/hr for the next 16 hours. At 24 hours, we can change to $D_5W \cdot$ ½NS + 20 mEq/KCl at 140 ml/hr and adjust the rate depending on the patient's urine output. Daily review of the serum electrolytes (especially sodium and bicarbonate) will guide changes in this regimen. The complications sustained by the patient were due to hyponatremia: paralytic ileus, muscle irritability, and seizures. These would have been prevented had the calculations obtained been used instead.

3 NUTRITION

GIDEON P. NAUDE

EDWARD PASSARO, JR.

The advent of nutritional support, both enteral and parenteral, has made possible the successful management of otherwise lethal diseases and complications. This chapter reviews the basis of nutritional support, indications, and complications.

CASE 1
ENTERAL FEEDING

A 68-year-old male had an esophagogastrectomy for adenocarcinoma of the cardia. He had lost some thirty lb before his operation, and his serum albumin was 3.0 g/dl. When first seen, he could swallow liquids with some difficulty, but not solids. His operation was considered urgent because of his severe degree of esophageal obstruction. At operation a catheter was placed in the proximal jejunum and brought out on the outer abdominal wall for enteral feeding. On the fifth postoperative day, he passed flatus, and enteral feedings were begun. He was initially given 50 ml/hr of D_5W and then progressed within 36 hours to a high calorie, high protein liquid meal totaling 2,400 ml. On the seventh postoperative day, a water soluble contrast study showed a small contained anastomotic leak. He was continued on the enteral diet until the 14th postoperative day, when a repeat study showed no leaks, at which time he was started on an oral diet.

CASE 2
PARENTERAL FEEDING

A 44-year-old white female presented to the emergency department for the 14th time in 1 year complaining of abdominal pain. The source of the pain was easy to determine, since she had had Crohn's disease from adolescence. The condition was discovered when a doctor removed her appendix for what ultimately proved to be Crohn's disease. Over the next 28 years she frequently had experienced abdominal pain and diarrhea. Her weight fluctuated initially, but she later became very thin and weak. Feelings of nausea swept over her, but she did not vomit. Her weight was 88 lb and she was 5 ft 9. The emergency physician made a diagnosis of a small bowel obstruction complicating Crohn's disease and she was admitted to the surgery service.

Having had so many intravenous catheters in the past that she had no easily accessible veins, a central line was placed for hyperalimentation. Total parenteral nutrition consisted of 25% dextrose, intralipid, and amino acid solutions.

GENERAL CONSIDERATIONS

Each individual maintains a unique body weight that is rather finely controlled despite considerable day-to-day variations in diet and activity. Disease, injury, and operations profoundly affect this exquisite balance, or homeostasis. Common causes of dysfunction are starvation, anorexia, vomiting, diarrhea, and ileus, leading to weight loss. Adverse effects are mediated principally through two mechanisms:

1. Decreased nutritional input
2. Change in the body's chemistry (e.g., release of catecholamines, decreased insulin secretion, and utilization) producing a catabolic state

The extent and nature of these changes depend primarily on the disease process. The patient described in Case 1 had a profound weight loss both because of his inability to eat and because of the cachectic effects of the cancer adversely affecting his homeostasis. The second patient had a chronic inflammatory condition of the intestines (Crohn's disease); in addition to producing bouts of obstruction, this condition led to changes in the intestine's ability to absorb nutrients, leading to malabsorption.

While there are many ways to express the degree of malnutrition (percentage of usual weight, percentage of ideal weight, time frame of weight loss), the usual and most practical approach is to obtain a careful history of the patient's normal eating habits and body weight, as well as the changes that have occurred since the onset of disease. Weight loss, even in the obese, is a reflection of catabolism and negative nitrogen balance.

Nitrogen balance is the best indication of the need for nutritional support. It can be estimated by history, or it can be measured by obtaining a 24-hour collection for urine urea nitrogen (UUN):

$$\text{Nitrogen balance (g/day)} = \frac{\text{protein intake (g/day)}}{6.25}$$

$$- (\text{UUN [g/day]} + 4)$$

where UUN is obtained in a 24-hour sample. Since the UUN is reported in terms of protein, the protein content is divided by 6.25 to obtain nitrogen. A positive result of greater than +2 g/day is indicative of anabolism, while a negative value indicates catabolism and demonstrates the need for nutritional supplementation. A good estimate can also be made by measuring the serum creatinine and measuring the 24-hour urinary creatinine excretion. The 24-hour urine creatinine is divided by the ideal creatinine for height. The result is expressed as a percentage: mild malnutrition = 60–80%, moderate = 40–60%, severe = less than 40%.

Other measurements of malnutrition are the mid-arm muscle circumference and the triceps skin fold, which is an indirect measurement of the body's store of fat and total muscle mass. The immune response to a standard stimulus such as PPD may be helpful as well.

The best indicator of malnutrition is the serum albumin. A value below 2.7 g% is indicative of severe malnutrition. The serum albumin value is a very strong predictor of both mortality and morbidity in surgical patients. Below levels of 3.5 g%, every 0.1-g decrease in the serum albumin is attended by a significant increase in both mortality and morbidity. Serum albumin levels are therefore useful guides in assessing the progress of the disease or the efficacy of nutritional support.

Nutritional support is directed at supplying the necessary nutrients either through the gut (oral or enteral feeding) or intravenously (parenteral), readjusting the body's chemistry toward anabolism (positive nitrogen balance). This is accomplished by diminishing catecholamine release by correcting hypotension and sepsis and by increasing the release of endogenous insulin and improving its peripheral utilization. Insulin is the sine qua non of anabolism. Once appreciated, it is simple to deduce the efficacy of various forms of nutritional support. Insulin is added to total parenteral nutrition (TPN) to enhance glucose uptake and utilization in cases in which hyperglycemia and glucose loss in the urine occur.

Eating is the most prompt and potent way to induce insulin secretion. Frequent ingestion of nutrient-rich foods produces weight gain in healthy individuals and patients alike, assuming that insulin utilization is not thwarted by blocking of the cells' insulin receptors, which occurs in sepsis and extensive malignancy. When a patient is unable to ingest food, the next best option is to place food in the gastrointestinal tract through a catheter in the stomach or intestine (feeding jejunostomy, Case 1). Among the various routes, entry through the stomach or duodenum (Figs. 3.1 and 3.2) is preferable to jejunostomy (Fig. 3.3), since the duodenum is the most active site for absorption of nutrients in the alimentary tract.

Parenteral or intravenous feeding is the least desirable route of nutrition, although it is often the only recourse. Hence, while oral glucose causes a brisk and potent insulin response, intravenous glucose initially causes no insulin secretion. This explains why patients receiving TPN require 2–3 weeks of treatment before they become anabolic and begin to gain weight. Sustained insulin secretion begins two weeks after the institution of TPN. Without the insulin response, anabolism is not achieved.

KEY POINTS

- Changes in homeostasis are caused by starvation, anorexia, vomiting, diarrhea, and ileus, leading to weight loss, through decreased nutritional support and a change in the body's chemistry, producing a catabolic state

- Degree of malnutrition generally ascertained by careful history of patients's normal eating habits and body weight, as well as changes since onset of disease

- Nitrogen balance is best indication of need for nutritional support

- Positive result of greater than +2 g/day indicates anabolism, negative value catabolism requiring nutritional support

- Good estimates of malnutrition made by measuring serum creatinine and 24-hour urinary creatinine excretion, mid-arm muscle circumference and triceps fold, and immune response; best indicator is serum albumin (<2.7 g% indicates severe malnutrition)

- Aim of nutritional support is to supply necessary nutrients through gut (oral or enteral feeding) or by intravenous route

- Insulin sine qua non of anabolism; it is added to total parenteral nutrition

- Insulin secretion induced by three routes: (1) eating (prompt and potent), (2) placement of food in the GI tract through catheter in the stomach or intestine, or (3) parenteral or intravenous feeding (least desirable)

DIAGNOSIS

Malnutrition and the need for nutritional support are not difficult to discern clinically. A good history is generally all that is required. Patients with chronic disabling diseases (Case 2) are more difficult to assess. A simple graph plotting the patient's weight changes over time, with intervening events such as operations, therapy, and hospitalizations, will bring the current state of the patient's condition into sharper focus.

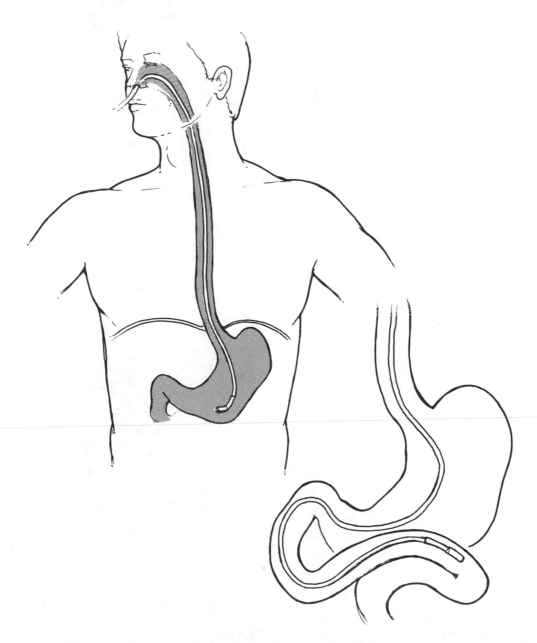

FIGURE 3.1   *When a patient is not able to eat, but the gastrointestinal tract still functions normally, a nasogastric tube can be placed, which allows enteral feeding. The disadvantages of nasogastric feeding are that the tube may cause erosion of the nasal alae, the feedings may reflux and cause aspiration pneumonia, and gastric distention may result. Longer tubes may be advanced through the pyloric sphincter into the duodenum (inset). This helps reduce the incidence of reflux and aspiration pneumonia.*

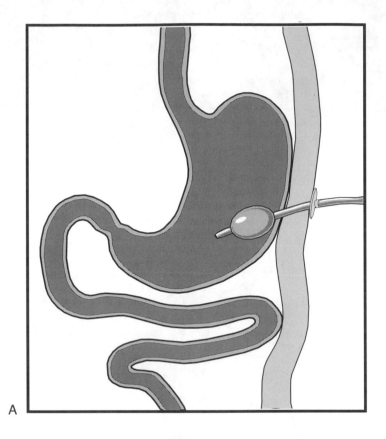

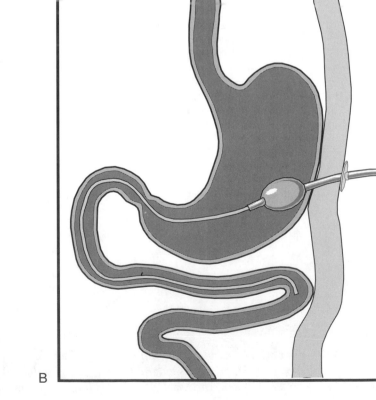

FIGURE 3.2 *(A) When long-term enteral nutrition is required, a permanent gastrostomy can be placed percutaneously. The first step requires placement of a catheter through the abdominal wall into the stomach under endoscopic guidance. (B) After the gastrostomy has been placed, a smaller catheter is threaded into the duodenum and jejunum. This allows feeding from a more distal point and effectively reduces the chances of aspiration pneumonia.*

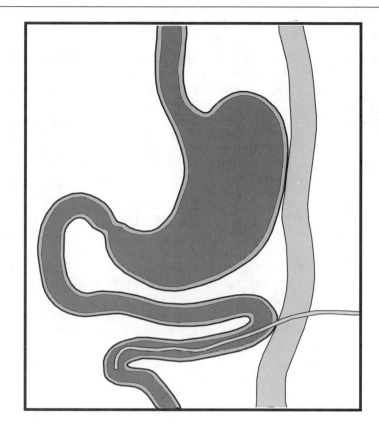

FIGURE 3.3 *A jejunostomy can be placed at the time of laparotomy. The catheter is secured to the bowel and then to the abdominal wall to prevent displacement. The relatively small size of the catheter requires meticulous care to prevent occlusion. Because the catheter lies in the jejunum, reflux and aspiration pneumonia do not occur.*

Physical examination invariably shows signs of wasting. The overall appearance or demeanor of the patient is depressed and muted. Speech is slow, soft, and minimal. The skin is cool and pale as the blood volume is contracted, and the patient is dehydrated. Wasting is evident in the temples, supraclavicular areas, and upper arms.

Anemia is common, although it may be masked by the hemoconcentration. While a number of specific body constituents can be accurately measured in a malnourished patient (iron, vitamin B_{12}), such information is seldom useful.

The most important laboratory determination is the serum albumin concentration. Although prealbumin has a shorter half-life (7 versus 18 days), and theoretically should be more sensitive to acute changes, it has not been shown to have any advantages over the more the readily available serum albumin concentration.

KEY POINTS

- A good history is generally all that is required for diagnosis
- Simple graph plotting weight changes over time brings patient's condition into sharper focus
- Physical examination will show signs of wasting
- Serum albumin concentration most important laboratory determination

DIFFERENTIAL DIAGNOSIS

Decreased intake of food may be the result of socioeconomic problems. The amount, type, volume, and frequency of meals must be ascertained. Substance abuse frequently leaves people without adequate resources to feed themselves or their dependents properly, resulting in malnutrition. Psychological conditions such as anorexia nervosa and bulimia must be sought and not confused with other organic causes of weight loss and cachexia. Difficulty in swallowing may be attributable to pain, neurological abnormalities interrupting the swallowing reflex, or mechanical obstruction due to swelling or a tumor.

Increased fluid loss may be due to vomiting, diarrhea, or a high output fistula. Malignant tumors, metabolic conditions such as diabetes and adrenal insufficiency, and chronic infections such as tuberculosis are potent causes of weight loss.

KEY POINTS

- Differential diagnosis includes socioeconomic problems, substance abuse, psychological conditions, difficulty in swallowing, increased fluid loss, malignant tumors, metabolic conditions (diabetes, adrenal insufficiency), and chronic infections

TREATMENT

The guiding principle of nutritional support, by whatever route, is to provide the patient with a slight excess of all nutritional factors. Therefore, in adults, it is not useful to attempt calculation of depleted nutritional stores with a view to replacing them precisely.

Enteral feeding is the preferred method of nutritional support. It has fewer complication and costs far less. Enteral nutrition is given when postoperative conditions and complications do not allow for normal feeding (Case 1) or when the patient is incapacitated, as after head injury or major surgery of the head and neck. Some patients with severe malnutrition benefit from enteral feeding to supplement whatever they are able to take orally.

Enteral formulas can be separated into three groups: polymeric, elemental, and modular. Polymeric diets consist of large molecular proteins, carbohydrates, and fats. These diets are the most physiologic, maintain the bowel mucosa best, and are the least expensive. They are given to patients whose bowel is normal, but for whom feeding is hindered by injury or surgery of the face or throat (including the esophagus), or in an unconscious patient. Elemental diets are predigested to yield amino acids, mono- and disaccharides, and fatty acids. These are given if bowel pathology is present or if the bowel is shortened (a segment has been removed or is not functioning). They are less physiologic than polymeric diets, do less to maintain the intestinal mucosa, and are considerably higher in cost. Modular diets are elemental diets that have been separated into the different constituents. They can be mixed in various combinations to suit specific needs, such as for diabetes, liver failure, renal failure, and certain metabolic abnormalities. Special formulations of enteral diets are available (e.g., amino acids, simple sugars) to enhance absorption in the proximal bowel without stimulation of the pancreas. These special enteral formulas tend to be very expensive and of little proven value. The major limitation of enteral diets is that about one-third of patients develop diarrhea, further aggravating fluid and electrolyte deficiencies. The usual causes are bolus feeding, cold fluids, and hypertonic solutions.

When no functional gastrointestinal tract is available, TPN must be used. TPN provides water, electrolytes, carbohydrates, lipids, amino acids, vitamins, and trace elements such as zinc, cobalt, and manganese (Tables 3.1 and 3.2). These materials are combined to a final concentration of about 25% dextrose, 3% amino acid, and 5% lipids. The lipids contain long chain and essential fatty acids; deficiency of lipids causes a dry scaly skin and hair loss. This hypertonic solution can only be given through the central venous system, where dilution and adequate mixing of the nutrients will take place. This is achieved by placing a central venous catheter inserted percutaneously through the subclavicular or transjugular routes. When TPN is used, the needs of the patient must be calculated. The free water requirement is 30–35 ml/kg/day—more if the patient is dehydrated and less if overloaded as in renal or cardiac failure. Electrolytes are needed for maintenance and to replace losses (see Ch. 2). Calories are derived from carbohydrates and fats. To maintain weight, 30–35 cal/kg is needed. In the presence of stress, such as massive trauma, sepsis, or major surgery, the need increases 1.2–1.8 times, depending on the type of stress. The basal caloric requirement should be multiplied by the stress factor, to determine how many calories are required. Carbohydrate, in the form of dextrose, is normally given at a dose of 2–4 g/kg of the patient's ideal weight and may go as high as 5 g/kg. Fat is given in the form of long chain fatty acids. Before lipids are administered, the serum triglycerides should be measured. If increased, intralipid infusion is contraindicated, because it may cause pancreatitis. Fats are begun at 0.5 g/kg and increased every 2 days in 0.5 g/kg increments, to a maximum of 2.5 g/kg. Several factors determine the ratio of carbohydrate to fat. Oxidation of carbohydrate produces one-third more carbon dioxide than is produced by fat. The respiratory quotient (RQ) of carbohydrate is 1 and the RQ of fat is only 0.7. The patient on a ventilator benefits by combining dextrose and fat to obtain a lower RQ and subsequently less energy expenditure to exhale the carbon dioxide produced. Protein is given in the form of amino acids at 1–1.5 g/kg of the ideal weight and may go as high as 3 g/kg. Vitamins and trace elements are added (Tables 3-1 and 3-2). For example, the patient discussed in Case 2 would require a volume of 30 ml × 40 kg = 1,200 ml. Calories required would be 35 kcal/kg × 40 kg = 1,400 kcal. This can then be multiplied by the patient's stress factor (moderate), that is, 1.4, 1,400 kcal × 1.4 = 1,960 kcal and the corresponding amount of carbohydrate and fat calculated. If rounded off to 2,000 kcal, one-half could come from carbohydrate and one-half from fat. The ratio of carbohydrate to fat could vary from 50:50 to 80:20, to virtually any ratio suitable for the patient, with 1,000 kcal from each. Carbohydrate amounts to 4 kcal/g, 1,000 kcal = 250 g, at 25% dextrose, which would be 1 L. Fat is 9 kcal/g, thus, 1,000 kcal = 111 g or 555 ml of a 20% solution or 1,110 ml of a 10% solution. These volumes may be rounded off to the nearest convenient number, taking standard packaging into account.

The major complications of TPN are sepsis, pneumothorax, and bleeding from catheter placement. With long term TPN, thrombosis of the superior vena cava can occur at tip of the TPN catheter.

KEY POINTS

- Guiding principle of nutritional support is to provide patient with slight excess of all nutritional factors
- Enteral feeding preferred method of nutritional support
- Polymeric diets consist of large molecular proteins, carbohydrates, and fats

TABLE 3.1 *Vitamins*

Vitamin	Daily Requirement	Action and/or Signs of Deficiency
Water soluble		
B$_1$ (thiamine)	5 mg/day IV	Necessary in carbohydrate metabolism; shortages present with peripheral neuropathy and encephalopathy
B$_2$ (riboflavin)	5 mg/day IV	Coenzymes in redox system; skin inflammation and visual disturbances
B$_3$ (niacin)	50 mg/day IV	Important in NADP system; pellagra displays skin, gastrointestinal, and neurologic abnormalities
B$_6$ (pyridoxine)	5 mg/day	Coenzyme in protein and lipid metabolism; dermatitis, neuropathy, and calcium oxalate stones
B$_{12}$ (cyanocobalamin)	12 µg/day, parenterally IM or IV	Nucleic acids synthesis; deficiency causes megaloblastic anemia and neurologic abnormalities
Biotin	60 µg/day	Cofactor in amino acid, fat, and carbohydrate metabolism; dermatitis, myalgia, and neurologic abnormalities
C (ascorbic acid)	50–300 mg	Collagen synthesis, wound healing, and immune system; scurvy: gums, periosteal, skin, and internal hemorrhage
Folic acid	600 µg/day	Nucleic acid synthesis; megaloblastic anemia and glossitis
Pantothenic acid	15 mg/day	Component of coenzyme A
Fat soluble		
A	2,500 IU/day	Maintains epithelial surfaces; deficiency: dermatitis, night blindness, and increased susceptibility to infection
D	250 IU/day	Rickets in children and osteomalacia in adults
E	10–50 IU/day	Antioxidant; deficiency: hemolysis, myonecrosis, and cardiomyopathy
K	10 mg/day to 10 mg/wk	Formation of clotting factors II, VII, IX, and X; deficiency causes a bleeding disorder

TABLE 3.2 *Trace elements*

Trace Element	Dosage	Action and/or Deficiency
Chromium	10 µg IV, 200 µg enterally	Facilitates insulin binding to membrane receptors; deficiency causes glucose intolerance
Cobalt (vitamin B$_{12}$)	12 µg/day	Nucleic acid synthesis; megaloblastic anemia and neurologic abnormalities
Copper	0.15–0.5 mg IV, 2–3 mg enterally	Several enzyme systems, including cytochrome oxidase; deficiency causes pancytopenia
Iodine	150 µg/day	Essential for thyroid hormone production; myxedema in adults and cretinism in infants
Iron	2 mg IV, 10 mg/day PO	Essential for hemoglobin and respiratory cytochromes; anemia and cerebral, muscular, and immune abnormalities
Manganese	0.2–0.8 mg IV, 2–5 mg orally or enterally	Cofactor for enzymes; gluconeogenesis and antioxidant capability of cells; nausea, weight loss, low fats, hair pigment changes
Selenium	20–40 µg IV, 50–200 µg enterally or orally	Part of glutathione peroxidase enzyme; deficiency causes cardiac failure and proximal neuromuscular weakness
Zinc	2.5 mg IV, 15 mg PO	Several enzyme systems and protein production; plasma proteins, growth, wound healing, and cellular immunity

- Elemental diets are predigested to yield amino acids, monosaccharides, disaccharides, and fatty acids

- Modular diets are elemental diets separated into the different constituents

- Major limitation of enteral diets is that about one-third of patients develop diarrhea

- If no functional gastrointestinal tract available, TPN must be used

- This hypertonic solution can only be given through the central venous system, where dilution and adequate mixing of the nutrients will take place

- Free water requirement is 30–35 ml/kg/day

- Calories are derived from carbohydrates and fats; 30–35 cal/kg needed

- Requirement increases 1.2–1.8 times in presence of stress (massive trauma, sepsis, major surgery)

- Basal caloric requirement is multiplied by the stress factor to determine caloric requirement

- Carbohydrates given as dextrose at 2–4 g/kg of ideal weight; fats given in form of long chain fatty acids

- Before lipid administration, serum triglycerides should be measured

- Oxidation of carbohydrate produces one-third more carbon dioxide than produced by fat

- Protein given as amino acids at 1–1.5 g/kg of ideal weight; vitamins and trace elements are added

- Major complications of TPN are sepsis, pneumothorax, and bleeding from catheter placement

FOLLOW-UP

The end point of nutritional support is the conversion of catabolism to anabolism. Weight gain is difficult to evaluate, as malnourished patients are commonly dehydrated. Measurements of creatinine clearance and serum albumin concentrations provide additional support for anabolism. Clinically, when patients begin to feel better, they become physically stronger and more animated. Chronically intubated patients who were previously difficult if not impossible to wean from the ventilator are now capable of breathing on their own.

KEY POINTS

- Conversion of catabolism to anabolism is end point nutritional support

- Measurements of creatinine clearance and serum albumin concentrations provides additional support for anabolism

SUGGESTED READINGS

Apelgren KN, Dean RE: Enteral Feeding in Long-Term Care. Precept Press, Chicago, 1990

   A comprehensive guide to enteral nutrition.

Barker LR, Burton JR, Zieve PD: Ambulatory Medicine. 4th Ed. Williams & Wilkins, Baltimore, 1994

   A concise discussion of oral, enteral, and parenteral nutrition.

Bell SJ, Pasulka PS, Blackburn GL: In Skipper A (ed): Dietitian's Handbook of Enteral and Parenteral Nutrition. Aspen, Rockville, MD, 1989

   Detailed information on enteral and parenteral nutrition is given in this useful reference work.

Civeta, JM, Taylor RW, Kirby RR: Critical Care. 2nd Ed. Lippincott-Raven, Philadelphia, 1992

   Comprehensive work on enteral and parenteral nutrition for the clinician and particularly the intensivist.

QUESTIONS

1. *The most important element in converting catabolism to anabolism is?*
   - A. Elimination of hypovolemia and sepsis and tumor burden.
   - B. Providing adequate quantities of nutrients.
   - C. Release of endogenous insulin.
   - D. All of the above.

2. *Enteral feeding in contrast to total parental nutrition is?*
   - A. Not nearly as effective.
   - B. More susceptible to septic complications.
   - C. Safer, easier, cheaper, and more effective.
   - D. None of the above.

3. *A course of TPN should be considered in patients who will require nutritional support?*
   - A. For 3 weeks or more.
   - B. 1 week to 10 days preoperatively.
   - C. Immediately postoperatively and until the patient is fully recovered (14–17 days).
   - D. As a precaution in patients at high risk of operative intervention.

4. *Complications of total parenteral nutrition are?*
   - A. Phlebitis.
   - B. Hyperglycemia.
   - C. Pancreatitis.
   - D. All of the above.

(See p. 603 for answers.)

4 SHOCK

FRED S. BONGARD

Shock is defined as the failure of adequate oxygenation of end organs. The clinical patterns are varied, but must be recognized expediently if patients are to be treated appropriately. The aims of this chapter are to (1) describe the different types of shock and correlate their underlying physiology with clinical manifestations, (2) elucidate the common etiologies of shock, (3) discuss the hemodynamic patterns associated with the different kinds of shock, and (4) describe the appropriate means of resuscitation and subsequent therapy. Although the hemodynamic patterns ascribed to the different kinds of shock may appear rigid, patients often present with cardiovascular profiles that do not fit any of the customary patterns. More than one etiology may be present, causing a mixed pattern that defies simple categorization.

CASE 1
HYPOTENSION AFTER A MOTOR VEHICLE ACCIDENT

A 23-year-old male was brought to the emergency room after being involved in a motorcycle accident. According to paramedics, the nonhelmeted patient was turning when he was struck broadside by a car moving 45 mph. He was thrown from the motorcycle and landed about 25 feet away. On initial evaluation by the paramedics at the scene, he was awake but confused. Blood pressure was 90/60 mmHg with a heart rate of 125 bpm. Contusions were apparent about the head and upper extremities. Severe angulation of the left leg was noted with massive swelling of the left thigh. Breath sounds were equal and full bilaterally. An intravenous infusion of lactated Ringer's solution was begun through a large intravenous catheter placed in the right forearm.

En route to the emergency room, his blood pressure declined to 70/50 mmHg. This was accompanied by an increase in heart rate to 150 bpm. He became progressively more disoriented and sleepy. Several rapid infusions of 500 ml of intravenous fluid were required to keep the systolic blood pressure above 80 mmHg.

Initial assessment in the emergency room found a barely arousable male whose skin was diaphoretic and ashen in color. Blood pressure was 75/50 mmHg with a heart rate of 140 bpm. An endotracheal tube was inserted to assist in ventilation while another large intravenous catheter was placed in the left arm. A Foley catheter returned 250 ml of clear yellow urine. The initial Hct was 35%. In response to the rapid infusion of 3 L of intravenous fluid, the blood pressure rose to 110/80 mmHg and the heart rate fell to 90 bpm. Small amounts of urine began to accumulate in the Foley collection bag. A second Hct returned at 25%. Continued administration of intravenous fluid and blood increased the blood pressure to 130/80 mmHg during which time he regained consciousness and began to complain of abdominal and right leg pain. A third Hct, obtained after the administration of 2 units of packed RBCs, was 23%.

CASE 2
PERFORATED COLON CANCER

A 72-year-old female presented to the emergency room complaining of 12 hours of abdominal pain. The presence of free air under the diaphragm on an upright chest x-ray, and a tender abdomen prompted immediate abdominal exploration. At the time of operation, a perforated cancer of the sigmoid colon with extensive soilage of the peritoneal cavity was found. The perforated colon was resected and a proximal colostomy performed.

Postoperative convalescence was uneventful for the first 2 days. On the morning of the third day, she was noted to be confused and lethargic. Shortly thereafter, her blood pressure declined to 80/40 mmHg with an increase in heart rate to 110 bpm. Rapid intravenous fluid infusion increased her blood pressure to 110/60 mmHg. Urine output remained depressed as did the level of consciousness. A flow-directed pulmonary artery catheter was inserted, which demonstrated pulmonary artery pressures of 25/10 mmHg, with a PCWP of 13 mmHg. CO was 9 L/min with a systemic vascular resistance of 500 dynes·sec^{-2}·cm^5. $S\bar{v}O_2$ was 85% with an (a-v)DO_2 of 3 ml/dl.

The patient was started on an intravenous infusion of dopamine at a rate of 5 µg/kg/min. Blood pressure did not increase until the dopamine infusion reached 13 µg/kg/min, at which point the CO was 12 L/min and the systemic vascular resistance was 700 dynes·sec^{-2}·cm^5. Antibiotic therapy was expanded. Over the next several hours, progressively greater amounts of dopamine were required to support her blood pressure. An infusion of norepinephrine was begun with a return of blood pressure to 100/60 mmHg. In spite of the pressor infusion, her blood pressure continued to deteriorate until she ultimately experienced a cardiac arrest and could not be resuscitated.

GENERAL CONSIDERATIONS

Shock may be grouped into three broad physiologic categories: (1) hypovolemic shock, (2) distributive shock, and (3) cardiac shock. Hypovolemic shock is the most common type among surgical patients and typically results from acute blood loss following trauma (Case 1). Distributive shock occurs when the cardiac output (CO) is redistributed so that oxygen delivery (DO_2) to critical visceral beds, such as the liver and kidneys, is insufficient (Case 2). Cardiac shock results from inadequate CO due either to cardiac failure or to mechanical restriction (pericardial tamponade), which prevents the heart from filling and emptying properly.

Hypovolemic shock is caused by loss of intravascular volume. This may be due to internal or external hemorrhage, or to severe dehydration without adequate volume replacement. Body water constitutes approximately 70% of total body weight and exists in three major compartments in equilibrium. Circulating blood, or intravascular volume, constitutes only 7% of total body weight, but is responsible for the distribution of oxygen and nutrients throughout the body. Extravascular (interstitial) fluids are in the interstices between blood vessels and cells, and constitute 14% of total body weight. Intracellular volume accounts for 42% of total body weight, and is the largest reservoir of fluid in the body. About 1% of fluid is sequestered in areas such as the vitreous humor, and does not normally participate in fluid exchange.

The cardiovascular system responds to intravascular volume loss with reflex mechanisms that maintain CO and blood pressure. The two primary responses are increased heart rate and peripheral vasoconstriction (Case 1). Blood pressure is directly proportional to peripheral vascular resistance and CO. CO, in turn, is dependent on heart rate and stroke volume. When intravascular volume decreases, cardiac filling declines, and the amount of blood ejected with each cardiac cycle (stroke volume) falls. An increase in heart rate will return CO toward normal by increasing the number of cycles per minute. Tachycardia can maintain CO, provided that some critical residual volume remains, and that the heart does not beat so fast that the chambers do not have time to fill during diastole. Blood pressure is also supported by peripheral vasoconstriction. Adrenergic discharge results in constriction of large capacitance venules and small veins. Because 60% of the circulating blood volume is normally in the venous circuit, this action moves blood back toward the heart, thereby augmenting venous return and increasing stroke volume.

When blood is lost acutely (Case 1), the hydrostatic pressure (in this case, blood pressure) within the vasculature decreases. When this occurs, the relative gradient of hydrostatic pressure between the interstitial and intravascular compartments changes, allowing fluid to move from the interstitial into the intravascular space. The extent of this fluid translocation is somewhat limited because volume leaving the interstitial compartment causes an increase in that compartment's osmotic pressure, which partially offsets the hydrostatic effect. Approximately 1–2 L of fluid can move into the intravascular space through this mechanism, although the process requires approximately 30–60 minutes to complete. This vascular refill is responsible for the initial decline in hematocrit (Hct) observed in hypovolemic patients.

The systemic consequences of hypovolemic shock are related to decreases in the global DO_2. DO_2 is dependent on the content of oxygen in arterial blood (CaO_2) and on CO. The major determinants of CaO_2 are the concentration of hemoglobin (Hb) and its oxygen saturation. Following hemorrhage and resuscitation with blood-free fluids, the Hb concentration may decline precipitously. However, unless pulmonary injury or respiratory embarrassment has occurred, gas exchange is usually not severely impaired, and Hb oxygen saturation remains normal. Systemic oxygen is defined as follows:

$$DO_2 \ (ml/min) = CaO_2 \ (ml/dl) \cdot$$
$$CO \ (L/min) \cdot 10$$

$$CaO_2 = [Hb \ (g/dl) \cdot 1.34 \cdot HbSat]$$

where CaO_2 is arterial oxygen concentration; CO is cardiac output; Hb is hemoglobin; and HbSat is fractional hemoglobin saturation (e.g., 0.98).

Examination of the equation indicates that following hemorrhage, DO_2 to tissue can fall due to (1) decreased CO, (2) decreased Hb concentration, and/or (3) decreased arterial HbSat. Peripheral consumption of oxygen ($\dot{V}O_2$) usually remains constant under these circumstances (approximately 225 ml/min of O_2) because most tissue beds are able to increase their extraction of oxygen. The brain and heart typically extract large amounts of oxygen normally, and hence are unable to increase their extraction significantly when delivery is limited. This explains why changes in mental status appear early in shock when the brain fails to receive its normal supply of oxygen rich blood.

Hypovolemic shock induces a number of associated systemic effects and compensatory mechanisms. Adrenergic discharge and the secretion of vasopressin and angiotensin combine with decreased blood flow to reduce renal glomerular filtration and urine production (Case 1). Salt and water retention assist in maintaining adequate circulating blood volume, producing highly concentrated urine. Sustained hypotension may cause acute tubular necrosis. Immunologic effects include the production of tumor necrosis factor (TNF), neutrophil stimulation, the production and release of oxygen free radicals, lysozomal enzymes, and leukotrienes C_4 and D_4. These latter mediators disrupt the integrity of the vascular endothelium and promote leakage of fluid into the interstitial space ("third spacing"). Hypotension also causes a decrease in splanchnic blood flow, which weakens the intestinal mucosal barrier to gut flora and promotes the translocation of micro-organisms from the gut lumen into the portal venous and lymphatic systems. This mechanism may explain why some patients develop septicemia following hypovolemic shock.

Distributive shock is so named because of the redistribution of blood flow to the viscera. The three most common types of distributive shock are septic, neurogenic, and anaphylactic. Among these, septic shock is the most common, and carries a mortality of between 40% and 60%. Aerobic gram-negative bacillary infections with *Escherichia coli* and *Klebsiella* are most common. Gram-positive organisms and fungi may also be responsible for septic shock. It is likely that interactions between bacterial products and host defenses are responsible for septic shock, rather than the bacteria themselves. Endotoxin is a lipopolysaccharide component of the cell wall of gram-negative bacteria that is released when the organisms die. It has effects on several homeostatic systems, including complement, kinins, coagulation factors, plasma phospholipases, cytokines, β-endorphins, platelet-activating factor, and prostaglandins. When endotoxin interacts with macrophages, a number of proteins, referred to as cytokines, are produced. These include tumor necrosis factor (TNF) and interleukins (IL)-1, -2, and -6. The cytokines induce counterregulatory hormones such as glucagon, epinephrine, and cortisol, which also play a part in the septic response. These products are responsible for increased vascular permeability and the release of toxic oxygen metabolites, which can cause extensive tissue destruction. Recent work has focused on nitric oxide (NO) as an important mediator of vascular dilatation and hypotension.

Septic shock manifests with elevated CO, decreased systemic vascular resistance, and decreased blood pressure (Case 2) (Table 4.1). Reflex increases in heart rate are responsible for maintaining blood pressure. Earlier investigators postulated that the opening of small but numerous arteriovenous shunts in the skin and subcutaneous tissue were responsible for decreasing systemic vascular resistance while maintaining blood flow to the skin. In contradistinction to hypovolemic shock where cutaneous blood flow declines, resulting in cool extremities, the open shunts were thought to explain the retained warmth of septic shock. Subsequent investigations have failed, however, to confirm the presence of such shunts. Rather, *redistribution* with mismatching of DO_2 and metabolic demand likely accounts for the observed hemodynamic alterations. Unlike hypovolemic shock, peripheral consumption and extraction of oxygen decrease in septic shock, although the overall metabolic rate is markedly elevated (Case 2).

TABLE 4.1 *Diagnostic criteria of the systemic inflammatory response syndrome*

Clinical evidence of an infection site

Hypothermia (<35.5°C) or fever (>38.3°C)

Tachycardia (>90 bpm)

Tachypnea (>20 bpm)

Inadequate organ perfusion or dysfunction as evidenced by *one* of the following:

   Poor or altered cerebral function

   Hypoxemia (PaO_2 <75 mmHg)

   Elevated plasma lactate

   Oliguria (urine output <30 ml/hr or <0.5 ml/kg body weight/hr)

(From Bongard FS, Shock and Resuscitation. p. 13. In Bongard FS and Sue DY: Current Critical Care Diagnosis and Treatment. Appleton & Lange, E. Norwalk, CT, 1994, with permission.)

Anaphylactic shock and anaphylactoid reactions are due to the sudden release of preformed inflammatory mediators from mast cells and basophils. The most common agents responsible are penicillin, hymenoptera (bee) stings, and contrast agents. Anaphylactic shock is a true amnestic response that occurs when a sensitized individual contacts an antigen resulting in the release of IgE. Histamine and platelet-activating factor are released into the circulation resulting in vasodilatation, bronchoconstriction, pruritis, bronchorrhea, platelet aggregation, and increased vascular permeability, which may lead to laryngeal edema and airway obstruction. Anaphylactoid reactions cause direct release of these compounds without mediation by IgE. The vasodilatation and vascular permeability result in decreased blood pressure and shock, while airway obstruction produces hypoxemia.

Neurogenic shock occurs when loss of peripheral vasomotor tone produces redistribution of intravascular volume. Blood pools in the periphery, venous return is decreased, and CO falls. Neurogenic shock occurs after high spinal cord interruption or following an improperly placed spinal anesthetic. Reflex tachycardia occurs to maintain CO, but if the cardiac sympathetic outflow is affected, bradycardia results. Because sympathetic flow to cutaneous blood vessels may also be interrupted, warm extremities, similar to those observed with septic shock, are present.

Cardiac shock occurs when the heart is unable to pump the blood volume presented to it. Cardiogenic shock develops when the heart loses its ability to function properly as a pump, and can occur after an acute myocardial infarction, with low output syndromes, and in end-stage cardiomyopathy. Other causes include rupture of the intraventricular septum, mitral or aortic insufficiency, papillary muscle rupture, and aortic valvular stenosis. Cardiocompressive shock occurs when the great veins and cardiac chambers are compressed, restricting normal filling and emptying. Cardiac compressive shock develops chronically, as the result of diseases that cause pericardial effusions, or acutely, as the result of a penetrating cardiac injury that allows the heart to pump blood into the pericardial sac.

Cardiogenic shock may occur semiacutely or over a prolonged period. When more than 45% of the left ventricular myocardium malfunctions, cardiogenic shock becomes clinically evident. Like hemorrhagic shock, cardiac shock results in decreased flow and DO_2 to the periphery. The significant differentiating feature is that patients with cardiac shock tend to be hypervolemic, rather than hypovolemic. Stage I (compensated hypotension) invokes the normal compensatory mechanisms (tachycardia and vasoconstriction), which are able to restore blood flow to normal levels. Stage II (decompensated hypotension) occurs when CO falls to the point that peripheral vasoconstriction is no longer able to maintain blood pressure. Stage III

(irreversible shock) results in activation of the ischemic mediators that cause cellular membrane injury. Bradycardia (<50 bpm) and arrhythmias are common during this final stage.

Cardiac compressive shock is a low output state that results from compression of the heart and great vessels. Common acute causes include penetrating cardiac injuries and tension pneumothorax. High levels of positive end-expiratory pressure from mechanical ventilators may collapse the intrathoracic vasculature and decrease cardiac filling, thereby simulating cardiac compressive shock. Decreased CO results and causes a decline in peripheral DO_2.

KEY POINTS

- Three physiologic categories of shock: (1) hypovolemic, (most common) from acute blood loss following trauma (Case 1), (2) distributive, occurring when CO is redistributed and DO_2 to critical visceral beds is insufficient, and (3) cardiac, resulting from inadequate CO due to cardiac failure or mechanical restriction (pericardial tamponade) that prevents the heart from filling and emptying properly

Hypovolemic shock

- Circulating blood, or intravascular volume, constitutes only 7% of body weight but responsible for distributing O_2 and nutrients throughout body

- Cardiovascular system responds to intravascular volume loss with reflex mechanisms that maintain CO and blood pressure; primary responses are increased heart rate and peripheral vasoconstriction

- Vascular refill responsible for initial Hct decline observed in hypovolemic patients

- Systemic consequences of hypovolemic shock related to decreases in DO_2

- Following hemorrhage, DO_2 can fall due to (1) decreased CO, (2) decreased Hb concentration, and/or (3) decreased arterial HbSat; peripheral consumption of VO_2 usually remains constant (225 ml/min of O_2) because most tissue beds increase O_2 extraction

- Salt and water retention assist in maintaining blood volume, producing highly concentrated urine

Distributive Shock

- Most common types of distributive shock are septic, neurogenic, and anaphylactic

- Septic shock (most common) with mortality of 40–60%, manifests with elevated CO, decreased systemic vascular resistance, and decreased blood pressure; aerobic gram-negative bacillary infections with *E. Coli* and *Klebsiella* most common

- Redistribution with mismatching of DO_2 and metabolic demand likely accounts for hemodynamic alterations

- Anaphylactic shock and anaphylactoid reactions due to sudden release of preformed inflammatory mediators from mast cells and basophils

• Neurogenic shock occurs when loss of peripheral vasomotor tone redistributes intravascular volume; blood pools in periphery, venous return is decreased, and CO falls

Cardiac Shock

• Cardiac shock occurs when the heart is unable to pump blood; cardiogenic shock develops when the heart loses ability to function as pump; cardiocompressive shock occurs when great veins and cardiac chambers are compressed, restricting normal filling and emptying

• Cardiac shock results in decreased flow and DO_2 to periphery; unlike hemorrhagic shock, patients tend to be hypervolemic, not hypovolemic

DIAGNOSIS

The diagnosis of shock depends on recognizing inadequate tissue supply of oxygen and nutrients. The specific type of shock responsible can usually be deduced from the clinical situation. Patients with acute blood loss are most likely to have hypovolemic shock, while postoperative patients with severe infections are most likely to have septic (distributive) shock.

The findings associated with hypovolemic shock are listed in Table 4.2. Although blood pressure is low, the extent of hypovolemia may not necessarily be severe. Young people can maintain their blood pressure in the face of moderately severe hypovolemia through vasoconstriction and minimal increases in heart rate. Older patients may develop hypotension with far less blood loss. Orthostatic blood pressure testing can clarify the extent of volume loss. Normally, transition from the supine to the sitting position will result in a decrease in blood pressure of less than 10 mmHg. When hypovolemia is present, the decline is greater. Older patients, who are minimally hypovolemic with normal blood pressures in the supine position, may exhibit hypotension when tested upright. When multiple injuries are present, orthostatic testing should be done with extreme caution because of the possibility of aggravating potentially unstable skeletal injuries.

Hypovolemia-induced reduction in CO manifests as coolness of the skin and pallor, collapse of cutaneous veins, and oliguria (<0.5 ml/kg/hr) (Case 1). Measurement of central venous pressure is usually not necessary. Placement of a central venous monitoring catheter in hypovolemic patients is dangerous because the subclavian and internal jugular veins are collapsed and difficult to cannulate. Ill-advised attempts may result in lethal consequences such as subclavian artery laceration, venous injury, or tension pneumothorax. If a pre-existing catheter is present, decreased central venous and pulmonary capillary wedge pressures (PCWPs) along with depressed CO will be observed. Because peripheral oxygen extraction is increased, mixed venous oxygen saturation ($S\bar{v}O_2$) is decreased. Pulmonary function is usually normal, as is arterial Hb oxygen saturation (SaO_2) and partial pressure (PaO_2). However, because venous HbSat is decreased due to increased peripheral extraction, the gradient between the arterial and venous oxygen contents [$(a-v)DO_2$] is increased typically to greater than 6 ml O_2/dl.

The Hct may be normal, low, or high, depending on the etiology and the duration of shock. In a patient with chronic Hb-free volume loss from diarrhea or from a gastrointestinal fistula, the Hct will be high. When hemorrhage is responsible, and some time has elapsed since the injury or the patient has received intravenous fluid,

TABLE 4.2 *Clinical findings associated with shock*

| | CARDIOGENIC SHOCK | CARDIAC COMPRESSIVE SHOCK | HYPOVOLEMIC OR TRAUMATIC SHOCK | | | HIGH-OUTPUT SEPTIC SHOCK | NEUROGENIC SHOCK |
			MILD	MODERATE	SEVERE		
Skin perfusion	Pale	Pale	Pale	Pale	Pale	Pink	Pink
Urine output	Low	Low	Normal	Low	Low	Low	Low
Pulse rate	High	High	Normal	High	High	High	Low
Blood pressure	Normal	Low	Normal	Normal	Low	Low	Low
Mental status	Anxious	Anxious	Normal	Thirsty	Anxious	Anxious	Anxious
Neck veins	Distended	Distended	Flat	Flat	Flat	Flat	Flat
Oxygen consumption ($\dot{V}O_2$)	Low	Low	Normal	Normal	Low	Low	Low
Cardiac index	Low	Low	Low	Low	Low	High	Low
Cardiac filling pressures	High	High	Low	Low	Low	Low	Low
Systemic vascular resistance	High	High	High	High	High	Low	Low

(From Holcroft J, Robinson MK: Shock: identification and management of shock states. In: Care of the Surgical Patient. Scientific American, New York, 1992, with permission.)

the Hct will be low. Of great importance, however, is that the Hct is normal when measured shortly after acute hemorrhage. Confirmatory studies include elevated lactic acid and depressed bicarbonate concentrations.

Patients with distributive shock have an increased CO in the face of decreased blood pressure. On physical examination, they have warm dry extremities and tachycardia, and may be confused or disoriented. When the etiology is sepsis, the systemic inflammatory response syndrome (SIRS) may appear before hemodynamic compromise occurs (Table 4.1). Septic shock is said to occur when the mean blood pressure is less than 60 mmHg or when there is more than a 40-mmHg decline in systolic blood pressure from premorbid baseline. If a pulmonary artery catheter is present, an increased CO with decreased systemic vascular resistance will be noted (Case 2). If decreased CO is present, concomitant hypovolemia should be suspected. PCWP is usually low or normal. Because of redistribution of blood flow, decreased $\dot{V}O_2$ results in an increase in $S\bar{v}O_2$, which is typically higher than 75%. The $(a-v)DO_2$ is decreased to less than 4 ml O_2/dl. Pulmonary dysfunction is common and is reflected by a decrease in PaO_2 and SaO_2. Pulmonary compliance decreases as the respiratory distress syndrome worsens, and patients require support with a ventilator.

Leukocytosis is common, although neutropenia may be present and portends a poor outcome. Disseminated intravascular coagulation (DIC) with increased prothrombin time (PT), elevated fibrin split products, and decreased fibrinogen concentration may occur. Hyperglycemia is common and is caused by the actions of the stress hormones, including epinephrine, glucagon, and cortisol. Serum glucose levels fall when liver failure occurs as a preterminal event. Hepatic dysfunction is reflected by increases in bilirubin, aminotransferase, and alkaline phosphatase concentrations. Positive blood cultures are obtained in only 45% of patients diagnosed with the SIRS or septic shock. Other organisms such as *Candida albicans* may be causative. The absence of micro-organisms in blood cultures should in no way exclude the diagnosis of septic shock.

Anaphylactic shock and anaphylactoid reactions occur after exposure inciting antigen. The first symptoms include cutaneous flushing and pruritis, followed by laryngeal edema and bronchospasm, bronchorrhea, and pulmonary edema. Other signs include seizure, lacrimation, abdominal distention, diarrhea, rinorrhea, and nasal congestion. If treatment is not given quickly, hypotension is followed by circulatory collapse.

Neurogenic shock is typically preceded by trauma or spinal anesthesia and presents with hypotension and tachycardia. Signs and symptoms of spinal cord injury and spinal shock will be present. Blood pressure may fall to very low levels, and is due to peripheral venous pooling. Like sepsis, neurogenic shock may present with cutaneous warmth in the denervated area. Laboratory studies are not helpful. A pulmonary artery catheter will show decreases in central venous pressure, PCWP, CO, and systemic vascular resistance.

The findings associated with cardiac shock depend on the underlying cause. When cardiogenic shock is responsible, physical examination will reveal findings consistent with the pathologic process. In acute presentations, precordial chest pain may be the most significant physical finding. Signs of hypervolemia such as presacral and pretibial edema, jugulovenous distention, hepatojugular reflux, and pulmonary congestion are present in the face of hypotension and oliguria. Tachycardia is usually present, except in terminal stages. The extremities are cool due to vasoconstriction and decreased flow.

A pulmonary artery flotation catheter will reveal elevated central venous pressure and PCWP. CO is decreased and systemic vascular resistance is increased. Because flow to the viscera is limited, peripheral oxygen extraction is increased, resulting in a decreased $S\bar{v}O_2$ of less than 75%. Similarly, the $(a-v)DO_2$ is increased to greater than 6 ml O_2/dl. Laboratory studies indicate a decrease in serum bicarbonate and an increase in lactate.

When cardiac compression is responsible, findings are similar and careful physical examination is necessary to elucidate the cause. For patients who are breathing spontaneously, inspiration may increase the degree of venous distention (Kussmaul's sign). A paradoxic pulse is noted and consists of a decline in systolic blood pressure of more than 10 mmHg with inspiration. When tension pneumothorax is present, tracheal deviation and hyperresonance of one chest cavity are pathognomonic findings. Because the increased pleural pressure displaces the mediastinum and all of its associated structures, the trachea and mediastinum will be displaced away from the involved hemithorax.

Pericardial tamponade may follow penetrating chest trauma, making the history of critical importance in establishing the diagnosis. Muffled heart sounds are common but may be difficult to assess.

In both cases, central venous or pulmonary artery catheters will indicate an increase in central venous pressure. CO decreases with apparent hypervolemia. Systemic vascular resistance is increased. When pericardial tamponade is present, central venous, pulmonary artery diastolic, and pulmonary capillary wedge pressure may all be equal.

Chest x-ray is useful in exhibiting a widened cardiac shadow when pericardial tamponade is present. When tension pneumothorax is responsible, a shifted mediastinum with a pneumothorax is noted. However, because tension pneumothorax is an immediately life-threatening condition, decompressive thoracostomy should *never* be delayed while radiography is obtained to confirm the diagnosis.

DIFFERENTIAL DIAGNOSIS

The principal physical findings and hemodynamic patterns associated with each type of shock are detailed in Table 4.1.

Shock due to hypovolemia produces findings similar to those associated with cardiac shock, with the important exception being that the latter has signs of hypervolemia such as neck vein distention. Alcohol intoxication may make the diagnosis of hypovolemic shock difficult because ethanol produces skin that is warm, flushed, and dry. Additionally, inebriated patients typically produce dilute urine. Orthostatic testing brings on a pronounced drop in blood pressure in intoxicated hypovolemic patients. Hypoglycemia is occasionally confused with hypovolemia, since these patients are also cold, clammy, oliguric, and tachycardic. When available, a history of insulin use should arouse suspicion. After obtaining a blood sample for analysis, a rapid intravenous infusion of 50 ml of 50% glucose will establish the differential.

Septic shock is rarely confused with other etiologies, although differentiation from SIRS (systemic inflammatory response syndrome) is a matter of degree. Among the other forms of distributive shock, neurogenic shock requires special attention. In patients presenting after trauma with spinal cord injuries and evidence of spinal shock, hypotension must not be attributed to a neurogenic mechanism until hypovolemia has been excluded. Many of these patients will have sustained multiple injuries and the potential for hemorrhage must be appreciated. Because of peripheral venous pooling, relative hypovolemia is present and is corrected in the same way as for patients with hemorrhagic shock. *Always attribute shock in a trauma patient to hypovolemia until proved otherwise.*

Cardiogenic shock should be suspected in patients with prior cardiac disease whose symptoms worsen. Acute abdominal pain accompanying the onset of shock should prompt consideration of a ruptured aortic aneurysm as a cause of hypovolemia. The absence of distended neck veins and a declining Hct are keys to the differential. Cardiac compressive shock usually follows acute penetrating trauma and is rare after blunt injury. The two most important etiologies—pericardial tamponade and tension pneumothorax—can usually be differentiated on physical examination of the chest. The findings of a deviated trachea, hyperresonance over one chest cavity, and distended neck veins are pathognomonic for tension pneumothorax.

• Shock in trauma patient always attributed to hypovolemia until proved otherwise

TREATMENT

The primary goal of the treatment of shock is the return of normal tissue function. This relies on the accurate diagnosis of shock and identification of the underlying cause. Common to the treatment of all types of shock is assessment of the patient's airway status and breathing. It cannot be overemphasized that any and all attempts at resuscitation will be futile unless the patient has a patent airway and is either breathing spontaneously or with assistance from a mechanical ventilator or assisted breathing unit such as an AMBU (assisted mechanical breathing unit) bag. Details of airway control and ventilatory assistance can be found in Chapters 8 and 10.

Among surgical patients, hypovolemic shock most commonly follows trauma with acute hemorrhage. In uninjured patients, the same priorities apply, although a more deliberate resuscitation may be possible. After initial airway concerns have been addressed, resuscitation begins with the placement of large bore intravenous catheters in the upper extremities. Central venous catheters have relatively small lumens and are not adequate for resuscitation. Rapid fluid infusion is the guiding principle of therapy for hypovolemic shock (Case 1). Isotonic fluid should be infused at a rate sufficient to correct the deficit rapidly. In younger people, fluid should be infused at the maximum rate that the delivery system can achieve. In older patients, or in those with a history of cardiac disease, infusion should be slowed once a response is detected, in order to prevent hypervolemia and congestive heart failure. The end points of resuscitation include (1) normalization of blood pressure, (2) decrease in heart rate, (3) increase in urine output to more than 1 ml/kg/hr, and (4) return of mental status.

The optimum resuscitation fluid is still debated among surgeons, but several general principles apply:

1. Because intravascular refill moves Hb-free fluid from the interstitium into the intravascular space, the interstitial volume must be replaced. Refill occurs early in resuscitation and is usually complete after the first 2 L of Hb-free solution have been administered. Hence, resuscitation should be initiated with balanced salt solution (crystalloid) at a rapid rate in an attempt to replace lost volume and increase blood pressure. Isotonic balanced salt solution such as normal saline or lactated Ringer's solution should be used. Because the electrolytes and water partition themselves according to the body's extracellular water content, most of the volume administered will leave the intravascular space. When these solutions are used for resuscitation in place of blood, approximately three to four times the estimated blood deficit is required to account for the redistribution between the intra- and extravascular spaces. Because this movement occurs within 30 minutes of administration, less than 20% of the infused balanced salt solution remains in the bloodstream after 2 hours.

2. If blood has been lost, oxygen-carrying capacity must be restored. Blood replacement usually begins after the second liter of balanced salt solution has been infused, unless arterial pressure, heart rate, and urine output have normalized. Typed and cross-matched packed red blood cells (RBCs) are preferred. However, they are usually not available on such short notice, and either type-specific or type O-negative blood must be given. The amount of blood required is dictated by the trend of the Hct during the resuscitation. Patients with low initial Hct will require relatively more blood than those with higher initial values. A general guideline is that 1 unit (approximately 250 ml) of packed RBCs will increase the Hct level by 3–4% if the patient is no longer hemorrhaging and if the infusion of balanced salt solutions has been reduced to maintenance levels (1.5–2 ml/kg/hr). A continued downward trend of the Hct should prompt continued investigation for the cause of the bleeding, with surgical intervention as needed.

3. Other fluids are occasionally used for resuscitation, including albumin, dextrans, starch, and mannitol. As a group, these "colloids" rely on high molecular weight species for their osmotic effect. Because the barrier between the intra- and extravascular spaces is only partially permeable to these molecules, colloids tend to remain in the intravascular space for longer periods of time. No specific advantages, with respect to crystalloids, have been demonstrated for colloid solutions.

4. A search should be made for the source of hemorrhage or volume loss and corrected. This frequently requires operative intervention to control hemorrhage, close a fistula, or relieve a bowel obstruction.

The initial therapy for septic shock is restoration of adequate circulating blood volume. Because fluid is lost through capillary leaks and sequestration, these patients are effectively hypovolemic. Balanced salt solutions are preferred to replace volume loss. A pulmonary artery flotation catheter should be inserted to guide therapy. Administration of volume is best titrated against PCWP and CO. Filling pressures should be elevated to higher than normal levels to compensate for the myocardial depression that accompanies sepsis. Typically, a PCWP of between 10 and 15 mmHg will be necessary, and may require the administration of several liters of balanced salt solution (Case 2). Hemodilution will result from the use of such fluids and may necessitate blood administration.

If intravascular volume resuscitation fails to restore blood pressure, pharmacologic support with pressors is required. Dopamine is the most commonly used inotropic agent. Its effects are due to the release of norepinephrine from the sympathetic nerves and the direct stimulation of α, β, and dopaminergic receptors. At lower doses (2–5 μg/kg/min), dopamine increases cardiac contractility and CO without increasing heart rate, blood pressure, or systemic vascular resistance. Renal blood flow and urine output increase in response to doses of 0.5–2.0 μg/kg/min. At doses at and above 10 μg/kg/min, dopamine has chronotropic as well as inotropic effects and causes α-adrenergic stimulation with resultant vasoconstriction. Dobutamine has relatively minor chronotropic effects and exerts its major action on β-adrenergic inotropic receptors. Dobutamine is a better choice for long-term infusion than dopamine, because the latter depletes myocardial norepinephrine stores. The dose of dobutamine typically ranges from 5–15 μg/kg/min. Infusion starts at 2–5 μg/kg/min and is titrated to the desired effect. Increased urine output is due to increased renal perfusion from elevated CO.

Other pharmacologic agents that may be used in the treatment of septic shock include isoproteronol, phenylephrine, and norepinephrine. Isoproterenol is a positive inotrope and chronotrope that can be used in patients who fail to respond to dopamine and dobutamine. Treatment begins with an intravenous infusion at a rate of 0.01 μg/kg/min and is increased until the desired effect is obtained. Norepinephrine poses both α- and β-adrenergic activity. In low doses, it increases both cardiac contractility and heart rate. At higher doses, peripheral vasoconstriction, cardiac contractility, and cardiac work are all increased. The initial dose is 0.05–0.1 μg/kg/min.

In addition to maintenance of blood pressure, other measures are required in the treatment of septic shock. These include respiratory support, nutritional support, antimicrobial therapy, and a diligent search for the underlying cause (Case 2). Identification of the septic source is critically important. If the offending tissue is not drained, debrided, or excised, sepsis will continue in the face of otherwise optimal treatment. When a likely source cannot be identified, empiric broad spectrum therapy should be instituted with drugs known to be effective against gram-positive, gram-negative, and anaerobic organisms. Corticosteroids have not been shown to increase survival in patients with septic shock, and should only be used in those with clinical or laboratory evidence of adrenal insufficiency.

Adequate fluid resuscitation is required to offset the effects of peripheral venous pooling in *neurogenic shock*. In some patients, this may be all that is required to treat hypotension, while others may require infusion of an α-adrenergic agent such as norepinephrine. Titration of norepinephrine is guided by the return of blood pressure and urine output.

The most important initial step in treatment of *anaphylactic shock and anaphylactoid reactions is to ensure that an adequate airway is present*. These patients require early emergent intubation to protect their airway before laryngeal edema develops. Intravenous fluid administration is required to offset fluid loss from capillary leakage. Drug therapy should begin with a subcutaneous dose of epinephrine (0.3–0.5 ml of 1:1000). This may be repeated every 5–10 minutes. Diphenhydramine is a histamine antagonist that should be given as quickly as possible (1 mg/kg). If hypotension persists, further fluid resuscitation is warranted, followed by dopamine at 5 μg/kg/min. If dopamine fails to increase the blood pressure, norepinephrine should be started at 3–4 μg/min and titrated until the mean arterial blood pressure is between 60 and 80 mmHg.

Cardiogenic shock may be accompanied by pain and anxiety if the patient is awake. Sedation with morphine in small intravenous bolus doses of 2–4 mg will calm the patient and help reduce right ventricular preload through its vasodilatory effect. Placement of a pulmonary artery flotation catheter is mandatory in a patient with cardiogenic shock to assess filling pressures and response to therapy. Although these patients may be grossly edematous, they are effectively hypovolemic. If PCWP is less than 10–12 mmHg, balanced salt solution should be administered to increase filling pressures. CO should be reassessed after each increase of 2–3 mmHg in PCWP. A PCWP as high as 20 mmHg may be required before optimum CO is obtained. Nitroglycerin reduces both right ventricular preload as well as left ventricular afterload, allowing the heart to pump against decreased resistance. The early use of nitroglycerin both decreases infarct size and reduces early mortality. β-Blockers decrease myocardial oxygen consumption, antagonize catechols, and have antiarrhythmic activity. The greatest effect is achieved if they are started within 2 hours after infarction.

Once an optimum volume status has been achieved, inotropes, vasodilators, and/or diuretics may be required. Dobutamine is the drug of choice for the management of cardiogenic shock because it has minimum chronotropic and peripheral vasoconstrictive effects. It may be given in doses up to 40 μg/kg/min without significantly increasing heart rate. Dopamine has a dose dependent effect with the disadvantage of increasing peripheral vasoconstriction and decreasing renal and splanchnic blood flow at higher infusion rates. Doses averaging 17 μg/kg/min are required to optimize perfusion. Unfortunately, doses this high increase myocardial oxygen demand, produce tachycardia, and limit renal perfusion.

Other inotropic drugs that may be used include isoproterenol and norepinephrine. Isoproterenol increases myocardial contractility and decreases peripheral vascular resistance by stimulating β$_1$ and β$_2$ receptors. Isoproterenol dramatically increases myocardial oxygen consumption and should only be used in patients with bradycardia or aortic valvular insufficiency. Norepinephrine has both α- and β-adrenergic effects. At higher doses, it increases blood pressure by increasing peripheral vascular resistance through its α-adrenergic effects. If cardiogenic shock proves resistant to both dobutamine and dopamine, norepinephrine may be used in doses of 1–2 μg/min and titrated to effect.

Vasodilators may be required to lower peripheral vascular resistance and decrease left ventricular afterload. Nitroprusside decreases both afterload and preload. Treatment should be started with a dose of 5–10 μg/min and increased in increments of 2.5–5 μg/min until an increase in CO is observed. The dose should be reduced if the systolic blood pressure falls below 90 mmHg. Nitroglycerin has its greatest effect on preload, which reflexly decreases left ventricular filling. It also dilates the coronary vasculature and should be used when cardiogenic shock is due to ischemia. The normal starting dose is 10 μg/min, which can be increased to a total dose of 100 μg/min.

Other considerations in the treatment of cardiogenic shock include correction of electrolyte abnormalities and management of arrhythmias.

The management of cardiac compressive shock relies on rapid and accurate diagnosis. Rapid fluid infusion may transiently increase blood pressure; however, surgical decompression of a tension pneumothorax or pericardial tamponade is the only definitive therapy.

KEY POINTS

• Attempts to resuscitate futile unless patient has patent airway and is breathing spontaneously or with mechanical assistance

Hypovolemic Shock
• Rapid fluid infusion is the guiding principle of therapy
• Isotonic fluid infused rapidly enough to correct the deficit
• End points of resuscitation: normalization of blood pressure, decrease in heart rate, increase in urine output to more than 1 ml/kg/hr, and return of mental status
• Resuscitation initiated with isotonic balanced salt solution such as normal saline or lactated Ringer's solution rapidly to replace lost volume and increase blood pressure
• Three to four times estimated blood deficit required to account for redistribution between intra- and extravascular spaces
• Blood replacement begins after second liter of solution infused, unless arterial pressure, heart rate, and urine output normalized

Distributive Shock
• Initial therapy is restoration of adequate circulating blood volume
• Patients often hypovolemic due to volume lost through capillary leaks and sequestration
• Dopamine most commonly used inotropic agent
• Dopamine effects due to release of norepinephrine from sympathetic nerves and direct simulation of α, β, and dopaminergic receptors

• At lower doses (2–5 μg/kg/min), dopamine increases cardiac contractility and CO without increasing heart rate, blood pressure, or systemic vascular resistance
• Dobutamine has relatively minor chronotropic effects, exerts its major action on β-adrenergic inotropic receptors, and is a better choice for long-term infusion than dopamine, which depletes myocardial norepinephrine stores
• If offending tissue not drained, debrided, or excised, sepsis remains despite otherwise optimal treatment

Neurogenic Shock
• Adequate fluid resuscitation is required to offset the effects of peripheral venous pooling

Cardiac Shock
• Placement of a pulmonary artery flotation catheter mandatory in cardiogenic shock to assess filling pressures and response to therapy
• Patients may be grossly edematous, but are effectively hypovolemic
• PCWP of 20 mmHg may be required before optimum CO obtained
• Once optimum volume status achieved, inotropes, vasodilators, and/or diuretics may be required
• Dobutamine drug of choice for cardiogenic shock due to minimum chronotropic and peripheral vasoconstrictive effects
• Surgical decompression of tension pneumothorax or pericardial tamponade definitive therapy—rapid fluid infusion only transiently increases blood pressure

M FOLLOW-UP

Most patients treated for shock have completed therapy before they leave the hospital. The notable exceptions are those with cardiac shock and congestive failure who are at risk of acute decompensation. Similarly, those with chronic pericardial tamponade due to underlying medical disorders may present with acute-on-chronic cardiac compressive shock.

SUGGESTED READINGS

Bone RC et al: Sepsis syndrome. A valid clinical entity. Crit Care Med 17:389, 1989

The classic paper on septic syndrome, which is now referred to as SIRS. A good basis for understanding the evolution of septic shock.

Bongard FS: Shock and Resuscitation. p. 13. In Bongard FS, Sue DY (eds): Current Critical Care: Diagnosis and Treatment. Appleton & Lange, E. Norwalk, CT, 1994

An expanded version of this chapter. Reviews in greater detail the pertinent physiology and treatment. Lengthy review of drug selection and dosing recommendations is included.

Holcroft JW, Robinson MK: Shock: identification and management of shock states. In: Care of the Surgical Patient. Scientific American, New York, 1992

This monograph is part of the American College of Surgeons' series published in loose-leaf form. It covers the basic science of shock in great detail and is a valuable resource.

QUESTIONS

1. The initial decrease in Hct that follows hypovolemic shock is due primarily to?

    A. Blood loss.
    B. Refill of the intravascular space.
    C. Osmotic gradient.
    D. Volume retention by the kidneys.

2. The hallmark of distributive (septic) shock is?

    A. Increased WBC count.
    B. Decreased Hct level.
    C. Increased CO.
    D. Increased systemic vascular resistance.

3. Which of the following findings is most consistent with a diagnosis of cardiogenic shock?

    A. CO = 6 L/min, $S\bar{v}O_2$ = 86%, normovolemia.
    B. CO = 3 L/min, $S\bar{v}O_2$ = 65%, hypervolemia.
    C. CO = 3 L/min, $S\bar{v}O_2$ = 65%, hypovolemia.
    D. CO = 3 L/min, $S\bar{v}O_2$ = 85%, hypervolemia.

4. The drugs of choice for the initial pharmacologic management of septic shock: cardiogenic shock are?

    A. Norepinephrine: nitroprusside.
    B. Dobutamine: dopamine.
    C. Dopamine: nitroglycerin.
    D. Dopamine: dobutamine.

(See p. 603 for answers.)

5 INFECTION

F R E D   S .   B O N G A R D

Infections present to the surgeon as both primary problems and as complications. In the first case, identification and localization are required before definitive management. When infections present as complications, they can vary from simple wound infections to complex intraabdominal or widespread septic foci. In these cases, localization and drainage form the keys to management. This chapter discusses the common types of surgical infections, the approach to diagnosis, and optimal management.

CASE 1
WOUND INFECTION

A 64-year-old female presented to the emergency room with symptoms of obstipation and increased abdominal girth. On evaluation, she was found to have a completely obstructing lesion in her sigmoid colon and was operated on within several hours. Before her operation, she received a single dose of a cephalosporin.

At exploration, a large sigmoid cancer was found and a left hemicolectomy was done with primary anastomosis of her distal transverse colon to the rectum. Her fascia and skin were closed. Postoperative antibiotic therapy consisted of a twice daily dose of the cephalosporin. On the fourth postoperative day, she began having fevers to 39°C with an elevated WBC count. There was a brownish purulent exudate issuing from the superior aspect of the wound, which had partially separated. When the skin sutures were removed, a foul smelling collection of fluid was found beneath the subcutaneous tissue. The fascial sutures could be seen at the base of the wound and were intact. Moistened gauze sponges were placed in the wound and allowed to dry before they were removed several hours later (wet-to-dry dressing). Culture of the wound exudate found *E. coli* as well as several anaerobic species.

Over the next 10 days, the dressings were changed every 8 hours, and the wound debrided with a scalpel to remove necrotic tissue. The base of the wound began to heal (granulate) slowly and eventually started to close. The patient was instructed on how to dress the wound herself and was discharged on the 14th postoperative day.

CASE 2
HEMORRHAGIC GASTRITIS
AFTER GUNSHOT WOUNDS

An 18-year-old male was shot three times in the abdomen and once in the right thigh. On arrival at the emergency room, he had a blood pressure of 70/50 mmHg and a heart rate of 130 bpm. He was resuscitated with several liters of balanced salt solution and 500 ml of type O-negative blood. Secondary survey found that he had no pulse or sensation in his right lower extremity below the groin. At operation, he was found to have 1,500 ml of blood in the abdomen, most of which was coming from a large laceration of the left lobe of the liver, which required partial resection for control. He also had injuries of the stomach and colon, both of which were leaking contents into the abdomen. The stomach was repaired primarily, while the colon lesion was treated with resection, diverting colostomy, and creation of a Hartmann's pouch. The abdominal portion of the operation required 5 hours and over 3,000 ml of blood.

Exploration of the right thigh wound found that the superficial femoral artery had been transected. By this time the right foot was cold and mottled. The artery was repaired using a segment of saphenous vein from the contralateral leg. A fasciotomy of each compartment of the calf was performed after flow was restored to the leg. The entire operation took 8 hours and required 5,200 ml of blood.

He required continued intubation with mechanical ventilation after operation because of poor gas exchange and hypoxemia. By the third postoperative day, chest x-rays began to exhibit diffuse pulmonary congestion bilaterally. His temperature was consistently elevated with peaks to 39°C. Antibiotic treatment included coverage for gram-positive and negative aerobes, as well as anaerobes.

On the fifth postoperative day, he became hyperglycemic after several days of normal glucose tolerance on his hyperalimentation regimen. Later that afternoon, he became hypotensive, and required over 2,500 ml of crystalloid to restore his blood pressure. A pulmonary artery catheter was inserted and provided evidence of septic shock. He was started on dopamine for blood pressure support. Over the next 2 days, urine output fell as increasing levels of pressors were required to support his blood pressure. On the ninth postoperative day, he began bleeding around his nasogastric tube, and bloody sputum was suctioned from the endotracheal tube. By the 10th day, bleeding worsened, and endoscopy was performed, which revealed diffuse hemorrhagic gastritis. Laboratory studies found a PT more than twice normal, and evidence of platelet consumption.

Despite aggressive management, the patient could not be resuscitated from an episode of hypotension on the 11th postoperative day. An autopsy revealed multiple infected sites, including the lungs, liver, and brain.

GENERAL CONSIDERATIONS

The immune response to infection consists of humoral and cellular responses. The major components of humoral immunity are natural antibodies, antigen-specific immunoglobulins (IgM, IgG, IgA, IgE), complement, coagulation factors, products of arachidonic acid, cytokines, and acute phase reactants. Among these, the antigen-specific immunoglobulins are particularly important. Exposure to bacterial, fungal, and viral antigens initially causes a nonspecific IgM antibody response. Eventually, longer lived IgG, IgA, or IgE antibodies are produced that

are capable of amnestic responses to the antigen. A principal effect of antibody binding to the antigen is opsonization, which allows recognition by phagocytic cells. This may result in inactivation or neutralization when the target is a virus or an endotoxin. The antibody-antigen complex causes the release of complement, which ultimately results in lysis of the offending organisms. In the case of endotoxins, such binding induces changes in the structure of the compound making it ineffective.

Metabolites of arachidonic acid play important roles in the inflammatory response. Arachidonic acid is part of the cell membrane of most cells. When stimulated by reactants such as endotoxin, phospholipase A and phospholipase C cause arachidonic acid to be metabolized through either the cyclo-oxygenase pathway or through the lipoxygenase pathway. The cyclo-oxygenase pathway leads to the production of eicosanoids such as thromboxane A_2 and prostacyclin. These mediators affect vasomotor tone, platelets, and the clotting cascade. The lipoxygenase pathway occurs mainly in fixed macrophages and gives way to a number of leukotrienes such as LTB_4, which is a potent chemotactic agent. Other products include LTC_4 and D_4, which are vasodilators and inducers of vascular permeability, allowing neutrophils and antibodies to gain access to areas of inflammation. The coordinated response between complement, coagulation, and arachidonic acid permits a broad-based attack on the offending agent.

The cytokines are inflammatory mediators produced by tissue-fixed macrophages throughout the body. These humoral agents have a number of actions but generally serve to amplify the inflammatory response. Tumor necrosis factor (TNF) primes the macrophage response, activates neutrophils, enhances T-cell responsiveness, and activates the proinflammatory state in endothelial cells. TNF is produced by macrophages in response to a number of stimuli including bacterial endotoxin. Interleukins (IL)-1, -6, and -8 are also particularly important in the inflammatory response. IL-1 resets the hypothalamic thermostat and induces fever. It is often referred to as the universal pyrogen. IL-1 also stimulates neutrophil maturation and release. Granulocyte colony stimulating factor (G-CSF) induces maturation and release of neutrophils and monocytes/macrophages from the bone marrow. IL-6 causes a shift in hepatocyte production from structural protein synthesis to acute phase reactants. IL-8 acts in a similar fashion to aid in coordinating the inflammatory response.

The humoral mechanisms, acting in concert, achieve the following functions:

1. Induce vasodilation and increase blood flow to areas of inflammation, which aids in the delivery of the various components of the immune response

2. Increase the production of mediators that cause endothelial cell retraction, increased capillary permeability, and improved delivery of immune mediators

3. Cause the production and release of chemotactic mediators, which aid in attracting the cellular components of the immune system to the site of inflammation

4. Cause simultaneous production of a number of activators of the coagulation cascade to cause stasis and thrombosis in the area of inflammation

The cellular portion of the inflammatory response includes both phagocytic and nonphagocytic components. The mobile phagocytic cells include the neutrophil and the circulating monocyte. The tissue-fixed macrophage and the proinflammatory mast cells, platelets, and endothelial cells also participate in the response.

The neutrophil is the most efficient phagocytic cell. Its effect occurs in a number of steps:

1. Activation and recruitment to the area of inflammation (chemotaxis)

2. Adherence of the activated neutrophil to the endothelial surface

3. Diapedesis of the neutrophil through the endothelial monolayer and basement membrane

4. Migration into the interstitial space

5. Recognition, phagocytosis, and neutralization of the offending agent

Neutrophil microbicidal activity takes place through a number of mechanisms, many of which involve production of oxygen radical species that are highly toxic. These include superoxide anion (O_2), hydrogen peroxide (H_2O_2), hydroxyl radical ($\cdot OH$), singlet oxygen ($O\cdot$), and halide acids. Oxygen independent mechanisms include acid proteases, lactoferrin, lysozyme, cationic proteins, elastase, and collagenase.

Macrophages also play an important part in the cellular cascade. They are the major source of chemotactic agents for neutrophils, monocytes, and other inflammatory cells.

KEY POINTS

Humoral Immunity
• Exposure to baterial, fungal, and viral antigens initially causes nonspecific IgM antibody response

• Eventually, longer lived IgG, IgA, or IgE antibodies are produced, which are capable of amnestic responses to antigens

• Cytokines are inflammatory mediators produced by tissue-fixed macrophages, which amplify the inflammatory response

• IL-1, -6, and -8 important to inflammatory response

Cellular Defense Mechanisms
• Both phagocytic and nonphagocytic components

• Neutrophil microbicidal activity takes place through mechanisms that involve production of highly toxic oxygen radical species

• Macrophages major source of chemotactic agents for neutrophils, monocytes, and other inflammatory cells

DIAGNOSIS AND TREATMENT

Urinary tract infections are the most common infection. Bacteriuria occurs at a rate of 5–10% per catheter day, with bacteremia and sepsis occurring in 2–4% of catheterized patients. Nearly all patients will have bacteriuria by the 10th day of catheterization. The organisms obtained most commonly include *Escherichia coli*, *Klebsiella pneumoniae*, *Proteus mirabilis*, *Pseudomonas aeruginosa*, *Staphylococcus epidermidis*, and enterococci.

Most patients with catheter-induced bladder colonization are asymptomatic. When fever and flank tenderness are noted, an ascending infection may be present. Diagnosis is based on urine culture, although microscopic examination of the urinary sediment may be helpful. Infection is present when more than 100,000 colony forming units/ml are found. Urinary sediment should also be inspected for white blood cell (WBC) count and tested for nitrite, which indicates WBC activation. A Gram stain of the urinary sediment will reveal the predominance of one type of organism. Gram stain of the sediment should be performed as a screening measure before a sample is sent for culture and sensitivity.

Patients who are asymptomatic should not receive antibiotic therapy, since bacteriuria should resolve when the catheter is removed. Symptomatic patients may be treated with trimethoprim-sulfamethoxazole, a quinolone, or a second- or third-generation cephalosporin. Antibiotics that are both excreted and concentrated in the urine, such as ampicillin, are excellent choices. Aminoglycoside therapy is needed occasionally. In uncomplicated cases, only 7 days of treatment are required. Repeat cultures of the urine after cessation of therapy may be helpful.

Pneumonias are responsible for about 15% of all nosocomial infections. The mortality rate for nosocomial pneumonias ranges from 5–20%, depending on the underlying physiologic status of the patient and on the infecting organism (Case 2). Pneumonias develop as a result of (1) inhalation of infectious organisms, (2) hematogenous seeding of the lung from remote sites, and (3) aspiration of oropharyngeal flora.

Among surgical patients, inhalation and aspiration of bacteria are the most common routes of infection. Seeding of the lung from sources such as skin and soft tissue infections, endocarditis, hepatic and splenic abscesses, and indwelling monitoring catheters occurs, but is uncommon. *Staphylococcus aureus* is the most common pathogen in these cases. Inhalation of microorganisms, either from the environment or through a ventilator circuit, is a frequent source of infection. Although ventilators are cleaned after each use, incomplete asepsis exposes the patient to a number of organisms such as *Mycobacterium tuberculosis*, *Chlamydia* spp, *Legionella*, and influenza virus. Aspiration of oropharyngeal secretions is the most common route of infection. This particularly affects trauma patients who have altered states of consciousness from their injury and cannot adequately protect their airway. Similarly, patients who require endotracheal intubation under emergent conditions frequently aspirate oropharyngeal and gastric contents. Although aerobic gram-negative bacilli are not normally part of the upper respiratory flora, colonization by these bacteria is common among hospitalized patients. Up to 50% of intensive care unit (ICU) patients will have such colonization by the 10th day of their stay in the ICU. Similarly, those receiving broad spectrum antibiotics may be colonized with highly resistant virulent organisms. Patients who are colonized are at risk of developing pneumonia. Recent work has shown that the routine use of H_2 antagonists increases the gastric pH, allowing the growth of microorganisms, including gram-negative bacilli, which when aspirated, produce severe pneumonia.

The diagnosis of postoperative pneumonia depends on clinical suspicion, physical examination, bacteriologic evaluation of sputum samples, and radiographic evidence. Persistence of fever past the first few days following surgery should suggest pneumonia. A fever of 38°–39°C is typical. Leukocytosis may be prominent, with a shift toward immature forms. Physical examination will reveal decreased breathing sounds over the involved lung. Tachypnea and tachycardia are common. If the pneumonia is severe, dyspnea may be prominent. Such findings must be differentiated from fluid overload and congestive heart failure. In the latter, systemic evidence of hypervolemia is present. Furthermore, cardiac examination will reveal a third heart sound (S_3). When pneumonia is present, sputum production is increased or changed in nature. When obtained by suction through the endotracheal tube it will become thicker and exhibit a change in color to yellow or green. Chest radiographs will show consolidation of previously normal areas. Pleural effusions may be present, as well as obscure anatomic landmarks such as the costophrenic recess and the heart borders.

Diagnosis and management depend on culture of the sputum and antibiotic sensitivity testing. Good quality sputum samples must be obtained, and may require bronchoscopy if the patient is not able to expectorate an adequate sample, or if endotracheal suction does not produce suitable material. Gram stain should be performed as soon as possible, and guides initial therapy (Table 5.1). Empiric antibiotic treatment for nosocomial pneumonia should be based on clinical, host, and microbiologic factors. Patients with compromised immune status require more aggressive therapy, while those with

TABLE 5.1 *Sputum gram stain to guide empiric therapy for sepsis*

Gram-positive cocci	*Streptococcus pneumoniae*
	Staphylococcus aureus
Gram-negative coccobacilli	*Haemophilus influenzae*
	Moraxella catarrhalis
Gram-negative bacilli	Enteric bacilli *(Klebsiella, Enterobacter)*
	Pseudomonas
Mixed bacteria	Oral contamination
	Mixed aerobes and anaerobes
No organisms present	Viruses
	Mycobacteria
	Fungi
	Mycoplasma
	Chlamydia
	Coxiella burnetii
	Legionella
	Pneumocystis carinii

(From Quenzer R, Allen S: Infections in the critically ill. In Bongard FS, Sue DY (eds): Current Critical Care Diagnosis and Treatment. Appleton & Lange, E. Norwalk, CT, 1994, with permission.

only minor findings who are otherwise in good health may be treated more conservatively. Additionally, the hospital's flora and resistance patterns must be considered. If a particular organism is known to be common, its sensitivity should be considered when choosing an antibiotic regimen. Table 5.2 provides a guide to antibiotic selection for the initial treatment of postoperative pneumonias. It should be modified as necessary to account for patient and local factors. Supportive care consists of vigorous pulmonary toilet (e.g., postural drainage), repeat bronchoscopy as needed, lateral rotation beds, bronchodilators, and supplemental oxygen. Once treatment has begun, the patient's overall status,

TABLE 5.2 *Initial therapy of nosocomial pneumonia*

CLINICAL SITUATION	DRUGS OF CHOICE
Cultures pending	Third-generation cephalosporin + aminoglycoside
Aspiration of gastric contents	Clindamycin + third-generation cephalosporin
Neutropenia or other sign of immunocompromise	Aminoglycoside + antipseudomonal penicillin or cephalosporin[a] or aztreonam + vancomycin

[a]Ceftazidime, cefoperazone.
(From Quenzer R, Allen S: Infections in the critically ill. In Bongard FS, Sue DY (eds): Current Critical Care Diagnosis and Treatment. Appleton & Lange, E. Norwalk, CT, 1994, with permission.

chest x-rays, and sputum cultures should guide subsequent treatment.

Wound infections are among the most common surgical complications. Their frequency ranges from less than 2% to more than 40%. The chance of developing a postoperative wound infection is dependent on many factors, including inherent patient risks, the type of surgery being performed, and the patient's preparation for the procedure. Some of the patient- and operation-dependent factors that increase the risk of infection are listed in Table 5.3. Of particular importance is preoperative preparation of the patient. The duration of preoperative hospitalization is important because the patient is exposed to flora that may not be present in the community setting. Such bacteria frequently have broad antibacterial resistance patterns and can become major sources of postoperative morbidity. Preparation of the patient and the operative site are also important. Because the colon is a rich source of bacteria, those undergoing elective colonic surgery should have both mechanical as well as antibacterial preparation. This begins the day before surgery when the patient drinks a polyethylene glycol solution that causes mechanical cleansing. This is followed by oral administration of erythromycin and neomycin in nonabsorbable forms. These further reduce the flora of the colon and leave a residue that reduces the number of bacteria present when the colon is subsequently resected.

Preparation of the operative site usually requires hair removal and skin coating with an antiseptic solution. Previously, patients were shaved the night before the operation to reduce time spent in the operating suite. Studies have shown, however, that shaving hair the night before operation increases the risk of wound infection because the small nicks and cuts produced by shaving become colonized with hospital pathogens. Optimal preparation now consists of hair removal, either with depilatory agents, clipping, or shaving, immediately before the operation begins. After hair has been removed, the skin is scrubbed with an antiseptic solution and then painted with povi-

done-iodine solution, which leaves an antimicrobial residue. The duration of the operation itself affects the incidence of wound infections, since surgery in excess of 2 hours has been shown to have an increased incidence of such infections.

The risk of a postoperative wound infection is related to the type of surgery performed (Table 5.3). In general, procedures are divided into four categories: clean, clean-contaminated, contaminated, and infected. Additionally, operative technique is important and includes such factors as the placement of the incision, shielding during the procedure to prevent contamination with flora, debridement of devitalized tissue, duration and extent of retraction, and method of closure. Wounds should always be closed without tension and with the minimum amount of suture required to effect adequate approximation. Drains should generally be routed away from wound edges and should not be placed unless there is a specific indication, because they may actually increase the wound infection rate. When skin is left open because of contamination, the wound should be packed lightly with saline soaked gauze that is changed regularly. Wounds should not be inspected until the second or third day to prevent contamination. When examined, care should be taken to change the dressing with sterile gloves and gauze sponges to prevent introducing new pathogens into the wound.

Antibiotic administration can reduce the incidence of wound infections. The use of such drugs should be chosen by general principles and by the site involved (Table 5.4).

Wound infections usually present between the 4th and 10th days after operation (Case 1), although some rare synergistic bacterial infections may be apparent within several hours after operation. Wound infections are accompanied by subjective symptoms of pain and heat, and by the objective signs of swelling, erythema, and occasionally seropurulent or frankly purulent exudate. Temperature elevation and leukocytosis are common. In the first few days after surgery, minor elevations in temperature and complaints of wound discomfort are normal and

TABLE 5.3   *Classification of surgical wounds and incidence of wound infection*

CLASS	CHARACTERISTICS	INCIDENCE (%)
Clean	Nontraumatic; no inflammation encountered; no break in technique; respiratory, alimentary, or genitourinary tracts not entered	<2
Clean-contaminated	Gastrointestinal or respiratory tract entered without significant spillage; appendectomy; oropharynx or vagina entered; genitourinary or biliary tract entered in absence of infected urine or bile; minor break in technique	2–8
Contaminated	Major break in technique; gross spillage from gastrointestinal tract	8–15
Dirty and infected	Acute bacterial inflammation encountered; transection of "clean" tissue for the purpose of surgical access to a collection of pus; traumatic wound with retained devitalized tissue, foreign bodies, fecal contamination, or delayed treatment, or all of these, or from dirty source	12–40

(Adapted from Meakins JL: Elective care. Infection. Guidelines for prevention of wound infection. In Wilmore DW et al (eds): Care of the Surgical Patient. Scientific American, New York, 1989, with permission.)

TABLE 5.4   *Prevention of wound infection and sepsis in surgical patients*

Nature of Operation	Likely Pathogens	Recommended Drugs	Adult Dosage Before Surgery[a]
Clean			
Cardiac			
Prosthetic valve, coronary artery bypass, other open heart surgery, pacemaker implant	*Staphylococcus epidermidis, S. aureus, Corynebacterium,* enteric gram-negative bacteria	Cefazolin or cefuroxime OR vancomycin[c]	1–2 g IV[b] 1 g IV
Noncardiac thoracic	*S. aureus, S. epidermidis,* streptococci, enteric gram-negative bacilli	Cefazolin or cefuroxime OR vancomycin[c]	1–2 g IV 1 g IV
Vascular			
Arterial surgery involving the abdominal aorta, a prosthesis, or a groin incision	*S. aureus, S. epidermidis,* enteric gram-negative bacilli	Cefazolin OR vancomycin[c]	1–2 g IV 1 g IV
Lower extremity amputation for ischemia	*S. aureus, S. epidermidis,* enteric gram-negative bacilli, clostridia	Cefazolin OR vancomycin[c]	1–2 g IV 1 g IV
Neurosurgery			
Craniotomy	*S. aureus, S. epidermidis*	Cefazolin OR vancomycin[c]	1–2 g IV 1 g IV
Orthopaedic			
Total joint replacement, internal fixation of fractures	*S. aureus, S. epidermidis*	Cefazolin OR vancomycin[c]	1–2 g IV 1 g IV
Ophthalmic	*S. aureus, S. epidermidis,* streptococci, enteric gram-negative bacilli, *Pseudomonas*	Gentamicin or tobramycin or neomycin-gramicidin-polymyxin B Cefazolin	Multiple drops topically over 2–24 hr 100 mg subconjunctivally at end of procedure
Clean contaminated			
Head and neck			
Entering oral cavity or pharynx	*S. aureus,* streptococci, oral anaerobes	Cefazolin OR clindamycin ± gentamicin	1–2 g IV 600–900 mg IV 1.5 mg/kg IV
Abdominal			
Gastroduodenal	Enteric gram-negative bacilli, gram-positive cocci	*High risk only:* cefazolin	1–2 g IV
Biliary tract	Enteric gram-negative bacilli, enterococci, clostridia	*High risk only:* cefazolin	1–2 g IV
Colorectal	Enteric gram-negative bacilli, anaerobes	Oral: neomycin + erythromycin base[d] Parenteral: cefoxitin or cefotetan	1–2 g IV
Appendectomy	Enteric gram-negative bacilli, anaerobes	Cefoxitin or cefotetan	1–2 g IV
Gynecologic and obstetric			
Vaginal or abdominal hysterectomy	Enteric gram-negatives, anaerobes, group B streptococci, enterococci	Cefazolin or cefotetan or cefoxitin	1 g IV
Cesarean section	Same as for hysterectomy	*High risk only:* cefazolin	1 g IV after cord clamping
Abortion	Same as for hysterectomy	*First trimester, high risk only:* aqueous penicillin G OR doxycycline 300 mg PO[f] *Second trimester:* cefazolin	1 million units IV 1 g IV

Continues

TABLE 5.4   *Continued*

Nature of Operation	Likely Pathogens	Recommended Drugs	Adult Dosage Before Surgery[a]
Dirty surgery			
Ruptured viscus[g]	Enteric gram-negative bacilli, anaerobes, enterococci	Cefoxitin or	1–2 g IV q6h
		cefotetan	1–2 g IV q12h
		± gentamicin	1.5 mg/kg IV q8h
		OR clindamycin	600 mg IV q6h
		+ gentamicin	1.5 mg/kg IV q8h
Traumatic wound	*S. aureus,* group A streptococci, clostridia	Cefazolin[g,h]	1–2 g IV q8h

[a]Parenteral prophylactic antimicrobials can be given as a single IV dose just before the operation. For prolonged operations, additional intraoperative doses should be given q4–8h for the duration of the procedure.

[b]Some consultants recommend an additional dose when patients are removed from bypass during open heart surgery.

[c]For hospitals in which methicillin-resistant *S. aureus* and *S. epidermidis* frequently cause wound infection, or for patients allergic to penicillins or cephalosporins. Rapid IV administration may cause hypotension, which could be especially dangerous during induction of anesthesia. Even if the drug is given over 60 minutes, hypotension may occur; treatment with diphenhydramine (Benadryl, and others) and further slowing of the infusion rate may be helpful (Maki DG, Bohn MJ, Stolz SM et al: Comparative study of cefazolin, cefamandole, and vancomycin for surgical prophylaxis in cardiac and vascular operations. A double-blind randomized trial. J Thorac Cardiovasc Surg 104:1423, 1992). For procedures in which enteric gram-negative bacilli are likely pathogens, such as vascular surgery involving a groin incision, cefazolin should be included in the prophylaxis regimen.

[d]After appropriate diet and catharsis, 1 g of each at 1 PM, 2 PM, and 11 PM the day before an 8 AM operation.

[e]Patients with previous pelvic inflammatory disease, previous gonorrhea, or multiple sex partners.

[f]Divided into 100 mg 1 hour before the abortion and 200 mg 30 minutes after.

[g]For "dirty" surgery, therapy should usually be continued for 5–10 days.

[h]For bite wounds, in which likely pathogens may also include oral anaerobes, *Eikenella corrodens* (human), and *Pasteurella multocida* (dog and cat), some Medical Letter consultants recommend use of amoxicillin/clavulanic acid (Augmentin) or ampicillin/sulbactam (Unasyn).

(From Anonymous: Antimicrobial prophylaxis in surgery. Med Lett Drugs Ther 37:79, 1995, with permission.)

usually do not warrant examination of the wound. However, if the fever exceeds 38.5°C or if the patient appears toxic, the wound should be examined because of the possibility of a necrotizing soft tissue infection. The presence of a thin watery exudate and/or crepitus around the wound supports this diagnosis and mandates examination.

Most wound infections are treated by removing the skin closure (staples or sutures) to allow the wound to drain. These infections are typically caused by *S. aureus,* which produces a thick creamy fluid. In all cases, the wound exudate should be Gram stained and sent for microbial culture and sensitivity testing. The wound should be packed lightly with a gauze sponge that has been moistened with normal saline or water. The dressing should be changed every 8 hours after the gauze has dried thoroughly. Such wet-to-dry dressings mechanically debride the wound only if they have dried thoroughly. Changing the dressing more frequently (before the sponge has dried completely) defeats the purpose of mechanical debridement. Contrary to commonly held belief, wet-to-dry dressing changes are not painless if done properly. Dilute acetic acid (0.1%) may be used to wet the dressing when *Pseudomonas* is present. Higher concentrations of acetic acid and other chemical agents are toxic to fibroblasts and may actually inhibit healing. The wound will heal by second intention at a rate dependent on its depth and width. Mechanical aids to debridement such as seaweed extracts may be useful in wounds that are particularly exudative, although they must be used with care to prevent disruption of the normal healing process. Systemic antibiotics are usually not needed for simple wound infections unless invasive pathogens are present (hemolytic streptococci), the patient is immunocompromised, prosthetic material is present, or there is evidence of systemic spread. Antibiotic therapy should be dictated by findings on the wound Gram stain and by microbial culture and sensitivity reports. Early necrotizing infections require *immediate* return to the operating room for debridement. Such wounds can be rapidly fatal if not treated aggressively with removal of affected tissue and antibiotics. Multiple redebridements over several days are usually required.

A cutaneous or soft tissue infection is a localized collection of pus surrounded by hyperemia and inflammation. It has a necrotic center that consists of bacteria, tissue debris, and leukocytes. A *furuncle* is an abscess that begins in a hair follicle or sweat gland and occludes the pilosebaceous apparatus. When a furuncle extends and becomes multilocular, it is referred to as a *carbuncle*. These typically occur on the back, back of the neck, hands and fingers, and hair-bearing portions of the abdomen and chest. Hidradenitis suppurativa is a chronic infection of the apocrine skin glands, and typically occurs in the axilla and groin. In its chronic state, hidradenitis suppurativa produces multiple skin nodules surrounded by fibrous tissue. Cellulitis, which is a superficial skin infection characterized by blanching erythema, is caused by *Streptococcus*. Unlike carbuncles and furuncles, cellulitis does not contain areas of fluctuance and necrotic centers.

Most superficial abscesses of the trunk, head, and neck are caused by *S. aureus* and are characterized by pain, erythema, and localized swelling. Systemic signs are uncommon, although regional lymph nodes are typically enlarged. The WBC count may be elevated with a shift to the left. Leukocytosis is more common with carbuncles and hidradenitis suppurativa than with furuncles or small areas of cellulitis. Cultures of drainage obtained directly or via needle aspiration should be sent for Gram stain and culture.

Incision and drainage is required for treatment of all but the smallest furuncles. Under local anesthesia using 1.0% lidocaine, a linear incision is made over the area of maximum fluctuance to express the underlying purulence. Packing with a small gauze wick may be required for larger carbuncles. The packing should be changed every 8 hours when the wound is cleaned. Simple furuncles usually resolve with incision and drainage alone, while more complex carbuncles require the use of systemic antibiotics (usually oral) that cover *S. aureus*. Most wounds treated with incision and drainage contract to a small scar. Larger wounds may require skin grafting. Cellulitis is best treated with oral penicillin VK since *Streptococcus* is almost always sensitive to this drug. The use of more expensive or broader spectrum antibiotics is not warranted in simple skin infections. When antibiotic therapy is required for abscesses or furuncles (large or deep processes with elevation or severe pain), agents with good coverage of *S. aureus* should be used. Since this organism is usually resistant to penicillin, agents with β-lactamase inhibitors should be used to prevent bacterial inactivation of the drug.

Necrotizing soft tissue infections spread rapidly and cause necrosis of the skin, subcutaneous fat, fascia, and muscle. Immunocompromised patients with diabetes, malignancy, steroid dependency, or acquired immunodeficiency syndrome (AIDS) are at highest risk, although such infections do occur routinely in the general population. Early on, signs and symptoms may be identical to those of superficial soft tissue infections except for severity and speed of spread. They are characterized by four cardinal signs: (1) edema beyond the area of erythema, (2) skin vesicles or bullae, (3) crepitus or subcutaneous air seen on radiography, and (4) the absence of lymphangitis or lymphadenitis. Hyperpyrexia and leukocytosis are common although late findings.

Meleney's synergistic gangrene most commonly occurs 2 or more weeks after trauma or surgery for an infection. It is characterized by edema, erythema, and tenderness, which progresses to three characteristic zones: (1) central necrosis with ulceration, (2) violaceous undermined edges, and (3) surrounding erythema.

Streptococcal gangrene is characterized by the rapid development of fever, marked erythema, pain, and swelling. Vesicles and bullae appear within 48 hours, followed by ecchymoses and gangrene of the skin by the fifth day. Similarly, clostridial cellulitis develops rapidly, and may appear within several hours after a laceration or a surgical procedure. It presents with a high fever, foul smelling seropurulent discharge, crepitus, and severe pain.

Necrotizing fasciitis develops rapidly and is accompanied by high fevers and signs of systemic toxicity. It progresses so quickly that its borders appear to change within 15–20 minutes. Because of the continuity between the scrotal and surrounding superficial fascia, Fournier's gangrene (dermal gangrene of the scrotum) may develop in the presence of necrotizing fasciitis. Necrosis of the skin and subcutaneous tissue is due to bacterial exotoxins that lead to thrombosis of afferent arterioles.

Clostridial myonecrosis (gas gangrene) presents with pronounced wound pain, swelling, and systemic toxicity. Crepitus, cutaneous necrosis, vesicles, and gangrene are late findings. Other organisms may cause a similar picture and result in nonclostridial myonecrosis.

The diagnosis of necrotizing soft tissue infections is made by clinical observation of the affected area. Leukocytosis is usually pronounced, and is accompanied by a significant number of immature forms. Hemolysis and coagulopathies are associated findings. Metabolic acidosis, hypocalcemia, and elevated creatine kinase are frequent. Exudate or aspirates should be obtained from the wound, Gram stained, and sent for microbiologic culture and antibiotic sensitivity testing. When radiographs are obtained, air may be present in the subcutaneous tissue or fascial planes.

Patients with necrotizing soft tissue infections are extremely ill and require immediate and aggressive resuscitation. Because of tissue necrosis and hyperthermia, they are very dehydrated and may be hypotensive from systemic sepsis. Intravenous antibiotic therapy should be started with high dose penicillin (20 million units/day), an aminoglycoside, and metronidazole. Once culture results become available, the antibiotics should be tailored as indicated. Early and thorough debridement and drainage of the affected area are lifesaving. This should include the overlying skin, subcutaneous tissue, and affected fascia and muscle. The wound should be packed open and inspected every few hours for evidence of ongoing necrosis. Amputations are common and may involve an entire extremity or more in extensive cases. Hyperbaric oxygen therapy may be beneficial in some cases (those with anaerobic bacteria such as *Clostridium perfringens*), but only after or in conjunction with thorough surgical debridement. Reconstructive plastic procedures are frequently required after the infection has been eliminated.

Tetanus continues to be a problem in poor rural areas and in developing countries. *Clostridium tetani* is an anaerobic bacillus found within the human gastrointestinal tract, soil, and many other areas. Although the organism itself is generally noninvasive, it produces an extremely potent exotoxin that blocks neuromuscular synaptic inhibition, resulting in severe spasms and rigidity. The usual initial sign is trismus (lockjaw) and stiffness of the back, neck, and abdomen. Spasms of the facial muscles (risus sardonicus), dysphagia, and laryngospasm are later findings. Involvement of the chest wall and diaphragm ultimately leads to respiratory embarrassment. Treatment includes neutralization of the exotoxin with tetanus immunglobulin (TIG, 3,000–6,000 units IM) followed by extensive wound debridement and antibiotic therapy with either penicillin, erythromycin, clindamycin, or metronidazole. Prophylaxis against tetanus following acute injuries depends on the patient's immunization status. For clean minor wounds, tetanus toxoid (Td) is usually given. For all other wounds, Td should be given if the patient was last immunized within 5 years. TIG, administered intramuscularly (250 units), should also be given if the immunization status is unknown or thought to be incomplete.

The peritoneal cavity is lined by semipermeable mesothelial cells that participate in bidirectional fluid and solute exchange. The surface area of the peritoneum is approximately equal to the total body surface area (1.7 m^2), of which 1 m^2 participates in fluid exchange. Under normal conditions, there is less than 50 ml of peritoneal fluid. In response to inflammatory stimuli, mast cells and macrophages release histamine and prostaglandins, which increase the vascular permeability of the peritoneum. Additionally, the omentum responds to the inflammation by localizing and sealing the area. Despite these defenses, bacterial inoculation can result in either generalized (peritonitis) or localized (peritoneal abscess or phlegmon) infection. One-third of intra-abdominal abscesses develop following containment of a generalized peritonitis. Contamination may occur from intrinsic sources such as bowel perforation, or from external trauma and seeding. When such abscesses develop, they are most likely to occur in the dependent portions of the peritoneal cavity (bilateral lower quadrants and pelvis), although the pumping action of the viscera may propel them cephalad and produce a subphrenic or subhepatic abscess. Secondary intra-abdominal infections are usually polymicrobial and may include *E. coli*, *Klebsiella* spp, *Proteus* spp, enterococci, *Bacteroides fragilis*, anaerobic cocci, and *Clostridia*.

The physical findings associated with intra-abdominal infections depend on the virulence of the infecting organisms, the duration and extent of the contamination, and the underlying physiologic status of the host. In advanced cases, patients are extremely toxic and may progress through septic shock to frank cardiovascular collapse. Patients display involuntary guarding and evidence of an acute abdomen. When an abscess is present, localized tenderness may be noted. This is particularly true with pelvic abscesses that are palpable on rectal examination and produce diarrhea or urinary urgency. Psoas muscle abscesses present with hip pain on passive or active motion. Subphrenic abscesses may present with dyspnea (due to diaphragmatic irritation), referred shoulder pain, hiccups, basilar atelectasis, pleural effusions, and/or tenderness over the tip of the 12th rib. Patients usually appear quite ill and have a high fever that is either continuous or intermittent. Leukocytosis is present until the late stage of septic shock when neutropenia occurs. Supporting findings include elevation of liver transaminases, azotemia, and metabolic acidosis on blood gas testing.

Imaging studies are usually required to determine the location of the abscess. Computed tomography (CT) scanning is the preferred modality because of its overall accuracy of greater than 95%. CT scanning is aided by the use of both oral and intravenous contrast. The drawbacks of CT scanning are that it requires movement of a potentially unstable patient to the CT scanner, uses ionizing radiation, and is expensive. Ultrasound is a diagnostic option but is limited by the fact that tissue/air interfaces interfere with the ultrasound beam. This limitation is particularly important in the upper quadrants, where the abscess may be obscured by overlying lung, and in the midabdomen, where it may be masked by surrounding bowel. Ultrasonic scanning of the pelvis can be improved by filling the bladder with water to improve sound transmission. The scanner is portable and can be brought to the bedside, precluding the need for patient transportation. Unfortunately the device is limited in its ability to provide exact anatomic information about the location of the abscess, and is highly operator dependent. Its overall accuracy in this application is 80–90%. Radionuclide scanning is occasionally used as an adjunct to CT and ultrasound. Indium-111 is a radiolabel that is incubated with the patient's WBCs and reinjected intravenously. The labeled leukocytes travel to the area of infection and are detected by a portable external counter. The study requires about 24 hours to complete and has an accuracy of about 80%, although anatomic information is poor. Both false-negative and false-positive results are common.

KEY POINTS

Postoperative infections

- Urinary tract infections most common nosocomial infection

- Bacteriuria occurs at 5–10% per catheter day, and bacteremia and sepsis occur in 2–4% of catheterized patients

- Most common organisms include *E. coli*, *K pneumonias*, *P. mirabilis*, *P. aeruginosa*, *S. epidermidis*, and enterococci

- Diagnosis based on urine culture and microscopic examination of urinary sediment

- Infection present with more than 100,000 colony forming units/ml

- Asymptomatic patients do not receive antibiotic therapy—bacteriuria should resolve when catheter removed

• Symptomatic patients treated with trimethoprim-sul-famethoxazole, a quinolone, or a second- or third-generation cephalosporin

Pneumonia
• Responsible for 15% of all nosocomial infections

• Nosocomial infection mortality rate is 5–20%, depending on patient's underlying physiologic status and on the infecting organism

• Aspiration of oropharyngeal secretions is most common route of infection

• Patients who require emergency endotracheal intubation often aspirate oropharyngeal and gastric contents

• Aerobic gram-negative bacilli colonization common among hospitalized patients

Wound Infections
• Dependent on inherent patient risks, type of surgery, and patient preparation

• Shaving the night before operation increases risk of wound infection

• Optimal preparation is to remove hair with depilatory agents, hair clipping, or shaving, immediately before operation

• Drains increase wound infection rate and are not placed unless specifically indicated

• Most wound infections treated by removing staples or sutures to allow wound drainage

• Systemic antibiotics only needed if invasive pathogens are present (hemolytic streptococci), the patient is immunocompromised or has a prosthesis, or there is evidence of systemic spread

• Early necrotizing infections can be fatal if patient not returned to operating room immediately for removal of affected tissue and antibiotics

Superficial cutaneous and soft tissue infections
• Cellulitis is a superficial skin infection characterized by blanching erythema caused by *Streptococcus*

• Most superficial abscesses of trunk, head, and neck caused by *S. aureus* and characterized by pain, erythema, and localized swelling—systemic signs uncommon, but regional lymph nodes enlarged

• Incision and drainage required for treatment of all but smallest furuncles

• Simple furuncles resolve with incision and drainage, while more complex carbuncles require systemic antibiotics (usually oral) for *S. aureus*

Necrotizing Soft Tissue Infections
• Four cardinal signs: edema beyond the area of erythema, skin vesicles or bullae, crepitus or subcutaneous air seen on radiography, and absence of lymphangitis or lymphadenitis

• Hyperpyrexia and leukocytosis common, but late findings

• Streptococcal gangrene characterized by rapid development of fever, marked erythema, pain, and swelling. Vesicles and bullae appear within 48 hours, followed by ecchymoses and gangrene of the skin by day 5

• Clostridial cellulitis also develops rapidly, often within several hours of laceration or surgery

• Necrotizing fasciitis develops rapidly and is accompanied by high fevers and systemic toxicity, progressing so quickly that borders appear to change within 15–20 minutes

• Diagnosis made by clinical observation of affected area, leukocytocis, hemolysis, coagulopathies, metabolic acidosis, hypocalcemia, and elevated creatine kinase

• Exudate or aspirates are obtained from wound, Gram stained, and sent for micropbiologic culture and antibiotic sensitivity testing

• On radiographs, air may be present in subcutaneous tissue or fascial planes

• Patients require immediate and aggressive resuscitation

• Intravenous antibiotic therapy started with high-dose penicillin (20 million units/day), aminoglycoside, and metronidazole

• Early and thorough debridement and drainage should include overlying skin, subcutaneous tissue, and affected fascia and muscle

• Hyperbaric oxygen therapy may be beneficial but only after or with thorough surgical debridement

Intra-abdominal Sepsis (Peritonitis)
• Usually polymicrobial and may include *E. coli, Klebsiella* spp, *Proteus* spp, enterococci, *B. fragillis*, anaerobic cocci, and *Clostridia*

• Physical findings depend on virulence of infective organisms, duration and extent of contamination, and underlying physiologic status of host

• Subphrenic abscesses may present with dyspnea (due to diaphragmatic irritation), referred shoulder pain, hiccups, basilar atelectasis, pleural effusions, and/or tenderness over tip of 12th rib

• CT scanning preferred diagnostic modality with 95% overall accuracy

• Ultrasound limited by tissue/air interfaces interfering with beam, particularly important in upper quadrants where abscess may be obscured by overlaying lung, and in mid-abdomen by surrounding bowel

SUGGESTED READINGS

Bleiweiss MS, Klein SR: Surgical infections. p. 156. In Bongard FS, Sue DY (eds): Current Critical Care: Diagnosis and Treatment. Appleton & Lange, E. Norwalk, CT, 1994

An excellent review of surgical infections for the house officer. Contains greater detail on many of the items discussed here.

The Medical Letter

Every year, The Medical Letter has at least one issue dedicated to nosocomial infections. This can be used as the stan-

dard for deciding on empiric therapy. The student is strongly encouraged to review the most recent issue containing this information

QUESTIONS

1. The humoral portion of the immune response has several components. Which of the following is not part of this mechanism?

    A. IL-1.
    B. G-CSF.
    C. TNF.
    D. Kupfer cells.

2. The most common nosocomial infection is?

    A. Pneumonia.
    B. Urinary tract infection.
    C. Wound infection.
    D. Cholecystitis.

3. The most important part of the management of necrotizing soft tissue infections is?

    A. Debridement.
    B. Antibiotic selection.
    C. Hyperbaric oxygen therapy.
    D. Antitetanus immunoglobulin.

4. The best diagnostic modality in the evaluation of a suspected intra-abdominal abscess is?

    A. Gallium scan.
    B. Ultrasound.
    C. MRI scan.
    D. CT scan.

(See p. 603 for answers.)

6

HEMORRHAGE, COAGULATION, AND TRANSFUSION

GIDEON P. NAUDE

Hemorrhage is defined as the abnormal loss of blood or the loss of abnormal quantities of blood. Small amounts of blood are lost physiologically in the gastrointestinal tract and during menstruation.

Blood loss may be acute and in large volumes, leading to shock and death if untreated, or chronically in small amounts, causing no hemodynamic instability, but eventually producing anemia.

CASE 1
FACTOR VIII DEFICIENCY

A young man was spending his apprenticeship in the carpentry workshop. He was new at the work and decided to put the long planks through the large rotating saw. He had never done this before. A loud voice boomed from behind, "Who told you to cut the beams?" Startled, he turned and the saw grazed the side of his left forearm. The skin was lifted in one place and absent over about 1 in., just above the wrist.

After the wound was bandaged, he excused himself. Going to the hospital was necessary, but he could not tell them he was a "bleeder." His grandfather had died after a tonsilectomy at the age of 36, when the patient's mother was 9 years old. When he had started work he lied on the form concerning his health, stating that his health was excellent and ticking 'no' to the question on blood disease. Well, he was strong and fit, but he required a factor VIII transfusion when teeth were extracted and on two occasions when he had been injured.

By the time he finished work, the bandage had been soaked with blood four times and he was feeling dizzy. At the hospital, factor VIII was given, causing the bleeding to stop quickly.

CASE 2
TRAUMA VICTIM

A 22-year-old athlete and college student was involved in a motorcycle accident, sustaining multiple limb fractures and a scalp laceration. The paramedics resuscitated him with several liters of balanced salt solution while he was being taken to the county trauma center. On arrival, he had a normal blood pressure and pulse and was producing adequate amounts of urine. Closed reduction of the fractures and suture of his laceration was performed in the emergency room and more crystalloid given. His Hct stabilized at 21% and it was decided not to transfuse, as his oxygen saturation was 100% and he could compensate with an increased cardiac output to maintain adequate

DO_2. During surgery for the placement of an internal fixation device, several hundred milliliters of blood were lost and transfusion was begun with cross-matched blood. Ten minutes later the anesthesiologist reported that his blood pressure had become extremely labile. Diffuse hemorrhage was noted in the operative field, with bleeding coming from areas that had previously been dry.

GENERAL CONSIDERATIONS

Hemostasis depends on the interaction of blood vessel walls, cellular blood elements (platelets), plasma procoagulant proteins (clotting factors), and regulatory mechanisms (fibrinolytic system and the anticoagulant proteins). In normal situations, the vascular endothelium resists the formation of thrombi, largely due to the actions of antiadhesive actions of prostacycline. Following injury, procoagulant proteins are produced, causing the adhesion of platelets to the subendothelium. The plug thus formed is a loosely organized collection of platelets referred to as a white clot. This primary phase of hemostasis serves to occlude the vessel and initially control the bleeding process.

Secondary hemostasis involves stabilization of the platelet plug, and requires activation of the *intrinsic* or *extrinsic* clotting cascades. The clotting factors are a group of circulating procoagulant factors whose activation results in the formation of an insoluble protein gel called fibrin. Two pathways are classically described, depending on the clotting factors involved and the mechanism of activation. Both pathways terminate in a common sequence (beginning with the conversion of factor X to activated factor Xa), which results in the conversion of prothrombin to thrombin. Factor XIII stabilizes the fibrin clot once formed. Calcium is required for most of the reactions. The extrinsic, or contact system begins when factor VII is activated by exposed tissue thromboplastin. Factor VIIa then activates factor X and the final pathway begins. The intrinsic pathway consists, in order, of factors XII, XI, IX, and VIII. Once generated, factor VIII activates factor X of the final pathway.

If coagulation were permitted to proceed unchecked, the thrombin in 2 ml of blood would be sufficient to clot the entire blood volume. Regulatory systems exist to prevent this catastrophic situation from developing. Activated factors are cleared by the reticuloendothelial system, and hepatocytes through phagocytosis. Plasmin causes fibrinolysis, and antithrombin III and protein C act directly on activated factors, rendering them inactive. Activated factor XII (XIIa) converts prekallikrein to kallikrein, kallikrein converts plasminogen to plasmin. Kallikrein also stimulates activation of factor XII to amplify this production. Tissue plasminogen activator (t-PA), produced by the vascular endothelial wall, activates plasminogen in the presence of fibrin.

Streptokinase (produced from bacteria) and urokinase (from urine and fetal kidney) both activate plasminogen, leading to fibrinolysis. For this purpose they are used clinically in thromboembolic disease. After plasmin digests fibrin, D-dimer is formed, which can be quantified and is an indicator of fibrinolysis. Plasmin, if left unchecked, can lead to consumption of the fibrinogen stores. This is avoided by α_2-antiplasmin and α_2-macroglobulin, which inactivate excess plasmin in the circulation. C1 esterase inhibits the activation of plasminogen by kallikrein.

KEY POINTS

- Blood loss may be acute and in large volumes, leading to shock and death if untreated; or chronically in small amounts, causing no hemodynamic instability, but eventually producing anemia

- Hemostasis depends on interaction of blood vessel walls, cellular blood elements (platelets), plasma procoagulant proteins (clotting factors), and regulatory mechanisms (fibrinolytic system and the anticoagulant proteins)

- Following injury, procoagulant proteins are produced, causing adhesion of platelets to subendothelium in a loosely organized plug referred to as a white clot; this primary phase of hemostasis occludes the vessel and initially controls the bleeding process

- Plasmin causes fibrinolysis, while antithrombin III and protein C act directly on activated factors, rendering them inactive

- Activated factor XII (XIIA) converts prekallikrein to kallikrein, kallikrein converts plasminogen to plasmin; kallikrein also stimulates activation of factor XII to amplify this production

- Tissue plasminogen activator (t-PA), produced by vascular endothelial wall, activates plasminogen in presence of fibrin

DIAGNOSIS

Abnormalities in primary hemostasis can be due to defects in the platelet or the vessel wall, leading to impaired platelet adherence to the subendothelial surface.

History is the single most important part of the diagnosis and evaluation of bleeding disorders. A family history of bleeding tendencies is particularly important. Congenital bleeding disorders are far less common than those that are acquired from drugs (such as aspirin or nonsteroidal anti-inflammatory drugs) or from concurrent illnesses (such as uremia). Even though the term *congenital* implies that these defects are present from birth, many such problems do not manifest until the patients are older. The history can suggest a platelet deficiency if there have been repeated incidents of prolonged bleeding with minor trauma or surgery, or easy bruising and capillary oozing from cuts and abrasions. On examination, petechial bleeds are evident. Splenomegaly could suggest hypersplenism or idiopathic thrombocytopenia.

Bleeding time is measured by making a small incision on the forearm using a template and timing the bleeding. This is nonspecific and will exhibit abnormality if platelet disorders (qualitative and quantitative), von Willebrand's deficiency, fibrinogen deficiency, and vascular collagen abnormalities are present. Normal bleeding time is less than 10 minutes. Coagulation (clotting factor) disorders do not usually affect the bleeding time.

Platelet counts give a quantitative assessment (normal, 150,000–400,000/mm³). The size of the platelets may also suggest their longevity, as young platelets are larger and denser. Bone marrow biopsy may be required in some cases to assess platelet production.

History is of great importance in diagnosing secondary hemostasis and may reveal a congenital defect in the quantity or quality of a clotting factor. Because factors II, VII, IX, X, and proteins C and S depend on fat soluble vitamin K for their synthesis, malnourished patients, those receiving antibiotics, and those with pancreatic insufficiency or obstructive jaundice may be deficient. Similarly, because many of the factors are made in the liver, patients with cirrhosis or other liver disease may have decreased concentration of these factors. Abnormalities of secondary hemostasis present with larger vessel bleeding, leading to intramuscular hematomas and hemarthroses and are usually due to specific clotting factor deficiencies.

The laboratory evaluation usually consists of the following:

Prothrombin time (PT): this test is a reflection mainly of factor VII activity, and hence should be used primarily to assess the extrinsic pathway. Because it also depends on factors II, V, and X, the common pathway is also tested. The PT is used primarily to monitor the efficacy of treatment with warfarin, which reduces the production of vitamin K-dependent factors, thrombin and fibrinogen, (extrinsic pathway).

Activated partial thromboplastin time (PTT): this study assesses coagulation via the intrinsic pathway and activation of factor X. It is used to monitor the effect of heparin infusion.

Thrombin time (TT): this assesses the availability and/or function of the conversion of fibrinogen to fibrin. Because heparin markedly increases the ability of antithrombin III to inhibit several of the conversion steps (especially factor X to factor Xa), its administration will prolong TT.

Reptilase (derived from snake venom): this assesses fibrinogen function, but is unaffected by heparin.

Individual factor assays (quantitative) can be performed for specific deficiencies.

Increased fibrinolysis is not easy to test for, as the usual coagulation profile (PT, PTT, TT) is not sensitive to fibrinolytic activity. Euglobin clot lysis time is a rough indicator of fibrinolytic activity. A time of less than 3 hours indicates increased fibrinolysis. D-dimer increase in the plasma is also an indicator of increased fibrinolysis.

KEY POINTS

- History most important part of diagnosis and evaluation of bleeding disorders, particularly family history of bleeding tendencies
- Congenital bleeding disorders far less common than those acquired from drugs such as aspirin or nonsteroidal anti-inflammatory drugs or from concurrent illnesses such as uremia; congenital defects, although present from birth, often do not manifest until patients are older
- History can suggest platelet deficiency if repeated incidents of prolonged bleeding with minor trauma or surgery, or easy bruising and capillary oozing from cuts
- Bleeding time measured by making small incision on forearm using template and timing bleeding; this is nonspecific and exhibits abnormality in platelet disorders, von Willebrand's deficiency, fibrinogen deficiency, and vascular collagen abnormalities
- Normal bleeding time is less than 10 minutes
- Coagulation disorders do not affect bleeding time
- Because factors II, VII, IX, X, and proteins C and S depend on fat soluble vitamin K for synthesis, those receiving antibiotics and those with pancreatic insufficiency or obstructive jaundice may be deficient
- PT used primarily to monitor efficacy of treatment with warfarin, which reduces production of vitamin K-dependent factors, thrombin and fibrinogen, to assess extrinsic pathway
- PTT used to monitor the effect of heparin

MANAGEMENT

Management of coagulation disorders in surgical patients centers largely around the perioperative period. Bleeding tendencies will lead to excessive blood loss at surgery, while hypercoagulability may cause deep venous thrombosis and pulmonary embolism during postoperative convalescence when the patient is relatively sedentary. Most disorders are acquired rather than congenital and can be managed with little difficulty once identified.

Aspirin and nonsteroidal anti-inflammatory drugs are the major acquired causes of platelet dysfunction. Aspirin, once bound to a platelet, causes permanent dysfunction. Hence, patients should be advised to stop aspirin use several weeks before surgery so that a pool of normally functioning platelets can be established. Among cardiac surgery patients, use of the bypass pump may cause mechanical platelet disruption resulting in thrombocytopenia. Transfusion of more than several units of blood is a common cause of dilutional thrombocytopenia among surgical patients. It is especially prevalent among trauma victims who have large blood losses that have been replaced with balanced salt solutions.

Platelet disorders, both quantitative and qualitative, are treated with platelet transfusions, which are indicated when the count falls below 50,000/µl to prevent bleeding at surgery, or below 20,000/µl to prevent spontaneous bleeding. Each unit contains about 5.5×10^{10} platelets and is good for about 5 days. Chills, fever, and allergic reactions occasionally occur. The usual dose for thrombocytopenic bleeding in an adult is 6–10 units. Desmopressin releases factor VIII, von Willebrand's factor (vWF), and plasminogen activator from endothelial cells and improves platelet function. Desmopressin is effective in patients with uremia and those who have undergone extensive surgical procedures such as cardiopulmonary bypass. It is given in doses of 0.3 µg/kg IV over 20 minutes. Maximal response usually occurs within 30 minutes.

Congenital secondary disorders of coagulation include von Willebrand's disease, hemophilia A (factor VIII deficiency), and hemophilia B (factor IX deficiency). von Willebrand's disease is inherited as an autosomal dominant and manifests as a bleeding tendency due to a decrease in vWF, which normally binds to factor VIII. Platelet adhesion to the vessel wall is dependent on vWF; therefore, platelet plug formation is adversely affected. The disease is diagnosed by decreased concentrations of vWF and factor VIII. Mild to moderate cases are treated with desmopressin, while severe forms are treated with fresh frozen plasma. Concentrates of factor VIII are available.

Hemophilia A is due to reduced concentration of factor VIII caused by a sex-linked abnormality. Those with more than 10% of normal concentration are mild hemophiliacs. Those with 2–10% of normal levels will bleed abnormally with minimal trauma, while those with less than 1–2% will bleed spontaneously. Desmopressin may be used in those with mild or moderate deficiency, while lyophilized factor VIII concentrate or cryoprecipitated antihemophilia factor (AHF) is needed in those with a severe deficiency. Levels should be increased to at least 25% before elective surgery.

Hemophilia B presents in a similar fashion to classic hemophilia. Desmopressin and cryoprecipitated AHF are not effective. Rather, the condition should be treated with the infusion of fresh frozen plasma or lyophilized factor IX concentrates that also contain factors II, VII, and IX.

Deficiencies of vitamin K-dependent factors (II, VII, IX, X, proteins C and S) should be treated with vitamin K administration. Fresh frozen plasma may be used when correction is needed urgently or for active bleeding. The administration of vitamin K corrects the problem within 12–36 hours. Patients with liver disease who are not able to synthesize the factors should be treated with fresh frozen plasma.

Thrombocytosis (thrombocyte count >600,000) can be primary as a bone marrow proliferative disorder, or part of associated conditions such as polycythemia vera, myeloid metaplasia, or chronic myeloid leukemia. If the count exceeds 1,000,000 in a symptomatic patient, plateletpheresis or hydroxyurea can be used to lower it. Asymptomatic patients with a count above 1,500,000 require treatment. Secondary thrombocytosis occurs after splenectomy; with bleeding and anemia, certain tumors, or infection; and postoperatively. Physicians should treat the underlying cause and use compressive stockings, exercise, and anticoagulation prophylaxis (usually heparin). Aspirin is of use in these cases. Hyperfibrinogenemia (>800 mg/dl) is associated with thrombotic events. Antithrombin III and protein C and S deficiencies all lead to increased thrombosis. These should be treated with warfarin administration.

Free thrombin (activated) is the cause of disseminated intravascular coagulation. It may occur in surgical patients following significant injury or in the face of sepsis. Once free thrombin is present, tissue factor is released, which causes further endothelial damage and more platelet and coagulation factor activation. Bleeding occurs due to consumption of platelets, fibrinogen, and factors V and VIII. Treatment should be aimed at the inciting process, which may be an undrained abscess or ischemia. Heparin may be used to prevent further conversion of prothrombin to thrombin. When bleeding is due to consumption of factors and platelets, transfusion of fresh frozen plasma, cryoprecipitate, and/or platelets may be required.

KEY POINTS

• Bleeding tendencies will lead to excessive blood loss at surgery, while hypercoagulability may cause deep venous thrombosis and pulmonary embolism during postoperative convalescence when patient is relatively sedentary

• Most disorders acquired rather than congenital and can be managed with little difficulty once identified

• Aspirin and nonsteroidal anti-inflammatory drugs major acquired causes of platelet dysfunction

• Aspirin causes permanent dysfunction; patients should be advised to stop aspirin use several weeks before surgery so that a pool of normally functioning platelets can be established

• Among cardiac surgery patients, use of the bypass pump may cause mechanical platelet disruption resulting in thrombocytopenia

• Platelet disorders are treated with transfusions; indicated when count falls below 50,000/µl to prevent bleeding at surgery, or below 20,000/µl to prevent spontaneous bleeding; each unit contains 5.5×10^{10} platelets and is good for 5 days

• Hemophilia A due to reduced concentration of factor VIII caused by sex-linked abnormality: those with more than 10% of normal concentration have mild hemophilia, those with 2–10% of normal levels will bleed abnormally with minimal trauma, those with 1–2% will bleed spontaneously

• Hemophilia B presents similar to classic hemophilia; desmopressin and cryoprecipitated AHF are not effective, rather, treat with infusion of fresh frozen plasma or lyophilized factor IX concentrate that also contains factors II, VII, and IX

TRANSFUSION

Transfusion becomes necessary when life-threatening hemorrhage occurs or when the oxygen content of the blood is decreased due to a low hemoglobin (Hb) concentration. There is no Hb concentration at which all patients will require blood transfusion.

Hb-oxygen affinity depends on the presence of 2,3-diphosphoglycerate (2,3-DPG) in the red blood cell (RBC), which decreases the Hb-oxygen affinity and allows oxygen to be released to the tissues. The concentration of 2,3-DPG rapidly decreases in liquid, stored blood. After 2 weeks, it is present in small amounts only and can take up to 48 hours to be replaced after transfusion. Patients in shock, with decreased cardiac output, require oxygen delivery and fresh blood or frozen RBCs (adequate 2,3-DPG is present).

Products currently available for transfusion consist of human blood and blood products (Table 6.1). Artificial blood substitutes are still experimental. Human blood is obtained from donors (homologous), from the patient before transfusion (autologous), or from the bleeding site during a procedure and autotransfused back to the patient. Donor-recipient compatibility is of paramount importance in homologous transfusions.

Transfusion reactions occur predominantly as a result of labeling and clerical errors and usually are not due to laboratory inability to cross-match correctly. ABO incompatibility occurs when the A or B antigen is infused into a patient with an anti-A or anti-B antibody. Group A has an anti-B antibody, group B has an anti-A antibody, group O has anti-A and anti-B antibodies, and group AB has no antibodies. Consequently, blood group AB can receive any blood, and group O can receive only O. Group A can receive A and O, and group B can receive B and O. Rhesus (Rh) and Kell are other important antigens. Many other groups exist but rarely cause reactions.

Reactions can occur after as little as 50 ml of blood has been infused. When ABO incompatibility is present, conscious patients complain of chills and fever, backache, and chest pain. Hemoglobinuria, renal failure, disseminated intravascular coagulopathy and bleeding, shock, and anaphylaxis can occur. When this incompatibility is diagnosed or suspected, the transfusion must be stopped immediately and the transfused blood along with a sample of the patient's blood should be sent to the blood bank for analysis. The urine should be analyzed for free Hb. Mannitol (25 g) and/or a loop diuretic (ethycrinic acid or furosemide) should be administered. During an anesthetic, the classic signs are masked and patients may present with blood pressure instability and diffuse oozing as first signs of an incompatible blood transfusion.

Delayed transfusion reactions may occur up to 3 weeks after transfusion. They present with fever, malaise, and hemolytic anemia. Indirect bilirubin is increased and the Coombs reaction is positive. Several types of delayed reaction may occur.

Antileukocyte febrile reactions occur after 5–10% of transfusions, particularly if multiple previous transfusions have been given. These reactions are usually self-limited. Patients complain of chills, fever, tachycardia, tachypnea, and occasionally hypotension. The transfusion is stopped and the blood retested. Future transfusions should use leukocyte-poor blood, and antihistamines or aspirin should be administered.

TABLE 6.1 *Products currently available for transfusion*

Product	Volume	Hemoglobin	Hematocrit	Other components	Functional life (days)
Whole blood + 60 ml CPD	500 ml	60 g	40	Plasma ± 250 ml White blood cells Platelets nonviable	CPD at 4°C (21) CPDA at 4°C (35) Adsol (42)
Red cells	300 ml	60 g	70	Plasma ± 80 ml White blood cells Platelets nonviable	CPD at 4°C (21) CPDA at 4°C (35) Adsol (42)
Cryopreserved cells	180 ml	54 g	90	No plasma No white cells No platelets, 2,3–DPG adequate	More than 20 years at –80°C After thawing, 3 days at 4°C
Frozen plasma	220 ml	0	0	Coagulation factors present Fibrinogen 400 mg, complement	4°C (1)–18°C (1 yr)
Platelets—several donors	50 ml	0	0	Platelets 5×10^{10}	22°C (5)
Platelets—one donor	300 ml	0	0	Platelets 5×10^{11}	Use in 1 day or freeze

Abbreviations: CPD, citrate, phosphate, dextrose; CPDA, CPD plus adenine; Adsol, CPDA plus glucose, mannitol, and sodium chloride; 2,3-DPG, 2,3-diphosphoglycerate.

Allergies to donor medications or other substances in the blood can occur if the antigen (e.g., penicillin) is transfused into an allergic individual.

Graft-versus-host disease occurs when an immunocompromised individual receives immunocompetent cells (leukocytes in blood or bone marrow) that initiate rejection of the host's normal tissue. This presents a few days to 1 month after the transfusion with fever, a rash, and gastrointestinal, hepatic, and bone marrow dysfunction. Mortality is associated with bone marrow suppression. Graft-versus-host disease is avoided by giving frozen blood or irradiated or washed RBCs in which the leukocytes have either been inactivated or removed before transfusion.

Thrombocytopenia, presenting with purpura and mucous membrane bleeding, occurs about 1 week after transfusion. Recovery can take up to 2 months.

Fluid overload can occur if significant volumes of fluid are administered. In those with cardiac or renal failure, the patient is at particularly high risk of fluid overload.

Cold blood transfused rapidly or administered rapidly (primarily for resuscitation) can cause ventricular arrhythmias. Because of the change in temperature, the oxygen dissociation curve is left-shifted, thereby decreasing oxygen release to the tissues. Furthermore, coagulation is adversely affected by decreased temperature.

Infections are infrequent but serious complications of transfusion. Screening for hepatitis B and C has markedly reduced the incidence of transfusion-related hepatitis. It has not reached zero yet, as donors are infective before the serologic tests become positive. All donor blood is routinely tested for human immunodeficiency virus (HIV). The incidence of transfusion-acquired HIV has decreased to about 1 in 150,000 transfusions. Unfortunately, blood is infective before serologic tests are positive. New tests are being developed that could further reduce the incidence.

A number of viral infections may be transmitted, including Epstein-Barr virus (EBV) and cytomegalovirus (CMV). These are of particular importance among immunocompromised recipients. CMV is the most commonly transfused infective agent.

Bacterial contamination occurs infrequently and is due to poor technique in obtaining, storing, and administering blood. It can also occur if a bacteremia is present in the host at the time of donation. Usually gram-negative, endotoxin producing, cold growing organisms are the cause. Clinically, the recipient presents with fever, chills, shock, and renal failure. This condition carries a high mortality. Syphilis is very rarely transmitted through transfusion. The spirochete dies if it is cooled and can only be transferred if fresh, warm blood is transfused or in a platelet transfusion (platelets are stored at room temperature).

Immunosuppression occurs after whole blood or RBC transfusion; the exact etiology is unclear at present. This has positive and negative aspects. Renal transplants have an improved survival after blood transfusion. Cancer patients, by contrast, have experienced increased tumor recurrence and decreased survival. Massive transfusion is associated with a higher incidence of anastomotic leak after colonic resection and anastomosis.

Several electrolyte abnormalities may occur after transfusion of more than several units of blood. Hypocalcemia occurs when citrate in stored blood complexes circulating calcium. This is dependent not only on the absolute volume of transfusion but on the rate as well. Muscle twitching, cardiac abnormalities, and ventricular fibrillation can occur. The diagnosis is made by laboratory evaluation and suspected by an increased ST segment and a T-wave delay. Hyperkalemia can occur after a large transfusion of relatively old blood in which the red cell wall fails to maintain the sodium-potassium pump, and the extracellular potassium rises. Repeated transfusions may lead to iron deposition in the liver, endocrine glands, and heart. Chronic or symptomatic iron deposition is treated by the chelating agent disferroxamine.

KEY POINTS

- Transfusion becomes necessary when life-threatening hemorrhage occurs or when oxygen content of blood is decreased due to a low Hb concentration

- Transfusion reactions occur predominantly as a result of labeling and clerical errors and usually not due to laboratory inability to cross-match correctly

- ABO incompatibility occurs when A or B antigen infused into a patient with anti-A or anti-B antibody; group A has anti-B antibody, group B has anti-A antibody, group O has anti-A and anti-B antibodies, and group AB has no antibodies

- Blood group AB can receive any blood, and group O can receive only O, group A can receive A and O, and group B can receive B and O

- Rhesus and Kell are other important antigens

- Reactions can occur after as little as 50 ml of blood has been infused

- When ABO incompatibility present, conscious patients complain of chills and fever, backache, and chest pain

- Hemoglobinuria, renal failure, disseminated intravascular coagulopathy and bleeding, shock, and anaphylaxis can occur as part of a transfusion reaction

- When incompatibility diagnosed, transfusion must be stopped and blood analyzed; urine must be analyzed as well for free Hb; mannitol and/or loop diuretic should be administered

- Delayed transfusion reactions may occur up to 3 weeks after transfusion and present with fever, malaise, and hemolytic anemia; indirect bilirubin is increased and Coombs reaction is positive

- Antileukocyte febrile reactions occur after 5–10% of transfusions, particularly if previous transfusions have been given; patients complain of chills, fever, tachycardia, tachypnea, and occasionally hypotension

• Cold blood transfused or administered rapidly can cause ventricular arrhythmias; because of change in temperature, oxygen dissociation curve is left-shifted, thereby decreasing oxygen release to tissues; coagulation is adversely affected by decreased temperature

• Infections infrequent but serious complications of transfusion; screening for hepatitis B and C has markedly reduced the incidence of transfusion-related hepatitis

• Viral infections may be transmitted, including Epstein-Barr virus and CMV; these are important among immunocompromised recipients

• CMV most commonly transfused infective agent

• Several electrolyte abnormalities may occur after transfusion of more than several units of blood; hypocalcemia occurs when citrate in stored blood complexes circulating calcium

SUGGESTED READINGS

Pisciotto PT (ed): Blood Transfusion Therapy. American Association of Blood Banks, Bethesda, MD, 1993

One of our favorite references on the topic. This paperback pocketbook is only 128 pages, but contains virtually everything about transfusion and hemostasis that most clinicians need to know. It can be obtained from a hospital blood bank or from the American Association of Blood Banks (8101 Glenbrook Road, Bethesda MD, 20814). It has information that will take years to appear in most textbooks.

Thompson AR, Harker LA: Manual of Hemostasis and Thrombosis. FA Davis, Philadelphia, 1983

A good general guide to the biochemistry of thrombosis and coagulation. Contains detailed information that would be useful in the preparation of a report or for teaching rounds.

QUESTIONS

1. The laboratory test most useful in monitoring the efficacy of heparin for anticoagulation is?

   A. TT.

   B. PTT.

   C. PT.

   D. Bleeding time.

2. An abnormality in the ability of platelets to aggregate and form a hemostatic plug will primarily affect which one of the following tests?

   A. TT.

   B. PTT.

   C. PT.

   D. Bleeding time.

3. Which of the following items is most important in the preoperative evaluation of a patient for abnormal coagulation?

   A. PTT.

   B. History.

   C. Bleeding time.

   D. Ristocetin inhibition time.

(See p. 603 for answers.)

7

ANESTHESIA AND PAIN CONTROL

TAI-SHION LEE

The development and evaluation of anesthesia represents important progress in medical history and patient care. Many operations have become possible because of improvements in anesthesia. Its fundamental purpose is to provide comfortable conditions that free the patient from pain, fear, and anxiety, thereby facilitating operation. Since almost all anesthetic techniques and agents have potential risks and produce adverse effects, it is essential to have a thoughtful plan for the perioperative period, when the patient is subjected to additional surgical trauma and stress.

The purpose of this chapter is to present the basic concepts and principles of anesthesiology.

GENERAL CONSIDERATIONS

Since each patient's condition is unique and anesthesia can be performed in a number of ways, planning for the best outcome is very important. When determining a mode of anesthesia, the anesthesiologist must ask pertinent questions. For example:

1. What is the scheduled operation?
2. What will be the patient's position on the operating table?
3. How long will the operation last?
4. What is the anticipated blood loss?
5. Is blood transfusion needed and how much?
6. Is there a heart problem, coronary artery disease, myocardial infarction, angina (and how long ago), or congestive heart disease?

7. Is there any need for a pacemaker before operation?
8. Is coronary angiography or echocardiography required?
9. Has hypertension been under good control?
10. Can hypotension be rapidly resuscitated?
11. How good is the pulmonary function?
12. Is there a possibility of respiratory infection or reactive airway disease?
13. Is the patient in acute renal failure?
14. How is the fluid and acid-base electrolyte status?
15. Is diabetes mellitus under good control and what is the blood sugar level?
16. Are there signs of uropathy, liver dysfunction, bleeding diathesis, or carotid artery disease?
17. What are the patient's current medications, and is there a history of alcohol or drug abuse?
18. How significant is the difficult airway? Is the patient's spine mobile?
19. Finally, what is the patient's anesthesia preference?

Anesthesia can be categorized into two major modes: general and regional. General anesthesia produces a state of unconsciousness, while regional anesthesia provides analgesia to one specific portion of the body. There are a variety of anesthetic agents and techniques available to achieve these goals, each with its own advantages and disadvantages.

General anesthesia produces an altered physiologic state of unconsciousness, analgesia, and amnesia. Muscle relaxation and areflexia of the autonomic nervous system are also considered essential components of general anesthesia. General anesthesia is induced pharmacologically through inhalation, intravenous, intramuscular, transcutaneous, or enteral administration of an anesthetic agent. There is wide variation in the degree of general anesthesia. Light anesthesia implies anesthesia with minimum depression of bodily functions, whereas deep general anesthesia induces total body depression to just before the point of significant deterioration of vital signs. The depth of anesthesia required depends on the dosage of anesthetic, the level of surgical stimulation, and the patient's condition.

Anesthesia affects many physiologic and metabolic functions. During general anesthesia, depressed myocardial contractility, vasodilatation, decreased venous return, loss of autonomic response, and maldistribution of blood flow can lead to significant changes in hemodynamics as well as tissue perfusion. Major respiratory problems include airway patency, decreased functional residual capacity, ventilation/perfusion maldistribution, central nervous system depression, and disruption of peripheral neuromuscular transmission. Suppression of the nervous system involves disturbances of somatic as well as autonomic nervous functions. Many important protective and regulatory mechanisms are lost, including decreases in renal and hepatic function, depression of gastrointestinal motility, immunosuppression, and endocrine derangements.

A state of general anesthesia is generally produced by administration of volatilized pharmacologic agents to the lungs via mask or an endotracheal intubation. Currently available and commonly used inhalation anesthetics include nitrous oxide, halothane, enflurane, isoflurane, desflurane, and sevoflurane. These agents are delivered by a complex and sophisticated anesthesia machine, which converts volatile liquids into anesthetic vapors that cross the alveolar-capillary membrane to enter the circulation where they are rapidly transported to the brain.

During inhalational anesthesia, MAC is defined as the minimum alveolar anesthetic concentration (at one atmosphere pressure) required to induce a lack of movement response to a standard skin incision in 50% of subjects tested. MAC reflects minimum concentration in the brain and is useful in titrating anesthesia. Clinically, a MAC of 1.2–1.3 can prevent movement in about 95% of patients. MAC varies for different anesthetics and can be influenced by various physiologic and pharmacologic factors (Table 7.1). MAC is a widely accepted method for comparing the potency of inhalation agents. The MAC is re-

TABLE 7.1 *Factors affecting MAC*

Age

Temperature

Atmospheric pressure

Ethanol abuse/intoxication

Hypotension

Hypoxemia, hypercarbia

Pregnancy

Hyper- or hypothyroidism

Medications (opioids, barbituates, benzodiazepines, phenothiazines, ketamine, monoamine oxidase inhibitors, cocaine, ephedrine, clonidine, methyldopa, reserpine)

duced when nitrous oxide (N_2O) is used in combination with a volatile anesthetic. A similar concept, MAC BAR, is the anesthetic necessary (at one atmosphere) to block adrenergic response to a standard skin incision.

A general anesthetic state may also be created by intravenous administration of anesthetic agents such as barbiturates, propofol, ketamine, or etomidate. Even though the use of intravenous anesthesia has expanded with newly introduced agents and delivery technology, the technique is usually only used for surgical procedures of short duration.

General analgesia is induced with intravenous administration of narcotics such as morphine, fentanyl, sufentanil, or alfentanil, supplemented with N_2O or small doses of inhalation agents to produce an anesthetic state (Table 7.2). It is commonly used in cardiac surgery and patients with unstable hemodynamics.

Balanced anesthesia combines different anesthetics such as inhalation vapors, intravenous agents, or mixtures of the two. The term implies a common technique combining muscle relaxants, intravenous barbiturates, narcotics, and N_2O/O_2 with or without other vapors.

Regional anesthesia induces anesthesia in just one designated part of the body. It results from application of local anesthetics in the vicinity of the nerve endings or nerve pathways. Regional anesthesia may be used for most surgical procedures done below the level of the di-

TABLE 7.2 *Commonly used opioids*

	Equivalent Potency	Elimination Half-Life (hr)	Duration of Action (hr)
Meperidine	1/10	3–4	2–4
Morphine	1	1.5–2.2	4–5
Afentanil	10	1–1.5	
Fentanyl	100	3–4.5	0.5–1.5
Sufentanil	1,000	2.5–3	

aphragm. It is particularly useful for operations on lower extremities or the inferior abdomen. Contraindications include bleeding tendency or preoperative use of anticoagulants, skin infections of the back, backache, and neurologic deficits.

Spinal anesthesia is a type of regional anesthesia induced by injection of a local anesthetic into the intrathecal (subarachnoid) space of the spinal canal. Spinal anesthesia produces sensory and motor blockade. It also blocks sympathetic nerves to cause vasodilatation and hypotension.

Epidural anesthesia is a form of regional anesthesia produced by blocking the spinal nerve trunks as they pass through the epidural (extradural) space. The anesthesia results from direct contact with the nerve roots and diffusion of the agent through the dura. As compared with spinal anesthesia, it is not as reliable and requires a much larger volume of anesthetic. It also has a slower onset and produces fewer problems with hypotension.

Caudal anesthesia is a variant of epidural anesthesia in which a local anesthetic is applied to the sacral region at the caudal end of the spinal column. It is used for rectal and perineal procedures, particularly in pediatric patients.

A regional anesthetic may also be produced by injection of a local anesthetic solution into an extremity artery with a proximal tourniquet. This (Bier) block is particularly useful for upper extremity procedures.

Local anesthesia is produced when anesthetics are infiltrated into a localized area of skin or subcutaneous tissues (Table 7.3). This may be extended to produce a field block in which an area is anesthetized by infiltrating a surrounding perimeter with local anesthetics.

Although local and regional techniques are generally safe and effective, several complications can occur. Excessive cephalad spread of a spinal/epidural anesthetic can affect the cardiopulmonary system significantly by blocking neural pathways. Involvement of intercostal nerves can lead to agitation, nausea and vomiting, bradycardia, paradoxical respiration, and apnea. The treatment of these problems requires the use of vasopressors, atropine, and mechanical ventilation.

A frontal or occipital headache, with or without tinnitus, may result from paraspinal anesthesia. It is believed to be caused by decreased pressure resulting from leakage of cerebrospinal fluid through the puncture site. This has been shown to be related to the size of the needle used. Treatment is with analgesics and an epidural blood patch.

Systemic toxicity is most commonly caused by accidental overdose of anesthetics. Seizures may occur as the major manifestation of toxicity. The excessive excitatory output may result from the action of local anesthetics on inhibitory fibers or centers in the brain and myocardial depression leading to circulatory collapse.

Advantages of regional anesthesia include less cardiovascular depression, fewer respiratory complications, excellent muscular relaxation and minimum doses of drug. Dis-

TABLE 7.3 *Commonly used local anesthetics*

Agent	Half-Life (HR)	Use	Maximum Single Dose
Amides			
Bupivacaine	3.5	Epidural, spinal infiltration	3 mg/kg
Etidocaine	2.6	Epidural, caudal infiltration, nerve block	3 (4)[a] mg/kg
Lidocaine	1.6	Epidural, caudal infiltration, nerve block	4.5 (7)[a] mg/kg
Mepivacaine	1.9	Epidural, caudal infiltration, nerve block	4.5 (7)[a] mg/kg
Esters			
Procaine	0.14	Spinal infiltration, nerve block	12 mg/kg

[a]Maximum dose with epinephrine.
(From Bongard FS: Critical Care, Diagnosis, and Treatment. Appleton & Lange, E. Norwalk, CT, 1994, with permission.)

advantages are less patient comfort, more stress, false sense of security, incomplete block, drug toxicity, and that it is not suitable for all operations. The choice between general or regional anesthesia is one for which there are no rigid rules. Many operations can be performed using either technique or a combination of the two. Besides the type, site, and duration of surgery, the choice will be determined by the needs and preferences of the surgeon, the personality and desires of the patient and the skill and experience of the anesthesiologist. Combined techniques take advantage of the benefits of regional anesthesia, augmented by a light general anesthetic. This has real potential because it combines the merits of regional anesthesia with substantially diminished amounts of general anesthetic to provide a comfortable, less stressful environment for surgery.

KEY POINTS

• Anesthesia categorized into two modes: general produces state of unconsciousness; regional provides analgesia to specific portion of body

• General anesthesia produces analgesia, amnesia, muscle relaxation, and areflexia of autonomic nervous system

• Hemodynamics and tissue perfusion can change significantly during general anesthesia, because of depressed myocardial contractility, vasodilatation, decreased venous return, loss of autonomic response, and maldistribution of blood flow

• During inhalational anesthesia, MAC is the minimum alveolar anesthetic concentration required to induce a lack of movement response to a standard incision in 50% of subjects tested

• Epidural anesthesia results from direct contact with nerve roots and diffusion of agent through dura; not as reliable as spinal anesthesia and requires much more anesthetic, has slower onset, but causes fewer hypotension problems

• Excessive cephalad spread of a spinal/epidural anesthetic can block neural pathways and affect cardiopulmonary system; involvement of intercostal nerves can lead to agitation, nausea and vomiting, bradycardia, paradoxical respiration, and apnea

• Regional anesthesia causes less cardiovascular depression, fewer respiratory complications, excellent muscular relaxation, and enables minimum drug doses; but also entails less patient comfort, more stress, a false sense of security, incomplete block, drug toxicity, and is not suitable for all surgery

A PREOPERATIVE EVALUATION

A preanesthetic visit by the anesthesiologist is important to evaluate the patient's status, improve rapport, and relieve anxiety. Since etiologies of perioperative complications and mortality are multifactorial and involve not only anesthesia itself but also surgery and the patient's condition, it is sometimes difficult to assess anesthetic risk preoperatively. Nevertheless, a classification of general condition has been developed by the American Society of Anesthesiologists and is commonly used to define risk.

Class I—A normal, healthy patient

Class II—A patient with mild systemic disease

Class III—A patient with a moderately severe systemic disease that limits activity, but is not incapacitating

Class IV—A patient with an incapacitating systemic disease that is a constant threat to life

Class V—A moribund patient not expected to survive 24 hours with or without an operation

Class E—A patient who requires emergency operation

Currently, because of increased knowledge of the pathophysiology disease and the effects of anesthetic agents, as well as improvements in anesthetic management, many diseases for which anesthesia and surgery were once precluded can now be performed. The anesthesiologist should be acquainted with the patient's status and medical problems beforehand in order to judge whether the patient is in optimal condition for the planned surgery and anesthesia.

When planning anesthetic management it is essential that the anesthesiologist have complete knowledge of the surgical requirements. These include type of surgery, approximate duration of operation, patient's position on the table, required level of muscle relaxation, anticipated blood loss, need for extra equipment or medications, and presence of any associated hazard.

In the past, certain empirically preset requirements for laboratory tests and values were recommended before patients were considered for anesthesia. Many are unnecessary or unhelpful. The history and physical examination are essential in determining the necessity of such tests. Requests should be individualized. Special tests should concentrate on pertinent evaluation of cardiopulmonary, hepatic, and renal function. Commonly ordered tests include hematocrit (Hct), electrocardiogram (ECG), chest x-ray, electrolytes, blood glucose, urea nitrogen, and creatinine.

Drugs may be given before surgery to facilitate induction, maintenance, and recovery from anesthesia. They should be prescribed only when necessary and on an individual basis, rather than routinely. In general, they are used for the following reasons: (1) to reduce fear and anxiety (sedatives such as tranquilizers and/or barbiturates), (2) to avoid adverse autonomic reflexes secondary to anesthesia or operative manipulations (sympatholytic or vagolytic agents), (3) to decrease secretions in the airway (drying agents such as atropine, glycopyrrolate, and scopolamine), (4) to enhance analgesia during light anesthesia (narcotics such as morphine, fentanyl, and meperidine), (5) to reduce the risk of aspiration by decreasing the volume and increasing the pH of gastric secretion (H_2 blockers or antacids), and (6) to decrease the incidence of nausea and vomiting (antiemetics). The effects and interactions of concomitant drug therapy should always be taken into consideration during administration of anesthesia.

Before anesthesia, the anesthesiologist, as well as the surgeon, must optimize the patient's condition. If not possible, modification of the planned surgery or anesthesia may be necessary. Since morbidity and mortality are expected to be greater in cases with significant physiologic derangements, if time allows, it is important to correct or improve them to the best level possible before operation. Extra effort should be given to the cardiopulmonary system and fluid status of the patient. Additional tests and appropriate consultation may be required.

Before starting any case, the anesthesia equipment, drugs, and other necessary items must be thoroughly checked, and required intravenous fluid (including blood) should be prepared. When the patient arrives, the anesthesiologist must first confirm the identity of the patient and the scheduled operation. Quick review of the patient's status is needed to ascertain any new changes and administration of premedications. The vital signs should be documented. Depending on the type of operation, one or more intravenous lines may be required. National standards for monitoring during anesthesia include the following: (1) ventilation (precordial stethoscope, capnography), (2) oxygenation (pulse oximeter, blood gases), (3) circulation (blood pressure, ECG, arterial catheter, central venous pressure (CVP), and (4) temperature (core or peripheral thermometer). In addition, muscle relaxation is assessed with a peripheral nerve stimulator. More sophisticated monitors such as a pulmonary artery catheter, electroencephalogram, and evoked potentials may be needed. Constant vigilance to maintain adequate circulation and respiration is the core of a safe anesthetic.

The patient must be properly positioned as required for the operation. It is important to provide comfort while avoiding any injury. Damage to the brachial plexus, radial, ulnar, sciatic and common peroneal nerves as well as pressure necrosis of the skin can occur during anesthesia due to malpositioning. Because of suppression of the compensatory autonomic response, it is essential to be gentle in positioning the patient, or a sudden circulatory collapse might result.

To start general anesthesia, the desired depth of the anesthetic state is produced by a variety of methods. This is commonly accomplished by inhalation or intravenous administration of anesthetic agents. Intramuscular, transcutaneous, or gastrointestinal administration are available but rarely used. The techniques employed may or may not include endotracheal intubation. Routine induction is conducted in a controlled, incremental manner. Bolus, stepwise titration, or steady infusion of the anesthetics are used depending on the situation. Crash induction (rapid sequence induction) is a special technique in which the anesthesiologist gains control of the patient's airway and anesthetic state as rapidly as possible. It commonly involves a large dose of intravenous anesthetic, a rapidly acting muscle relaxant, and endotracheal intubation. It is indicated in patients at high risk of pulmonary aspiration of gastric contents. Induction refers to the period that begins with the administration of the first anesthetic until the desired depth of the anesthetic state is reached. It represents a critical time in anesthesia, since many significant physiologic alterations occur.

In most circumstances, general anesthesia is conducted using endotracheal intubation to ensure a patent airway. The procedure is performed orally or nasally. Currently used endotracheal tubes are single-use and are made of polyvinylchloride or silastic. The high volume, low pressure cuff permits a tight fit for positive pressure ventilation and prevention of aspiration. Cuffless tubes are commonly used in pediatric anesthesia.

It is important to place the endotracheal tube in the trachea properly. Esophageal intubation, resulting in hypoxia and death, can be detected by auscultation and by expired carbon dioxide monitoring. Exhaled carbon dioxide can be measured through a properly placed endotracheal tube, while a tube that lies in the esophagus will produce virtually no carbon dioxide. Endobronchial intubation, except for special indications should be avoided. Precautions should be exercised during endotracheal intubation to prevent aspiration in full stomach cases, stress response in coronary heart disease, and increased intracranial pressure in head injury cases.

The "planes" of anesthesia described during diethyl ether anesthesia are not applicable or appreciated for modern anesthetic agents. The depth of anesthesia can usually be assessed from clinical signs, particularly cardiovascular and respiratory. Depending on surgical requirements, anesthesia can be maintained at light, moderate, or deep levels.

Relaxation of skeletal muscles may be required during surgery to facilitate operative procedures. Neuromuscular blocking agents cause skeletal muscle relaxation by blocking the neuromuscular transmission ability of acetylcholine to activate the postsynaptic nicotinic cholinergic receptors of the muscle fiber. There are two types of neuromuscular blocking agents, depolarizing and nondepolarizing. Drugs that produce membrane depolarization and initiate muscle contraction (fasciculation) are called depolarizing agents. They structurally resemble acetycholine and have a rapid onset and short duration of action. They are competitive and are only inactivated by serum pseudocholinesterase. Succinylcholine is the only such agent available in the United States. No antagonist is available.

Nondepolarizing neuromuscular blocking agents block neuromuscular transmission by competing with acetylcholine for the nicotinic receptors. They usually have a slower onset and longer duration of action than depolarizing agents. Depending on the duration of action, they can be classified as short-acting (mivacuronium), intermediate (vecuronium, atracurium), and long-acting (pancuronium, pipecuronium, doxacurium) (Table 7.4). Muscle paralysis produced by nondepolarizing agents can be reversed by cholinesterase inhibitors (neostigmine, pyridostigmine, edrophonium), which increase acetylcholine concentrations.

Using a peripheral nerve stimulator, the adequacy of neuromuscular blockade can be assessed and monitored. The twitch response measures the strength of muscle contraction following a single electrical stimulation to its motor nerve. At least 75% of the receptors must be blocked to produce a significant decrease in twitch strength. Clinically, a nearly complete suppression of twitch response indicates adequate surgical relaxation. Normally, continuous contraction is produced following rapid, repeated electrical stimulation of a motor nerve. This tetanic response fades with continuous stimulation when there is blockade at the neuromuscular junction. The rate of fade is related to the depth of blockade. The *train of four* is a commonly used technique to monitor the degree of neuromuscular blockade. A twitch response is produced following four consecutive supramaximal electrical stimulations given at 0.5-second intervals. The ratio of the height of the fourth twitch to the first twitch is used to assess the level of blockade. Since it has its own control, it is a reliable technique. The degree of muscle relaxation can also be assessed by physical examinations such as hand squeeze on command, ability to raise and hold the head for 5 seconds, and various respiratory measurements such as vital capacity and inspiratory and expiratory force.

At the termination of anesthesia and surgery, while the anesthesia wears off, partial pressures of anesthetics in the

TABLE 7.4 *Commonly used neuromuscular blocking agents*

	DURATION (MIN)	ONSET (MIN)	INTUBATION DOSE (MG/KG)	SUPPLEMENTAL DOSE (MG/KG)
Depolarizing				
Succinylcholine	5–10	0.5–1	0.15–1.5	
Nondepolarizing				
Mivacurium	10–20	2–3	0.15	
Atracurium	20–35	3–5	0.5	0.07–0.10
Vecuronium	20–35	3–5	0.1	0.015–0.02
Pipecuronium	60–90	3–5	0.15	
Doxacurium	60–90	4–6	0.08	
Pancuronium	60–90	3–5	0.1	0.007–0.015
Metocurine	60–90	3–5	0.4	0.04–0.07
D-Tubocurarine	60–90	3–5	0.6	0.05–0.1

arterial blood and brain fall rapidly and reequilibrate. The patient emerges from unconsciousness and the body starts to readjust and recover. Recovery is relatively rapid when the anesthesia was not prolonged. Hyperventilation usually facilitates elimination of anesthetic vapors. This is also a period when significant physiologic change can occur due to a reversal of muscle relaxation, termination of ventilatory support, and the perception of nociceptic stimulation from surgical trauma. Efforts to maintain hemodynamic stability and assure a secured airway and adequate spontaneous respiration are mandatory. Cardiopulmonary mishaps may occur during transport of the patient to the recovery room.

Malignant hyperthermia is a complication uniquely associated with anesthesia. It is characterized by a paroxysmal fulminant hypermetabolic crisis. Massive heat is generated and overwhelms the dissipation mechanisms of the body. Malignant hyperthermia may occur at any time perioperatively. Halothane and succinylcholine are the most common offenders, although almost any anesthetic agent or muscle relaxant may be responsible. The precise mechanism has not been fully elucidated. The main pathophysiologic event is believed to be a sudden increase in intracellular calcium concentration in skeletal (and perhaps cardiac) muscle triggered by causative agents. The excessive myoplasmic calcium activates adenosine triphosphatase and phosphorylase, thus causing muscle contraction and a massive increase in oxygen consumption, carbon dioxide production, anaerobic metabolism, and heat generation. As a result, severe respiratory and metabolic acidosis develop followed by dysrhythmias, and in severe cases, cardiac arrest. Rhabdomyolysis, hyperkalemia, and myoglobinuria are common consequences of muscle damage. Clinically, a sudden marked increase in end-tidal carbon dioxide is the best early clue to the diagnosis, which can be confirmed by a muscle biopsy. Early diagnosis and prompt aggressive treatment cannot be overemphasized. All possible triggering agents must be discontinued and hyperthermia controlled immediately. The patient should be intubated and hyperventilated with 100% oxygen. Most importantly, intravenous administration of dantrolene must be given as soon as possible (1–2 mg/kg every 15–30 minutes, up to 10–20 mg/kg if necessary). With early diagnosis and aggressive effective treatment, the mortality is now approximately 5%.

KEY POINTS

- Commonly ordered tests include Hct, ECG, chest x-ray, electrolytes, blood glucose, urea nitrogen, and creatinine

- National standards for monitoring anesthesia: (1) ventilation (precordial stethoscope, capnography), (2) oxygenation (pulse oximeter, blood gases), (3) circulation (blood pressure, ECG, arterial line, central venous pressure), and (4) temperature (core or peripheral thermometer)

- Muscle relaxation assessed with peripheral nerve stimulator

- Neuromuscular blocking agents cause skeletal muscle relaxation by blocking neuromuscular transmission ability of acetylcholine to activate postsynaptic nicotinic cholinergic receptors of the muscle fiber

- Depolarizing neuromuscular blocking agents produce membrane depolarization and initial muscle contraction (fasciculation), resemble acetylcholine, have a rapid onset and short duration of action, and are competitive and only inactivated by serum pseudocholinesterase; succinylcholine is the only such agent available in the United States

- Nondepolarizing neuromuscular blocking agents block neuromuscular transmission by competing with acetylcholine for nicotinic receptors; have slower onset and longer duration of action; 75% of receptors must be blocked to decrease twitch strength significantly

- Continuous contraction is produced following rapid, repeated electrical stimulation of motor nerve; this tetanic response fades with continuous stimulation when blockade exists at neuromuscular junction; rate of fade related to depth of blockade

• Hyperventilation facilitates elimination of anesthetic vapors, and significant physiologic change can occur due to reversal of muscle relaxation, termination of ventilatory support, and perception of nociceptic stimulation from surgical trauma

• Malignant hyperthermia, a complication of anesthesia, characterized by paroxysmal fulminant hypermetabolic crisis; may occur anytime postoperatively, and most commonly with halothane and succinylcholine

• Malignant hyperthermia results in severe respiratory and metabolic acidosis, dysrhythmias, and cardiac arrest; rhabdomyolysis, hyperkalemia, and myoglobinuria are common consequences of muscle damage

• Marked increase in end-tidal carbon dioxide is best early clue to diagnosis, and is confirmed by muscle biopsy; intubate patient, hyperventilate with 100% oxygen, and most importantly, administer intravenous dantrolene as soon as possible

TABLE 7.5 *Commonly used parenteral analgesics*

Drug	Bolus (mg)	Lockout Period (min)
Afentanil	0.05–0.2	3–10
Buprenorphine	0.03–0.2	5–20
Fentanyl	0.015–0.075	3–10
Meperidine	5–30	5–15
Morphine	0.5–3	5–20
Nalbuphine	1–5	5–15
Sufentanil	0.002–0.01	3–10

FOLLOW-UP

The importance of adequate pain management in postoperative patients has long been appreciated and emphasized. Over the last decade, advances in technology, better understanding of pathophysiology, and improvements in pharmacologic agents have greatly changed the practice of pain control in postoperative patients. In a sense, acute pain serves as one of the body's protective mechanisms. Physiologically, however, pain aggravates central hypothalamic neuroendocrine reactions and triggers the stress response. Persistent pain, if not corrected, can be detrimental and can lead to a catabolic state and negative nitrogen balance.

Clinically, pain causes tachycardia, peripheral vasoconstriction, hypertension, and increased myocardial oxygen consumption, along with anxiety, confusion, fear, and sleeping disturbances. Pain may produce splinting and reflex spasm of the abdominal and thoracic muscles, limit diaphragmatic excursions, and inhibit cough. Functional residual capacity and sputum clearance are reduced. Areas of atelectasis may result from regional hypoventilation and lead to hypercarbia, and ultimately, pneumonia. Pain also promotes immobilization, deep vein thrombosis, and increases the risk of pulmonary embolism. Pain relief in the postoperative period is not only humanitarian but also therapeutic. An aggressive approach to pain management can improve patient comfort and hemodynamics, decrease morbidity and mortality, and reduce hospital stay and costs.

Pain starts with the release of algogenic (pain producing) substances such as serotonin, histamine, bradykinin, and prostaglandins, from injured and damaged tissue. The transduced neural impulses sensitize nerve endings and initiate the nociceptive pathway. Somatic and visceral pain are transmitted through A-delta and C fibers to the neuraxis at the dorsal horn of the spinal cord. These fibers synapse in laminae I and V and in the substantia gelatinosa. The nociceptive impulses then ascend through the neospinothalamic and the paleospinothalamic tracts to the reticular activating system, thalamus, and somatosensory cortex of the parietal lobe. When the efferent pathway is elicited, endogenous opiate-like substances (endorphins and enkephalins) are released to attenuate the release of neurotransmitters into the synaptic clefts. The final net perception of pain from the afferent and efferent modulated impulses is completed and interpreted by the cortex.

Theoretically, pain can be blocked or attenuated at different sites of transduction, transmission, modulation, and perception in the nociceptive pathway. Many agents are available to serve this purpose, including local anesthetics, narcotics, nonsteroidal anti-inflammatory drugs (NSAIDs), antiserotonergics, and antihistamines (Table 7.5).

It is important to realize the significant discrepancy in perception of pain between the patient and the physician. The physician should not assume and exclude the presence of significant pain just because obvious pain expression is absent. Other than direct complaint from the patient, muscle spasm, hyperventilation, tachycardia, and other autonomic and endocrine responses (confusion, paranoia, delirium, agitation, sleep deprivation, and fear) are common manifestations. They all can significantly exaggerate sympathetic nervous system activity. Pain may sometimes present with depression, withdrawal, and immobility.

Techniques for postoperative pain relief have improved dramatically over the past several years and now center largely around patient controlled analgesia (PCA).

Advances in technology, such as the development of computerized infusion pumps, make this mode of delivery popular in the management of postoperative pain. Aside from intermittent bolus doses controllable by the patient, most pumps also allow for continuous basal infusion. The maximal dose per time period and lockout interval can be set to avoid overdose. The advantage of PCA is that the patient is able to titrate the medication to individual needs so that better pain control is obtained. It has been shown that PCA produces satisfactory pain relief with less medication and improves pulmonary function and general mobility. It decreases overall postoperative complications and hospital stay. It should be started at a lower dosage and titrated upward as needed. The combination of PCA with continuous infusion has the advantage of providing a baseline plasma level of analgesia while allowing titration of boluses to overcome varying acute changes in the threshold of pain perception. Whenever an opioid infusion is used in a spontaneously breathing patient, respiratory function should be monitored closely. Naloxone, an opioid antagonist, must be available for reversal in cases of significant depression.

Regional analgesia may also be used for postoperative pain management. Administration of local anesthetics or opioids at different levels of the spine produces good control of pain following thoracotomy, laparotomy, and operations involving the lower extremities, without affecting the patient's alertness. The major advantage of opioids over local anesthetics is that sympathetic and motor nerves are not blocked. Conversely, regional analgesia with local anesthetic agents generally provides better pain relief than opioids because anesthetic agents block both the afferent and efferent pathways of the reflex arc, which minimizes neuroendocrine and metabolic responses to noxious stimuli. Using local anesthetics in low concentrations may avoid hypotension and paralysis. The vasodilatory effect may be beneficial to decrease myocardial oxygen demand by reduction of preload and afterload, thereby improving peripheral circulation in cardiovascular cases. Increase in gastrointestinal motility may cause nausea and vomiting. Depending on the levels of blockade, respiratory function can be improved because of relief of pain and muscle spasm. Using opioids provides excellent, long-lasting pain control without direct effects on hemodynamics and motor function. However, the adverse effects include nausea, pruritus, urinary retention, and biphasic respiratory depression. In epidural morphine analgesia, the earlier phase reflects the rise of serum levels through absorption from epidural veins. It commonly occurs 20–45 minutes after an injection. The second phase coincides with rostral spread and appears approximately 5–10 hours later. Respiratory impairment is rare but can be delayed and is very serious. The risk of infection is another problem of the paraspinal approach. A proper combination of opioids and local anesthetics may achieve the ideal goal of adequate analgesia with minimum metabolic and physiologic changes.

Similar to intravenous PCA, paraspinal analgesia can be patient administered. This method of analgesia, combined with continuous infusion, may provide better pain control in most instances. Using opioids and/or local anesthetics has recently gained popularity in postoperative pain management. Paraspinal opioid analgesia provides highly effective pain relief with no direct effects on hemodynamics and motor function. However, it may be less effective than regional analgesia in blocking nociceptive perception and the associated metabolic and neuroendocrine reactions.

Other modalities such as intercostal blocks, intrapleural blocks, and peripheral nerve blocks are also useful for special indications. Less predictable pain relieving methods such as cryoanalgesia, transcutaneous electrical nerve stimulation, and hypnosis are available but not commonly used for control of postoperative pain.

NSAIDs are a group of agents with heterogeneous structures that decrease inflammatory reactions, reduce fever, and relieve pain. The mechanism remains unclear, but may involve the inhibition of prostaglandin synthesis. Clinically, they are commonly used for the treatment of mild to moderate pain. NSAIDs cause no change of sensorium, respiratory depression, or dependence. Adverse effects include platelet dysfunction, gastric erosion and bleeding, and interstitial nephritis. Currently, ketorolac is the only approved parenteral NSAID.

Ketamine, a phencyclidine derivative, produces dissociative anesthesia with profound analgesia. It is useful for pain control in relatively short bedside diagnostic and surgical procedures such as dressing changes in burn patients.

KEY POINTS

- Pain causes tachycardia, peripheral vasoconstriction, hypertension, increases oxygen consumption, and reduces functional residual capacity and sputum clearance; causes anxiety, fear, and sleeping disturbances

- Pain may produce splinting and reflex spasm of abdominal and thoracic muscles, limit diaphragmatic excursions, and inhibit cough

- Areas of atelectasis may result from regional hypoventilation and lead to hypoxemia, hypercarbia, and ultimately, pneumonia

---

SUGGESTED READINGS

Clinton JE, Ruiz E: Emergency airway management procedures. In Hedges R (ed): Clinical Procedures in Emergency Medicine, 2nd Ed. WB Saunders, Philadelphia, 1991

Do not be fooled into thinking that endotracheal intubation is the only way to provide ventilation. This chapter reviews several important alternatives to emergency airway management.

Lee TS: Intensive care anesthesia and analgesia. p. 214. In Bongard FS, Sue DY (eds): Current Critical Care Diagnosis and Treatment. Appleton & Lange, E. Norwalk, CT, 1994

A more in-depth review of the material presented here. Contains a number of useful and hard-to-find tables.

QUESTIONS

1. MAC is the alveolar concentration of an anesthetic agent required to?

    A. Prevent fasciculation in response to nerve stimulation.

    B. Prevent α-wave burst patterns with painful stimuli.

    C. Prevent spontaneous respiration.

    D. Prevent movement in response to a standard skin incision.

2. When compared with spinal anesthesia, epidural anesthesia?

    A. Requires a smaller volume of agent.

    B. Produces less hypotension.

    C. Has a faster onset.

    D. Is generally more reliable.

3. Which of the following paired statements is true regarding muscle relaxing agents?

    A. Depolarizing: pancuronium.

    B. Nondepolarizing: rapid onset.

    C. Competitive blockade: succinylcholine.

    D. Reversible: succinylcholine.

4. Which of the following is not true with regard to malignant hyperthermia?

    A. It may be caused by any anesthetic agent or muscle relaxant.

    B. It is best treated with dantrolene.

    C. The anesthetic agent may be continued.

    D. It is heralded by an increase in carbon dioxide production.

(See p. 603 for answers.)

8

W O U N D

H E A L I N G   A N D

M A N A G E M E N T

R. KENDRICK SLATE

Wound healing is essential for survival. Improperly managed wounds can be life threatening, functionally disabling, and cosmetically devastating. The aims of this chapter are to (1) describe the phases of wound healing, (2) review the process of wound closure, (3) describe the factors influencing wound healing, (4) discuss the management of wounds, and (5) describe abnormal scars and their treatment.

CASE 1
FACIAL LACERATION

A 5-year-old white male presented to the emergency room 6 hours after sustaining a right cheek laceration on a piece of window glass. The laceration was 5 cm long and irregular, running from the right zygoma to the angle of his jaw. The injury was filled with clotted blood and dirt. Physical examination revealed normal right facial movements indicating that the lower branches of the right facial nerve were intact. Examination of the right parotid duct was performed by dilating the orifice of Stensen's duct with a small lacrimal dilator. The duct was uninjured.

The wound was anesthetized locally with 1% lidocaine with 1:100,000 epinephrine, and copiously irrigated with sterile saline. The surrounding skin was cleaned with an iodine solution and the wound debrided. Clot, debris, and necrotic tissue were removed and the wound irrigated again. Irregular skin edges were trimmed, debriding only as much as necessary to ensure a clean bed. The skin was

gently undermined to relieve tension. Using atraumatic technique, the dermis was approximated and the skin closed. A sterile dressing was applied. The sutures were removed after 5 days to avoid suture scars. The patient healed well with the scar slowly changing color from pink to more normal over the next 12–18 months.

GENERAL CONSIDERATIONS

The three phases of wound healing form an overlapping continuum. These include the inflammatory phase, the proliferative phase, and the maturation phase.

The inflammatory phase (lasting 1–4 days) begins with the injury, and is marked by cellular and vascular response. Initially there is a brief 5–10-minute period of vasoconstriction followed by active vasodilatation. Vasoactive amines and kinins are released into the wound. Cells migrate into the wound, including neutrophils, monocytes, fibroblasts, and endothelial cells. The venules become dilated and the lymphatics become clogged. The wound develops redness, heat, swelling, and pain. The cellular response helps remove clot, debris, and bacteria from the wound.

The proliferative phase (lasting 3–40 days) follows the inflammatory phase. Fibroblasts that have migrated into the wound begin to produce glycosaminoglycans, which eventually form fibrillar collagen. There is an increased rate of collagen production for the next 3–6 weeks. Collagen accumulates in the wound until the rate of collagen production equals its rate of degradation.

Wound tensile strength increases rapidly during the proliferative (fibroblastic) phase. The tensile strength is a measurement of the wound strength per unit area. There is a rapid increase with the peak ultimately occurring at around 60–80 days postinjury, when the wound tensile strength achieves 70–80% of normal skin and then plateaus, never quite reaching normal skin strength.

The maturation or remodeling phase (3–6 weeks onward) is a time of increased collagen production and degradation. Collagen fibers reassemble into a more organized pattern. Intermolecular cross-linking of collagen matures the scar, causing it to be less raised and indurated. This phase lasts 9–12 months or longer in an adult and still longer in a child. The maturation process is dynamic and depends on many variables, such as age, genetics, type of wound, wound location, and the amount of inflammation.

Wounds close by primary, secondary, or tertiary healing. Primary healing (first intention) is the closing of a wound directly by suturing, grafting, or using a flap. The wound is debrided and cleaned as necessary to reduce inflammation. The dermis should be closely approximated with sutures until adequate tensile strength is achieved. The original scar is red and raised during maximal collagen synthesis, but then flattens and lightens in color over time.

Secondary healing (secondary intention) occurs when the wound heals openly and spontaneously with a prolonged inflammatory phase without being closed by suture. Wound closure depends on epithelialization and contraction. Epithelialization includes the sequence of mobilization, migration, mitosis, and cellular differentiation. Epithelial cells mobilize, migrate as they lose contact inhibition, and flow to cover the wound until they meet cells from the opposite side. As the cells migrate, they increase in number by mitosis. Once the wound is covered with cells, cellular differentiation occurs, restoring normal basal to surface layers. Epithelialization proceeds at approximately 1 mm/day. Contraction of the wound is probably provided by myofibroblasts and is an active normal process that decreases the size of the wound. Contracture is a result of the healing process and is due to contraction of a scar. The end result may be undesirable and cause a functional deformity (e.g., across a joint), which often requires release.

Tertiary healing (third intention) is delayed primary wound healing after several days. This occurs when the process of secondary intention is intentionally interrupted and the wound is mechanically closed. This usually occurs after granulation tissue has formed. When delayed closure is planned, tissue cultures should be obtained if there is possible infection (100,000 or more bacteria per gram of tissue). If the wound is infected, further debridement must be performed before closure.

Conditions in the wound and environment should be optimized to enhance healing. One of the most important factors for proper wound healing is oxygen. Fibroblasts are oxygen sensitive and produce collagen if the arterial partial pressure of oxygen (PaO_2) is above 40 mmHg. If tissue oxygenation is inadequate, there is also a higher risk of wound infection. For adequate oxygen delivery (DO_2), there must be adequate inspired oxygen, hemoglobin (Hb), and vascular perfusion of the tissues. Smoking increases the risk of hypoxia.

Steroids and vitamins can greatly affect wound healing. Steroids inhibit inflammation and appear to inhibit wound macrophages, wound closure, and contraction. Vitamin A helps restore the anti-inflammatory effects of steroids. Vitamin C is a cofactor for collagen production, while high doses of vitamin E have been found to inhibit healing. Zinc is also an important factor for normal healing.

Growth factors are polypeptides that promote cell proliferation. Some of these factors include fibroblast growth factors, platelet derived growth factors, epidermal growth factors, transforming growth factors, and monocyte/macrophage derived growth factors.

As one ages, the wound healing phases last longer, and wound strength and closure rates tend to decrease. This delayed healing may be secondary to a decreased tolerance of ischemia rather than to a defect in the healing process.

Nutrition and hydration are critical. If serum albumin levels fall below 2 g%, inflammation and fibroplasia are impaired. Methionine, an essential amino acid, is especially critical to reversing the effects of depleted proteins. Hydration is important for the epithelialization of wounds. Therefore, occlusive dressings increase epithelial repair.

Infection can devastate wound healing. An infection is present when the bacteria count is greater than 100,000 per gram of tissue. Infection decreases tissue oxygen, prolongs inflammation, decreases leukocyte function, and retards epithelialization.

Appropriate wound healing occurs when environmental temperatures are optimum and not hypothermic. Keeping the wound warm enhances healing.

Chemotherapy and radiotherapy can inhibit wound healing. Chemotherapeutic agents decrease fibroblast proliferation and wound contraction. Radiotherapy can cause occlusion of small blood vessels and damage fibroblasts. Skin may be damaged in chronic radiation ulcers.

Diabetes mellitus affects the microcirculation and stiffens red blood cells. It affects the microvasculature, promoting atherosclerosis, and produces lower extremity high venous back pressures, causing impaired phagocytosis. These patients are also more susceptible to infections.

Wound healing is also affected by surgical technique. Tissue must not be traumatized or overly cauterized. Hematomas should be avoided. Tight sutures and tissue ischemia can result in necrosis with prolonged and poor healing.

KEY POINTS

• The three phases of wound healing form an overlapping continuum—inflammatory, proliferative, and maturation

• The inflammatory phase (1–4 days) begins with injury, and is marked by cellular and vascular response; wound develops redness, heat, swelling, and pain

• Wound tensile strength increases rapidly during proliferative (fibroplastic) phase; achieves 70–80% of normal skin and then plateaus, never quite reaching normal skin strength

• The maturation or remodeling phase (3–6 weeks) is a time of increased collagen production and degradation

• Wounds close by primary, secondary, or tertiary healing

• Primary healing (first intention) is closing of a wound directly by suturing, grafting, or a flap; dermis should be closely approximated with sutures until adequate tensile strength is achieved

• Secondary healing (secondary intention) occurs when the wound heals openly and spontaneously with a prolonged inflammatory phase without suture. Wound closure depends on epithelialization and contraction

• Tertiary healing (third intention) is delayed primary wound healing after several days, when secondary intention is intentionally interrupted and the wound is mechanically closed; usually occurs after granulation tissue has formed

• Steroids inhibit inflammation and appear to inhibit wound macrophages, wound closure, and contraction

• Infection is present when the bacteria count is greater than 100,000 per gram of tissue

---

WOUND MANAGEMENT

The goal of wound management is to close the wound as soon as possible. The patient should be in a comfortable position and may be given sedation if needed to decrease anxiety. For smaller wounds, local anesthesia using 1% lidocaine with 1:100,000 epinephrine is injected using a 25 gauge or smaller needle (Case 1). More dilute concentrations of local anesthesia may be used if covering larger areas, to provide a greater volume of anesthetic. Epinephrine is contraindicated in some situations, such as a pre-existing medical condition or vulnerable area of the body (e.g., a digit that is supplied by an end artery). The anesthesia is injected slowly and given 5–7 minutes to become effective.

Following anesthesia, the surrounding skin and wound should be cleansed, irrigated, and debrided of devitalized tissue and foreign bodies. The tissue should be handled gently with only minimal debridement necessary in the head and neck area since these areas are very vascular. The wound edges should be trimmed and if the wound is in the hairline, the edges should be parallel to the hair shafts. There should be meticulous hemostasis before closing the wound.

Excellent surgical technique is important in order to achieve a good scar. Atraumatic technique is used to approximate the tissues that should be closed in layers. These can include the periosteum, fascia, dermis, and skin. Undermining of the edges may be necessary to decrease tension. Absorbable suture is used for deeper layers, and nonabsorbable suture is used for the skin. A monofilament nonabsorbable suture, such as nylon, is usually preferred for the skin because it is less reactive than multifilament suture.

The skin edges should be exactly approximated and everted. Steristrips may be placed over the closed wound with a dressing that is absorptive and protective. Most surgeons usually wait 2–3 days before allowing gentle washing of the wound.

Surgical sutures are removed at different postoperative periods, depending on the location. Sutures in the head and neck area may be removed in 3–5 days. They can be removed in 7–10 days from the rest of the body, but may require longer than 10 days in the extremities. Suture marks are the result of delayed suture removal and too much tension. The resulting scar depends more on the type of injury and closure than on the type of suture or needle, or method of suture used (e.g., running versus interrupted). Scars look their worst during the first 2–3 months following injury. As the scar matures, it tends to flatten, soften, and lighten in color, which usually takes 1–2 years. Scar revision is performed after 1 year, but may be performed earlier or later depending on the maturation of the scar. Some wounds require specialized management. These include abrasions, contusions, lacerations, avulsions, and puncture wounds. Abrasions should be cleaned, irrigated, and debrided. Dirt and foreign material should be removed as soon as possible with a scrub brush or dermabrasion to help prevent traumatic "tattoos" from healing over dirt and pigment.

Contusions should be evaluated and hematomas evacuated. In the first 2 days after injury, ice may be used locally to reduce swelling and bleeding. Afterwards, the contused area should be warmed to increase absorption of blood and edema. Lacerations and small partial avulsions should be trimmed and closed while larger partial avulsions should be revised and sutured if possible. Partially avulsed tissue should be sutured without tension. If the tissue is totally avulsed it should be replaced with a skin graft.

Puncture wounds can often be misleading and should not be underestimated. The wound may need to be explored and x-rayed for retained foreign bodies. Animal bites should be cleaned, debrided, and closed, or left open, depending on the severity, time since the bite, and the presence or absence of contamination. Human bites contain a variety of bacteria that can potentially cause severe infections. Therefore, most human bites should be cleaned and left open. Broad spectrum antibiotics should be used with bites and the wounds closely observed for signs of infection.

The majority of wounds may be closed after they are cleaned and debrided. Pulsatile lavage is an excellent way to irrigate and clean the wound before closing. However, some wounds should be left open. These include human bites, severely contaminated wounds, those with a lengthy time since injury (>6–8 hours), severely crushed tissue, wounds in patients on high steroid dosages, and those in markedly obese patients.

Contaminated wounds, if closed, should be debrided and closed without tension with only skin sutures. Skin sutures should be monofilament. Steristrip tapes may be used to close small wounds. The wound should be checked for infection within 48 hours after closure. If unsure about closing a wound, it is better to delay and close it at a later time.

Chronic wounds tend to have granulation tissue. The management goal is to convert the chronic contaminated wound into an acute clean wound. This is performed by debridement, topical antibacterial preparation, and the use of biologic dressings. Biologic dressings include allografts, xenografts, and some synthetic dressings. These dressings help clean the wound and lessen pain. After multiple debridements, tissue samples can be taken to estimate bacteria counts. Before closure, the wound should have bacteria counts of less than 100,000 per gram of tissue and appear clean, healthy, and well vascularized. The wound may then be closed directly with a skin graft, or with a pedicle or free flap.

KEY POINTS

- The goal of management is to close the wound as soon as possible

- For smaller wounds, local anesthesia (1% lidocaine with 1:100,000 epinephrine) is injected, using a 25 gauge or smaller needle

- Epinephrine contraindicated in some situations, such as a pre-existing medical condition or vulnerable area of the body

- Absorbable suture used for deeper layers and nonabsorbable suture for skin; a monofilament nonabsorbable suture is preferred for skin because it is less reactive than multifilament suture

- Sutures in the head and neck area may be removed in 3–5 days, and in 7–10 days from the rest of the body; may require

longer in the extremities; suture marks result from delayed suture removal and too much tension

- Abrasions should be cleaned, irrigated, and debrided

- Human bites are cleaned and left open, broad spectrum antibiotics administered, and wounds closely observed for infection

- Biologic dressings include allografts, xenografts, and some synthetic dressings, which help clean the wound and lessen pain

ABNORMAL SCARS

Abnormal scarring may occur with wound healing. These scars are called hypertrophic scars. They are thick scars that contain excess collagen, which remains within the wound borders. They usually occur in young, dark-skinned people. Keloids are also thick scars that may continue to grow and coalesce. They usually occur in patients 10–30 years of age, and are most frequent in blacks. Widespread scars are flat, wide, and often depressed.

Treatment depends on the type of scar. Widespread scars can be treated with scar excision and a layered closure. Hypertrophic scars are improved with corrective surgery, while keloids return or even worsen after surgery alone. Combination therapy, with surgery and intralesional steroid injections, is more effective than any single treatment method. The intralesional steroid is triamcinolone and is administered to adults according to scar size. In adults, for 1–2-cm lesions, the maximum dose is 20–40 mg; for 2–6-cm lesions, the maximum dose is 40–80 mg; and for lesions 6–10+-cm, the maximum dose is 80–120 mg. The intralesional injections may be repeated monthly for 4–6 months. The maximum doses for children are 40 mg for ages 1–5 years, and 80 mg for ages 6–10 years. Steroids are probably more effective in preventing abnormal scars than in resolving them. Pressure and irradiation can also serve as surgical adjuncts when given immediately after keloidectomy. Other less used treatments include exogenous electric current, colchicine, tetrahydroquinone, asiatic acid, retinoic acid, zinc oxide, silicone gel, and antineoplastic agents such as thio-TEPA and methotrexate.

KEY POINTS

- Hypertrophic scars are thick scars that contain excess collagen, which remains within the wound borders

- Usually occur in young, dark-skinned people

SUGGESTED READINGS

Irvin TT: The healing wound. p. 3. In Buchnall TE, Ellis H (eds): Wound Healing for Surgeons. Bailliere Tindell, London, 1984
  A detailed review of the physiology and biochemistry of wound healing, written largely for surgeons

Kucan JD, Brown R, Hicherson B et al: Wounds in Plastic and Reconstructive Surgery—Essentials for Students. Plastic Surgery Educational Foundation, Arlington Heights, IL, 1993

A concise outline of wound healing and management

QUESTIONS

1. Wounds reach the plateau of their tensile strength during which phase of healing?

    A. Inflammatory.
    B. Proliferative.
    C. Remodeling.
    D. Reductional.

2. Wounds usually do not reach their final appearance until how long after closure?

    A. 3–4 weeks.
    B. 3–4 months.
    C. 9–12 months.
    D. 2–3 years.

3. Epinephrine should not be used in combination with a local anesthetic in which of the following areas?

    A. Finger.
    B. Head and neck.
    C. Buttock.
    D. Abdominal wall.

4. A wound is generally considered infected when a biopsy reveals a bacteria count greater than?

    A. 10,000 bacteria per gram tissue.
    B. 50,000 bacteria per gram tissue.
    C. 100,000 bacteria per gram tissue.
    D. Quantitative counts are not important as long as the wound shows red granulation tissue.

(See p. 603 for answers.)

CRITICAL

CARE

FRED S. BONGARD

As our ability to support sicker patients improves, the practitioner will be called on to care for more complex patients with large numbers of physiologic derangements. Such efforts are largely confined to the critical care unit, where an impressive and intimidating array of diagnostic and therapeutic devices are in routine use. This chapter discusses the more common of these, including pulmonary artery catheters and mechanical ventilators. Specifically, it reviews the interpre

tation of central hemodynamic parameters, calculations, oxygen delivery (DO2) data, and the fundamentals of ventilator management.

CASE 1
CAR ACCIDENT WITH MULTIPLE INJURIES

An 85-year-old female's car was struck on the left side causing significant damage. Her injuries included a ruptured spleen, partial avulsion of the mesentery of the transverse colon, rib fractures, and a large pulmonary contusion. After splenectomy and repair of her colon, she was brought to the ICU. Her ventilator settings were as follows: mode, assist control; FIO_2, 0.50; tidal volume, 500 ml (she weighed 50 kg); rate, 12 breaths/min; PEEP, 5 cmH_2O. Her arterial blood gases were as follows: pH, 7.340; PCO_2, 46 mmHg; PaO_2, 160 mmHg; and SaO_2, 100%.

The following morning, she was awake and alert, but was complaining of pain from her rib fractures. Her ventilator mode was changed to SIMV at a rate of 10 breaths/min. Her spontaneous respiratory rate was 8 breaths/min, resulting in 12.5 L/min of ventilation. Over the day, attempts to decrease the ventilator's rate met with agitation and com-

plaints of shortness of breath. After several days, it became clear that the pain associated with her rib fractures would not permit weaning from the ventilator.

Attempts to reduce the ventilator rate below 5 breaths/min proved impossible. Despite good arterial blood gas results (pH = 7.400, $PaCO_2$ = 43 mmHg, PaO_2 = 120 mmHg), she became progressively more agitated. To reduce the work of breathing, pressure support ventilation was attempted. A support pressure of 15 cm H_2O allowed reduction in the frequency of her mechanical breaths to below 5 breaths/min for the first time. Over the next 2 days, her SIMV rate was reduced to zero, and she was able to breathe spontaneously. Gradually, her pressure support was weaned and she was successfully extubated on the 13th postinjury day.

CASE 2
POSTOPERATIVE PATIENT

A 63-year-old male underwent operation for gangrenous cholecystitis. On the second postoperative day, he became agitated and developed a fever of 39°C and a leukocytosis. The next day, he had an episode of hypotension and tachycardia that corrected with intravenous fluid administration. Later that afternoon, his blood pressure fell again, this time without response to 1 L of lactated Ringer's solution. He was transferred to the ICU for hemodynamic monitoring. Initially, his BP was 110/50 mmHg, with a CVP of 5 mmHg. Crystalloid administration increased the CVP to 9 mmHg without effect on the systemic BP, which progressively declined to 85/55 mmHg. Dopamine was begun to support the blood pressure and a pulmonary artery flotation catheter was placed, which revealed a pulmonary artery pressure of 16/6 mmHg; PCWP of 9 mmHg; and a CO of 7.5 L/min.

Over the next several hours, he became dyspneic and required endotracheal intubation and mechanical ventilation. Initial ventilator settings were as follows: mode, assist control (rate = 10 breaths/min); FiO_2, 0.75; tidal volume, 750 ml; PEEP, 5 cmH_2O. Blood gases on these settings were

	ARTERIAL	MIXED VENOUS
pH	7.280	7.150
PO_2 (mmHg)	80	55
PCO_2 (mmHg)	40	47
HCO_3^- (mg/L)	19	17
Base excess	−6.7	−11.6
Hb saturation (%)	94.1	78.4

An urgent CT scan revealed a large fluid collection in the right upper quadrant, which was drained percutaneously and produced 200 ml of seropurulent material. Antibiotic therapy was optimized based on the gram stain and subsequent culture results.

Over the next several days, his blood pressure stabilized with less dependence on dopamine infusion. CO fell to 5.8 L/min and systemic vascular resistance increased to 980 dynes·s·cm^{-5}. Mean BP stabilized at 90 mmHg. The ventilator was switched to intermittent mandatory ventilation and weaning was begun. On the seventh postoperative day, bedside respiratory mechanics revealed tidal volume (spontaneous), 7 ml/kg; vital capacity, 20 ml/kg; respiratory rate, 16 breaths/min; and arterial blood gases as follows: FiO_2, 0.21; pH, 7.380; PaO_2, 88 mmHg; and $PaCO_2$, 47 mmHg. The patient was extubated that day without difficulty and was transferred from the ICU the subsequent morning.

GENERAL CONSIDERATIONS

Critically ill patients frequently require continuous blood pressure monitoring. For most applications, this is accomplished with an indwelling catheter/transducer system. For systemic arterial blood pressure, a small 20-gauge plastic catheter is inserted into a radial artery and connected through nondistensible tubing to a pressure sensitive transducer. The transducer has a thin membrane that responds to changes in pressure by altering the electrical characteristics of an associated circuit. These changes are sensed by a physiologic amplifier to which the transducer is connected. Because the result obtained is dependent on differential pressures (arterial-atmospheric), it is important that the transducer system be calibrated and adjusted so that a zero pressure reference point (usually the right atrium) is used. If the transducer is incorrectly calibrated *above* the reference point, all pressures obtained will be lower than actual; they will be greater than actual if the catheter/transducer system is referenced *below* the zero point.

Three systemic arterial pressures are usually recorded: systolic, diastolic, and mean. The mean pressure is calculated as follows:

$$\frac{Systolic + (2 \times diastolic)}{3}$$

Mean arterial pressure (MAP) represents the standing pressure in the arterial circuit after the phasic component is removed. Pulse pressure is the difference between the systolic and diastolic pressure. Pulse pressures less than 30 mmHg are commonly associated with severe hypotension, tachycardia, and aortic stenosis, while widened pulse pressures are found in aortic regurgitation, arteriovenous fistulas, and patent ductus arteriosus.

Central venous pressure (CVP) reflects the balance between venous return and right-sided cardiac output (CO) (Case 2). The use of CVP to estimate left ventricular preload is problematic because CVP primarily reflects changes in right ventricular end-diastolic pressure and only secondarily reflects changes in pulmonary venous and left heart filling pressures.

A central venous catheter is placed either through a subclavian or an internal jugular vein so that its tip lies in the superior vena cava, just above the right atrium. The catheter is then connected to an electronic transducer/display apparatus. The normal range of CVP is between 5 and 15 mmHg. When CVP is low, hypovolemia is present. When CVP is elevated, hypervolemia, congestive heart failure, or pericardial tamponade may be present.

In patients without pre-existent cardiac or pulmonary disease, CVP is useful as an indicator of volume status. A rapid infusion of 5–10 ml/kg of crystalloid is employed to aid in determining whether decreased blood pressure is due to hypovolemia or to cardiogenic failure. If CVP rises initially and then declines, severe hypovolemia is present. If CVP rises initially and then slowly declines, moderate hypovolemia is indicated (Case 2). However, if CVP increases rapidly and remains elevated, cardiac failure or pericardial tamponade is present.

The flow directed pulmonary artery flotation catheter (Swan-Ganz catheter) is a multilumen device inserted like a CVP catheter, but is advanced through the right heart into a terminal pulmonary capillary. The balloon on the tip of the catheter is filled with 0.5–1.5 ml of air. The inflated balloon carries the catheter through the right ventricle into a terminal pulmonary vessel. The tip of the catheter is positioned so that the distal lumen "looks through" the pulmonary capillary into the left heart. This pulmonary capillary wedge pressure (PCWP) correlates with the left atrial and ventricular filling pressures. Normal PCWP is between 5 and 10 mmHg (Case 2). Several conditions that adversely affect the ability of PCWP to reflect left-sided pressures include mitral stenosis, aortic regurgitation, and positive end expiratory pressure (PEEP) applied during mechanical ventilation. The latter is of particular concern because PEEP is commonly used in critically ill patients. In these cases, a portion of the PEEP adds to left ventricular pressure, and the PCWP gives a falsely elevated estimate of left ventricular preload. When the distal balloon is deflated, the catheter returns to a more proximal position in the pulmonary artery and records pulmonary artery systolic and diastolic pressures. When PCWP cannot be obtained, pulmonary artery diastolic pressure serves as a good estimate of left ventricular and diastolic pressure. Normal pulmonary artery systolic pressure is between 5 and 20 mmHg, while normal pulmonary artery diastolic pressure is between 3 and 10 mmHg.

Right heart CO is obtained with a pulmonary artery catheter. The principle of indicator dilution is used to measure the flow of blood past the catheter. The thermal indicator (a bolus of cold saline) is injected into the proximal catheter. A sensing thermistor is located near the tip of the catheter. The change in blood temperature over time is proportional to the CO. Care must be taken to ensure that the correct amount of saline (typically 10 ml) is injected, or the results will be erroneous. Too much saline will produce too low a result, while too little will produce a falsely elevated CO. The results of CO measurements may be divided by the patient's body surface area to obtain a normalized result referred to as the cardiac index. Typical values for the cardiac index range between 2.8–4.2 L/min/m^2. Additionally, the CO index may be combined with other measured values to obtain hemodynamic parameters useful in diagnosis and management.

The pulmonary artery catheter may also be used to withdraw blood from the distal pulmonary artery to measure mixed venous hemoglobin oxygen saturation (Case 2). Withdrawal from the distalmost part of the pulmonary artery is required to ensure that satisfactory mixing of coronary sinus and systemic blood has occurred. Blood from the myocardium is highly desaturated and returns to the right atrium through the coronary sinus. Failure to account for the influence of the coronary circulation will result in erroneously high values of mixed venous oxygen saturation (S$\bar{v}$O$_2$). Normal S$\bar{v}$O$_2$ is between 70 and 80% saturation. Lower values imply increased peripheral extraction of oxygen from the blood before it returns to the

heart. This occurs in low flow states such as hemorrhage and cardiogenic shock. Elevated S$\bar{v}$O$_2$ occurs when peripheral oxygen consumption falls, as in septic shock or with large arteriovenous fistulas (Case 2).

Respiratory failure is the inability of the respiratory system to maintain a normal state of gas exchange between the atmosphere and the tissues. This is measured by alterations of the arterial blood gases, partial pressure of oxygen (PO$_2$), carbon dioxide pressure (PCO$_2$), and pH. Respiratory failure may be due to compromise of the pulmonary parenchyma itself, which occurs with pneumonia or the adult respiratory distress syndrome (ARDS), or failure of the surrounding chest wall and neuromuscular system to provide adequate ventilation of the lungs. Diseases of the lungs themselves usually present with hypoxemia (decreased arterial blood oxygen), while those of the respiratory system other than the lungs usually cause hypercapnia (increased arterial blood carbon dioxide).

Respiratory failure is defined as (1) arterial PO$_2$ (PaO$_2$) less than 60 mmHg while breathing room air (FIO$_2$ [fraction of inspired carbon dioxide], 0.21), or (2) arterial PCO$_2$ greater than 45 mmHg. Normally, almost all the oxygen in the alveoli diffuses across the alveolar-capillary interface to oxygenate the blood. The partial pressure of oxygen in the alveoli (PAO$_2$) may be calculated using the alveolar gas equation:

$$PAO_2 = (FIO_2 \times P_B) - PaCO_2/R$$

where P$_B$ is the atmospheric pressure (corrected for water vapor) and R is the respiratory gas exchange ratio or respiratory coefficient (typically 0.8). Under normal circumstances, virtually all the venous blood entering the lung is fully oxygenated. However, when deoxygenated venous blood reaches the arterial circulation without equilibrating the alveolar gas, venous admixture is said to occur, and an alveolar-arterial gradient [(A-a)DO$_2$] is produced that results in hypoxemia.

The alveolar gas equation is of particular importance because it allows us to quantitate how well the lungs are oxygenating the blood. For example, the second patient presented was breathing 75% oxygen. His arterial carbon dioxide (PaCO$_2$) was 40 mmHg. Using the alveolar gas equation, we can calculate what the partial pressure of oxygen in a typical alveolus should be. If the atmospheric pressure is 760 mmHg and the vapor pressure of water is 47 mmHg, then the equation becomes PAO$_2$ = (760 – 47) × 0.7 – (40/0.8), which simplifies to (713) × 0.7 – 50, or 450 mmHg. Notice the notation PAO$_2$ (not PaO$_2$) is used, since this represents the partial pressure of alveolar, not arterial, oxygen. The partial pressure of arterial oxygen (PaO$_2$) was 80 mmHg, making the alveolar-arterial oxygen gradient [(A-a)DO$_2$] equal to 450 – 80, or 370 mmHg. While breathing room air, this gradient normally is 5–10 mmHg, and increases to about 50 mmHg while breathing pure oxygen. The large A-a gradient tells us that the patient is relatively hypoxemic for the amount of oxygen he is breathing and therefore has pulmonary dysfunction.

A second cause of hypoxemia due to venous admixture is ventilation/perfusion ($\dot{V}/\dot{Q}$) mismatching. This mechanism is the most frequent cause of hypoxemia and occurs when blood flow to the lung and ventilated gas are not properly matched. Some blood is exposed to collapsed alveoli, which have no gas in them, resulting in a "shunt" of blood through the lung. Other areas of adequate gas ventilation may not be exposed to blood at the alveolar-capillary interface, resulting in "dead-space" ventilation. The effects of $\dot{V}/\dot{Q}$ mismatching on gas exchange are complex, but for practical purposes, any lung disease that alters the distribution of ventilation or blood flow results in $\dot{V}/\dot{Q}$ mismatching. Hypoxemia due to $\dot{V}/\dot{Q}$ mismatch occurs in asthma as well as in pulmonary vascular disease such as pulmonary embolism, where the distribution of blood flow is altered. Following a pulmonary embolism, blood flow to the lungs is altered such that blood no longer reaches normally ventilated alveoli. Although ventilation is relatively normal, perfusion is decreased and the $\dot{V}/\dot{Q}$ ratio increases. This is an example of increased dead space and wasted ventilation in which alveolar gas does not interface with pulmonary capillary blood. ARDS is characterized by obliteration of the alveolar-capillary interface such that blood reaching the exchange surface does not equilibrate with alveolar gas. In this situation, blood flow is wasted because ventilation is decreased. The $\dot{V}/\dot{Q}$ ratio decreases and blood shunts through the lung without proper gas exchange. Although dead space ventilation ($\dot{V}/\dot{Q} \to \infty$) and shunt ($\dot{V}/\dot{Q} \to 0$) appear to be opposites, many disease states produce both effects in different parts of the lung. Increases in dead space tend to effect ventilation with increased $PaCO_2$, while increases in shunt tend to lower PaO_2.

When respiratory failure is present, mechanical ventilation may be indicated, if an easily reversible cause is not found. Before the institution of mechanical ventilation, the airway must be intubated to permit airflow to and from the lungs. Such intubation may be accomplished either through an orotracheal or nasotracheal route. Nasotracheal intubation usually produces less patient discomfort, is less awkward, and permits better stabilization of the tube. Endotracheal tube size depends upon body habitus and sex. Most adult women will require a 7.5- to 8.0-mm inner diameter tube, while most men will tolerate an 8.5- to 9.0-mm tube. The resistance of flow through the tube is inversely proportional to its cross-sectional diameter. Hence, the largest tube possible should be used to reduce airway pressures, and to reduce the patient's work of breathing when weaned from the mechanical ventilator.

Indications for airway intubation and mechanical ventilation are usually divided into two categories, physiologic and clinical. Physiologic indications include hypoxemia, which persists in spite of supplemental oxygen administra-

tion, $PaCO_2$ of 55 mmHg or more with pH less than 7.25, and vital capacity less than 15 ml/kg, such as may occur in the face of neuromuscular disease. Clinical indications include altered mental status with impaired ability to protect the airway, respiratory distress (Case 2), upper airway obstruction, and a high volume of secretions that cannot be cleared by the patient and require frequent suctioning.

Mechanical ventilation is designed to decrease the work of breathing and assist in providing adequate gas exchange. Ventilators can broadly be divided into two categories, pressure controlled and volume controlled. The ventilators are so named because they are designed primarily to deliver a set volume or to deliver a predetermined pressure. Volume controlled ventilators have been preferred until recently, when pressure controlled devices were shown to offer some advantages.

Volume controlled ventilators can be understood by imagining a simple device that has only two controls, one for tidal volume (amount of gas delivered per breath) and one for rate (number of breaths per minute). The minute volume ($\dot{V}_E$) that the patient receives is calculated by multiplying the respiratory rate by the tidal volume (Case 1). Because there are no other controls, there are no provisions for managing patient breaths in between ventilator breaths, for limiting the maximum pressure developed with each breath, or for allowing the patient to initiate a breath. Such a simple ventilator would deliver the preset volume at a preset interval regardless of the response. Such ventilators exist and are similar to those used by anesthesiologists when patients are fully paralyzed and facilities to assist in breathing are not required. This mode is referred to as continuous mandatory ventilation (CMV), because the patient does not interface with the ventilator's operation. If the volume control dial was exchanged for a pressure dial, the ventilator would now deliver the set pressure at the predetermined rate. While the first ventilator produced a certain amount of *volume* (irrespective of pressure), the new device delivers a certain amount of *pressure* (irrespective of volume) at the predetermined interval. Although both are continuous mandatory ventilators, the first is volume controlled (the pressure developed depends upon the resistance of the airways) and the second is pressure controlled (the volume delivered depends upon how much gas flows through the device at the preset pressure level).

Clearly, neither of the two rudimentary devices described would have much practical use in the critically ill patient. The volume cycle ventilator could develop dangerously high pressures before the preset amount of volume was delivered, while the pressure controlled machine provides no information on the volume that is being delivered. To limit pressures, most volume controlled ventilators include special pressure limiting devices ("pop-off" valves) to prevent overdistention of the lungs (barotrauma). Similarly, pressure controlled machines have gauges that indicate how much volume is being delivered. In both cases, however, the machines described are unable to adjust to the patient's intrinsic breathing pattern.

Let us now assume that the ventilator is refined to allow the patient to breath between the preset mechanical cycles. Hence, the patient can now breathe at the patient's own rate, with the ventilator cycling at a predetermined frequency. The respirator would simply ensure that the patient intermittently receives mandatory breaths. This mode, known as intermittent mandatory ventilation (IMV), is useful both for full ventilatory support as well as for weaning. When trying to reduce the level of mechanical ventilation, IMV assures the physician that the patient who stops breathing would still receive the minute ventilations preset on the ventilator. Either volume controlled or pressure controlled IMV can be used, with the latter regulated by the preset pressure per breath, rather than by the volume. In general usage, most IMV ventilators are synchronized (SIMV) to the patient's breathing so that the ventilator will not cycle when the patient is breathing and thereby create high levels of airway pressure and potential barotrauma. Such SIMV devices are easy to set, and constitute the mainstay of ventilator use. It should be noted, however, that since the patient is allowed to breathe between mechanical cycles, the work of breathing may remain high, especially if the patient is taking small volume breaths. SIMV does not respond to the patient's intrinsic respiratory rate, other than to synchronize with it.

If the ventilator were redesigned with a facility that allowed it to cycle in response to a patient initiated breath, we would say that the machine assists ventilation. Furthermore, if it had the ability to deliver breaths at a predetermined rate (if the patients were to stop breathing) we would have designed an assist control (AC) ventilator. Again, either pressure or volume can be preset, so that when a patient begins to breathe, the machine responds by delivering the required pressure or volume. AC ventilators are useful for patients who have normal respiratory rates but very small tidal volumes. Although the machine senses the patient initiated breath, the work of breathing is not completely eliminated because the mechanical device still requires the use of valves and tubes. Patients who are tachypneic will often develop a respiratory alkalosis because they will receive a full ventilator breath each time they initiate a breath.

Although SIMV and AC are the principal modes of ventilation, other refinements have been introduced to help wean difficult patients. Of particular importance is pressure support ventilation, which supplies a given amount of initial pressure and then stops, allowing the patient to finish the inspiratory effort. Because the greatest portion of the work of breathing occurs during the early phase of inspiration, this mode is particularly helpful in weak or older patients who rapidly tire when breathing on their own (Case 2).

When mechanical ventilation is no longer required, support is weaned in a number of ways. The rate of the ventilator may be reduced, assist mode may be changed to IMV, inspired oxygen may be reduced, and pressure support may be withdrawn. The usual criteria for weaning from ventilation include spontaneous minute volume less than 10 L/min; tidal volume more than 5 ml/kg; spontaneous rate less than 25 breaths/min; and maximum negative inspiratory pressure less than -25 cmH$_2$O (Cases 1 and 2). Before extubation, continuous positive airway pressure (CPAP) may be applied to the endotracheal tube after mechanical assistance has been withdrawn. CPAP compensates for the normal positive pressure produced in the airway by glottic closure, and prevents the collapse of alveoli. Brief trials of CPAP should be used before extubation to determine whether a patient is able to breathe independently of the mechanical ventilator while still maintaining adequate blood gases. However, since the work of breathing is increased because of the relatively small lumen and greater length of the endotracheal tube compared to the trachea, such trials should not be allowed to exceed 30 minutes.

These values represent optimum goals, but not absolute requirements for removing a patient from mechanical ventilation. The patient's spontaneous breathing rate should not be excessively rapid or the patient will tire quickly and require reintubation. Additionally, inspiratory force should be sufficient (<25 cmH$_2$O) to overcome the recoil forces of the chest wall and lung. Minute volume should be adequate to provide normal ventilation and PaCO$_2$. Most patients are not removed from ventilators while breathing room air, since most still require supplemental oxygen. Rigid requirements for PaO$_2$ are therefore unhelpful. In general, patients should have a PaO$_2$ of near 100% or less than 50% inspired oxygen.

KEY POINTS

• Mean arterial pressure represents the standing pressure in the arterial circuit after the phasic component is removed

• CVP reflects the balance between venous return and right-sided CO

• Normal range of CVP is 5–15 mmHg; when low, hypovolemia is present, when high, congestive heart failure or pericardial tamponade exists

• Rapid infusion of 5–10 ml/kg crystalloid determines whether decreased blood pressure is due to hypovolemia or cardiogenic failure; if CVP rises and declines, severe hypovolemia is present; if rises and slowly declines, moderate hypovolemia is present; if CVP increases rapidly and remains high, cardiac failure or pericardial tamponade is present

• PCWP correlates with left atrial and ventricular filling pressures, and is normally 5–10 mmHg

• When PCWP cannot be obtained, pulmonary artery diastolic pressure (normally 3–10 mmHg) is a good estimate of left ventricular and diastolic pressure

- Typical values for the cardiac index range from 2.8–4.2 L/min/m^2; normal S$\bar{v}$O$_2$ is 70–80% saturation

- Hypoxemia due to venous admixture is most frequently due to $\dot{V}/\dot{Q}$ mismatching, when blood flow to lung and ventilated gas not properly matched

- Any lung disease that alters distribution of ventilation or blood flow results in $\dot{V}/\dot{Q}$ mismatching

- Physiologic indications for airway intubation and mechanical ventilation are hypoxemia, PaCO$_2$ <55 mmHg, PCO$_2$ >55 mmHg and pH <7.25, and vital capacity <15 ml/kg (as in neuromuscular disease)

- Clinical indications for mechanical ventilation include altered mental status with impaired ability to protect airway, respiratory distress, upper airway obstruction, and a high volume of secretions not cleared by patient and requiring frequent suctioning

- Mechanical ventilation decreases work of breathing and assists in providing adequate gas exchange

- IMV is useful for full ventilatory support and weaning; when reducing mechanical ventilation, IMV assures physician that patient will receive preset minute ventilation if patient stops breathing

- SIMV does not respond to patient's intrinsic respiratory rate; synchronizes with it

- Assist control (AC) ventilation provides a full breath every time a patient initiates a breath; respiratory alkalosis (hypocapnia) may result in agitated tachypneic patients

- Continuous positive airway pressure compensates for normal positive pressure produced in airway by glottic closure

SUGGESTED READINGS

Bongard FS: Critical care monitoring. In Bongard FS, Sue DY (eds): Current Critical Care Diagnosis and Treatment. Appleton & Lange, E. Norwalk CT, 1994

This chapter reviews the state-of-the-art in critical care monitors. It also explains the basics behind each measurement.

Swan HCJ et al: Catheterization of the heart in man with use of a flow-directed balloon-tipped catheter. N Engl J Med 283: 447, 1970

The classic article on pulmonary artery catheterization. A useful look into the past that discusses, for the first time, the use of this device.

Sue DY: Respiratory failure. In Bongard FS, Sue DY (eds): Current Critical Care Diagnosis and Treatment. Appleton & Lange, E. Norwalk CT, 1994

A detailed review of respiratory failure and ventilator management.

QUESTIONS

1. Central venous pressure monitoring is most useful in patients?

    A. Without valvular heart disease.

    B. With pulmonary artery hypertension.

    C. With left ventricular failure.

    D. With isolated cardiac ischemia.

2. Which of the following values is not measured directly by a pulmonary artery flotation catheter?

    A. Cardiac output.

    B. Pulmonary capillary wedge pressure.

    C. Pulmonary artery systolic pressure.

    D. Systemic vascular resistance.

3. Unlike SIMV, the AC mode for mechanical ventilation?

    A. Can only be volume cycled.

    B. Can only be used in patients who are fully paralyzed.

    C. Assists patients once they have initiated their own breath.

    D. Can be used for weaning.

(See p. 603 for answers.)

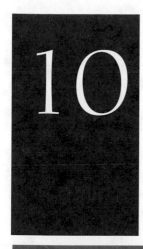

10 SURGERY IN PATIENTS WITH AIDS

CASE 1
KAPOSI'S SARCOMA

A 27-year-old male presented with diffuse abdominal pain. He had been diagnosed with AIDS 6 months previously, when he was found to be HIV positive and had biopsy-demonstrated cutaneous Kaposi's sarcoma. Three months before admission, he developed cryptococcal meningitis, which was treated with amphotericin B and flucytosine for more than 1 month. One week before admission, he had crampy abdominal pain, poorly localized, but usually worse in the left upper quadrant and the mid-abdomen. He had several episodes of vomiting and low grade fever, resulting in loss of weight. He was admitted due to dehydration and severe cramping pain. He was hepatitis B surface antigen positive. He had no previous operation.

The patient appeared thin and chronically ill. Several violaceous macules were noted consistent with Kaposi's sarcoma of the skin. The neck had shotty lymphadenopathy. The abdomen was mildly distended, with minimal tenderness to palpation, but without guarding or rigidity. On rectal examination, no masses were found. The stool was trace guaiac positive.

The Hb was 12 g/dl, Hct 36%, WBC count 12,000/mm³, with 77 neutrophils, 5 bands, 11 lymphocytes, and 7 monocytes. Electrolytes were normal, although liver chemistries were mildly elevated.

The patient was hydrated. A right upper quadrant ultrasound examination was normal. He continued to have intermittent crampy abdominal pain and occasional diarrhea. Two days after his admission, abdominal pain suddenly increased, associated with a temperature to 38.5°C and the development of abdominal rigidity and rebound tenderness. Blood cultures grew *Bacteroides fragilis* and *Clostridia*. At operation extensive inflammation of the transverse colon with an area of perforation was noted. The transverse colon was resected with a diverting colostomy of the right colon and mucous fistula of the descending colon created. The resected colon showed ulceration with loss of mucosa and underlying granulation tissue with many small thrombosed blood vessels. Prominent vasculitis with extreme acute and chronic inflammation and fat necrosis was observed. The vascular changes were suggestive but not fully diagnostic of CMV vasculitis. No typical CMV inclusion bodies were identified.

The patient was started on antibiotics, which were continued for 1 week. He had evaluation of his colon with water soluble contrast medium on postoperative day 10, which was normal. A colonoscopy through the mucous fistula on postoperative day 11 was performed, showing no typical ulceration or exudate suggestive of CMV. He was discharged from the hospital after one month.

As an outpatient he developed more extensive Kaposi's sarcoma tumors for which he received chemotherapy. A CMV retinal vasculitis resulted in blindness. He expired 6 months after the colon resection. At autopsy he was found to have extensive Kaposi's sarcoma of the skin involving the gastric mucosa, duodenal and peritoneal serosa, rectal mucosa, and liver. Also noted were CMV destruction of the adrenal glands and CMV infection of the lungs and gastrointestinal tract.

GENERAL CONSIDERATIONS

Human immunodeficiency virus (HIV) is an RNA retrovirus transmitted through sexual contact, parenteral exposure to blood and blood products, and maternal-fetal pathways. The virus attaches to the surface of CD4+ T lymphocytes, also called T-helper lymphocytes, destroying them and causing progressive immunologic dysfunction, eventually culminating in the acquired immunodeficiency syndrome (AIDS). Patients with AIDS develop disseminated opportunistic infections and unusual malignancies that are generally managed by primary care physicians or infectious disease consultants. Among the most difficult problems presented to the surgeon by the patient with AIDS is evaluation of acute abdominal pain, as described in this case.

The usual clinical indications for abdominal exploration require reconsideration in the AIDS patient. Multiple opportunistic infections may be present simultaneously; these infections commonly produce fever, but this may be unrelated to the abdominal process. Leukocytosis may be unreliable in evaluation of common conditions, such as appendicitis, because a normal count in these patients may be present even in the face of acute intra-abdominal inflammation. However, in the event of bowel perforation, leukocytosis is generally observed. In the general population, the combination of abdominal pain and diarrhea is usually interpreted as gastroenteritis. However, in AIDS patients, diarrhea is extremely common and should not prompt dismissal of a complaint of abdominal pain as simple gastroenteritis.

Thrombocytopenia is observed in one-third of patients infected with HIV. Those with severe thrombocytopenia who fail medical treatment may require splenectomy for treatment, which is generally well tolerated and causes no additional immunocompromise.

Many surgeons faced with a patient with AIDS who requires operation are concerned that the risk of postoperative complications is high. CD4+ cells are not involved in wound healing, so there is no theoretical rationale for impairment of wound healing due to HIV infection. This appears to be confirmed by clinical findings. Elective surgical procedures in AIDS patients are not associated with a greater risk of complications than in the general population. However, emergency operations in AIDS patients do have a high rate of morbidity and mortality (Case 1).

Many patients with AIDS have chronic cramping abdominal pain, usually due to colitis. Diarrhea is common and may be attributed to many organisms, including *Shigella, Campylobacter, Giardia, Entamoeba histolytica, Blastocystis hominis, Cryptosporidium,* or cytomegalovirus (CMV). However, of all the common infections involving the gastrointestinal tract, CMV is the most likely infection to result in emergency surgical consultation (Table 10.1).

KEY POINTS

- In AIDS patients, multiple opportunistic infections may be present simultaneously; can produce fever but may be unrelated to abdominal process

- Diarrhea extremely common; should not prompt dismissal of abdominal pain as simple gastroenteritis

- CD4+ cells are not involved in wound healing, so wound impairment not due to HIV infection

- Elective surgical procedures not associated with greater risk of complications than in non-AIDS population

- CMV the most likely infection to result in emergency surgical consultation

---

TABLE 10.1   *Common operative complications in the gastrointestinal tract*

Organ Involvement	Perforation	Obstruction	Hemorrhage
Oropharynx		Kaposi's sarcoma	Kaposi's sarcoma
Esophagus	Candida, CMV, Kaposi's sarcoma	Kaposi's sarcoma	Kaposi's sarcoma
Stomach and small bowel	CMV, *Mycobacterium avium-intracellulare, Cryptosporidium,* Kaposi's sarcoma, lymphoma CMV, Kaposi's sarcoma, lymphoma	CMV, Kaposi's sarcoma, lymphoma	CMV, Kaposi's sarcoma, lymphoma
Liver, hepatobiliary tract, and gallbladder	Kaposi's sarcoma, lymphoma, CMV, *Cryptosporidium*	Kaposi's sarcoma, lymphoma	Kaposi's sarcoma
Appendix	CMV, Kaposi's sarcoma		
Colon	CMV, *Mycobacterium avium-intracellulare, Cryptosporidium,* Kaposi's sarcoma	CMV, *Mycobacterium avium-intracellulare,* Kaposi's sarcoma	CMV, *Mycobacterium avium-intracellulare,* Kaposi's sarcoma
Anotectum		Condylomata acuminatum, Kaposi's sarcoma, lymphoma, squamous cell carcinoma, cloacogenic carcinoma	Ulcers, Kaposi's sarcoma, lymphoma, squamous cell carcinoma, cloacogenic carcinoma

(From Fry DE: HIV: pathogenisis, risks, and safety for the surgeon. Surg Rounds 331:899, 1993, with permission.)

DIAGNOSIS

Abdominal problems arise from the complications of AIDS, predominantly CMV infection and Kaposi's sarcoma. CMV is one of the five members of the herpesvirus family and may be found somewhere in the body in more than 50% of AIDS patients. *Candida* and *Pneumocystis carinii* are more frequent opportunistic infections in AIDS patients, but CMV infects the endothelial cells of capillaries in the gut mucosa and leads to diffuse ulcerative gastroenteritis. CMV colitis is identified endoscopically by well circumscribed ulcerations with overlying fibrinous exudate. Biopsy shows either CMV inclusions in the endothelial cells or a vasculitis (Case 1). The vasculitis of the mucosal and submucosal capillary beds in the gut may lead to necrosis and perforation.

Kaposi's sarcoma is a neoplasm derived from the endothelial cell of the lymphatics in skin and mucosal surfaces. The characteristic violaceous color is due to extravasation of hemosiderin into false vascular channels in the tumor (Case 1). Lesions that are few in number or confined to the skin or mouth are usually left untreated. However, Kaposi's sarcoma may progress to involve the gastrointestinal tract in approximately 40% of AIDS patients. It carries a poor prognosis.

KEY POINTS

- CMV colitis identified endoscopically by well circumscribed ulcerations with overlying fibrinous exudate

- Biopsy shows either CMV inclusions in endothelial cells or a vasculitis

- Kaposi's sarcoma may lead to involvement of gastrointestinal tract in about 40% of AIDS patients; carries a poor prognosis

DIFFERENTIAL DIAGNOSIS

Malignant lymphoma of the non-Hodgkin's variety may also involve the gastrointestinal tract and lead to obstruction. A palpable mass on abdominal examination in the AIDS patient with intermittent obstructive symptoms suggests the presence of a non-Hodgkin's lymphoma. When these tumors are treated with chemotherapy, it is not uncommon for bleeding or perforation to result. If bleeding cannot be controlled endoscopically or angiographically, or if there is perforation, the operative strategy should be to remove the tumor and create a primary anastomosis, barring significant contamination of the peritoneal cavity.

The nature of gastrointestinal lymphomas in patients with AIDS is aggressive, but prognosis for these patients is better than for those with CMV perforation or extensive gastrointestinal Kaposi's sarcoma. Survival beyond 1 year after resection has been reported. Multiagent chemotherapy may result in remission, but there is a high recurrence rate and a short disease free interval.

AIDS patients develop the same surgical problems observed in the general population. Acute calculous cholecystitis and peptic ulcer disease are common problems in patients infected with HIV. Symptoms of right upper quadrant pain or epigastric pain are identical to those in patients without AIDS.

HIV-associated cholangitis has been described. This syndrome is believed to be related to CMV and to *Cryptosporidium* infection. Liver function tests are elevated, and single or multiple areas of narrowing and dilatation of the intrahepatic or extrahepatic bile ducts are observed. Papillary stenosis and strictures of the distal common bile duct may be treated by endoscopic sphincterotomy. Surgical intervention is rarely required.

Acalculous cholecystitis may develop in AIDS patients due to *Cryptosporidium*, CMV, or *Candida* infection, as well as lymphoma, Kaposi's sarcoma, or following extended periods of total parenteral nutrition (TPN). Management of calculous or acalculous cholecystitis in the AIDS patient should be the same as in the general population. Laparoscopic techniques should be strongly considered because of decreased risk to the operative team.

Right upper quadrant pain in AIDS patients may also be due to hepatitis or pacreatitis. Hepatitis B infection is common in AIDS patients (Case 1). Hepatitis may also be caused by CMV, *Mycobacterium avium-intracellulare*, or *Pneumocystis carinii*. Some of the medications given for treatment of AIDS, such as ddI (2',3'-dideoxyinosine) may cause hepatitis. Pentamidine, used in the treatment of *Pneumocystis carinii* pneumonia, may cause severe life threatening pancreatitis. Treatment consists of cessation of therapy and standard management of the complications of pancreatitis.

Right lower quadrant pain in the AIDS patient may be due to appendicitis, non-Hodgkin's lymphoma, lymphadenopathy, or *Mycobacterium avium-intracellulare*. Infection with this organism can lead to severe abdominal pain, fever, weight loss, and hepatosplenomegaly. A terminal ileitis resembling Crohn's disease may be observed endoscopically, or mycobacterial infection may present on computed tomography (CT) scan with multiple enlarged retroperitoneal lymph nodes. *Mycobacterium avium-intracellulare* may also cause an enterocolitis that results in perforation; in these cases, laparotomy with resection and fecal diversion will be required. The diagnosis of mycobacterial infection is made on the basis of biopsy or the presence of acid fast microorganisms in feces. Treatment of mycobacterial infection or abdominal *Mycobacterium tuberculosis* consists of multiple antibiotics.

KEY POINTS

- A palpable mass on abdominal examination in an AIDS patient with intermittent obstructive symptoms suggests presence of a non-Hodgkin's lymphoma

- Gastrointestinal lymphomas in AIDS patients are aggressive, but prognosis is better than for those with CMV perforation or extensive gastrointestinal Kaposi's sarcoma

- Syndrome of HIV-associated cholangitis believed to be related to CMV and to *Cryptosporidium* infection; liver function tests are elevated, and single or multiple areas of narrowing and dilatation of intrahepatic or extrahepatic bile ducts observed

- Pentamidine, used in treatment of *Pneumocystis carinii*, may cause life-threatening pancreatitis

- *Mycobacterium avium-intracellulare* infection may lead to severe abdominal pain, fever, weight loss, and hepatosplenomegaly

- Diagnosis of mycobacterial infection made on basis of biopsy or presence of acid fast microorganisms in feces

TREATMENT

Proper management of CMV infection of the gut with perforation or bleeding is based on an understanding of the underlying vasculitis. Perforations should not be treated by simple oversewing or patching. This approach does not provide adequate treatment of the vasculitis, which is similar to areas of localized bowel ischemia or infarction. As with infarcted bowel, areas involved must be resected. Primary anastomosis is discouraged. Areas of perforation and obvious ulcers with inflammation should be completely resected and an ileostomy or colostomy with a mucous fistula created. Less aggressive procedures frequently lead to repeat perforation, peritonitis, sepsis, wound disruption, and death. The prognosis is invariably worsened by delay in operation. In patients with AIDS and severe CMV colitis requiring surgery who have advanced disease, the postoperative mortality rate ranges from 37% to 71%, increasing to 86% after six months. Prompt surgical management with complete resection of areas of bowel affected by CMV vasculitis should reduce postoperative mortality.

CMV infection of the colon may also produce bleeding from the ulcers. Endoscopic attempts at control should be considered first. CMV infection of the esophagus may lead to ulcers and dysphagia or bleeding. Operation of the CMV infected esophagus should only be considered in cases of perforation.

The gastrointestinal submucosal lesions of Kaposi's sarcoma can cause obstruction, perforation, or massive bleeding; surgery is required. Simple resection or bypass may be considered in the case of obstruction. Radiotherapy may also be used to shrink the tumor and control local symptoms.

KEY POINTS

- Areas of perforation and obvious ulcers with inflammation require complete resection

- Ileostomy or colostomy with mucous fistula should be created

FOLLOW-UP

Any surgical procedure in an AIDS patient should be considered palliative. The stage of progression of AIDS, the magnitude of the operative procedure planned, and the functional and nutritional status of the patient should be carefully evaluated before attempting surgery. Elective resection of a gastrointestinal lymphoma or cholecystectomy by laparoscopic or open technique may be very well tolerated by the patient with AIDS who has good functional status and a controlled opportunistic infection. By contrast, the cachectic debilitated patient with multiple active opportunistic infections who presents with an acute abdomen presents a much more challenging picture. Operative risk, prognosis, and expected quality of life should be discussed fully with the patient.

Concern regarding an uncertain diagnosis or risk to the operative team should not delay surgery for peritonitis, uncontrolled bleeding, or other standard emergency indications. Universal precautions for the prevention of blood exposure should be observed. Eye shields and double gloving should be used liberally; trunk and lower extremity reinforcement is advisable in the event of significant blood loss or when large volumes of irrigation are anticipated. Every effort should be made to minimize the use of sharp instruments and needles. Careful technique will prevent injury and risk of HIV infection to the operative team and help ensure the best care for the patient (Table 10.2).

TABLE 10.2 *Recommendations of the American College of Surgeons with respect to surgeons and HIV infection*

Surgeons have the same ethical obligations to render care to HIV-infected patients as they have to care for other patients.

Surgeons should use the highest standards of infection control involving the most effective knowledge of sterile barriers, universal precautions, and scientifically accepted infection control practices. This practice should extend to all sites where surgical care is rendered.

To date, there have been no documented incidents of transmission of HIV from a surgeon to a patient and no transmission of the virus to a patient in sterile operating room environment. Therefore, HIV infected surgeons may continue to practice and perform invasive procedures, unless there is clear evidence that a significant risk of transmission of infection exists through an inability to meet basic infection-control procedures or the surgeon is functionally unable to care for patients. These determinations are to be made by the surgeon's personal physician and/or an institutional panel designated for confidential counseling.

(From Fry DE: HIV: pathogenisis, risks, and safety for the surgeon. Surg Rounds 133, 1993, with permission.)

SUGGESTED READINGS

Burack JH, Mandel MS, Bizer, LS: Emergency abdominal operations in the patient with acquired immunodeficiency syndrome. Arch Surg 124:285, 1989

Consten E, van Lanschot J, Henny CH et al: General operative aspects of human immunodeficiency virus infection and acquired immunodeficiency syndrome. J Am Coll Surg 180:366, 1995

Fry DE: HIV: pathogenesis, risks, and safety for the surgeon. Surg Rounds 331, 1993

Wilson SE, Robinson G, Williams RA et al: Acquired immune deficiency syndrome (AIDS); indications for abdominal surgery, pathology and outcome. Ann Surg 210:428, 1989

QUESTIONS

1. Which of the following statements is not true?

    A. Elective surgery in AIDS patients carries a greater risk than a similar procedure in normal patients.

    B. Thrombocytopenia is present in about one-third of AIDS patients.

    C. A normal WBC count may be observed even in the face or severe infection.

    D. Diarrhea is common in AIDS patients even without intestinal pathology.

2. Which of the following infectious agents is most likely to result in emergency surgical consultation and operation in AIDS patients?

    A. *Shigella.*

    B. *Candida albicans.*

    C. Cytomegalovirus.

    D. *Cryptosporidium.*

3. A palpable abdominal mass in an AIDS patient who presents with pain and symptoms of intermittent bowel obstruction most likely has?

    A. Kaposi's sarcoma.

    B. Non-Hodgkin's lymphoma.

    C. Adenocarcinoma of the colon.

    D. Bowel perforation due to cytomegalovirus.

4. The diagnosis of Mycobacterium avium-intracellulare *is best confirmed by?*

    A. Chest x-ray.

    B. Sputum culture.

    C. Presence of acid fast organisms in the stool.

    D. Skin testing.

(See p. 603 for answers.)

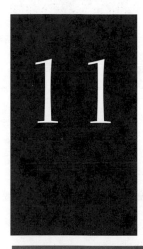

11

PRINCIPLES

OF SURGICAL

ONCOLOGY

HERNAN I. VARGAS

STANLEY R. KLEIN

Cancer is a group of diseases with different manifestations. Their common characteristic is disordered cell growth and regulation. By definition, these tumors have the potential to metastasize. Benign neoplasms may manifest as tumors, but do not typically invade adjacent tissues and do not metastasize. The aim of this chapter is to define the principles underlying the treatment of all forms of malignancy.

CASE 1
BREAST CANCER

A 44-year-old female presented with a 4-month history of a progressively enlarging mass in the right breast. She denied any nipple discharge or pain. Her older sister died of breast cancer at 46 years of age; her younger sister is alive with bilateral breast cancer; her mother also died of breast cancer. Her last mammogram was 18 months ago.

She appeared in good health. On physical examination, there was a 2- by 2-cm mass in the upper outer quadrant of the right breast. There were no skin changes. Examination of the opposite breast, both axillae, and the supraclavicular fossa was normal. Blood counts and liver chemistries were normal. Chest x-ray was unremarkable. Bilateral mammography showed a spiculated mass corresponding to the palpable mass and a separate cluster of microcalcifications in the lower inner quadrant of the right breast.

Fine needle aspiration cytology study of the palpable mass showed adenocarcinoma cells. She had an ex-

cisional biopsy of the mammographically localized area of microcalcifications that revealed infiltrating ductal carcinoma.

A modified radical mastectomy of the right breast was performed. No residual carcinoma was found in the area of the excisional biopsy. Of 30 axillary lymph nodes, 3 were positive for carcinoma. She received adjuvant chemotherapy and is currently doing well 5 years after surgery. She is taking tamoxifen and has no evidence of recurrence. She has had yearly mammograms without any evidence of a tumor in the opposite breast.

CASE 2
SOFT TISSUE MASS

A 48-year-old Hispanic female presented with a 16-month history of a progressively enlarging mass over the sacrum. One year ago, an incisional biopsy revealed fibroadipose tissue. She was told that she had a "lipoma" and not to worry. Her prior medical history and family history were unremarkable.

On examination, she had a 8 × 8-cm mass located over the sacrum. This was hard, but not fixed to the underlying bone. An MRI of the sacrum and pelvis was obtained, revealing a mass of high attenuation separate from the bone, consistent with a soft tissue tumor, not consistent with fatty tissue. Core needle biopsy showed sarcoma.

A subperiosteal resection and wide excision of the tumor with adjacent normal tissue was done. The surgical margins were free of tumor. The wound was closed with advancement flaps and drains were placed. Final pathology confirmed the original diagnosis with a close deep margin at 0.8 cm. She has subsequently received radiotherapy to the tumor bed and drain sites. She was doing well 3 years postoperatively without any evidence of recurrence.

GENERAL CONSIDERATIONS

In the United States, over 1.2 million cases of newly diagnosed cancer are reported each year; approximately 500,000 deaths were due to cancer in 1992. Cancer is second only to heart disease as a cause of death.

Recent advances in the understanding of cancer biology have facilitated the approach to the cancer patient. Following a diagnosis, the goal is to establish the extent of the disease (staging). Treatment of cancer is based on four modalities: operation, chemotherapy, radiotherapy, and immunotherapy.

KEY POINTS

• Cancer is a group of diseases with different manifestations, whose common characteristic is disordered cell growth and regulation; by definition, these tumors can metastasize

• Cancer is second only to heart disease as a cause of death

DIAGNOSIS

The evaluation of a patient with cancer starts with a carefully taken history and a thorough physical examination. Most symptomatic patients present with complaints of a palpable mass, cough, weight loss, bleeding, or gastrointestinal symptoms. Fewer cases are identified at an asymptomatic stage as a result of screening practices such as an abnormal mammogram, abnormal uterine cervical cytology, guiac-positive stool, abnormal colonoscopy, or an enlarged prostate.

A properly taken family history may reveal a familial trait for breast, colon, or other cancer (Case 1). Other risk factors—including age, smoking, exposure to ionizing radiation, polycyclic hydrocarbons, or aromatic amines—are associated with certain cancers.

A diagnosis of cancer should be substantiated with a pathologic diagnosis. Careful attention should be devoted to the planning and performance of the biopsy procedure. Any time a tissue sample is obtained, the incision or needle tract is considered contaminated and should be placed in an area that will be subjected to cancer treatment to eliminate any potential seeding of cancer cells.

The following are accepted means of obtaining a tissue sample:

1. *Excisional biopsy*—consists of excision of the tumor mass. It should only be done when the mass is small and further resection of adjacent tissue, if needed for definitive treatment, will not be compromised.

2. *Incisional biopsy*—an incision is placed over the tumor and a portion of the tumor is excised. It is often the preferred modality in larger tumors for which histological diagnosis directs subsequent treatment. It provides a large specimen, but there is risk of bleeding and breakdown of the suture line by tumor or infection.

3. *Core needle biopsy (tru-cut biopsy)*—is equivalent to an incisional biopsy; percutaneously, with a special large bore needle, a fragment of tissue is obtained. There is risk of bleeding and spread of cancer cells through tissue planes. This technique is most helpful in large tumors to avoid poor healing of an incisional biopsy.

4. *Fine needle aspiration cytology*—percutaneously, a "skinny" needle is introduced in the tumor; with gentle suction, fragments of tissue, but mostly cells, are aspirated into the hub of the needle.

Perhaps the cancer in the first patient could have been detected earlier if the patient had actively participated in a screening program, given her significant family history. Since the patient had a palpable mass, and epithelial cancers are easily identified on cytology, a cytologic diagnosis was adequate. A second suspicious area was detected on mammography and, not being palpable, mandated an excision of the area to confirm the suspicion of cancer.

In Case 2, the first biopsy revealed "fibroadipose tissue" that probably represents adipose tissue overlying the mass. The mass was missed due to a sampling error on the first biopsy. This emphasizes the importance of careful surgical technique. A tru-cut biopsy was chosen due to the large size of the mass, in order to avoid contamination of adjacent tissue planes and the risk of wound breakdown. Fine needle aspiration was not attempted because the cytologic characteristics of stromal tumors are not well defined. In both cases, the needle tracks and scars from previous biopsies were encompassed by the subsequent surgical resection.

STAGING

Staging is a system to define the extent of disease in a standardized fashion. It is a consequence of our understanding of the biology of cancer. Adequate classification and staging will help determine appropriate treatment, evaluate results of therapy more accurately, and compare the results of different modalities of therapy from different institutions more reliably.

Staging should start with a careful history and physical examination. Selective use of laboratory tests, like alkaline phosphatase for tumors that metastasize to liver or bone and carcinoembryonic antigen for colon cancer, are helpful. Radiographic studies should include a chest x-ray. Computed tomography (CT) scanning, magnetic resonance imaging (MRI), and radioisotope studies should be ordered judiciously and in a cost-effective manner.

The TNM classification of the Union International Contre Cancrum and the American Joint Committee on Cancer stratifies patients according to the following:

T—characteristics of the tumor

N—characteristics of the lymph nodes

M—presence of metastases

In addition, some patients are at risk of having a second cancer. This occurs with some frequency in patients with breast cancer (Case 1) and is called synchronous cancer if it is diagnosed within 6 months of the primary diagnosis. This finding is often significant (Case 1) because it may prompt a change in treatment, such as mastectomy instead of breast preservation. Synchronous cancers occur in about 5% of patients with colon cancer; therefore, preoperative colonoscopy is recommended.

Special studies are requested when there is a significant likelihood of providing information that would help clarify the prognosis of an individual patient, or information that would prompt a different treatment. In the case of sarcomas (Case 2), a chest CT is indicated due to the high incidence (20%) of pulmonary metastases. A bone scan was also requested in Case 2 to evaluate for direct bony involvement and to search for occult skeletal metastases (as high as 20%).

KEY POINTS

• Adequate classification and staging help determine treatment, evaluate therapeutic results, and compare results of different modalities from different institutions more reliably

---

TREATMENT

The treatment of the cancer patient should be individualized. The modality is selected according to the tumor histogenesis, the organ of origin, and the extent of disease. Often, multimodality treatment, including operation, chemotherapy, radiotherapy and, more recently, immunotherapy is required. An important question in planning therapy is to define whether the patient has known metastatic disease, or is at high risk of having metastases that are not large enough to be detected by physical examination or radiologic studies. Patients' physiologic status and wishes are also important in treatment selection.

Surgery and radiotherapy are modalities of treatment of local disease. Historically, operation was the first mode of therapy to be effective in the treatment of cancer. It has been the single most significant form of treatment since antisepsis and general anesthesias were introduced in the middle of the 20th century, and still is the single most definitive treatment for the majority of solid tumors. Unfortunately, approximately 70% of patients will fail surgical therapy alone, mostly due to systemic metastases.

The surgeon must define the role of the surgical procedure in the care of the individual patient:

1. *Surgery for diagnosis*
2. *Surgery for staging*—as depicted by Case 1, where clinical examination did not reveal any axillary adenopathy but the surgical specimen did. Pathologic confirmation provides more accurate assessment of the extent of locoregional disease than physical examination alone. Surgical staging is similarly considered the gold standard following laparotomy in patients with gastrointestinal malignancies.
3. *Surgery for cure*—failure to resect all locoregional disease will result in failure to cure. An oncologic en-bloc resection should encompass the primary tumor with clear margins (grossly and microscopically), including adjacent organs (if necessary), the regional lymphatics, and the biopsy site.

   Further understanding of tumor biology and familiarity with adjuvant modalities of treatment will temper the magnitude of surgical resection. Limited resection will be applicable in tumors that are responsive to chemotherapy and radiotherapy, allowing for a better functional and cosmetic result, like in soft tissue sarcomas (Case 2) or breast cancer.
4. *Surgery for debulking*—it is limited and only reserved for selected malignancies, to reduce the tumor burden. It is essential that other modalities are effective in controlling the residual disease (e.g., ovarian cancer).
5. *Surgery for palliation*—surgery is often necessary to relieve symptoms even when resection for cure is not feasible. For example, when a patient with colon cancer is found to have nonresectable liver metastases, segmental resection of the colon may be beneficial in the control of pain, bleeding, and/or obstructive symptoms.
6. *Surgery for prophylaxis*—the field of primary prevention originated from our ability to identify individuals at high risk of developing disease (in this case, to develop cancer). An example is prophylactic colectomy in persons with familial polyposis.

Radiotherapy is also a local modality of treatment. Its efficacy is dependent on the relative radiosensitivity of the tumor. When effective, it has the advantage of destroying tumors with preservation of function and form. It can be used as a primary modality of therapy as in Hodgkin's disease. As an adjuvant modality, it may limit the extent of necessary surgical resection, with preservation of a limb as in the case of sarcoma or with preservation of the breast as in mammary cancer. Palliative radiotherapy is used to control symptoms from metastases or a primary tumor.

Chemotherapy is the treatment of cancer with drugs. When drugs are used as the primary modality of treatment, it is called induction chemotherapy. Chemotherapy has been used as an adjuvant modality (to attack metastases at a microscopic state) with some success in patients with breast cancer and in selected patients with colon cancer. No benefit of adjuvant chemotherapy has been noted in other malignancies (gastric, pancreatic carcinoma, sarcomas). Neoadjuvant or primary chemotherapy entails the use of anticancer drugs before surgery for a solid tumor. The response of the primary tumor is followed, being used as an in vivo model for the sensitivity of the disease.

KEY POINTS

• Surgery and radiotherapy are modalities of treatment of local disease

• Approximately 70% of patients will fail surgical therapy alone, mostly due to systemic metastases

• Neoadjuvant or primary chemotherapy entails the use of anticancer drugs before surgery for a solid tumor

---

C FOLLOW-UP

Close follow-up is necessary in the care of cancer patients. The surgical oncologist must be willing to listen, be compassionate, and communicate with the patient, being realistic but always providing emotional support to the patient and relatives. Follow-up of the cancer patient should also emphasize rehabilitation after surgery (amputation, mastectomy) and return to a productive life.

Evaluation for follow-up must address the following questions:

1. Was the patient potentially cured?
2. Is there a locoregional recurrence?
3. Is there evidence of metastases?
4. Is there a metachronous lesion?
5. Is the patient at risk of other cancers?

The answers are provided after a carefully taken history and physical examination, and selective use of laboratory and radiologic examination. Specific tests may be required to detect metachronous lesions (colonoscopy, mammography).

SUGGESTED READINGS

Balch C, Bland K, Brennan M et al: What is a surgical oncologist? Ann Surg Oncol 1:2, 1994

A personal viewpoint of the role of the surgeon in treating patients with cancer.

Hall EJ: Radiation biology. CA Cancer, suppl. 55:2051, 1985

A history and overview of radiotherapy.

Rosenberg S: Principles of surgical oncology. p. 238. In De Vita V, Hellman S, Rosenberg S (eds): Cancer: Principles and Practice of Oncology. 4th Ed. Lippincott-Raven, Philadelphia, 1993

Outlines the basic tenets of surgical oncology.

QUESTIONS

1. Staging of a cancer is useful in?
   A. Establishing a prognosis before therapy.
   B. Determining the proper therapy.
   C. Retrospectively evaluating the success of therapeutic approaches.
   D. Comparing results from different institutions.
   E. All of the above.

2. Neoadjuvant therapy refers to?
   A. The newest experiment protocol.
   B. Therapy administered before surgical treatment.
   C. The first treatment the patient receives.
   D. Concurrent chemotherapy and radiotherapy.

(See p. 603 for answers.)

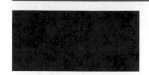

12

ACUTE

ABDOMEN

EDWARD PASSARO, JR.

Abdominal pain is one of the most common complaints of patients seen in the emergency room. Surgeons are frequently called to evaluate these patients to determine those who have an acute abdomen, or disease within the abdomen that may require hospitalization or a subsequent operation. This represents one of the greatest challenges in clinical medicine.

This chapter outlines an approach to the differentiation of the acute abdomen from the more common self-resolving episode of abdominal pain.

CASE 1
ABDOMINAL PAIN "IDK"

A 52-year-old male came to the emergency room because of abdominal pain of approximately 8 hours' duration and the recent onset of vomiting. He reportedly was in good health until 1 hour after lunch, when he noted the insidious onset of generalized upper abdominal pain. Initially he had no nausea or vomiting. He remained at work the rest of the afternoon despite his discomfort but was unable to do any work. Once home, he went to bed, but his abdominal pain remained unchanged. He did not eat supper but did take some sips of water. He was aware that he "could hear his bowels growling" but he did not have a bowel movement nor did he pass flatus. Early in the evening he suddenly became nauseated and within a few minutes had vomited a large quantity of sour fluid along with particulate matter that he recognized as his lunch. He was both cold and sweaty, but his abdomen felt better. He returned to bed, and 30 minutes later, had to vomit again. This time the contents were only a small quantity of bile-stained fluid. As his pain was not diminished and he felt generally ill, he came to the hospital.

His past history was unremarkable. He had no previous operations. He drank only an occasional beer with meals, and did not smoke. He had no food intolerance and reported no allergies except hay fever. He denied taking NSAIDs, antacids, or other medication. He had a customary bowel movement that morning shortly after breakfast. He recalled that 12–15 years ago he had a similar episode of abdominal pain but not as severe. He had not seen a doctor. On examination his temperature was 37.7°C. His abdomen was not distended but borborygmi was present. He had diffuse tenderness to palpation throughout the upper abdomen. The lower quadrants were less tender to palpation. There was no rebound or guarding. On rectal examination the stool guaiac was negative. A urinalysis was normal. His WBC count was 11,500 and a serum amylase was subsequently reported as normal. Plain films of the abdomen had been taken before the patient was seen by a physician. They showed small patches of gas without air fluid levels in the small intestine, but no other abnormalities.

He was started on intravenous fluids and a nasogastric tube was inserted in the stomach. His abdominal pain and physical findings were unchanged 4 hours after admission for observation. An ultrasound scan of the liver and gallbladder was made and no abnormalities were noted. After the pain eased, the patient fell asleep. The following morning he felt considerably better. He drank some liquids but was reluctant to eat solid food. He was afebrile.

He was discharged home and was instructed to call back 6 hours later, as well as the following day. He reported that he had remained free of abdominal pain, had a bowel movement, and returned to work.

CASE 2
RUPTURED CORPUS LUTEAL CYST

A 28-year-old married female was seen in the emergency room because of lower abdominal pain that she had for 8 hours. The pain was somewhat greater on the right than on the left. She had never experienced pain of this sort before, but did report that her menstrual periods were often accompanied by pain. Her last menstrual period was 2 weeks prior.

On physical examination her vital signs were normal. Her abdomen was not distended but was tender to palpation in both lower quadrants, right greater than left. There was no rebound or guarding. On pelvic examination, the cervical os appeared to be normal. The adnexa were free of masses or tenderness, but she was more tender on the right than the left. A WBC count returned as normal. Both urine and blood specimens were taken for pregnancy testing (β-human chorionic gonadotrophin), and subsequently returned as negative for pregnancy. The patient was released home without a specific diagnosis and was requested to call in 12 hours.

She returned to the emergency room 4 hours later. In the interim she noted that the pain had become more severe and constant, and was predominantly on the right side. She was slightly nauseated but experienced no vomiting. She had no bowel movement but had passed flatus. She had urinated without difficulty. On physical examination, the physician who examined her previously noted that there was an increase in her abdominal pain and discomfort on palpation. He was unsure whether she had rebound tenderness and a surgical consultation was obtained. The surgeon's examination confirmed the abdominal findings noted by the emergency room physician. A repeat pelvic examination showed some increased tenderness in the right lower quadrant. She remained afebrile but her WBC count had increased to 13,000.

Following discussion, she was admitted and brought to the operating room where a laparoscope was introduced into the abdomen. With only partial insufflation, the right lower quadrant was examined and the appendix was seen and found to be normal. The right ovary showed a clot and a small quantity of blood-stained fluid was found in the pelvis. A sample was taken for culture and the rest aspirated. The uterus appeared to be normal as did the colon. She was thought to have a ruptured corpus luteal cyst with hemoperitoneum. Two hours following the procedure, the patient noted relief of her abdominal pain, although she was sore. She proceeded to take liquids and solids and was discharged home 2 hours thereafter. The next day a telephone call confirmed that she was feeling better and was eating.

GENERAL CONSIDERATIONS

Abdominal pain of one type or another represents about 40% of all patient visits to emergency rooms. However, for every 1,000 patients with abdominal pain seen, only one-quarter (250) are admitted into the hospital, and of those admitted, approximately half (125) require an operation. The preoperative diagnosis in this group is correct only 70% of the time. Compounding this difficult triage is that in only half of the patients seen in the emergency department with abdominal pain will the etiology of the pain ever be known (Case 1). Since only a few patients seen with abdominal pain come to operation, the surgeon needs a practical and safe strategy to sort out patients with an acute abdomen from those with nothing more than abdominal pain.

It is difficult to define an acute abdomen. The term is used to signify an abdominal condition that needs immediate attention but does not necessarily require an operation. There are many factors, however, which delay the identification of patients with an acute abdomen. These factors include (1) the poor correlation between standard textbook descriptions of acute abdominal problems and an individual patient's complaints, (2) an undue reliance on laboratory tests and scanning studies, (3) a lack of appreciation for early signs and symptoms of the acute abdomen, and (4) an emphasis on early diagnosis or "labeling" that precludes an open, unbiased approach to this complex problem.

Although many medical and surgical diseases are often cited as causes of abdominal pain, what compels us to apply a label or diagnosis is that the label suggests a set of instructions as to what the physicians should do next. For example, if we are confronted with a patient with an acute abdomen of unknown etiology, and a consultant gives the patient the diagnosis of acute appendicitis, it is quite clear what the next steps will be. The patient's consent will be obtained to perform an appendectomy and the operating room will be notified. Similar situations exist if the label were "perforated peptic ulcer disease"; there would be a flurry of activity to have the patient prepared for operative closure of the perforation. But what happens if there is no label or diagnosis? Physicians become bewildered and anxious and occasionally irate. Their inability to achieve a diagnosis is taken as a measure of inadequacy or failure. This drives physicians almost immediately to apply a label to the patient, no matter how inappropriate. It is difficult for us to contend with a potentially threatening unknown. Unfortunately, we are more comfortable with the security of a wrong diagnosis than with the reality of an uncertain diagnosis. Actually, most patients will never have the etiology of their abdominal pain ascertained. Additionally, many patients are operated on to ascertain the diagnosis (Case 2). The demand for a quick, accurate diagnosis of the patient with an acute abdomen is both unrealistic and potentially dangerous. Alternatively, waiting or observing the patient without treatment may be inappropriate and dangerous. Physicians, to relieve the anxiety of the unknown, usually apply a working diagnosis to the patient (e.g., rule-out appendicitis).

KEY POINTS

- Abdominal pain is one of the most common complaints of patients seen in the emergency room

- For every 1,000 patients with abdominal pain seen, only 250 admitted to hospital, and of those, only 125 require operation

- Preoperative diagnosis in 125 patients is correct only 70% of the time

- In only half of patients seen in emergency department with abdominal pain will etiology of pain ever be known

- Surgeon needs practical and safe strategy to differentiate patients with acute abdomen from those with abdominal pain

- Many factors delay identification of patients with acute abdomen: (1) poor correlation between textbook descriptions and patient complaint, (2) undue reliance on laboratory tests and scans, (3) lack of appreciation for early signs and symptoms, and (4) emphasis on early diagnosis or labeling, precluding an open approach

- Many patients undergo operation to ascertain diagnosis

- Demand for quick, accurate diagnosis of patient with acute abdomen is unrealistic and potentially dangerous

A DIAGNOSIS

An effective method to deal with the problem is to apply the label IDK—"I don't know." Besides providing an appropriate and accurate label it suggests two prudent courses of action: (1) initiate resuscitation and (2) plot the clinical course of the patient over time to determine whether an acute abdominal problem is present.

Resuscitation early (intravenous fluid, gastric suction, type and cross-match, etc.) may subsequently prove unnecessary in many patients. However, its great virtue in patients whose clinical course in unknown is that it prevents further deterioration of the clinical state, and the patient is prepared if prompt operation is warranted. As experience has shown, the problem is not that too many patients are needlessly given intravenous catheters, but rather that patients in need of resuscitation do not receive it until late, when their clinical condition has deteriorated.

Two clinical patterns describe the course of all acute abdominal disease. The first is marked by a progressive worsening of the patient's clinical parameters. Such a disease pattern culminates in either prompt resolution (spontaneous detorsion of a sigmoid volvulus) or progression to death (strangulated bowel infarction, perforation, sepsis). The best example of such an inexorable disease process is appendicitis (Fig. 12.1A).

The other clinical pattern is a waxing and waning clinical course, or crescendo-decrescendo pattern. Biliary colic from cholelithiasis typically follows this pattern (Fig. 12.1B). Thus, when first seen, patients may appear to be worsening or improving depending on when they are seen during the clinical course. Importantly, such patients will often give a history of repeated episodes with a similar pattern.

When seen early in the clinical course, neither of these patterns may be discernible. Nevertheless, the strategy mentioned here will allow for the detection of either clinical course outlined above, or if the condition resolves spontaneously without a label other than "IDK."

Plotting the clinical course of the patient as a function of time allows an objective assessment as to whether the patient is improving or getting worse (Cases 1 and 2). The plot or graph should be at the patient's bedside so as to be readily available. Write the ordinate as dis-ease (i.e., the departure from ease). For most patients, the more numerous and reliable points on the curve are those obtained from a carefully taken history. In particular, when patients are seen early in the course of their dis-ease, detailed questioning will aid in determining when the disease began, that is, when there was a departure from ease. This transition point can be precipitous, as with a perforated duodenal ulcer, when the patient can recall to the minute when the dis-ease began. More commonly, however, acute abdominal disease begins as an insidious, almost imperceptible change, as in the patient who regularly eats two to three slices of toast and jelly for breakfast elected to have one slice that morning for reasons he or she was unaware of at the time. In fact, a subtle but progressive loss of appetite is the earliest and most consistent change in the patient developing an acute abdomen. However, all signs or symptoms that change should be plotted so that a pattern can be discerned.

Once a pattern of worsening clinical state becomes evident from the graph of the findings, the decision to operate or do an invasive test becomes clear. Under these circumstances further tests or studies are contraindicated. Every effort should be made to intervene and halt the progression of the disease process as well as determine its nature.

In summary, the approach outlined in this chapter:

1. Emphasizes a generic approach to be applied to all patients with a presumed acute abdomen

2. Emphasizes prompt resuscitation steps being taken in all patients, recognizing that many subsequently will be found not to require it

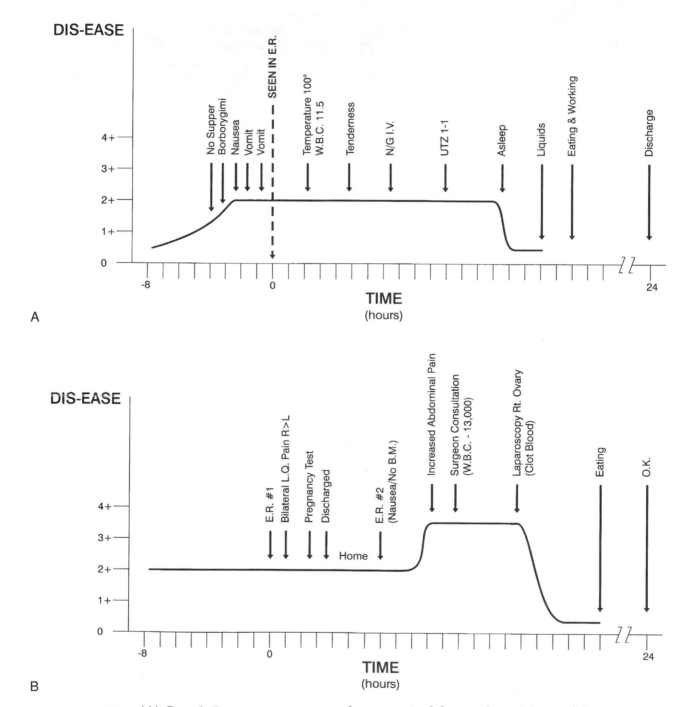

FIGURE 12.1 *(A) Case 1. Progressive worsening of symptoms and then resolution in case of IDK. (B) Case 2. Clinical course of ruptured corpus luteal cyst with progression of dis-ease leading to laparoscopy.*

3. Emphasizes a carefully taken detailed history, making particular note of the loss of appetite and changes in behavior that antedate the development of gastrointestinal-related complaints such as pain, vomiting, or diarrhea

4. Emphasizes the use of the label IDK as the safest and most appropriate diagnosis or label

5. Emphasizes avoiding quick diagnosis or labeling, as it prompts inappropriate testing and/or treatment

6. Emphasizes the plotting of the patient's dis-ease as a function of time to determine when intervention for diagnosis and/or treatment is required

---

KEY POINTS

- An effective method to deal with acute abdomen is to apply the label "IDK" (I don't know)

- IDK suggests two prudent courses of action: (1) initiate resuscitation and (2) plot clinical course of patient over time to determine if acute abdominal problem is present

- The problem is not that too many patients are needlessly given intravenous catheters, but that patients in need of resuscitation do not receive it until clinical condition has deteriorated

- Two clinical patterns describe course of all acute abdominal disease: (1) progressive worsening of patient's clinical parameters and (2) waxing and waning clinical course, or crescendo-decrescendo pattern

- Plotting the clinical course of the patients as a function of time allows objective assessment of whether patient is improving or getting worse

---

SUGGESTED READINGS

Brewer RJ: An analysis of 1000 consecutive cases in a university hospital emergency room. Am J Surg 131: 219, 1976

Excellent analysis of diagnostic problem of abdominal pain. Must be read to grasp the problem of differentiating the acute abdomen.

Simmens HP, Decurtins M, Rotzer A: Emergency room patients with abdominal pain unrelated to trauma. Hepatogastroenterology 28: 471, 1991

QUESTIONS

1. In what percentage of patients seen in an emergency room because of abdominal pain will the etiology of the pain become known?

   A. 20%.

   B. 40%.

   C. 60%.

   D. 80%.

2. The best approach to discern an acute abdomen from other causes of abdominal pain is?

   A. To observe the patient, allowing the disease to "declare itself."

   B. To carry out early selective testing to quickly establish a diagnosis.

   C. To obtain prompt consultation with general surgeons, a radiologist, and others to arrive at the diagnosis.

   D. To begin resuscitation in all suspected instances, apply the label IDK, and plot the patient's clinical course to determine if the disease is progressing.

3. The pattern of abdominal pain that usually gives a history of a similar attack is?

   A. Crescendo-decrescendo disease.

   B. Progressive inexorable disease.

   C. Both A and B.

   D. None of the above.

4. The most important parameter in recognizing an acute abdomen is?

   A. A skillful abdominal examination by a surgeon.

   B. A careful, detailed history.

   C. Selective radiographs or scans.

   D. Specific blood tests.

(See p. 603 for answers.)

13

GROIN AND ABDOMINAL HERNIAS

EDWARD PASSARO, JR.

Groin hernias are confusing and exasperating to most students. The anatomy of the groin region is usually presented in great detail and with a plethora of names. The anatomic elements are conceived of as disparate individual components and are not thought of as an integrated unit. Furthermore, the anatomy is just structural elements. Any functional component to the pieces, individ-

ually or collectively, is missing. There is an excessive use of eponyms, both anatomic and surgical, which adds to the confusion rather than providing clarity. Above all, no fundamental principle of groin hernia formation or treatment is ever enunciated. Lacking this basic insight into the problem, the student quickly forgets both the isolated, detailed anatomy and the eponyms.

It is as if someone who had never seen an automobile was exposed to the disassembled parts strewn on a garage floor. What could be gleaned about a car and how it works by looking at the pieces? How much better to first see a car moving down the street and then explain the relationship of the parts to one another and the principle of converting fuel into motion.

The aims of this chapter are to (1) review briefly and succinctly the pertinent anatomy of groin hernias, (2) delineate the principle of groin hernia formation and repair, and (3) describe surgical repairs in terms of anatomy for easy conceptualization. Other hernias of the abdominal wall are also described. Based on this knowledge, the student should be able to deduce the common signs and symptoms of groin hernias and their features on physical examination, ascertain their relative risk to the patient

(and the reasons for them), and describe the principles of the different repairs.

CASE 1
INDIRECT INGUINAL HERNIA

A 27-year-old male noted the progressive enlargement of a right inguinal bulge over the course of 1 year. Recently, it had extended downward into the scrotum and at presentation was associated with discomfort when the patient coughed, lifted objects, or strained. Although previously the bulge disappeared when lying down, at presentation it was always present. He tried to massage it in a effort to "reduce" it, but experienced discomfort and aborted the attempt.

CASE 2
SLIDING HERNIA

A moderate size left inguinal mass rapidly developed in a 60-year-old male. Concomitantly, he noted some constipation relieved in part by massage of the mass. On physical examination, bowel could be palpated within the mass. A barium enema showed no intrinsic colon lesion but did show a portion of the colon in the inguinal mass.

GENERAL CONSIDERATIONS

The relevant anatomy for groin hernias is pictured in Figure 13.1. Usually this anatomy is vaguely familiar but not integrated. The anatomic schema have been labeled with numbers as well as names. It will be useful to reproduce these simple schematic drawings on a piece of paper as a way to begin to conceptualize the three-dimensional aspects of the anatomy while engaged in depicting them on a two-dimensional surface. The numbering sequence should assist you in your efforts. Figure 13.1A is a frontal view of the relevant anatomy while Figure 13.1B is a transectional view in the plane X-X' perpendicular to the plane of the paper. This view is comparable to that which the surgeon sees while incising through the tissue layers during the course of an operation.

Figure 13.1A demonstrates that the muscle fibers of the external oblique are not present and that fibers of the internal oblique invest the spermatic cord. These are called the cremasteric fibers.

Hesselbach's triangle is an important eponym. The area of the triangle is important as it is an area of potential weakness because of a lack of muscle. After all, it is muscle that makes the abdominal wall strong. Its lack makes the wall weak.

Note the relationship of the internal and external inguinal rings (9) to the triangle. Direct hernias protrude through Hesselbach's triangle. Indirect hernias, as the name implies, protrude by passing indirectly through the internal ring, descending down the inguinal canal connecting the internal and external rings, and emerging through the external ring. They may enter the subcutaneous tissues of the groin, or descend further down into the scrotum. Recall that the testis is a retroperitoneal structure that descends behind the peritoneum into the scrotum. It occupies the dorsal and lateral aspects of the inguinal region. The inguinal canal, therefore, as it emerges through the internal inguinal ring, is both ventral and medial to the cord structures. This relationship is a consequence of the developmental aspects of the testis and cord structures. It is important for the operating surgeon to identify the indirect hernia sac quickly based on its anatomic position, ventral and medial to the cord structures.

A convenient way to illustrate these three-dimensional anatomic relationships is to imagine being in a room with a single door, which is then closed (Fig. 13.2). Imagine that you are a piece of small bowel in a large plastic bag (peritoneum) that fills the room. If the door were structurally weak, every time you (as intestine in the peritoneal sac) leaned against it, it would bulge into the corridor outside. You are mimicking a *direct hernia*. The door, be-

cause of its structural weakness, represents Hesselbach's triangle. Now imagine that, while you were leaning against the door, the room was suddenly rotated 90 degrees so that the wall opposite to the door had rotated below you. You would slide away from the bulging door and the door would return to its normal contour. This represents the course of events when a patient with a direct hernia stands erect (door bulges) or lies down (90 degrees rotation from the erect position). Furthermore, whether the door is small or large, there appears to be no intrinsic risk or damage to you (viscus, small bowel).

Now open the door to the room, so that it is ajar. The internal door jamb represents the internal inguinal ring. Note that the door is at one edge of Hesselbach's triangle. The outer door jamb (in the corridor) represents the external inguinal ring at the other margin of Hesselbach's triangle. The oblique passage from inside the room, past the internal door jamb, along the door to the external door jamb, and finally to the corridor outside, represents the passage of the inguinal ring obliquely through the abdominal wall. This is the path of the *indirect inguinal hernia*.

Now, try to pass through the narrow space between the slightly opened door and the door jamb. You might get started out of the door, but if pressure is applied from outside the room to close the door, you would be trapped (or as we say clinically, imprisoned or incarcerated). If you had gone beyond the external door jamb, into the corridor (surrounding tissues leading down to the scrotum) when the door was closed, you would not be able to get back into the room (an irreducible hernia).

In this simple way, it is easy to conceive of the mechanisms responsible for the formation of direct and indirect hernias. One can relate the anatomic features of the inguinal region to each other using the room and door as a three-dimensional model. It also allows us to understand some of the pertinent clinical features of the two different types of hernia, such as the usually easy reducibility of a direct hernia when lying down.

Given this information, which of these hernias would you rather have yourself, and why? To answer that question properly, one must know what the mechanism of hernia formation is and what the consequences of the mechanism might be. Clearly, you do not want a hernia that has a great potential to injure you. From what we have already discussed it is apparent that because an indirect hernia can become incarcerated in a confined oblique passage, it is more apt to lead to swelling of the trapped bowel, with resultant ischemia to its mucosa, gangrene, perforation, and sepsis (Case 1).

The direct hernia is far less apt to produce these changes and, therefore, is the "groin hernia of choice" between the two. To repeat, hernias that are small and in which a viscus (usually small bowel) can pass through a constricting passage or ring, have the potential to entrap the bowel (incarcerate it). Once it is caught in place, the

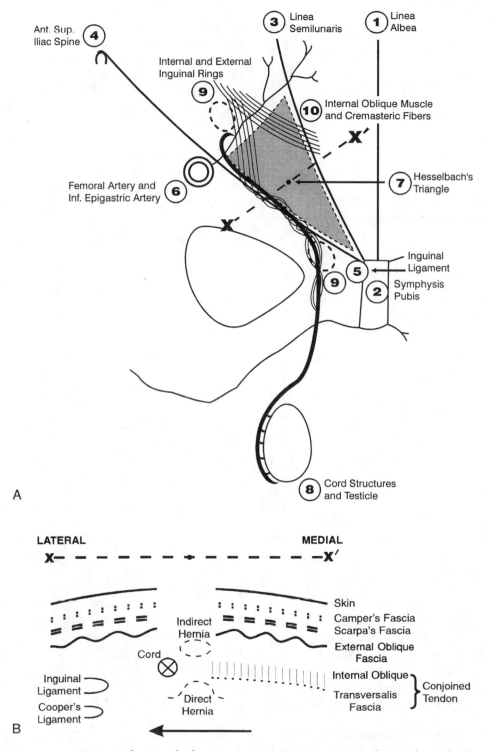

A

B

FIGURE 13.1   *(A) Frontal view of relevant anatomy. (B) Transectional view through plane X---X'.*

Additional hernias that are apt to incarcerate and strangulate the bowel are umbilical hernias and femoral hernias. The latter are particularly notorious. Femoral hernias occur along the femoral vessels in the groin (Fig. 13.3). Typically, the space (or potential space) along the medial aspect of the vessels is small. It is sharply and rigidly defined by the inguinal ligament above, by the femoral vessels above and laterally, and by the pubic ramus medially. The space, therefore, cannot readily expand to accommodate the intruding viscus. The result is that strangulation and perforation of the bowel are more common with this type of hernia than with any other. Furthermore, because this area is surrounded by generous layers of fat and is deep in the femoral crease, it is not easy to examine and discern the presence of a hernia therein. Furthermore, femoral hernias may entrap only one wall of the bowel (Fig. 13.4), in which case a Richter's hernia occurs. These hernias do not produce intestinal obstruction such as an incarcerated indirect her-

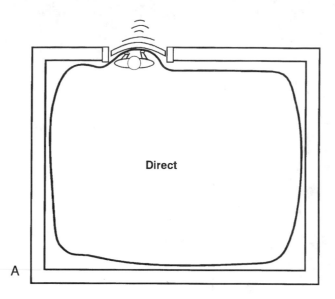

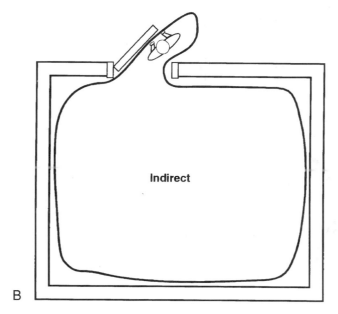

FIGURE 13.2   *(A & B) An analogy of a direct and indirect hernia (see text for details).*

bowel can experience other changes such as the intraluminal transudation of fluid and gases, which further contributes to its swelling and luminal obstruction. It presents to the physician as a form of intestinal obstruction. If the swelling from these processes increases the intraluminal pressure such that perfusion of the mucosa of the trapped bowel segment is impaired (strangulation), other changes quickly follow. Bacteria are no longer contained intraluminally but, because of the loss of mucosal integrity, readily pass through the bowel wall into the surrounding tissues. The passage of bacteria into the bowel wall coupled with the relative ischemia from the distended bowel leads to gangrene and perforation.

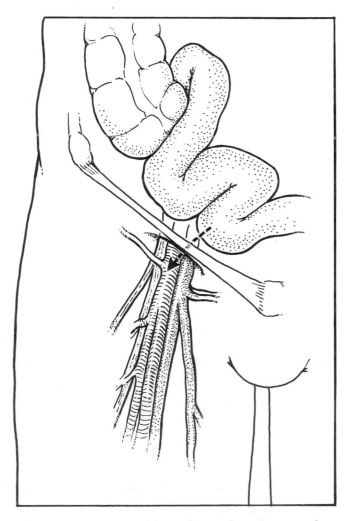

FIGURE 13.3   *Area of femoral triangle and course of a femoral hernia.*

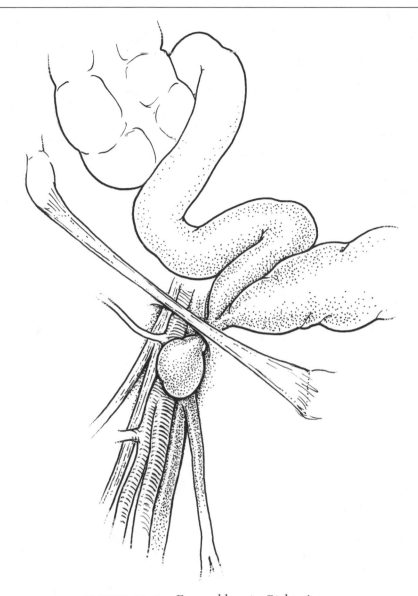

FIGURE 13.4 *Femoral hernia, Richter's type.*

nia might, because the lumen of the bowel remains patent. Femoral hernias are therefore difficult to recognize clinically because of their deep anatomic position and the lack of gastrointestinal symptoms until gangrene and sepsis ensue.

The principles behind the repair of an inguinal hernia can be understood by examining Figure 13.1B. Note the relationship of the indirect hernia sac medial and ventral to the cord structures. The operation begins by mobilizing this sac and ligating it at the level of the internal inguinal ring, after which it is amputated. The direct sac is merely pushed inward to return it to the abdomen. Laterally lie the inguinal ligament and Cooper's ligament, both tough immobile structures that serve as anchoring tissues. There are no other tissues in the immediate area that can be mobilized and brought medially. Medially lies the internal oblique muscle and the transversalis fascia, which forms the conjoined tendon. This tissue is supple and mobile, and serves as excellent material to buttress a weak area devoid of muscle. The principle of all uncomplicated inguinal hernia repairs, therefore, is to anchor the supple and mobile medial tissue to the immobile strong ligaments found laterally. The concept follows logically from a consideration of the anatomy. The other consideration is whether the tissues used for repair should pass beneath or over the cord structures (Fig. 13.1B), or whether the cord should be displaced to some other position (i.e., subcutaneous). The student is invited to reproduce Figure 13.1B in as many different ways as possible using variations of the above principle. Each of these repairs carries its own eponym and is listed in the Glossary and depicted in Figure 13.5.

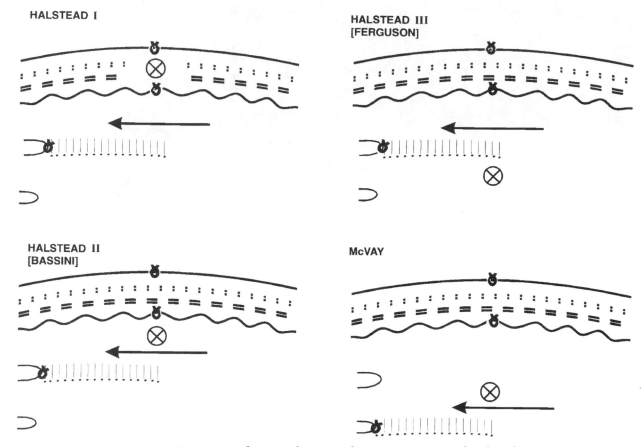

FIGURE 13.5   *Transectional views of common hernia repairs (see also the Glossary).*

Femoral hernias are repaired by reducing the bowel from the femoral canal and closing or obliterating the defect by approximating the tissues on either side of it.

Laparoscopic repair of groin hernias has provided a view from the inside out. The orifice of the internal inguinal ring can be readily seen and closed, and the femoral space inspected and closed, if necessary. To repair a direct hernia defect, the peritoneum overlying the area of Hesselbach's triangle is opened, a piece of synthetic mesh overlaid, and the peritoneum reapproximated over it. To use our earlier analogy, the weak door is buttressed by a piece of strong plywood tacked over it. A particularly confusing hernia is the so-called sliding hernia, in which a portion of the hernia sac is composed of a hollow viscus such as the colon or bladder. Think of an indirect hernia on the left side, which appeared rather suddenly in an elderly male and rapidly achieved a large size. In addition, the patient noted some difficulty in moving his bowels since the appearance of the hernia and massaged it during evacuation to assist in defecation (Case 2). On physical examination, you might readily appreciate bowel in the hernia, which is difficult if not impossible to reduce. All these findings are characteristic of a sliding hernia with sigmoid colon forming part of the hernia sac. Again, think of yourself in a plastic bag in a room with the door slightly ajar. This time,

however, between the plastic sac and the wall leading to where the door opens, there is a large horizontal collapsed tube at about waist height. As you and the plastic sac proceed out through the slightly opened door (internal inguinal ring) the tube beneath the plastic (retroperitoneal sigmoid colon) is dragged out as well. Seen from the outside, from the corridor looking at the external door jamb, there is a large plastic tube partially collapsed and behind it and to one side of it is the bulge of a plastic sac. The importance of recognizing a sliding hernia is to prevent inadvertent injury to the blood supply or inadvertent enterotomy during repair. Once properly identified, the hernia is repaired by reducing the bowel, closing the internal ring, and strengthening the area as with other inguinal hernias.

Hernias in other portions of the abdominal wall usually occur generally through defects in the fascia. These are either congenital, related to physical stress or exertion, or from previous operations. As a generalization, such hernias may produce pain or discomfort with physical activity, or may be an unsightly and occasionally disabling protrusion, but only rarely are they the cause of obstruction and gangrene of bowel and/or omentum. Their repair consists of reducing the hernia contents in the abdominal cavity and then closing and/or reinforcing the weakened fascial tissues.

KEY POINTS

- Useful to reproduce the simple, schematic drawings of Figure 13.1 to begin to conceptualize the three-dimensional aspects of the anatomy while depicting them on a two-dimensional surface

- Hesselbach's triangle is an important eponym; area of triangle is area of potential weakness because of lack of muscle, which makes abdominal wall strong

- Direct hernias protrude through Hesselbach's triangle

- Indirect hernias protrude by passing indirectly through internal ring, descending down inguinal canal connecting internal and external rings, and emerging through external ring

- Imagine stepping into a room with a single door, which is then closed (Fig. 13.2); if structurally weak, every time you (as intestine in peritoneal sac) leaned against the door, it would bulge into corridor outside; you're mimicking a direct hernia: the oblique passage from inside the room, past the internal door jamb, along the door to the external door jamb, and finally to the corridor outside, represents the passage of the inguinal ring obliquely through the abdominal wall; this is the path of the indirect inguinal hernia; you might get started out of the door, but if pressure is applied from outside the room to close the door, you would be trapped

- Hernias that are small and in which a viscus (usually small bowel) can pass through constricting passage or ring, have the potential to entrap bowel

- Additional hernias that are apt to incarcerate and strangulate bowel are umbilical hernias and femoral hernias

- Femoral hernias may entrap only one wall of the bowel (Fig. 13.4), in which case a Richter's hernia occurs; these do not produce intestinal obstruction such as an incarcerated direct hernia might, because lumen of bowel remains patent

- Principle of all uncomplicated inguinal hernia repairs, therefore, is to anchor the supple and mobile medial tissue to the immobile strong ligaments found laterally

LUMBAR HERNIAS

The lumbar region, divided into superior and inferior triangles, is also subject to weakness of presumed congenital origin. These rare hernias should be considered in patients complaining of lumbar pain and discomfort on exertion. The hernias are difficult to detect on physical examination in many instances because of the overlying tissues. The most common is a superior triangle (Grynfelt) hernia bounded by the sacrospinalis muscle, internal oblique muscle, and the inferior margin of the 12th rib. A lower triangle, or Petit's hernia, is bounded by the lateral margin of the latissimus dorsi, the medial margin of the external oblique, and the iliac crest. Repair of the weakened area is performed with synthetic mesh for coverage.

FASCIAL HERNIAS

These hernias are thought to arise from physical straining, producing defects in the linea alba or midline (preperitoneal or epigastric hernia) or linea semilunaris (lateral border of the rectus, spigelian hernia). The hernias tend to be small, with preperitoneal fat protruding through the defect. They produce pain and discomfort on effort limited to the small defect. Repair consists of simple closure of the defect.

UMBILICAL HERNIA

Although common in infancy, most umbilical hernias close with time. In the adult, umbilical hernias are associated with increases in intra-abdominal pressure, such as with pregnancy, obesity, and ascites. The defect is usually small, so that incarceration and strangulation are common. The principles of repair are to reduce the contents and simply close the defect.

INCISIONAL HERNIA

By far the most common of the abdominal wall hernias is related to previous operations. Often there is a history of wound infection or wound disruption ("popping of the sutures") followed by a gradually increasing bulge in the wound with associated discomfort. If the defect is small, incarceration and strangulation of the contents can ensue. Repair is done by opening the old incision, reducing the contents after ensuring their viability, removing old suture material in the area (presuming it to be infected), and rerepairing the fascia directly if possible. When direct repair is not possible, synthetic mesh is used to cover the defect.

SUGGESTED READINGS

Nyhus LM, Condon RE: Hernia. 2nd Ed. Lippincott-Raven, Philadelphia, 1978

A comprehensive and detailed text by experts on all aspects of hernia. The many different approaches to inguinal hernia repair by the proponents are presented. Useful in providing a broad background in surgical approaches to inguinal herniorrhaphy.

Ponka JL: Hernias of the Abdominal Wall. WB Saunders, Philadelphia, 1980

A very well-illustrated text on a wide range of hernia repairs. Excellent resource delineating the individual steps of a hernia repair.

QUESTIONS

1. *The indirect inguinal hernia is much more dangerous than the direct inguinal hernia because?*

   A. Direct hernia's occur in an area of weakness (Hesselbach's triangle) that has no areas of construction likely to trap bowel.

   B. Indirect hernia's protrude indirectly through the abdominal wall along the inguinal canal, a potentially narrow, confining region.

   C. Bowel entrapped (incarcerated) within the inguinal canal can become strangulated, leading to necrosis and sepsis.

   D. All of the above.

2. *The principle of all uncomplicated inguinal hernia repairs is?*

   A. Excision of the hernia sac.

   B. To anchor supple medial tissue to lateral immobile ligaments.

   C. To elevate the cord structures above the repair.

   D. None of the above.

3. *Femoral hernias are clinically difficult to detect because?*

   A. They are "deep seated" (i.e., in an anatomic region that is hard to examine).

   B. They may entrap only a small piece of bowel or only one wall of the bowel (Richter's hernia).

   C. They may produce few symptoms until late.

   D. All of the above.

(See p. 603 for answers.)

GLOSSARY

Halstead I: Cord is placed in subcutaneous position fascia, with external oblique closed beneath it. Conjoined tendon is then sutured to inguinal ligament. This procedure is no longer indicated.

Halstead II (Bassini): Conjoined tendon is brought beneath cord and anchored to inguinal ligament. Fascia of external oblique is closed over cord. This is a standard primary repair of indirect hernia (after ligation of sac at internal inguinal ring) and small direct hernias.

Halstead III (Ferguson): After high ligation of indirect hernia sac, conjoined tendon is brought over (ventral) to cord and sutured to inguinal ligament. This procedure is commonly done in infants.

McVay: Conjoined tendon is anchored to Cooper's ligament with cord above (ventral). This procedure is often employed in recurrent hernias.

14

ABDOMINAL

TRAUMA

FRED S. BONGARD

Trauma is the leading cause of death among all Americans less than 55 years of age and constitutes one of the major causes of preventable illness. Trauma has become a nationwide epidemic, claiming more young victims than heart disease, cancer, or human immunodeficiency virus (HIV). Although much injury is accidental, firearm violence is a particular problem among urban youth. A recent study came to the disturbing conclusion that firearms kill more children under 18 years of age than do motor vehicle accidents. Hospital and rehabilitation costs of trauma exceed several billion dollars per year. Although postinjury prehospital transport, acute care, and rehabilitation have improved dramatically over the past several years, injury prevention remains the great challenge.

This chapter reviews the general principles of trauma management, including immediate resuscitation, evaluation, and diagnosis. The guiding principles that separate penetrating injuries from blunt injuries are discussed. In addition, the postoperative and critical care aspects of trauma management are detailed.

CASE 1
GUNSHOT WOUND

A 19-year-old male was attending a rally when gunfire erupted. He was struck once in the mid-abdomen and collapsed onto the grass. When the paramedics arrived, his initial blood pressure was 110/70 mmHg with a heart rate of 110 bpm. A large bore intravenous catheter was inserted in his right arm. He was transported quickly to a local trauma center.

Upon arrival, he was undressed and placed on a gurney with his head between large sandbags. Nasogastric and urinary catheters were inserted. The nasogastric aspirate produced gross blood. Several radiographs were taken of his neck, chest, and pelvis. The initial Hct was 40%, which fell to 37% after he received 2,000 ml of lactated Ringer's solution.

Over the next few minutes, examination of his abdomen revealed that abdominal viscera could be seen through the bullet wound. At laparotomy, perforations of the stomach and small bowel were found. The defects were repaired primarily, and he made an uneventful recovery.

CASE 2
MOTOR VEHICLE ACCIDENT

A 23-year-old female was driving home from a party, where she had been drinking heavily. She drove through a stop sign and was struck on the driver's side by a pickup truck. Her car spun on impact and struck a tree near the intersection.

Before transport by the paramedics, she was placed in a hard cervical collar and on a firm back board. Her initial BP was 90/50 mmHg, with a heart rate of 120 bpm. Two large bore IV catheters were placed in her upper extremities; 1,000 ml of lactated Ringer's solution was infused during her trip to the hospital, where she arrived with a BP of 120/70 mmHg and a heart rate of 100 bpm.

The initial evaluation consisted of radiographs of her neck, chest, and pelvis, along with placement of a catheter in her bladder. Because she was awake and talking, endotracheal intubation was not required. The initial Hct was 40%, dropping over the next 15 minutes to 32%. Examination of her abdomen revealed moderate tenderness in the left upper quadrant. The third Hct was 30%. A deformity of her left thigh with significant swelling was noted.

She was taken for a CT scan, which showed free fluid around the spleen and a large fracture of the spleen itself. A splenectomy was done. The postoperative course was complicated by the need for repair of a femoral fracture. Pneumonia developed on the second postoperative day, requiring endotracheal intubation with mechanical ventilation for several days. Following extubation, she steadily improved and was ultimately discharged on postoperative day 13. She was charged with felony drunk driving.

GENERAL CONSIDERATIONS

Treatment of the trauma victim must be organized and deliberate in order to stabilize the patient, identify the injuries, and treat in an appropriate order. Although patients are usually categorized by mechanism into blunt (Case 2) or penetrating (Case 1), initial care is similar. It is divided into four stages: primary survey (ABCs), resuscitation, secondary survey, and definitive care.

The primary survey takes place immediately after the patient reaches the hospital. It is intended to identify life threatening conditions. The primary survey may be remembered as **A-B-C-D-E:**

A **A**irway management and cervical spine

B **B**reathing

C **C**irculation and control of hemorrhage

D **D**isability and neurologic status

E **E**xposure and environmental control

Airway control is the first and single most important step in the management of the trauma victim. Assessment of the airway includes talking to the patient (if awake) and examining the oropharynx for potentially obstructing foreign bodies, such as gum, food debris, and loose teeth. Those who can speak normally and who do not exhibit stridor do not have a compromised airway (Case 2). When patients are unconscious, the tongue falls posteriorly into the oropharynx and may occlude the airway. Placement of a simple rubber airway to reposition the tongue anteriorly may be all that is required in these spontaneously breathing patients.

Assessment of the cervical spine is included under airway management because attempts to secure a patent airway that requires flexion, extension, or rotation of the neck may dislocate unstable cervical vertebrae and cause permanent neurologic impairment. Cervical spine radiographs (Cases 1 and 2) are required to ensure that bony or ligamentous damage with misalignment has not occurred. This must be done before the patient's neck is unduly manipulated. Assessment requires radiographic visualization of the entire cervical spine and first thoracic vertebrae. An anterior, cross-table lateral, and open-mouth odontoid view are usually sufficient to ensure that alignment of the cervical spine is not compromised. Until such assessment has been completed, the patient's neck should be rigidly immobilized to prevent possible spinal cord injury. A cervical spine injury should always be suspected in a multisystem trauma patient or in a patient with an altered level of consciousness, until cervical spine injury has been excluded.

Breathing is required for pulmonary gas exchange. Chest injuries that compromise the normal breathing apparatus, as well as spinal cord injuries, hypotension, and altered consciousness from injury or inebriation, are common causes of impaired breathing. Mechanical ventilation is indicated when spontaneous breathing is inadequate, or when respiratory effort is compromised because of injury or paralytic agents used for endotracheal intubation.

Circulation is most often compromised by blood loss and hypovolemia (see Ch. 4). Following injury, hypotension must always be assumed to be due to hypovolemia, until proved otherwise. The level of consciousness, as well as skin color, and pulse rate are useful modalities for assessing circulatory compromise. External bleeding is usually not present, except in the case of major vascular injuries, scalp lacerations, or open fractures. Such bleeding should be controlled during the initial survey, with the application of direct pressure over the source, until definitive management is possible. Concealed hemorrhage in the abdomen, pelvis, or chest is far more common than gross external hemorrhage. The fascial compartments surrounding the muscles in the leg may sequester several hundred milliliters of blood after a long bone fracture (Case 2). This may also occur in the fascial compartments of the arm or buttock. The potential for such concealed hemorrhage should always be considered in the presence of major fractures, crush injuries, or soft tissue destruction that may accompany either blunt or penetrating trauma.

Disability may be rapidly assessed using the simple mnemonic:

A **A**lert

V Responds to **V**ocal stimuli

P Responds to **P**ainful stimuli

U **U**nresponsive

The Glasgow Coma Scale (see Ch. 82) provides a more detailed evaluation and may be substituted for this simple system as desired. Changes in the level of consciousness may be due to head injury, decreased oxygenation, shock, or the prior use of drugs and alcohol.

Exposure is required for adequate examination of the patient. The patient should be undressed fully and kept warm during examination. This is particularly important for those who also have major burns, as heat can be lost quickly. A patient with a potentially unstable spine should be rolled to one side in a coordinated effort ("log-rolled"), to prevent neurologic injury.

Resuscitation begins concomitantly with primary survey and addresses abnormal findings. Useful techniques for airway control include the chin lift and the jaw thrust. In the former approach, the physician's second and third fingers are placed in the patient's mouth around the the lower incisors, and the jaw brought forward. The jaw thrust requires placing the thumbs behind the angle of the patient's mandibles and lifting the jaw forward. Particular care must be exercised with these maneuvers, to stabilize the neck and prevent neurologic damage from an unstable cervical spine.

When the airway itself is compromised, or in a patient who is unconscious and unable to maintain a patent airway, endotracheal or nasotracheal intubation is indicated. Nasotracheal intubation may only be accomplished in a spontaneously breathing patient because of the need for synchronization with opening of the vocal cords. Immediately after the airway is placed, auscultation of both lung fields is required to ascertain that the tube has not inadvertently entered the esophagus or has not been advanced so far that its tip has passed into the right mainstem bronchus.

Tracheostomy or cricothyroidotomy is required for the patient with distorted anatomy or stridor. These maneuvers are typically used in gunshot wounds of the face or neck and in severe facial or cervical blunt trauma, when the airway is either not identifiable or may have been disrupted distal to the oropharynx. Patients with gunshot wounds of the neck who present with stridor or subcutaneous emphysema should be approached with extreme caution because they may have partial injuries of the trachea that could become complete transections if endotracheal intubation were attempted.

Cricothyroidotomy is the procedure of choice for orofacial trauma in a patient in respiratory distress. The cricothyroid membrane, which connects the thyroid and cricoid cartilages, can usually be palpated even in those with severe injury. Incision through the skin carried down to and through this membrane will permit rapid access to the trachea. A 7 French cuffed endotracheal tube can be inserted through the incision, furnishing good access for ventilation. When the patient is awake and breathing spontaneously, a tracheostomy is preferable. This is best performed in the operating room, where adequate ancillary support is available. A stridorous patient who is able to breathe spontaneously should be allowed to remain in a position of comfort (usually sitting up, leaning forward) until the airway can be addressed. Attempts to force the patient into the supine position may result in acute—often lethal—airway obstruction.

Breathing (gas exchange) may be compromised after head or chest injury; either a mechanical bag and mask or a ventilator may be required if the patient is unable to ventilate sufficiently. Supplemental oxygen should be provided to ensure adequate arterial oxyhemoglobin saturation. A tension pneumothorax (see Ch. 53) may compromise ventilation and must be decompressed immediately if present.

Circulatory support begins with the placement of two large bore IV catheters (Cases 1 and 2). These should be placed in the upper extremities to prevent extravasation through potential abdominal venous injuries. Balanced salt solutions should be infused at a rate determined by the severity of hypotension and the patient's size. Typically 2 L of solution is given over the first 15 minutes in an attempt to restore blood pressure (Case 1). When the catheters are placed, blood should be withdrawn and sent for cross-matching as well as basic laboratory studies which includes an hematocrit. Special studies may be required in the presence of head injuries. A toxicology screen is often helpful. Until type-specific or cross-matched blood is available, O-negative blood should be used for resuscitation. Hypovolemic shock should not be treated with vasopressors, steroids, or sodium bicarbonate.

Urinary (Cases 1 and 2) catheters and nasogastric catheters should be placed. Urinary catheterization should not be performed in patients with suspected urethral injury or transection because the catheter may cause further damage to the urethra. Urethral injury should be suspected if there is blood at the penile meatus or in the scrotum, or if the prostate is "high-riding" or cannot be palpated on rectal examination. The prostate is partially tethered in place by the urethra as it passes through the urogenital diaphragm; transection of the urethra will allow the prostate to retract superiorly into a "high-riding" position if downward traction is removed. If a urethral injury is suspected, a retrograde urethragram should be obtained prior to catheterization. Once the urinary catheter has been placed, urine should be examined for the presence of blood, which may indicate urogenital injury. Quantitation of urine output is a useful measure of circulatory status and may therefore be used to monitor resuscitation. A minimal 0.5 ml/kg/hr is indicative of satisfactory volume and cardiodynamic status in adult patients.

Nasogastric catheters are useful for evacuating stomach contents and relieving patient discomfort. Blood in the nasogastric aspiration may represent blood that has been swallowed, traumatic insertion, or trauma to the stomach (Case 1). A gastric suction tube should be inserted orally if a fracture of the (nasal) cribriform plate is possible or else the catheter may come to lie in the cerebral parenchyma.

Once resuscitation has begun, blood pressure, urine output, and pulse oximetry for arterial oxyhemoglobin saturation are useful measures for assessing the patient's response.

DIAGNOSIS

The secondary survey constitutes the principal diagnostic portion of initial trauma care. It is during this time that special radiography studies and diagnostic procedures are completed.

The diagnostic evaluation should begin with a history taken from the patient, family, or bystanders. The mechanism of injury and associated factors in blunt trauma include the use of seatbelts, vehicular damage, direction of impact, steering wheel deformation, presence of air bags, passenger space intrusion, and ejection from the automobile (Case 2). After penetrating injury, factors include caliber of the firearm used, distance from the weapon, trajectory, and type of gun (shotgun versus handgun). For stabbing victims, number of blows and length of the knife may be important.

A medical history should be obtained from the patient if conscious, or from the family if available. The following mnemonic may be used:

A	**A**llergies
M	**M**edications
P	**P**ast illnesses
L	**L**ast meal
E	**E**vents related to the injury

The complete physical examination performed during the diagnostic phase should begin at the head and progress distally. The following items should be addressed: visual acuity, use of contact lenses, pupil size and equality, hemorrhage, presence of penetrating injuries, associated head injury, palpable fractures, and scalp lacerations. Examination of the face should focus on orofacial trauma, changes in airway status, midface fractures, facial nerve injuries, and cervical spine injuries. Patients with maxillofacial or head trauma must be assumed to have an unstable cervical spine injury, until proved otherwise. Hence, the neck must be stabilized until such injuries can be excluded definitively. When penetrating trauma of the neck is present, injuries of the trachea or esophagus, or both, must be suspected. In these cases bronchoscopy and esophagoscopy along with contrast studies of the esophagus are mandatory. A missed tracheal injury may result in sudden airway compromise, while an undetected esophageal perforation may produce mediastinitis and overwhelming sepsis.

Evaluation of the chest and abdomen requires anteroposterior visualization. The patient must be "log-rolled" cautiously onto one side to permit posterior examination. The neck must be stabilized during this maneuver, to avoid potential cervical injuries. Lacerations and contusions should be noted. Paradoxic movement of one section of the chest constitutes a flail segment. Palpation of the entire rib cage for fractures and crepitance should arouse suspicion of underlying pulmonary parenchymal injury. Percussion, along with auscultation, should be performed to examine for the presence of a pneumothorax or tension pneumothorax. When a simple pneumothorax is present, breath sounds will be distant, and percussion will produce a dull beat. When the pleural cavity contains air under pressure (tension pneumothorax), the percussion beat will be hyperresonant, breath sounds distant, and the mediastinal structures (trachea and heart) displaced to the contralateral side. Although the primary survey includes evaluation for these entities, careful re-examination during the secondary survey is warranted.

Pericardial tamponade may occur when the cardiac chambers or coronary arteries are lacerated within a relatively intact pericardium. The cardiac chambers can no longer fill appropriately, and cardiac output is compromised acutely (see Ch. 4). Distended neck veins, tachycardia, and hypotension are hallmarks of pericardial tamponade.

Examination of the abdomen should include visualization, auscultation, and palpation. Pain may be poorly localized and of varying magnitude. Voluntary guarding may result from the patient's fear of pain on palpation. This finding should not be taken as indicative of significant injury. Involuntary guarding is usually indicative of severe intra-abdominal injury, however. Normal initial examination of the abdomen does not exclude a significant intra-abdominal injury, and careful re-examination after the primary survey is warranted. Special tests such as peritoneal lavage or computed tomography (CT) scanning may be required to exclude the possibility of solid organ rupture and intra-abdominal hemorrhage.

The pelvis and perineum should be examined for the possibility of pelvic fracture and associated injuries, such as perineal contusions, hematomas, lacerations, and urethral bleeding. A rectal examination with testing of the stool for occult blood is mandatory. Lack of anal sphincter tone may be indicative of severe spinal cord injury. Stability of the pelvis may be assessed crudely by pressing in on the iliac wings to determine whether laxity is present. Pelvic radiographs are required to evaluate the extent of such fracture.

The extremities should be inspected for deformity, hemorrhage, lacerations, and contusions. Fractures should be splinted and appropriate radiographic studies obtained. Distal pulses should be examined and recorded along with neurologic status. When a pulse is diminished, quality of the contralateral pulse should be determined to account for factors such as hypotension. When a pulse is absent, reduction of associated fractures may return the pulse to normal. Angiography is often required to determine the extent of the injury and to aid in planning definitive vascular repair.

Neurologic examination, including an abbreviated mental status assessment, is vital. The Glasgow Coma Score should be recorded at this time and repeated frequently in patients with multisystem injury (see Ch. 82). Any evidence of paralysis or paresis suggests injury to the peripheral nervous system and warrants further investigations. Complete immobilization of the patient's body is required until spinal injury is excluded. Changes in the patient's mental status may be due to intracranial bleeding and increased intracranial pressure. An emergent CT scan

of the brain is required to determine whether these lesions are present.

The trauma patient should be re-evaluated frequently during initial care to determine whether status has changed. This is particularly important when the level of consciousness is altered and/or when a head injury is present.

DIFFERENTIAL DIAGNOSIS

When the abdominal examination is equivocal or unreliable due to head injury or intoxicants, additional studies are required to diagnose injury and to differentiate between physical findings. Diagnostic peritoneal lavage and CT scanning are the two most common modalities used for multisystem injury in patients who have sustained blunt trauma (Case 2).

Because the abdomen may sequester large amounts of blood without outward signs of distention, diagnostic peritoneal lavage is a useful technique for determining the presence of intra-abdominal hemorrhage. The technique has a 98% sensitivity rate. The procedure is performed by making a small midline infraumbilical incision, under local anesthesia. It is carried through the skin and fascia to the peritoneum, which is opened to give free access to the celomic cavity. A soft plastic catheter is then inserted, under direct vision to avoid inadvertent injury to bowel and omentum; 1 L of balanced salt solution (10 ml/kg in children) is rapidly instilled. The fluid container is then placed on the floor, and the fluid allowed to return under its own pressure. At least 750 ml of return must be collected to make the study valid. Criteria for a positive diagnostic peritoneal lavage include any of the following: red blood cell (RBC) count greater then 100,000 cells/mm^3, white blood cell (WBC) count greater than 500 cells/mm^3, or the presence of bacteria or bile in the lavage fluid. Because of their retroperitoneal location, injuries to the kidneys and duodenum may not be detected by diagnostic peritoneal lavage unless the overlying peritoneum has been disrupted. Fractures of the pelvis frequently cause peritoneal injury and may allow blood to enter the abdominal cavity, resulting in a false positive lavage.

Relative contraindications to the performance of a diagnostic peritoneal lavage include previous operations (because of scarring and fibrous bands, which may increase the risk of iatrogenic injury and decrease the sensitivity of the test), morbid obesity, advanced cirrhosis, and established coagulopathy. The use of diagnostic peritoneal lavage in pregnant patients is controversial.

CT scanning may also be used for the differential diagnosis of intra-abdominal injury. Unlike diagnostic peritoneal lavage, it provides specific anatomic information about the location of injury and semiquantitates the degree of hemorrhage present. CT scan requires transportation of the patient away from the emergency department and mandates a hemodynamically and neurologically stable patient. Both oral (dilute Hypaque) and intravenous contrast are used to increase the accuracy of the study. However, CT may miss hollow viscus gastrointestinal injuries. Therefore, in the absence of liver or splenic injuries, the presence of free fluid in the abdominal cavity suggests an injury to the gastrointestinal tract.

KEY POINTS

- Diagnostic peritoneal lavage is a useful technique for determining presence of intra-abdominal hemorrhage, as abdomen may sequester large amounts of blood without outward signs of distention
- Criteria for positive diagnostic peritoneal lavage: RBC count greater than 100,000 cells/mm^3, WBC count greater than 500 cells/mm^3, or presence of bacteria or bile in lavage fluid

---

TREATMENT

The organs injured after blunt trauma are different from those damaged after penetrating trauma. The solid organs—liver, spleen, and kidneys—are involved most frequently (Case 2), although hollow viscera such as the small bowel, stomach, and colon may be affected, especially if they are caught between the spine and the source of the blunt injury (e.g., the steering wheel). Blunt tears may also occur in the diaphragm typically on the left, as well as posterolaterally. The position of the nasogastric tube on a plain chest radiograph is the best diagnostic tool; CT scans are notoriously insensitive for detecting diaphragmatic injury. At laparotomy, repair can usually be accomplished by simple approximation and suture of the defect.

Gastric injuries are usually in the form of "blowouts" that occur when the trauma occurred shortly after eating or drinking. Contamination of the peritoneal cavity with gastric contents occasionally leads to delayed peritonitis. Repair consists of debridement of any devitalized gastric wall, reapproximation, and suture. In some instances, a partial gastrectomy may be required. Duodenal rupture occurs after frontal impact or as a result of striking bicycle or motorcycle handlebars. Blood aspirated from the nasogastric tube should arouse suspicion and prompt an oral contrast-enhanced CT scan. As opposed to duodenal rupture, submucosal duodenal hematomas in

the first or second portion of the duodenum are common. Initial CT scanning may not demonstrate the lesion, which presents several days after the injury as a mechanical obstruction. Patients report bloating shortly after eating and frequently vomit. Although liquids are tolerated better than solids, patients are seldom able to take enough by mouth to maintain adequate protein/calorie balance and supplemental nutrition (hyperalimentation) is required. The lesion is usually self-limiting and resorbs within a few weeks.

Pancreatic injuries are not uncommon and most typically occur when a direct blow compresses the organ against a vertebral body. Contusions, lacerations, and complete transections may occur. CT scanning is usually diagnostic, although endoscopic retrograde cholangiopancreatography (ERCP) may be required. When a laceration or transection is present, partial (distal) pancreatectomy may be required. Fortunately, most injuries occur distal to the midportion of the gland and do not involve the mesenteric vessels.

Upper genitourinary injuries result from direct trauma to the back or flank and cause contusions and hematomas of the kidney. When the force is sufficiently severe, renal transection may occur. In general, isolated renal injuries do not require operation unless there is evidence of renal artery injury with ischemia of the kidney (see Ch. 77).

Injuries of the small bowel and colon take place when loops of the hollow viscus are trapped between the vertebral column and the offending force. While complete distruption of a bowel segment can occur, it is infrequent. More commonly, a portion of the bowel wall is contused, and a segment of its mesentery is avulsed, resulting in segmental ischemia. These lesions are very hard to diagnose preoperatively; patients usually come to operation because of progressive abdominal findings or severe pain out of proportion to their physical examination. When frank perforation occurs, diagnostic peritoneal lavage may be useful in making the diagnosis. Repair is straightforward and consists of segmental resection and primary repair of the small bowel. When the colon has been injured and stool spillage has occurred, most surgeons opt for resection with a diverting colostomy, which can be taken down and primary anastomosis created within several months. If minimal damage to the colon has occurred, primary repair may be possible, although this should not be attempted if the patient has been hypotensive or if there are associated intra-abdominal injuries.

The spleen is the most frequently injured solid abdominal viscus (Case 2). Splenic injuries are common following impact and should be suspected when left-sided rib fractures are present. Patients with frank splenic rupture are hypotensive and difficult to resuscitate. Less severe splenic injury may present with modest hypotension that is rapidly corrected with fluid infusion. Splenic injuries are graded I to V. A grade I splenic injury is a simple capsular laceration that usually has stopped bleeding by the time exploration is undertaken. Grades II to IV involve progressively greater degrees of splenic parenchymal disruption, while a grade V injury includes the splenic hilum and vessels. Nonoperative therapy is warranted for patients whose CT scans exhibit minor splenic injury and who remain hemodynamically stable. Splenic salvage (splenorrhaphy) at laparotomy consists of tamponade and repair of the injured spleen. It is typically used with lesser grades of injury in which bleeding can be controlled easily. Complete splenectomy is the treatment of choice for badly injured spleens (grades IV and V) and for patients with multiple associated injuries. It is unwise to attempt splenic repair when gastrointestinal injuries are present because of the danger of postoperative infection.

Liver injuries are similar to splenic injuries and have a comparable grading system. Nonoperative management of hepatic trauma is warranted for lower grades of injury when the patient is hemodynamically stable, as well as for children. In some instances, the hepatic veins that connect the liver to the inferior vena cava may be torn. In these cases, hemorrhage is profound, and hypotension may not be reversible during resuscitation. Hepatic vein injuries carry a mortality rate approaching 100%. When isolated segments of the liver are injured, segmental hepatic resection is undertaken with excellent results.

KEY POINTS

- In blunt trauma, solid organs—liver, spleen, and kidneys—most frequently involved

- With frank hollow viscus perforation, diagnostic peritoneal lavage may be useful in diagnosis

- Spleen most frequently injured solid abdominal viscus—patients may be hypotensive and difficult to resuscitate; less severe splenic injury may present with modest hypotension rapidly corrected with fluid infusion

- Nonoperative therapy warranted when CT scans show minor splenic injury and when patient hemodynamically stable

- Complete splenectomy treatment of choice for badly injured spleen

SUGGESTED READINGS

Advanced Trauma Life Support Student Manual. 5th Ed. American College of Surgeons Committee on Trauma, Chicago, 1993

The single best reference on the management of the trauma patient. This book is published by the American College of Surgeons as part of a training course for nonsurgical practitioners. Students interested in emergency medicine are urged to take this course and secure a copy of the manual.

Moore EE, Mattox KL, Feliciano DV (eds): Trauma. 3rd Ed. Appleton & Lange, E. Norwalk, CT, 1993

A lengthy detailed textbook on trauma written by a number of distinguished authors. It contains virtually everything you would want to know about the topic.

Trunkey DD, Lewis FR (ed): Current Therapy of Trauma. 3rd Ed. BC Decker, Philadelphia

A good, readable work on trauma that contains most of the basic needed by house officers.

QUESTIONS

1. *The single most important item to address in the initial management of a trauma patient is?*
   A. Airway.
   B. Breathing.
   C. Circulation.
   D. Head injury.

2. *Following injury, circulation is best restored with?*
   A. D_5W.
   B. Lactated Ringer's solution.
   C. D_5NS.
   D. Albumin.

3. *Blood at the tip of the urethral meatus in a man?*
   A. Indicates the need for immediate catheter placement.
   B. Dictates mandatory CT scan.
   C. May be indicative of a urethral injury.
   D. Is usually from a renal injury.

4. *Which of the following is not a criterion for positive diagnostic peritoneal lavage?*
   A. >100,000 RBC/mm^3.
   B. >500 WBC/mm^3.
   C. Amylase >150 IU.
   D. Presence of bile.

(See p. 603 for answers.)

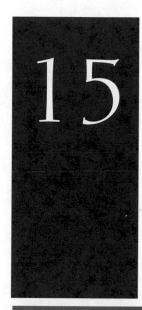

15

ESOPHAGEAL

MOTILITY

DISORDERS AND

DIVERTICULA

EDWARD PASSARO, JR.

Derangement of the propulsive activity or of the sphincteric mechanisms guarding the upper and lower ends of the esophagus leads to profound changes in individuals' ability to swallow and therefore nourish themselves. Dysphagia, or difficulty in swallowing, is an ominous complaint, very rarely exaggerated or misrepresented by the patient, and should alert the physician that there is a serious, if not life-threatening disorder involving the esophagus. A history of difficulty in swal-

lowing solids and/or liquids demands prompt and thorough investigation to find the cause so that prompt treatment may be started and adequate swallowing and food intake can be restored.

CASE 1
ZENKER'S DIVERTICULUM

A 75-year-old male complained of mild dysphagia. He noted from time to time that the "food didn't go down normally." He would occasionally choke or sputter while eating. The dysphagia was not accompanied by pain. Near the end of his meal he would occasionally regurgitate some food particles recently eaten. There was no associ-

ated nausea. He also noted that increasingly he would be awakened at night because of coughing. He found this particularly disturbing. Occasionally, food particles were present in the sputum. He had lost no weight and had not changed his eating habits. He did note that he was more careful to chew his food thoroughly before swallowing.

His physician found no abnormalities of the mouth or neck on physical examination. He was referred for an esophagoscopy, which was reported as normal. Next, a swallow of a thickened barium preparation under cinefluoroscopy showed a cricopharyngeal diverticulum (Zenker's diverticulum). Operation was advised to prevent further bouts of aspiration. The large diverticulum in the left neck was excised. Following discharge he experienced no further dysphagia or nocturnal coughing episodes.

CASE 2
ACHALASIA

A 55-year-old female was seen for progressive difficulty in swallowing solid foods over the past 4 months. She first noted that on eating the evening meal she would experience some lower substernal discomfort. Initially this would be relieved by drinking a glass of water. As her symptoms progressed she took to cutting her meat into smaller pieces, which initially helped. Gradually, however, they produced the same subxyphoid and substernal distress that was not adequately relieved by a drink of water. She was now convinced that her food could get down to here (pointing to her xyphoid) where it tended to get stuck. Her diet had changed imperceptibly to softer foods eaten in smaller meals. She had lost 25 lb of weight, for which she was in some ways grateful. Her energy and vitality were not appreciably altered.

Her physician could find no masses or lymphadenopathy on examination. He scheduled an esophagoscopy. The latter showed a thickened, dilated esophagus throughout with a reddened, slightly edematous mucosa at the distal end of the esophagus. The endoscope was advanced into the stomach, which was normal. Biopsies of the reddened distal esophagus showed only normal tissue with mild inflammation.

It was recommended that she have a Heller procedure done. At operation, esophagoscopy was done while the surgeon exposed the lower 8 cm of the esophagus and the gastric cardia through the laparoscope. A long esophageal myotomy was done, cutting across the cardioesophageal sphincter. Both the endoscopist and the surgeon noted the esophageal mucosa, which was not cut, to herniate or "pout" through the esophageal incision. The esophagus now appeared capacious. She was discharged the following day and 2 months later had regained 20 lb and experienced no further dysphagia.

GENERAL CONSIDERATIONS

The esophagus connects the mouth and the stomach beginning at about the sixth cervical vertebrae and ending just below the diaphragm, where it blends into the stomach. Most of the esophagus is intrathoracic, where it passes behind the bronchus just to the left of the carina. The esophagus is a muscular tube, a flattened H in shape in the resting state, lined by stratified squamous epithelium. Scattered throughout the epithelium are mucus glands serving as a lubricating mechanism. The surrounding muscle layer does not have a serosal covering like the remainder of the gastrointestinal tract. This lack of a serosal layer, among other things, is a major reason why operations on the esophagus involving an anastomosis are prone to leak or disruption.

The muscular coats of the esophagus give it distinct anatomic and physiologic features. Muscle fibers from the cricoid cartilage and pharynx covering the upper third of the esophagus are voluntarily controlled striated muscle. The distal two-thirds of the esophagus is smooth muscle under involuntary control. Thus, while we can initiate swallowing to a point (try swallowing more than 20 times!) the action is primarily involuntary (you can swallow as much liquid or food as your stomach can hold; your esophagus does not tire). This smooth, coordinated activity between striated and smooth muscle fibers to propel contents down the lumen into the stomach is only minimally understood. The inner circular muscle and outer longitudinal muscle layer, whether striated or smooth, act in an intricately coordinated fashion as a single physiologic unit.

Normally, when swallowing solid food, the tongue presses against the palate, pushing the food into the pharynx where a coordinated, voluntary swallowing action begins. There is closure of the glottis so as to protect the airway. Respiration is suspended and the normal high resting pressure at the pharyngoesophageal sphincter rapidly relaxes and the food bolus enters the esophagus. The food bolus initiates a complex peristaltic wave, relaxing the esophagus immediately in front of the bolus, while contracting the circular muscle fibers immediately behind the bolus. This propels the bolus of food toward the stomach at approximately 4–6 cm/sec. When we are upright, gravity causes liquids and many foods to fall more rapidly than peristalsis can propel them. However, peristalsis is sufficiently powerful to permit swallowing of solids and liquids even when we are standing on our heads, with gravity acting against the swallowing mechanism.

The wave of contraction—beginning with food entering the upper esophagus and sweeping down the entire length of the esophagus to the stomach—is called primary peristalsis. When food becomes lodged at some point in the esophagus, the local distention will stimulate a series of peristaltic waves beginning at that point, called secondary peristalsis. The latter is designed to aid in clearing the esophagus either of ingested food or of gastric contents, which may reflux back into the esophagus when there is relaxation or failure of the cardioesophageal sphincter. Such secondary peristaltic waves are generally perceived by the individual, while primary peristalsis does not occur unless the food bolus is unduly hot or cold. Nonpropulsive contractions, occurring locally or throughout the esophagus, are called tertiary and are considered to be abnormal. They may, however, be present in elderly patients who are asymptomatic.

The neural integration of swallowing and esophageal propulsion are only partially understood. The swallowing reflux originates in the medulla oblongata, while the pharyngeal and esophageal propulsion are innervated by motor branches from the 5th, 7th, 9th, 10th, 11th, and 12th cranial nerves. The relative importance of these nerves and the local myogenic mechanisms involved in peristaltic activity are unknown.

The major tool in understanding esophageal physiology is manometry. This is done by passing a bundle of three fine polyethylene catheters with open ports 5 cm apart. The catheters are constantly and gently perfused with a saline solution to ensure their patency and are connected to manometers and recording devices. By passing the bundle the length of the esophagus, normal high pressure zones at both the upper and lower ends can be seen, with an intervening lower pressure region in the intrathoracic portion of the esophagus. When the bundle is positioned in the mid-esophagus, and swallowing is initiated, a normal pressure tracing and transit can be ascertained (Fig. 15.1). Manometric studies help determine the location and type of peristaltic abnormality encountered. These studies are occasionally used in conjunction with cinefluorography. Endoscopy is almost always done to determine the nature of the pathologic process by obtaining visualization and by biopsies.

> ### KEY POINTS
>
> • Major tool in understanding esophageal physiology is manometry, done by passing bundle of three fine polyethylene catheters with open ports 5 cm apart; catheters constantly and gently perfused with saline solution to ensure patency and connected to manometers and recording devices
>
> • By passing the bundle the length of esophagus, normal high pressure zones at both upper and lower ends can be seen, with an intervening lower pressure region in intrathoracic portion of esophagus

DIAGNOSIS

Dysphagia from cricopharyngeal sphincter dysfunction occurs mainly in individuals over 60 years of age. The dysphagia develops immediately on swallowing, particularly solids. Coughing and sputtering are common, as the dysmotility causes minor degrees of aspiration of both food and saliva. The pathophysiology is related to either an incomplete relaxation of the cricopharyngeal sphincter, or incoordination between the swallowing mechanism and the sphincter. A cinefluoroscopic study of a barium swallow shows a hesitant passage of the contrast, often due to what appears to be a mechanical obstruction from the contracting pharyngeal musculature at the lower end of the pharynx. Aspiration may be seen. Manometry, which is more difficult at the proximal sphincter, confirms the lack of coordination between the swallow and the relaxation of the sphincter.

At the other end of the esophagus, achalasia, a primary failure of the cardioesophageal sphincter to relax in response to swallowing, can occur. This neuromuscular disorder's etiology is unknown. The dysmotility produces dilatation of the proximal esophagus and hypertrophy of the sphincter, particularly of the circular muscle.

Because of the dysmotility, which results in a functional but not in an organic obstruction, the patients experience dysphagia (Case 2). In particular, the history is one of a progressive difficulty, first in swallowing solid materials such as a bolus of meat or bread, and progressively in difficulty in handling large quantities of liquids. Patients can generally localize the pain or discomfort to the distal

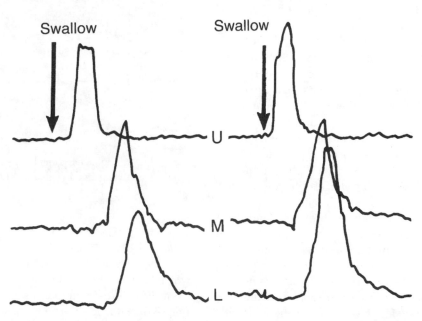

FIGURE 15.1 *Deglutition. Normal esophageal peristaltic waves and pressures during consecutive swallows. Note the orderly downward progression of the waves. U, upper; M, mid; L, lower.*

end of the esophagus by pointing to the area of the xyphoid or slightly above. Discomfort and pain from distention are common, and are usually followed by regurgitation. Obstruction may be accompanied by vigorous esophageal contractions, producing a substernal pain.

Passage of a nasogastric tube down the esophagus and into the stomach, if possible, should be the initial investigation. The presence of large quantities of fluid in the mid-esophagus with undigested food particles passing through the tube confirms the diagnosis of esophageal obstruction. The esophagus should be gently lavaged with saline, and endoscopy should be done. Esophagoscopy generally reveals a dilated esophagus with a smooth aperture at the lower esophagus through which the instrument can be advanced (Case 2). This distinguishes it as a physiologic obstruction, rather than a mechanical obstruction from a malignancy of either the distal esophagus or proximal stomach.

Although a barium esophagram is commonly done, it is less helpful than esophagoscopy and potentially dangerous due to the risk of aspiration. A very characteristic esophagram is that of a proximal dilated esophagus, which symmetrically tapers at its lower portion to a thin smooth stream entering into the stomach.

Manometry shows a very characteristic dysmotility pattern. The peristaltic activity in the body of the esophagus is disorganized if not absent. In particular, primary peristaltic waves are absent. One of the theories of achalasia formation is intrinsic autonomic denervation of the distal esophagus. These patients are sensitive to stimulation with bethanechol, which produces a strong contraction of the esophagus, often accompanied by brief but severe pain.

The pain from diffuse esophageal spasm is substernal and sustained; hence ischemic cardiac disease must always be considered in the differential diagnosis. Fluoroscopic and manometric studies are diagnostic for diffuse esophageal spasm. Esophagoscopy is done to rule out an inflammatory process such as esophagitis or a tumor responsible for the pain and dysmotility. Treatment varies according to the severity of the symptoms. Many patients can be managed with long-acting nitrates or anticholinergic drugs. Severe or refractory forms of the disease are treated by a long myotomy. Clinically esophageal motility disorders can be confused with reflux esophagitis and myocardial infarction.

Reflux esophagitis can produce chronic inflammatory changes at the lower esophagus. Patients experience dysphagia because of the dysmotility induced by the inflammation. A good history aids in the differential, as patients with chronic reflux esophagitis usually report improvement in their symptoms by avoiding alcohol, smoking, and certain foods and by taking antacid medications. Esophagoscopy shows the lower end of the esophagus to be severely inflamed and edematous. Biopsies will show severe

imflammatory changes and metaplasia of the luminal epithelium (Barrett's epithelium).

Not infrequently the esophageal disease is mistaken for angina, as diffuse esophageal spasm or pain mimics the substernal distress of angina. Sublingual nitroglycerin tablets cause the prompt relief of symptoms from angina but not esophageal disease. Most importantly, patients with esophageal motility disorders will have had several attacks in the past. Myocardial infarction will seldom occur as often, and the anginal attacks thereafter are generally treated with sublingual nitroglycerin successfully. Esophageal motility studies are of help in the differentiation.

The most important differential is between achalasia and cancer at the cardioesophageal junction. Esophagoscopy and biopsy is the most direct and expeditious route to diagnosis.

Scleroderma can also present as achalasia. Biopsy of the lower esophagus aids in the differential.

KEY POINTS

- Dysphagia from cricopharyngeal sphincter dysfunction occurs mainly in individuals over 60 years of age; develops immediately on swallowing, particularly solids

- Coughing and sputtering are common, as dysmotility causes minor degrees of aspiration of food and saliva

- Pathophysiology related to either incomplete relaxation of cricopharyngeal sphincter, or incoordination between swallowing mechanism and sphincter

- Passage of nasogastric tube down esophagus and into stomach, if possible, should be initial investigation

- Presence of large quantities of fluid in mid-esophagus with undigested food particles passing through the tube confirms diagnosis of esophageal obstruction

- Esophagus should be gently lavaged with saline, and endoscopy done

- Esophagoscopy generally reveals a dilated esophagus with a smooth aperture at the lower esophagus through which the instrument can be advanced

- Manometry shows very characteristic dysmotility pattern; peristaltic activity in the body of esophagus is disorganized if not absent

- Reflux esophagitis can produce chronic inflammatory changes at the lower esophagus; patients experience dysphagia because of dysmotility induced by inflammation

TREATMENT

The operation of choice is a Heller procedure, in which a longitudinal myotomy is carried out, extending from the inferior pulmonary vein down to the upper portion of the stomach. The approach can be through the thorax or the abdomen, but currently is being done with increasing frequency as a combined laparoscopic approach with esophagoscopy control. The esophageal incision is carried through all the muscle layers until the mucosa is seen "pouting" between the severed muscular ends. The object of the procedure is to render the cardioesophageal sphincter incompetent. Thus, esophageal reflux may occur postoperatively. For this reason, many surgeons incorporate a Nissen fundoplication in conjunction with the Heller procedure, in order to avoid the postoperative complication of reflux. The other complication is inadvertent perforation of the esophageal mucosa with a subsequent esophageal leak. However done, the Heller myotomy is effective in relieving the obstruction and giving good to excellent results in 85% of patients. When done through the laparoscopic approach, the postoperative morbidity is extremely low so that patients experience a near normal passage of food through the esophagus almost immediately.

Therapy is directed at relieving the physiologic obstruction by disrupting the abnormal sphincter. In the past, attempts at frequent dilatations with a variety of esophageal dilatators have been done. Although these produce transient relief of symptoms they have been consistently ineffective in permanent alleviation of the physiologic obstruction. More recently, forceful dilatation of the esophageal gastric junction with pneumatic balloon devices has provided longer relief of symptoms, but has failed in most patients. All prospective comparative studies have demonstrated the efficacy of surgery over other treatment modalities.

KEY POINTS

• Operation of choice is a Heller procedure, in which longitudinal myotomy is carried out, extending from inferior pulmonary vein down to upper portion of stomach

• Approach can be through thorax or abdomen, but currently done with increasing frequency as a combined laparoscopic approach with esophagoscopy control

• The esophageal incision is carried through all the muscle layers until the mucosa is seen "pouting" between the severed muscular ends

---

DIFFUSE ESOPHAGEAL SPASM

The motility disorder affecting the mid-portion (if not the entire esophagus) is diffuse esophageal spasm. The patients note dysphagia shortly after initiating swallowing.

Manometric studies show sustained forceful or high amplitude contractions that are not propulsive. Contrast fluoroscopic studies show areas of esophageal narrowing from spastic disordered contractions producing a "corkscrew esophagus" appearance. Some patients with diffuse esophageal spasm have a concomitant motility disorder of the cardioesophageal junction (achalasia), suggesting that a common pathologic mechanism is responsible for both disorders.

KEY POINTS

• The motility disorder affecting the mid-portion of the esophagus is diffuse esophageal spasm; patients note dysphagia shortly after initiating swallowing

---

SUGGESTED READINGS

Chakkaphak S, Chakkaphak K, Ferguson MK: Disorders of esophageal motility. Surg Gynecol Obstet 172:325, 1991

Massey BT, Dodos WJ, Hogan WJ et al: Abnormal esophageal motility: an analysis of concurrent radiographic and manometric findings. Gastroenterology 101:344, 1991

An excellent review of our current understanding of the etiology and interpretation of these diagnostic modalities.

QUESTIONS

1. An acute patient complaint of dysphagia is best managed by?

    A. A careful head and neck examination followed by CT.

    B. Indirect laryngoscopy.

    C. A barium swallow preferably with fluoroscopy.

    D. Esophagoscopy with biopsy of any lesions.

2. Complaints of pressure sensation and substernal pain can be found in?

    A. Esophageal disease.

    B. Cardiac disease.

    C. Peptic ulcer disease.

    D. All of the above.

(See p. 603 for answers.)

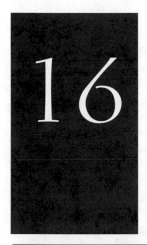

16

HIATAL HERNIA AND REFLUX ESOPHAGITIS

EDWARD PASSARO, JR.

Hiatal hernia and esophagitis are important conditions in both infants and adults. The pharmaceutical industry has directed much effort to treat these diseases because they are common.

This chapter presents the forms of hiatal hernia and esophagitis and their sequelae.

CASE 1
PARAESOPHAGEAL HERNIA

A 72-year-old male was seen because of substernal pain and pressure within an hour after eating. He also reported recent gas and bloating, but no nausea or vomiting. There had been no weight loss, and his vigor and exercise tolerance were not diminished. An ECG and creatinine phosphokinase enzymes were normal both in the basal state and postprandial. Because of a mild anemia and guaiac positive stools a total colonoscopy was done and was normal. A UGI showed a portion of the stomach present in the left chest; however, the gastroesophageal junction was noted to be below the diaphragm. Esophagoscopy revealed an inflamed lower esophagus. With some difficulty the scope was inserted into a shortened gastric lumen and then, guided by the findings on the UGI, the scope was turned back to look at the fundic portion herniated into the chest. The edge of a gastric ulcer was seen and biopsied at about the level of the diaphragm. When the scope entered into the herniated portion of the stomach, a moderate amount of "coffee ground" secretions were aspirated. Subsequently, the biopsies of the gastric ulcer were reported as benign. At operation, a portion of the posterior wall of the fundus was found herniated through a 5-cm defect in the diaphragm to the

left posterior lateral aspect of the cardioesophageal junction. On reducing the herniated stomach, a 1.5-cm ulcer was found where the stomach lay over the edge of the diaphragm. The ulcer was excised, the defect in the diaphragm repaired, and the stomach anchored to the anterior abdominal wall where a gastrostomy was fashioned. Following recovery from his operation he had no distress on eating and his Hct returned to normal levels.

CASE 2
REFLUX ESOPHAGITIS AND
BARRETT'S ESOPHAGUS

A 48-year-old female noted the gradual onset of substernal pain shortly after starting a meal. Coincidentally she noticed heartburn, primarily at night, after retiring to bed. Although she had gained some 20 lb following the onset of menopause 3 years earlier, she had begun to lose weight in the past 2 months. Her Hct was normal and her stools were guaiac negative. Ultrasonography of the gallbladder did not reveal any stones. Chest and abdominal films were normal. After a 4-week course of elevating the head of the bed administering H₂ receptor antagonists and liquid antacid therapy she had minimal relief of symptoms. There was no further weight loss. Esophagoscopy showed marked inflammation of the lower 6 cm of the esophagus. Biopsies of the inflamed region disclosed the presence of Barrett's epithelium and operation was advised. Preoperative esophageal manometry and pH monitoring showed the LES pressure to be approximately 5 mmHg and the pH to be 3. A Nissen fundoplication was done. At follow-up 6 months later the pressure was 12 mm Hg and pH 7. The patient was asymptomatic and the esophagus appeared to be grossly normal. Repeat biopsies, however, showed the presence of Barrett's epithelium and repeat EGD was recommended initially at 6-month intervals.

GENERAL CONSIDERATIONS

The lower esophagus has a physiologic sphincter mechanism to maintain a relatively high (15–20 mmHg) resting pressure. The sphincter is important in maintaining a barrier to gastric contents, so that food and/or acid secretions from the stomach do not reflux back into the esophagus. A number of agents including alcohol, tobacco, chocolate, and mints may cause the lower esophageal sphincter (LES) to relax and the pressure to fall, so that reflux of gastric contents into the lower esophagus may occur. In general, such LES relaxation is common and even beneficial, as for example, following eating. A few mints after a large meal can promote the eructation of swallowed air. This relieves the full or bloated sensation after a particularly large feast. Similarly, while reflux of food or acidic gastric contents into the lower esophagus occurs naturally several times during the course of a day, the pH is normally restored to neutral promptly by the swallowing of saliva and the peristaltic activity of the esophagus.

Hiatal hernias may present with symptoms of esophageal reflux and, conversely, esophageal reflux disease often is associated with hiatal hernia. Hiatal hernias mostly are asymptomatic. There are two types of hiatal hernia. The most common by far (90%) is a sliding hiatal hernia where, as the name implies, a portion of the proximal stomach has herniated or slid into the chest (Fig. 16.1A). As a consequence, the cardioesophageal junction is displaced into the chest as well. Sliding hiatal hernias are most often discovered incidentally during investigations for other causes. They are thought to occur with increasing age and obesity.

The rarer form of hiatal hernia is a paraesophageal hernia (Fig. 16.1B). Here the cardioesophageal junction may be below the diaphragm in its normal position and,

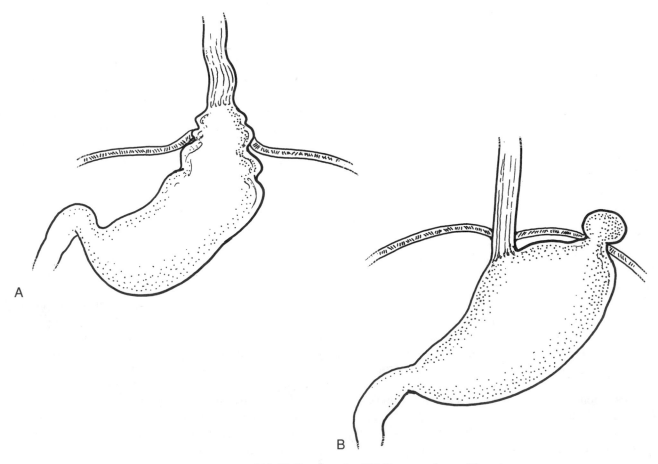

FIGURE 16.1   *(A) Sliding hernia. (B) Paraesophageal hernia.*

beyond it (*para* is Greek for "beyond"), a portion of the stomach is herniated through a diaphragmatic defect. The patient described in Case 1 has a typical paraesophageal hernia. These hernias may be present for long periods and can involve from only a small portion up to the entire stomach (the so-called upside-down stomach, as it is inverted about the horizontal axis when it comes to lie entirely in the chest), and can produce surprisingly little or no symptoms until a complication occurs. The usual complication is incarceration of the herniated stomach, producing symptoms of obstruction such as substernal pain and bloating (Case 1).

In turn, the incarceration of the herniated stomach produces distention, ischemia, and ulceration. The patient presented in Case 1 experienced these changes, culminating in the formation of a gastric ulcer, which was bleeding and responsible for his anemia. This complication may be severe, as when the ulcer perforates into the hernia sac found within the chest or when it erodes through the gastric wall into the diaphragm. In these instances the herniated stomach may be very difficult to reduce into the abdominal cavity. A symptomatic paraesophageal hernia is a surgical emergency.

Reflux esophagitis can occur without the presence of a hiatal hernia (Case 2). The reason for the apparent loss of the normal LES resting pressure and the reflux of gastric contents is not known; recognized provocative, if not causative, factors are alcohol, tobacco, and obesity, as noted above.

Chronic irritation of the esophageal mucosa by reflux of acid and pepsin (or even alkaline secretions) from the stomach can lead to the development of metaplasia of the epithelium. Whereas the normal esophagus is lined by a flattened, squamous epithelium, metaplastic changes produce a columnar glandular epithelia that resembles the lining of the stomach. In fact, following the initial description of these changes it was thought that there was a proliferation and progression of gastric endothelium up into denuded regions of the inflamed lower esophagus. Subsequent studies have shown instead that Barrett's epithelium represents a transformation of squamous epithelium into columnar epithelium. The involvement of metaplastic changes may range from minimal areas to the entire esophagus. Similarly, the histologic changes seen in biopsies may range from regular, well-organized cellular elements to marked dysplasia. Ultimately these changes can lead to the formation of malignancy (adenocarcinoma.) Barrett's esophagus or epithelium is therefore an important prognostic factor for subsequent malignant degeneration. That is why the patient in Case 2 was followed by repeat endoscopic examinations.

KEY POINTS

- Lower esophagus has a physiologic sphincter mechanism to maintain high resting pressure (15–20 mmHg)

- Although reflux of food and acidic gastric contents into lower esophagus occurs several times a day, pH is neutralized by swallowing saliva and peristaltic activity of esophagus

- Most common hiatal hernia (90%) is sliding hiatal hernia, which occurs when a portion of proximal stomach herniates, or slides, into chest, causing cardioesophageal junction to be displaced into chest as well

- Rarer hiatal hernia is paraesophageal (Fig. 16.1B); cardioesophageal junction may be below diaphragm in its normal position and, beyond it, a portion of stomach is herniated through diaphragmatic defect; a symptomatic paraesophageal hernia is a surgical emergency

- Reflux esophagitis can occur without hiatal hernia

- Chronic irritation of esophageal mucosa by reflux of acid and pepsin (or even alkaline bile) from the stomach can cause metaplasia of epithelium to develop

- Barrett's epithelium represents transformation of squamous epithelium into columnar epithelium; is an important prognostic factor for subsequent malignant degeneration

DIAGNOSIS

Reflux esophagitis is usually suggested by the history of substernal pain on eating associated with episodes of heartburn and the reflux of gastric contents ("water brash") or food. In particular, the relationship of reflux to positional changes such as lying down at night or bending over to tie one's shoes is very characteristic. Recent weight gain may exacerbate the symptoms. Symptoms associated with Barrett's epithelium are particularly difficult to treat medically and therefore suggest a severe chronic form of the disease. By contrast, the reflux esophagitis that accompanies a sliding hiatal hernia is milder in form and responds more favorably to simple medical measures for treatment.

The diagnosis is best established by esophagogastroscopy. All patients suspected of having reflux esophagitis should undergo esophagogastroduodenoscopy (EGD). EGD not only establishes the diagnosis based on the findings of a reddened, inflamed, distal esophageal mucosa but also is important in ascertaining the stage of the disease, both by biopsy and by noting the presence or absence of strictures or overt malignancy. Barrett's epithelium itself, however, is seldom recognized on inspection but should be suspected when the inflammatory process in the esophagus is severe, particularly after trials of medical therapy. Thus, biopsy should always be taken of the involved portions of the esophagus, as the incidence of malignancy is some 20-fold greater in patients with Barrett's esophagus than those without.

Esophageal manometry and pH measurements over a 24-hour period have been described and advocated by investigators of this disease. However, such a level of investigation is neither accepted nor tolerated by most patients and serves to confirm but hardly ever suggests the diagnosis. In a typical patient suffering from reflux, there is usually a lower resting LES pressure (Case 2) and when it is below 10 mmHg, Barrett's changes are more common. Additionally, the pH is below 5 for long periods throughout both the day and night, both with the patient erect and recumbent.

The presence or absence, as well as the differentiation of a sliding hernia from a paraesophageal hernia is best done by an upper gastrointestinal barium contrast study (UGI) series. Although endoscopy may suggest the presence of either a sliding or a paraesophageal hernia, it commonly misses the sliding hernia and it may be difficult to detect a paraesophageal hernia. The UGI series is helpful to the endoscopist in attempting to visualize and inspect the herniated portion of the stomach (Case 1).

Rare congenital forms of diaphragmatic hernia can occur behind the sternum (Morgagni) or in the dorsal lateral aspects of the diaphragm (Bochdalek's hernia). They are best diagnosed by UGI series.

KEY POINTS

• Symptoms associated with Barrett's epithelium difficult to treat medically, and suggest a severe form of this disease

• Diagnosis best established by esophagogastroscopy

• Biopsy always taken of involved portions of esophagus, as malignancy is 20 times greater in patients with Barrett's esophagus than those without

• Presence or absence, and differentiation of sliding hernia from paraesophageal hernia best done by UGI series

---

DIFFERENTIAL DIAGNOSIS

Patients with angina or evolving myocardial infarction can have symptoms identical to those in patients with reflux esophagitis. Thus, ruling out significant myocardial disease is the most important consideration when establishing the diagnosis of reflux esophagitis (Case 1). A carefully taken history of pain related to exercise and unrelated to eating, decreased vigor and exercise tolerance, arrythmias and episodes of dyspnea, suggest cardiac disease rather than primary esophageal disease. Serial ECGs and creatinine phosphokinase serum and enzymes may help differentiate the two conditions. The response to sublingual nitroglycerin tablets is equivocal in both cardiac patients as well as esophageal disease patients, as both may obtain transient but definite relief.

Rarely, when the diagnosis cannot be clearly established, perfusing the lower esophagus with a dilute solution of hydrochloric acid (Bernstein test) will reproduce the patient's symptoms, whereas a saline solution as a control does not.

Other diagnoses to be considered are biliary tract disease and peptic ulcer disease. The location of the pain and its temporal relationship to eating may be mimicked by biliary tract disease. In particular, stones in the common bile duct may produce epigastric pain rather than the more typical right upper quadrant pain produced by most gallbladder stones. Ultrasonography is helpful (Case 2).

Endoscopy, which is done to confirm the diagnosis of reflux esophagitis as well as to grade the severity of the disease, also serves to detect unsuspected peptic ulcer disease. Occasionally, gastric ulcers localized on the lesser curvature of the stomach but unrelated to either hiatal hernias or esophageal reflux may present with symptoms identical to those in patients with reflux disease. Such ulcers are easy to detect on endoscopy and biopsy. In Case 1, endoscopy was of particular value in uncovering an ulcer in the patient's herniated stomach that was responsible for bleeding and anemia.

KEY POINTS

• Ruling out myocardial disease most important consideration in establishing diagnosis of reflux esophagitis

• Also to be considered are biliary tract disease and peptic ulcer disease

• Endoscopy is done to confirm diagnosis of reflux esophagitis

---

TREATMENT

The treatment of reflux esophagitis is directed at correcting any identifiable defect and preventing further harmful changes in the esophageal mucosa.

Sliding hiatal hernias and associated reflux esophagitis generally respond well to medical therapies. These include controlled weight loss, elevation of the head of the bed to reduce nocturnal reflux, and combinations of antacids and acid inhibitors such as histamine (H_2) receptor blocking agents and omeprazole, a potent inhibitor of enzymatic processes responsible for acid production. Alcohol, caffeine, and tobacco use should be avoided. Repeat endoscopic evaluation of the esophagus should be done in 2–3 months to ensure that healing has taken place. Should esophagitis persist, antireflux procedures such as a Nissen fundoplication in which the lower 6 cm of the esophagus is wrapped with the gastric fundus (Fig. 16.2) should be offered. The procedure is highly effective (90%) in producing an increased LES resting pressure, and in markedly reducing if not eliminating reflux. When done by the laparoscopic technique the morbidity is very low.

The treatment of symptomatic paraesophageal hernias is urgent, as the complications from unattended hernias can be catastrophic. These patients should be admitted promptly to the hospital, and nasogastric decompression of the stomach instituted to prevent further distention of

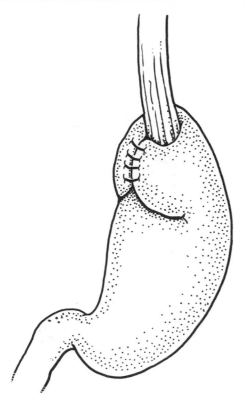

FIGURE 16.2 *Nissen fundoplication.*

the hernia, followed by operation. The herniated portion of the stomach, usually the posterior fundic wall, is reduced and then the defect sutured close (Case 1). The stomach is further anchored to the diaphragm and/or anterior abdominal wall to reduce recurrent herniation. Many surgeons will combine the reduction of the fundus with Nissen fundoplication.

Patients who do not respond to medical therapy or those with Barrett's epithelium present on biopsy should have an antireflux procedure to prevent continued damage to the esophageal mucosa. Although the Nissen fundoplication is the most widely utilized procedure, antireflux operations such as the Hill or Belsey repair achieve similar results, namely increased LES resting pressures. Although all the procedures are effective in preventing further esophageal reflux, none have been shown to cause reversal of Barrett's epithelium to normal. Thus, patients with this lesion require continued surveillance.

KEY POINTS

- Sliding hiatal hernias and associated reflux esophagitis respond well to medical therapy
- Nissen fundoplication highly effective (90%) in producing an increased LES resting pressure, and in markedly reducing if not eliminating reflux

- None of procedures effective in preventing esophageal reflux reverse Barrett's epithelium to normal

FOLLOW-UP

Outcome data on the careful follow-up of patients with Barrett's epithelium following operation are not available. Follow-up endoscopic surveillance, initially at 6 months and subsequently at yearly intervals, is necessary to detect and treat malignant changes in the mucosa. This can be done by repeat esophagoscopy and biopsy or brush cytology of the distal esophageal mucosa. What is clear is that with each passing decade Barrett's epithelium has a greater chance of being converted to an overt malignancy.

SUGGESTED READINGS

Spechler SJ: Comparison of medical and surgical therapy for complicated gastroesophageal reflux disease in veterans. N Engl J Med 326:786, 1992

This cautiously conducted multi-institutional study shows that carefully selected patients are best treated with surgery.

Stein HJ: Complications of gastroesophageal reflux therapy. Role of the lower esophageal sphincter, esophageal acid, and acid alkaline exposure and duodenogastric reflux. Ann Surg 216:35, 1992

Comprehensive comparisons of known etiological factors in the incidence of complications.

QUESTIONS

1. A paraesophageal hernia in contrast to a sliding hernia has?

A. The cardioesophageal junction located below the diaphragm.

B. A greater tendency to incarcerate the herniated stomach.

C. Become a surgical emergency when the patient develops symptoms.

D. All of the above.

2. Reflux esophagitis?

A. Can occur without the presence of a hiatal hernia.

B. Is associated with reduced LES pressure.

C. Can cause Barrett's epithelium.

D. All of the above.

(See p. 603 for answers.)

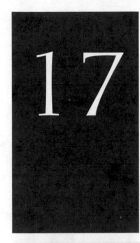

17

TUMORS

OF THE

ESOPHAGUS

EDWARD PASSARO, JR.

The esophagus is the conduit by which food reaches the stomach and continues for digestion. As a muscular, well defined channel, it tolerates obstruction poorly, whether partial or complete, transient or permanent. We can all recall an episode in life when either food or a foreign body transiently blocked our esophagus. We have difficulty in swallowing, dysphagia, and clearing our gullet. The feeling is terrible and never to be forgotten.

This chapter focuses on esophageal tumors that produce obstruction, initially partial in nature and increasing over time. The patient experiences dysphagia, albeit an insidious progressive form rather than the sudden severe dysphagia we have all experienced.

CASE 1
SQUAMOUS CELL CARCINOMA

A 67-year-old male was seen because of difficulty swallowing meat. The patient noted that insidiously over the past 3 months he had progressive difficulty, first in eating steaks, and subsequently other meats. He described the food as sticking or stopping immediately above his xiphoid, and he took to sipping water throughout his meals, as he felt this helped alleviate the food sticking. Gradually he altered his diet, substituting chopped foods and meats for solid portions.

During this 3-month interval he had had no pain, nausea, or vomiting. On one occasion because a "bite of meat became stuck" he attempted to induce vomiting by sticking his finger down his throat. After several retching episodes, the meat was expectorated and he immediately felt relief. He also reported a 20-lb weight loss during this time and a decrease in his usual energy.

A barium swallow showed an obstruction at the distal 4 cm of the esophagus with mild dilatation of the esophagus above it. At the point of obstruction there was an irregular shelving defect with a very narrow irregular "string" of barium outlining the narrow lumen emptying into the stomach. Esophagoscopy showed a dirty, gray, circumferential irregular mass at the distal esophagus, nearly blocking the entire lumen. The mass was friable and oozed when touched by the scope. The mucosa immediately above the mass was intact but slightly engorged. The mucosa in several areas appeared raised into small irregular mounds. Two biopsies were reported as showing invasive squamous cell carcinoma. He was started on total parenteral nutrition, and an initial course of radiotherapy (approximately 3,000 cGy) was given to the distal esophagus combined with 5-fluorouracil chemotherapy for six weeks. Two months later, at operation, the distal esophagus was shrunken and stiff. Distally, the upper fourth of the stomach was divided at a point approximately 8 cm from the gastroesophageal junction. Proximally, the esophagus was divided 4 cm above the mass. A circumferential rim of the proximal end of the esophagus was submitted for frozen section; no cancer was identified. Then, through the right chest, the stomach was brought up into the mediastinum and an esophagogastrostomy was done. His postoperative course was uneventful. Two months later he was able to eat steak and other meats without difficulty.

CASE 2
LEIOMYOMA

A 50-year-old female went to see her physician because of a recent bout of dysphagia while at a party. Careful questioning revealed that for the past 2 years she had had attacks of difficulty in swallowing and that she felt that "the food was not going down." After a moment or two of hesitation in eating she would experience no further difficulty. She was under the impression that the attacks occurred in particular when she was excessively tired or had been drinking alcoholic beverages. There had been no nausea, vomiting, food intolerance, or change in bowel habits. Her weight had not changed.

An esophagram showed a 2-cm smooth curvilinear defect in the mid-esophagus. A CT scan of the chest was seen. There was no invasion of the surrounding structures. In the mid-esophagus a smooth hemispherical protrusion into the lumen of the esophagus was seen on esophagoscopy. The mucosa over it was intact and normal in appearance.

The patient was told that she had a presumably benign tumor of the mid-esophagus that would either grow slowly or possibly not grow any further. Six months later she experienced another bout of dysphagia while at a party, after which she returned to her physician and operation was advised.

The surgeons found a 3-cm smooth, firm tumor embedded in the wall. It was excised with a rim of normal muscle surrounding it. The mucosa was not violated. The muscle layers were reapproximated. Histologic examination showed a benign leiomyoma. The following year she attended three major parties without any difficulty.

GENERAL CONSIDERATIONS

Tumors of the esophagus, whether benign or malignant, eventually produce dysphagia. Dysphagia (whether from tumor or other causes) is a serious complaint that should immediately alert the physician to carry out prompt, thorough inquiry into its cause.

Unfortunately the most common tumor of the esophagus is a malignant tumor, either squamous cell or adenocarcinoma. About one-half occur in the mid-third of the esophagus, the upper and lower one-third account for

about 25% each. When visualized (Case 1), the tumor appears as a grayish friable mass with areas of erosion. Spread is by direct invasion into the surrounding tissues; in most cases, tumor is found in the surrounding lymph nodes by the time the patient is seen. In addition, the tumor spreads by direct propagation within the wall of the esophagus itself. This is manifested by small irregularities in the contour of the esophageal wall as seen on endoscopy (Case 1). Esophageal carcinomas are notorious for their propensity to invade into the surrounding structures. In the middle third of the mediastinum, this includes vital structures (the aorta, trachea, and left main stem bronchus). Thus, many patients are inoperable at diagnosis. Distant spread of the tumor occurs by hematogenous spread, most commonly to the liver, lungs, and bone.

The unique geographic concentrations of tumors in certain regions of the world suggest that they are strongly influenced by environmental factors. In some of the northern provinces of China, carcinoma of the esophagus is the most frequent tumor encountered. The etiologic factors have not yet been identified despite intense investigations. In the United States, South Carolina has a very high incidence relative to the rest of the country and tobacco use, both smoking and chewing, is considered an etiologic factor.

Recognized inflammatory conditions of the esophagus include achalasia and reflux esophagitis, which can lead to metaplastic changes identified as Barrett's epithelium, a precancerous state. Both processes exhibit chronic inflammation of the esophagus, usually the lower portion, and a propensity for adenocarcinoma formation, rather than squamous cell cancer. Both processes require decades to become important risk factors. Achalasia produces inflammation by physiologic obstruction of the cardioesophageal sphincter (see Ch. 10), resulting in the retention of food and secretions. In turn, the chronic stasis of intraluminal contents produces inflammation of the mucosa with ulcer formation and thickening of the esophageal wall. Reflux esophagitis (see Ch. 13) is caused by acid and pepsin bathing the lower esophagus chronically. In severe cases, this may lead to inflammatory mucosal changes, culminating in metaplasia of the squamous lining into columnar epithelium. Continued inflammation leads to malignant transformation.

KEY POINTS

- The esophagus is a muscular, well defined channel; it tolerates obstruction poorly, whether partial or complete, transient or permanent

- Tumors of the esophagus, benign or malignant, eventually produce dysphagia, a serious complaint whose cause should be investigated immediately

- Inflammatory conditions include achalasia and reflux esophagitis, which can lead to metaplastic changes (Barrett's esophagus), a precancerous state

DIAGNOSIS

All patients presenting with dysphagia or in whom the diagnosis of esophageal tumor is suspected on clinical grounds, should undergo esophagoscopy as the initial, key diagnostic procedure. All too often (Case 1), the patient is first given a barium swallow and radiographs obtained. In the partially or totally obstructed patient, the barium study can lead to regurgitation and aspiration of the barium, along with retained esophageal contents from the obstruction.

By contrast, esophagoscopy is helpful in removing the retained secretions and food particles from the proximal obstructed esophagus and obtaining a clear view of the lesion. The appearance of a malignant tumor, whether squamous cell or adenocarcinoma, is characteristic (Case 1). Furthermore, an opportunity is provided not only to biopsy the tumor but also to evaluate the spread of the tumor, often submucosal, as in Case 1. In Case 2, esophagoscopy showed the mucosa to be intact and the lesion was submucosal in the midportion of the esophagus.

Esophagoscopy, but not a barium radiography study, permits inspection and biopsy of the mucosa in and around the lesion. This is important in patients with malignant tumors of the esophagus because many will have a degenerative mucosa (Barrett's mucosa), not only adjacent to the tumor but occasionally some distance from it. This altered mucosa should be excised in conjunction with the tumor; clearly, precise identification and localization at esophagoscopy are critical to subsequent therapy.

Dysphagia is the cardinal symptom in all esophageal diseases. Whatever the cause, it is an important sign that should prompt investigation by the physician. Thus, while a number of esophageal diseases can be considered, they are roughly divided into dysphagia accompanied by pain and that which is painless. As in achalasia (see Ch. 10) and reflux esophagitis (see Ch. 13), these conditions are accompanied by symptoms of substernal pain or discomfort, particularly related to eating. By contrast, patients with carcinoma of the esophagus may have no pain or pain related to eating accompanying symptoms of dysphagia, despite the erosions in the tumor, as malignant tumors are insensate (Case 1). Esophagoscopy is of particular help in identifying the presence or absence of any causative factor. Biopsy during esophagoscopy generally provides a definitive diagnosis. In some cases, the tumor has produced proximal obstruction of the esophagus so that the tumor may not be visualized directly. Cytologic examination of esophageal brushings and washings may help in these instances.

Benign tumors of the esophagus are almost impossible to diagnose on clinical criteria alone. A benign lesion is suggested or more likely when the symptoms of dysphagia are both intermittent and not pronounced (Case 2). The lack of weight loss, an important sign of constitutional homeostasis, also points to a malignant process. The diagnosis of benign conditions is best made by imaging techniques such as computed tomography (CT), in which the contour of the lesion and whether it is infiltrating in the surrounding tissues can be ascertained. Esophagoscopy for benign tumors is only helpful in that an intrinsic mucosal lesion is not seen and that the defect appears to be extrinsic. Endoscopic ultrasonography, a relatively new modality, is rapidly proving to be the test of choice for questionable lesions.

KEY POINTS

- Patients with dysphagia or with suspected esophageal tumor should undergo esophagoscopy as initial, key diagnostic procedure

- Esophagoscopy (but not barium radiography) permits inspection and biopsy of muscosa in and around lesion

- Dysphagia is cardinal symptom in all esophageal diseases, whether accompanied by pain or painless

- In patients with carcinoma of the esophagus, dysphagia may be accompanied by pain or no pain related to eating, despite erosions in tumor—malignant tumors are insensate

- Benign tumors of esophagus almost impossible to diagnose on clinical criteria alone; contour of lesion and whether it is infiltrating surrounding tissues best ascertained by CT

TREATMENT

Current recommended treatment for squamous or adenocarcinoma is a combination of preoperative (neoadjuvant) radiotherapy and chemotherapy (Case 1). The best results have been achieved after first administering a course of radiotherapy (3,000–4,000 cGy) to the esophagus in combination with or followed by a course of chemotherapy with such agents as 5-fluorouracil and cisplatin. The rationale is that chemotherapeutic agents are effective in preventing continued growth of the tumor, while radiotherapy is particularly effective at killing microscopic as well as macroscopic tumor deposits in the tissues surrounding the esophagus. Some shrinkage of the major tumor mass occurs with the combined therapy, facilitating subsequent excision of the tumor.

As these patients have invariably lost weight before diagnosis, and because both the radiotherapy and chemotherapy frequently produce additional weight loss because of anorexia and vomiting, patients will often require maintenance with nutritional supplementation (Case 1).

Operation is advised for patients who are found not to have disseminated disease or distant metastasis. Those who have more advanced disease are unlikely to live more than a few months. Although attempts to produce a lumen through the tumor with heater probes, lasers, and stents have all been used, such treatments are accompanied by a risk of serious complications, including bleeding, perforation, sepsis, and aspiration, and should be reserved for patients considered inoperable. Although seemingly benign and conservative treatment options, they are often otherwise. A simple tube gastrostomy to provide nutrition for the patient's remaining life may in most instances be simpler.

When disseminated tumor is not found and the patient's general condition indicates survival beyond 6 months, operation is advised. It offers not only the chance for cure, but provides excellent palliation.

> **KEY POINTS**
>
> • Current recommended treatment for squamous or adenocarcinoma is a combination of preoperative (neoadjuvant) radiotherapy and chemotherapy
>
> • In absence of disseminated tumor, and when survival beyond 6 months is likely, operation is advised

FOLLOW-UP

Patients are evaluated after treatment for either a complication of the treatment or recurrent tumor. In either instance, esophagoscopy is the optimal method for follow-up evaluation and is done generally at 3-month, 6-month, and 1-year intervals.

Complications of treatment, such as operation with or without radiotherapy and chemotherapy include esophageal structure formation or ulceration, or both. These complications are thought to be the aftermath of compromised submucosal blood flow leading to a focal area of ischemia. As the blood supply to the esophagus is neither extensive nor with collaterals, it is easily compromised both by surgical procedures and by radiotherapy and chemotherapy. Topical mucosal barrier agents such as sulcrufate are given for ulcers of the esophagus. Strictures are best treated early by dilatation, which can be done under direct vision during esophagoscopy and subsequently by the patient.

Recurrent tumor tends to occur at the suture line if a resection has been done or at the margins of the initial tumor site if the patient received radiotherapy and chemotherapy alone. CT and chest radiographs are of limited value in detecting small tumors recurrence shortly after treatment.

> **KEY POINTS**
>
> • Esophagoscopy is optional method for follow-up evaluation; done generally at 3-month, 6-month, and 1-year intervals

SUGGESTED READINGS

DeMeester TR, Zamimotto G, Johansson K: Sensitive therapeutic approach to cancer of the lower esophagus and cardia. J Thorac Cardiovasc Surg 95:42, 1988

Excellent evaluation of patients for operations.

Jacob P et al: Natural history and significance of esophageal squamous cell dysplasia. Cancer 65:2731, 1990

Careful study shows the premalignant potential of metaplastic changes.

QUESTIONS

1. *The major distinction between benign and malignant esophageal tumors is?*
   A. The former generally arise from the submucosal layers of the esophagus, whereas the latter invariably arise from the mucosal layer.
   B. The degree of esophageal obstruction is less in benign than in malignant tumors.
   C. Benign tumors occur in the upper portions of the esophagus and malignant tumors in the lower portion.
   D. None of the above.

2. *Adenocarcinoma and squamous cell carcinoma of the esophagus are histologically distinct?*
   A. And require specific treatment for each type of malignancy.
   B. And have vastly different biological behavior.
   C. And arise from different elements of the mucosa.
   D. But their treatment and prognosis are not too dissimilar.

(See p. 603 for answers.)

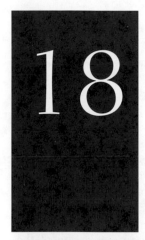

18

PEPTIC

ULCER

DISEASE

EDWARD PASSARO, JR.

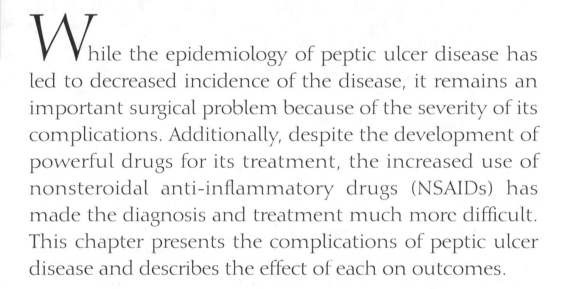

While the epidemiology of peptic ulcer disease has led to decreased incidence of the disease, it remains an important surgical problem because of the severity of its complications. Additionally, despite the development of powerful drugs for its treatment, the increased use of nonsteroidal anti-inflammatory drugs (NSAIDs) has made the diagnosis and treatment much more difficult. This chapter presents the complications of peptic ulcer disease and describes the effect of each on outcomes.

CASE 1
BLEEDING DUODENAL ULCER

A 78-year-old white female was admitted to the hospital because of melena and weakness of 24 hours' duration. She gave a history of having duodenal ulcer disease for approximately 25 years and has been taking anti-ulcer medicines more or less since that time.

Approximately 8 years previously she was admitted to her community hospital because of abdominal pain, abdominal distention, and a low grade fever. Her physicians reportedly were concerned that she had a perforated ulcer, although an upright chest radiograph and abdominal radiographs failed to show the presence of free air. She had recently increased her use of NSAIDs because of recurrent hip pain, but had lapsed in taking her antacid medications. A nasogastric tube was inserted, and she was given intravenous antibiotics. Over the ensuing 48 hours, abdominal pain and distention decreased and the fever resolved.

In addition to NSAIDs the patient was taking nitroglycerin for episodes of angina over the past 5 years and a β-blocker that effectively controlled her hypertension. She was admitted to the intensive care unit, where a nasogastric tube was inserted and returned approximately 500 ml of a "coffee ground" material. It was strongly guaiac positive, as were her stools. The hematocrit was 28%, and 2 units of packed red blood cells was given. EGD was done in the intensive care unit after she had received the blood transfusion. The pylorus was noted to be somewhat narrow and deformed. The scope was passed through with some difficulty. On the posterior wall of the duodenal bulb, a stationary clot was noted in what appeared to be an ulcer base. Attempts at gently washing off the clot proved unsuccessful.

Approximately 36 hours later, she experienced some nausea and substernal angina. When her physicians arrived, she had begun to vomit "coffee-ground" material and frank blood. Blood was rapidly given, and she was taken for operation. At operation the pylorus was noted to be scarred and slightly deformed. An ulcer in the posterior wall of the duodenum could be palpated through the anterior duodenal wall. A pyloroduodenotomy was made and large, dark red clots as well as bright arterial blood was aspirated. A 2-cm, posterior wall, deep, duodenal ulcer with spurting arterial bleeding was noted. The vessel in the ulcer base was ligated. The pyloroduodenotomy was closed in a vertical axis as a pyloroplasty and a parietal cell vagotomy done. After a convalescence of 12 days she was discharged, eating five small feedings a day.

CASE 2
CASTRIC ULCER

A 72-year-old male was seen by his physician because of epigastric distress shortly after eating a meal, and occasionally during the meal itself. He had lost some 10 lb during the past 2 weeks. He was told that he probably had ulcer disease and was given histamine receptor antagonists. On follow-up 6 weeks later, he reported feeling better, although not entirely normal. He had not regained any weight. Endoscopy was advised. In the fundus of the stomach, a 3-cm gastric ulcer was noted on the ventral wall; biopsies were taken from four quadrants of the ulcer's rim. The biopsies showed only chronic inflammatory changes. Another 6-week course of medical therapy was instituted and sulcrulfate, a mucosal barrier agent, was added. On return visit the ulcer was only partially healed, and operation was advised. The ulcer and the distal half of the stomach were excised and a gastroduodenostomy done. On follow-up 1 year later, he was asymptomatic and not taking any medications. His weight had returned to normal.

T GENERAL CONSIDERATIONS

The term *peptic ulcer disease* is used to connote the benign ulceration of both the stomach and duodenum, as these disease processes share many features in common, namely, symptoms of epigastric distress or pain related to meals and a favorable response obtained with antacid therapy. Duodenal and gastric ulcers share the same set of complications, including pain, intractability, perforation, obstruction, and bleeding. Beyond that, significant differences emerge. Each of these should be considered separately.

The cause of duodenal ulcers is unknown. It is often erroneously attributed to excessive acid production of the stomach. In fact, most patients with duodenal ulcer do not secrete excessive quantities of acid. Acid secretion deservedly receives attention because it can be effectively controlled by medication, and control of acid secretion leads to healing of the ulcer. Current therapy is so effec-

tive that earlier complications from ulcer disease, such as intractable pain, bleeding, perforation, and obstruction, are less frequently encountered.

Recently the bacterium *Helicobacter pylori* has been implicated in the development of duodenal ulcer disease. Precisely how the organism that colonizes predominantly the distal portion of the stomach is involved in duodenal ulcer formation is unknown. More importantly, a combination of three antibiotics—metronidazole, amoxicillin, and bismuth—given for a period of 1 month in conjunction with omeprazole is effective in eradicating the organism and in promoting healing. In particular, ulcer recurrence is invariably associated with recolonization of the stomach by *H. pylori*.

While the idea that peptic ulcer disease may be related to an infection is not new (although soundly rejected for many decades), long-term experience in the management of each of the complications of duodenal ulcer disease following antimicrobial therapy is unavailable. Anti-*H. pylori* therapy is a useful adjunct because of its safety and early promise. The development of complications leads to referral of patients to the surgeon for correction of these problems and for opportunity for cure. Surgery for duodenal ulcer disease and peptic ulcer disease, for that matter, are often spoken of in the singular, that is, one operation to treat any and all ulcer complications. Stated another way, does it make any difference which ulcer complication you might have? Are you sure? You might try picking a complication of ulcer disease for yourself and ask, for example, what difference might there be if you are to be treated by a surgeon for perforation rather than bleeding from your ulcer, as was evident in the patient in Case 1. We review the case here because it vividly illustrates many of the key features of some of the complications.

You recall that this patient had ulcer disease for approximately 25 years and was taking medications for the relief of pain or discomfort. The pain is generally chronic, goes away with adequate therapy, and is quick to return when therapy is stopped or interrupted. Pain itself does not constitute an emergency, and pain per se does not cause death. So, at first glance, it might seem that pain would be the preferred complication to have. The drawback is that operation for pain is not very successful, as pain is subjective and difficult to evaluate.

This patient was admitted on one occasion for abdominal pain, distention, and fever and was thought to have perforation. Free air was looked for but was not found. In fact free air is absent in anywhere from one-fourth to one-third of patients with a perforation. Nevertheless, this patient was hospitalized and appropriately treated as if she had a perforation. The presumed perforation occurred when she was taking NSAIDs and interrupted her medical therapy for ulcer disease. NSAIDs are an important and common cause of ulcer complications currently. As an example, as many as 50% of patients treated for perforation have been found to be taking NSAIDs. This episode also demonstrates that some forms of perforated duodenal ulcers can be treated conservatively. The patient's age, the fact that she was taking NSAIDs, and because the diagnosis was suspected but not proven, a nonoperative form of therapy was chosen and was successful. Other studies have shown that in carefully selected patients with significant comorbidity factors, such as heart disease, stroke, and general debility, perforated duodenal ulcer can be effectively treated medically.

Most patients with perforated duodenal ulcers are treated surgically. This is because morbidity and mortality in the average patient are reduced by prompt surgical treatment.

What procedure should be done is dependent on two important factors: whether there is a prior history of duodenal ulcer disease for 3 months or more, and evaluation of the patient's overall health, including the duration and degree of peritoneal contamination found at operation.

With regard to the first factor, those patients with no history of ulcer disease or with disease of less than 3 months' duration require only simple closure of the perforation. This is because most of these patients, for reasons that are not understood, will have no further difficulty from duodenal ulcer disease. This is particularly true if an acute exacerbating factor has been identified that can be eliminated (e.g., NSAID intake). By contrast, those patients with a history of greater than 3 months will have a highly likely (70–90%) chance of having further severe ulcer complications if the ulcer is simply closed.

For these reasons, surgeons have sought for prognostic factors that would suggest the safety and effectiveness of a definitive ulcer operation at the time of operation for perforation. These prognostic factors are age (<65), duration of perforation (<6 hours), and degree of contamination (minimal to moderate). Under these circumstances a definitive ulcer operation can be done. A parietal cell vagotomy with simple closure of the ulcer is best, as it has the lowest mortality and morbidity rate, while effectively curing the ulcer in 85–90% of patients.

Another major complication of duodenal ulcer disease is bleeding, as was experienced by the patient in Case 1. Bleeding is the deadliest complication of duodenal ulcer and of gastric ulcer, accounting for almost all mortality in the surgical treatment of this disease. The reason is simple: although humans tolerate external bleeding from a wound rather well, they are not designed to bleed internally. Bleeding internally, into the gut, brain, chest, abdomen, or soft tissues, carries both high mortality and complication rates. Furthermore, transfusion of blood, independent of the rate of bleeding, has a mortality and morbidity of its own, as it interferes with the body's defense mechanism against infection, immunologic response, and normal coagulation. As in the patient in Case

1, bleeding constitutes an emergency in many instances. Emergency surgery is intrinsically more hazardous to the patient than in the same procedure done under elective circumstances.

The last complication is that of obstruction at the pylorus from severe duodenal ulcer disease. This can occur because of extensive disease and subsequent scarring in the area, resulting in a mechanical blockage—gastric outlet obstruction. More often, the obstruction is physiologic, rather than mechanical. The propulsive element of the stomach, the antrum, becomes ineffective in efforts to evacuate the stomach because of the chronic impairment of the normal emptying process from inflammation.

Patients with gastric ulcers tend to be older than patients with duodenal ulcer disease. As with duodenal ulcer disease, there has been a gradual decrease in incidence. In contrast to duodenal ulcer disease, in which the stomach is grossly normal or supranormal in function (rapid emptying, increased acid secretion, gastrin release with meals), gastric ulcers can be thought of as one step in the progression of the degenerating gastric mucosa on its way to malignancy. Thus, while active duodenal disease excludes the presence of a gastric malignancy, gastric ulcers point to gastric malignancy in the ulcer, seen in almost 10% of patients. Gastric ulcers are typically located at the junction between normal gastric mucosa and mucosa undergoing inflammatory or degenerative changes. Although elderly patients have a high incidence of colonization with H. pylori, the role of this infection in gastric ulcer formation is unknown. The associated gastritis almost always accompanying gastric ulcer is now considered to be caused by the organism.

The specific complication of the ulcer disease is the major factor in determining the procedure indicated for treatment. For example, pain is associated with no mortality, but with considerable morbidity. The operation of choice would be a procedure with no or exceedingly low mortality and an acceptable morbidity. Exchanging the pain and discomfort of an active ulcer with an outcome of very frequent (and at times uncontrollable) diarrhea from some form of ulcer operation would not be acceptable to most patients. The operation that combines no mortality with no untoward side effects is highly selective or parietal cell vagotomy.

Bleeding is the most lethal complication of bleeding duodenal ulcer disease; treatment has therefore been directed at preventing ulcer recurrence. The collective experience has been that abdominal truncal vagotomy and antrectomy has been the most effective procedure in curing the ulcer and therefore reducing the risk of rebleeding. This is a major procedure. It is associated with side effects, such as diarrhea; "dumping," in which patients feel faint and sweaty after eating a meal with concentrated sweets; and early satiety. Surgeons have looked for the less morbid procedures, accepting a higher ulcer recurrence as part of the bargain. This is why a parietal cell vagotomy was done for the patient in Case 1. Faced with an elderly frail patient who recently suffered a major hemorrhage, the surgeons elected to ligate the bleeding vessel and to stop the bleeding and then do a parietal cell vagotomy to control the ulcer disease.

KEY POINTS

- Cause of duodenal ulcers unknown; often erroneously attributed to excessive acid production of the stomach; most patients with duodenal ulcers do not secrete excessive quantities of acid

- *Helicobacter pylori* recently implicated in development of duodenal ulcer disease; ulcer recurrence invariably associated with recolonization of stomach by this bacterium

- Development of complications leads to referral to surgeon for correction and for opportunity for correction

- You might try picking a complication of ulcer disease and consider what difference there might be if treated by a surgeon for perforation rather than for bleeding from the ulcer

- NSAIDs an important and common cause of ulcer complications, with as many as 50% of perforations found in patients taking these agents

- In carefully selected patients with significant morbidity factors (e.g., heart disease, stroke, and general debility), perforated duodenal ulcer effectively treated medically

- Most perforated duodenal ulcers treated surgically, to reduce morbidity and mortality

- Procedure selection based on (1) prior history of duodenal ulcer disease for 3 months or more, and (2) evaluation of overall health status (including duration and degree of peritoneal contamination—in absence of these factors, simple closure of perforation warranted

- Prognostic factors include age (<65 years), duration of perforation (<6 hours), and degree of contamination (minimal to moderate)

- Parietal cell vagotomy with simple closure of ulcer has lowest mortality and morbidity and effectively cures the ulcer in 85–90% of cases

- Deadliest complication of duodenal and of gastric ulcers is bleeding—accounts for almost all morbidity in surgical treatment

- Obstruction at the pylorus most often physiologic, rather than mechanical

- Gastric ulcers considered a step in progression of degenerating gastric mucosa toward malignancy (in contrast to duodenal ulcers, in which stomach is grossly normal or supranormal in function, e.g., rapid emptying, increased acid secretion, gastrin release with meals)

- Specific complication of ulcer disease is major factor in determining the procedure

- Bleeding most lethal complication of bleeding duodenal ulcer disease; therefore, treatment directed at preventing ulcer recurrence

---

DIAGNOSIS

Patients with gastric ulcers, in contrast to duodenal ulcer patients, experience pain with eating. Conversely, eating tends to alleviate the pain from duodenal ulcers. Thus, not uncommonly, duodenal ulcer patients may initially gain weight, whereas patients with gastric ulcers lose weight. The dull, aching, deep-seated pain is in the epigastrium. In addition to weight loss, not infrequently patients have anemia and chronic low grade blood loss in the stool because of the ulcer and associated gastritis.

The simplest and most direct way to establish the diagnosis is by esophagogastroduodenoscopy (EGD). In addition to ruling out other possibilities, direct visualization of the ulcer provides important information on its size, location, and surrounding gastric mucosa, as well as an opportunity to biopsy the ulcer and other areas suspicious of malignancy.

KEY POINTS

- Patients with gastric ulcers (in contrast to duodenal ulcers) experience pain with eating

- EGD simplest and most direct way to establish diagnosis

DIFFERENTIAL DIAGNOSIS

The pain associated with either gastric ulcer or gastritis is, for all practical purposes, identical. Gastritis is the main differential diagnosis. Malignant degeneration of the ulcer or obvious malignant tumor of the stomach is the other major differential diagnosis. All can be best identified by EGD examination. A barium gastrointestinal study has no advantages over endoscopic examination and is not indicated in most patients.

Chronic cholecystitis can be confused with duodenal ulcer disease. Oral cholecystography is a simple inexpensive but less and less used modality. Ultrasonography of the gallbladder will identify stones as well as the condition of the gallbladder wall, which is generally thickened.

Reflux esophagitis can occasionally be confused with ulcer disease. It is also found in conjunction with duodenal ulcers, particularly when there is some gastric retention from the ulcer. Endoscopy is an ideal method used to detect it and the ulcer disease.

KEY POINTS

- Gastritis, malignant degeneration of ulcer, or obvious malignant tumor of stomach (main differential diagnosis) can all be best identified by EGD examination

TREATMENT

The patient described in Case 2 demonstrates many of the therapeutic considerations in the treatment of gastric ulcer. You may recall that this patient was first treated empirically for peptic ulcer disease, on the basis of symptoms. A conventional course of 6 weeks of H_2 receptor blocker drug therapy was instituted. The medication was effective in alleviating some of his epigastric distress, but not his systemic complaints. Gastroscopy led to the finding of a gastric ulcer. The second course of therapy also failed to promote healing. At operation the ulcer was removed in continuity with the antrum, or distal half of the stomach. Removal of the antrum is empirical; that is, just why this approach causes gastric ulcers to heal is unknown, but it is extremely effective, with an ulcer recurrence rate of less than 2%. Even when the ulcer is not excised in continuity with the distal portion of the stomach, as with gastric ulcers located in the area of the cardioesophageal junction, antrectomy remains very effective treatment.

Biopsy, usually of the quadrants, should be routine for all gastric ulcers. Occult malignancy is present in 5–10% of cases. The finding of a malignancy in the ulcer would prompt early operation for removal, rather than an attempt at protracted drug therapy.

KEY POINTS

- Removal of antrum is empirical—causes healing but reason unknown
- Biopsy (usually of quadrants)—should be routine for all gastric ulcers

---

SUGGESTED READINGS

Graham DY: Effect of treatment of *Helicobacter pylori* infection on the long-term recurrence of gastric or duodenal ulcer: a randomized controlled study. Ann Intern Med 116:705, 1992

Demonstrates the role of H. pylori, *both in ulcer occurrence and in recurrence.* H. pylori *eradication is important in both cases.*

Ohme D, Brawner J, Hermann R: Surgery for duodenal ulcer. A study relating indications to the results of surgery. Am J Surg 1333:267, 1977

Establishes the importance of the specific complication of duodenal ulcer disease in influencing morbidity, mortality, and operation needed.

QUESTIONS

1. The most dreaded complication of peptic ulcer disease, duodenal or gastric, is?
   A. Perforation.
   B. Pain, intractability.
   C. Obstruction.
   D. Bleeding.

2. NSAIDs complicate both the diagnosis and treatment of the peptic ulcer disease because?
   A. These medications, often in conjunction with aspirin, are being taken by a large segment of the population.
   B. The drugs are irritating to the gastric mucosa independent of the presence of acid. They produce symptoms that can be readily mistaken for peptic ulcer disease.
   C. NSAIDs are capable of producing peptic ulcers, leading to perforation and bleeding.
   D. All of the above.

3. H. pylori *has recently been implicated in the development of gastritis and peptic ulcer disease. The main evidence to support the latter is?*
   A. *H. pylori* is to be found in the stomach of all patients with duodenal ulcer disease.
   B. Patients with diffuse gastritis and/or diffuse ulceration of the stomach and duodenum invariably are heavily colonized with *H. pylori*.
   C. *H. pylori* uniformly produced peptic ulceration in the experimented animal.
   D. Eradication of *H. pylori* in patients with duodenal ulcers is very effective in promoting healing of ulcers; in the event of recurrence, recolonization has taken place.

4. Optimal operative treatment for gastric ulcers is?
   A. Antrectomy or distal.
   B. Antrectomy with contiguous excision of the ulcer.
   C. Ulcer excision.
   D. Ulcer excision with highly selective vagotomy.

(See p. 603 for answers.)

19 TUMORS OF THE STOMACH

EDWARD PASSARO, JR.

Tumors of the stomach can arise from the mucosa or the muscular elements, or the stomach may be the site of a more systemic disease, as with lymphoma. This chapter reviews these broad classifications as well as discussing the biologic behavioral differences among tumors arising from the mucosa.

CASE 1
GASTRIC ADENOCARCINOMA

A 70-year-old male complained of early satiety, fatigue, and a 30-lb weight loss within the past 2 months. He had no palpable lymphadenopathy. His Hct was 30% and a stool guaiac was only weakly positive for occult blood. Endoscopy showed the antral region of the stomach to be filled for three-quarters of its circumference with a grayish, friable polyploid tumor. The tumor bled easily when it was brushed by the endoscope. The scope could not be passed beyond the tumor into the duodenum. The proximal portion of the stomach was flaccid and atonic but otherwise normal in appearance. The endoscopist believed that the stomach was fixed dorsally to the parieties as he could not move it. A biopsy of the tumor showed moderately well-differentiated adenocarcinoma. At operation the surgeon noted that the dorsal wall of the antrum was indeed stuck to the pancreas, much as the endoscopist had predicted. In addition, on the ventral wall of the body and antrum of the stomach, he noted whitish nodules that felt firm to palpation. There were several enlarged lymph nodes in the celiac axis. A frozen section was done on one of these excised celiac nodes, and metastatic gastric adenocarcinoma was found within. The stomach was transected at mid-body and the distal portion sharply dissected from the pancreas by cutting through the infiltrating cancer. A gastrojejudostomy reconstruction was done. Following recov-

ery the patient was able to eat normally, but approximately 6 months later he developed marked anorexia, inanition, and died.

CASE 2
BENIGN LEIOMYOMA

A 67-year-old female had an episode of vomiting, noting approximately 100 ml of dark blood. She had not lost weight, but noted that over the past year, particularly on eating a large meal, she had some "pains or cramps" in the upper gastric region. In the past 2 weeks she had had a sharp increase in the frequency and intensity of these pains. She had bought some liquid antacids to see if they would relieve her symptoms, but she noted no change. On palpation, no masses could be felt in the epigastrium. Her Hct was 42% and the stool was weakly guaiac positive. She was thought to have a gastric ulcer and a gastroscopy was done. The endoscopist noted a bulging submucosal mass 4 cm in diameter in the body of the stomach dorsally. There was a 1-cm ulceration in the central portion of the mass that was oozing blood. A biopsy taken at the edge of the ulcer showed mostly inflammatory reaction in the mucosa and submucosa with a small amount of abnormal muscle cells at the margin of the specimen. The pathologist considered the biopsy to be inadequate for a definitive diagnosis. A repeat endoscopy with biopsy was scheduled. However, the following day the patient vomited nearly 300 ml of dark blood, small dark clots, and some food particles. She was operated on urgently. A 5-cm, smooth, purplish colored tumor was found in the dorsal gastric wall in the mid-body region. The mass was excised with a rim of normal gastric wall and the gastrotomy closed. The final diagnosis was a benign leiomyoma.

CASE 3
GASTRIC LYMPHOMA

A 53-year-old construction worker developed early satiety. In addition, he noted a tightness or fullness in his abdomen on bending to pick up a piece of lumber or his tools. He had not lost weight, and in fact, was concerned that he "was getting a belly." He had been working steadily. On examination a mass with indistinct borders could be palpated in the epigastrium. The mass could be moved slightly, was firm to palpation, and nontender. The patient was unaware of the mass. On gastroscopy the mucosa appeared to be intact but was lifted in irregular contours producing a reduction in the lumen. The gastric walls were firm and not distensible. A biopsy at the peak of one of the lumps was taken as well as a brush washing from the antral region. The biopsy showed a gastric lymphoma. A CT study showed the stomach wall to be thickened throughout, but a greater degree of thickening was evident in the antral region. The patient was presented to the tumor board conference of the hospital, where opinions were divided as to whether a distal hemigastrectomy should be done first followed by chemotherapy and possibly radiotherapy, or whether the latter two should be given without operation. The patient elected not to undergo operation. His abdominal mass shrunk rapidly during the course of his treatment. Three years later he was asymptomatic and judged free of disease.

GENERAL CONSIDERATIONS

Gastric carcinoma in the United States has been decreasing in incidence for the past 30 years, for reasons that are not known. This observation and the wide variations in the incidence of the disease in different countries, suggest that environmental and dietary factors may be involved in gastric cancer development.

Tumors that arise from the mucosa (adenocarcinoma), in contrast to those that arise from the muscle (leiomyoma, leiomyosarcoma) or are found in gastric lymphoid tissue (lymphoma) are invariably malignant although they display a wide range of clinical behavior (Fig. 19.1). For example, superficial spreading adenocarcinoma seldom metastasizes; large bulky adenocarcinomas found in the distal stomach metastasize late; and a form known as linitis plastica spreads rapidly throughout all layers of the stomach and is invariably incurable by the time it is discovered.

Tumors that arise from the muscle layers of the stomach are the common benign leiomyomas and the rare, malignant leiomyosarcomas. Although their biologic behavior is very different, leiomyomas and leiomyosarcomas are similar histologically, except for the greater preponderance of mitotic figures in the latter.

Leiomyomas and leiomyosarcomas are relatively slow growing tumors, and expand both extra- and intraluminally. Due to their submucosal origin, they are not perceived by the patient until they erode into the mucosa and cause bleeding. Occasionally, the tumor remains submucosal but grows to such a size that there is a reduced gastric capacity and the patient experiences early satiety. Only rarely can these tumors be palpated.

The stomach is rich in stromal elements and these can be the site of development of gastric lymphomas (Fig. 19.2). Gastric lymphomas rarely produce the systemic manisfestation of lymphomas located elsewhere in the body (fatigue, night sweats, anemia). They tend to grow to a relatively large size before they produce pain, early satiety, and weight loss. Occasionally (Case 3), patients will have a palpable mass at the time they present to a physician.

Gastric lymphomas occur at an earlier age than other gastric tumors.

KEY POINTS

• The decreasing incidence of gastric carcinoma and wide variations in incidence in different countries suggest that environmental and dietary factors are involved

• Tumors arising from mucosa (adenocarcinoma)—in contrast to those arising from muscle (leiomyoma, leiomyosarcoma) or found in gastric lymphoid tissue (lymphoma)—are invariably malignant, although display wide range of clinical behavior

• Due to submucosal origin, leiomyomas and leiomyosarcomas are not perceived by the patient until they erode into mucosa and cause bleeding

• Gastric lymphomas rarely produce systemic manifestations of lymphomas located elsewhere in the body (fatigue, night sweats, anemia); tend to grow to relatively large size before produce pain, early satiety, and weight loss

DIAGNOSIS

Esophagogastroduodenoscopy (EGD) is the best way to investigate the symptoms (early satiety) and signs (melena, hematemesis) seen with gastric tumors. In addition, it allows for biopsy if a mass is seen (Case 1), and for identification of a mucosal-covered mass in the wall of the stomach (often with central ulceration), which is characteristic of leiomyomas, benign or malignant (Case 2). In

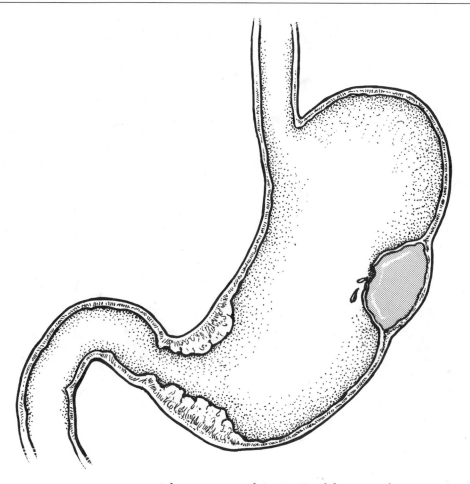

FIGURE 19.1   *Adenocarcinoma/leiomyoma of the stomach.*

Case 3, the findings of reduced gastric lumen with a grossly intact mucosa in a large and palpable stomach led to consideration of an infiltrating tumor.

EGD also provides information on the pliability and mobility of the gastric wall. In Case 1 the endoscopist was able to determine that the tumor was fixated to adjacent organs.

Upper gastrointestinal series (UGI) show silhouettes that are very characteristic for each of the lesions seen in the three patients presented. UGI, however, does not provide a tissue diagnosis. Most importantly, the barium contrast study cannot provide adequate information on motility of the gastric mucosa and gastric wall. Thus, superficial, spreading carcinoma and linitis plastica can be missed on x-ray studies.

CT scans are commonly used to look for the extent of the tumor and involvement of adjacent organs. However, patients with gastric tumors almost always require operation for relief of symptoms or attempts at cure. The CT examination rarely provides information not otherwise available at operation and lacks sensitivity and specificity for adjacent organ invasion. Celiac axis lymph node involvement, a common feature of metastatic gastric adenocarcinoma, is difficult to discern by CT examination.

KEY POINTS

• EGD the best way to investigate symptoms (early satiety) and signs (melena, hematemesis) of gastric tumors

• CT commonly used to look for extent of tumor and involvement of adjacent organs

DIFFERENTIAL DIAGNOSIS

The diagnoses of adenocarcinoma, leiomyoma, and gastric lymphoma as described are not usually difficult. Large benign gastric ulcers, particularly those that have penetrated the gastric wall, can produce a large inflammatory mass that resembles a malignant tumor. They produce symptoms similar to those in patients with gastric tumors. Also, gastric ulcers may be the site of tumor formation and contain occult malignant change within them.

Pancreatic pseudocysts can mimic the presentation of gastric tumors as the cysts grow and impinge on the posterior wall of the stomach. In addition to the mechanical ob-

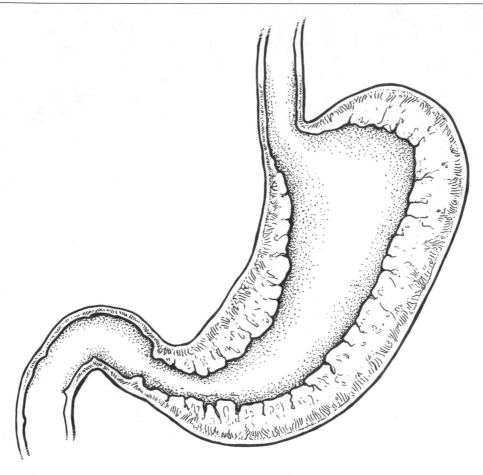

FIGURE 19.2   *Lymphoma of the stomach.*

struction, the inflammatory process produces gastric atony, further reducing gastric emptying.

Rarely, other stromal elements of the gastric wall undergo tumor development. These include neurofibromal and mixed stromal elements tumors. Aberrant pancreatic tissue, usually in the antral region, may resemble a leiomyoma, as can a metastatic melanoma to the stomach.

Benign giant hypertrophy of the gastric mucosa and wall (Ménétrier's disease) grossly resembles gastric lymphoma, and biopsy is required to differentiate them. The symptoms produced by benign giant mucosal hypertrophy very closely resemble those produced by lymphoma.

Gastric pseudolymphoma describes a benign focal lesion rather than the usual widespread infiltrating gastric lymphoma. However, the two lesions are histologically nearly identical and the source of considerable clinical confusion. Pseudolymphoma is treated by local excision rather than radiotherapy or chemotherapy.

KEY POINTS

• Gastric pseudolymphoma describes benign focal lesion rather than usual widespread infiltrating gastric lymphoma

TREATMENT

Gastric tumors are discovered because they produce bleeding, early satiety, and weight loss or gastric outlet obstruction. They require operation to alleviate these symptoms, which are not correctable by medical therapy. Additionally, attempting to cure the patient of the malignancy requires operation.

The treatment and rates of cure of gastric adenocarcinoma depend almost entirely on the biologic behavior of the tumor. Superficial spreading adenocarcinoma, while infrequently seen in the United States, has an 80% chance of cure by wide resection of the involved region of the stomach. Occult adenocarcinoma found in gastric ulcers similarly can be cured in many (40–60%) patients. Larger, bulkier tumors (Case 1) have usually spread beyond the confines of the stomach when first seen, and subsequently the cure rate is only 10–15% in this group. Adenocarcinoma of the stomach do not respond to either chemotherapy or radiotherapy. Extensive resections of the stomach, spleen, and adjacent lymphoid tissue have been attempted to improve the cure rate, but have not proved effective.

Leiomyomas can readily be treated by excision of the tumors as well as a margin of the surrounding gastric wall. If benign, they do not recur, whereas if malignant, they can seldom be cured even by very wide excision.

Controversy exists over the treatment of gastric lymphomas (Case 3). Some medical centers consider removal of the major portion of the lymphoma by gastric resection to make subsequent chemotherapy and radiotherapy more effective and safer, reducing the likelihood of gastric perforation from tumor necrosis during the course of combined therapy. Others believe that operation should be reserved to treat the complications of chemotherapy and radiotherapy (perforation and bleeding). The cure rate is approximately 70% with gastric lymphoma.

KEY POINTS

- Treatment and rates of cure of gastric adenocarcinoma depend almost entirely on biologic behavior of tumor
- Adenocarcinoma of stomach does not respond to either chemotherapy or radiotherapy

FOLLOW-UP

Patients with malignant lesions are followed at 6-month intervals for the following 2 years. Most recurrences will become apparent then. If patients become symptomatic, they need repeat endoscopy to provide palliation. Chemotherapy and radiotherapy are not effective in treating recurrent gastric adenocarcinoma.

SUGGESTED READING

Kim JP, Kim YW, Yang HK, Noh DY: Significant prognostic factors by multivariate analysis of 3926 gastric cancer patients. Med J Surg 18:872, 1994

Exhaustive analysis of prognostic factors in gastric cancer in all its forms.

QUESTIONS

1. Gastric tumors arise from?

    A. Mucosa.

    B. Muscle layers.

    C. Stromal elements.

    D. All of the above.

2. In treating adenocarcinoma the best predictor of the likelihood of cure is?

    A. The extent of the procedure to encompass all tumor and lymphoid drainage.

    B. The biologic behavior of the tumor.

    C. Postoperative chemotherapy and radiotherapy.

    D. The location of the tumor in the stomach, with antral lesion being more favorable than those of the cardioesophageal region.

2. Gastric lymphomas?

    A. Occur in younger patients then do other gastric tumors.

    B. Can be confused with gastric pseudolymphoma.

    C. Can be confused with giant benign gastric hypertrophy.

    D. All of the above.

(See p. 603 for answers.)

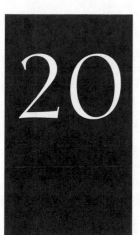

20

UPPER

GASTROINTESTINAL

HEMORRHAGE

EDWARD PASSARO, JR.

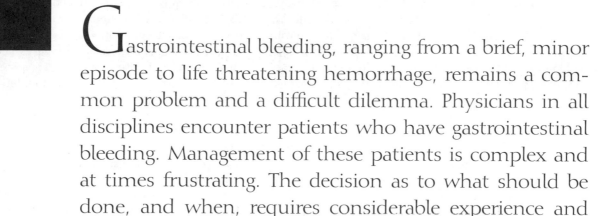

Gastrointestinal bleeding, ranging from a brief, minor episode to life threatening hemorrhage, remains a common problem and a difficult dilemma. Physicians in all disciplines encounter patients who have gastrointestinal bleeding. Management of these patients is complex and at times frustrating. The decision as to what should be done, and when, requires considerable experience and expertise. Morbidity and mortality are closely related and are affected by the way the problem is managed.

This chapter sets forth the early considerations in the initial evaluation and management of all gastrointestinal bleeding. Some of the more common specific causes of upper gastrointestinal bleeding, as well as methods of management, are then discussed in greater detail.

CASE 1
DUODENAL ULCER

A 60-year-old male was seen in the emergency room because of melena of 48 hours' of duration. The BP was 105/70 mmHg, pulse 110 bpm, and he complained of the recent onset of lightheadedness and dizziness. Rectal examination showed a black "tarry" stool that was strongly guaiac positive. He was given oxygen by face mask and two 16-gauge IV catheters were started in the arms. Blood was drawn for Hct (later returned as 24%) and for type and was matched for 6 units of blood. A nasogastric tube was passed and the gastric residual was approximately 100

ml of a clear acidic aspirate. Retching was induced by examining the back of the pharynx with a tongue blade. The aspirate then changed to a mixture of bilious fluid containing some dark obvious blood. Matched blood was transfused and a history taken. The patient admitted to "bouts of indigestion," usually following extended bouts of drinking for which he self-prescribed antacid tablets and liquids. He had never seen a physician for these symptoms. He admitted to having "2–5 drinks" daily as part of his business activity with clients. He took aspirin on occasion, both for headaches and for hangovers.

Three units of packed RBCs was given. His pulse was 90 bpm and BP 130/80 mmHg. Endoscopy was done; the stomach and esophagus were normal. The duodenum was found to have a 1.5-cm posterior ulcer with a clot in the base. Several small superficial erosions on the anterior wall of the bulb were seen.

The clot in the ulcer was lavaged off by the endoscopist and some bright red bleeding noted. A bipolar electrocoagulation of the ulcer base was done and the bleeding ceased. The patient was started on raditidine the following day, when the NG tube was withdrawn. The Hct remained at 30% following transfusion and his ulcer cleared. Follow-up endoscopy 1 month later showed that the ulcer had healed.

CASE 2
BILIARY OBSTRUCTION

A 64-year-old female was admitted because of fever, jaundice, and right upper quadrant pain. She had been given antibiotics. ERCP showed an incomplete obstruction of the common bile duct at the level of the confluence of the major ducts. Attempts by the endoscopist to pass a guidewire through the lesion for stenting of the obstructed region and relief of the proximal obstruction proved unsuccessful. At 12 hours, the patient had remained febrile with intermittent temperatures to 40°C, when she began vomiting blood. Repeat endoscopy was done after evacuation of a large quantity of dark clots as well as dark liquid blood. The entire stomach was noted to be covered with abrasions varying from a few millimeters to centimeters in diameter, actively oozing blood. Endoscopy was difficult and was limited to the stomach. The patient was intubated, and active blood transfusion through an IV catheter started. She was noted to be more jaundiced and coagulopathic. She was brought to the interventional radiology suite for percutaneous draining of her proximal dilated biliary system.

This was done and purulent bile aspirated. Bleeding of large quantities of dark liquid blood continued from the NG tube. Transfusions of fresh frozen plasma in addition to blood were given. Despite these measures, she remained coagulopathic, the jaundice deepened, and she became comatose. The patient expired the following day.

M GENERAL CONSIDERATIONS

ost bleeding from the gastrointestinal tract (85%) will stop spontaneously. This is of obvious great clinical significance in the management of all patients. Difficulty continues to arise, however, in distinguishing the 15–20% of patients who fail to stop bleeding or in whom rebleeding promptly occurs.

An important additional distinction is between bleeding sources in the upper gastrointestinal tract (esophagus, stomach, small bowel) and the lower gastrointestinal tract (colon). Of the two, we consider upper gastrointestinal tract bleeding the more serious because of the nature of the lesions (see below). Upper gastrointestinal tract bleeding is more frequent and is estimated to prompt 300,000 admissions annually in the United States.

A third major risk factor is age. The morbidity and mortality rates associated with gastrointestinal bleeding in the elderly (65 years or older) are significantly higher than those in younger patients, increasing nearly 10-fold for both elective and emergent procedures.

The last important variable is bleeding during hospitalization for other problems. For example, while the mortality rate may be within a range of 20–25% among outpatients examined because of bleeding, it rises to 70% among patients who are hospitalized for other reasons before bleeding begins. Bleeding while in hospital is almost exclusively from the upper gastrointestinal tract. Thus, elderly patients hospitalized for other reasons, who develop an unexpected upper gastrointestinal bleed, are at exceedingly high risk.

It is difficult, if not impossible in some circumstances, to determine which patients will stop bleeding and which will not, or in which patients bleeding will resume once it has stopped. Thus, it is important to consider all gastrointestinal tract bleeding, of whatever degree, as potentially life-threatening. A false sense of security and lack of preparedness compromises both the patient's chance of survival and the surgeon's opportunity to intervene when indicated.

Following resuscitation, the next important step is to determine whether the source is the upper or lower gastrointestinal tract. While this may become apparent during the course of the resuscitation itself, it is wise to have a uniform plan of investigation, applied to all patients so as not to be misled by the route of bleeding or the possibility of two or more lesions coexisting. Since the lesions and their treatment differ from bleeding from either end of the gastrointestinal tract, upper and lower gastrointestinal bleeding are considered in separate chapters.

KEY POINTS

- Most bleeding from the gastrointestinal tract (85%) will stop spontaneously

- Difficulty arises in distinguishing the 15–20% of patients in whom bleeding does not stop or in whom bleeding promptly recurs

- Upper gastrointestinal tract bleeding more serious (than lower gastrointestinal tract bleeding) because of nature of lesions

- Bleeding while in hospital almost exclusively occurs in upper gastrointestinal tract; thus elderly patients hospitalized for other reasons, developing an unexpected upper gastrointestinal bleed, are at exceedingly high risk

---

A TREATMENT

n outline for the emergency treatment of bleeding from the upper gastrointestinal tract is given in Table 20.1. An IV catheter in the upper extremity or neck vein should be established with a 16- or 18-gauge cannula. At least 30

TABLE 20.1 *Outline of resuscitation*

1. Start an IV catheter using a 30-ml syringe and an 18-gauge needle.

2. Obtain 30 ml of blood and separate into three tubes: one tube should be used for type and cross-matching for 4 units, one tube to be observed over a period of 1 hour to determine clotting time and ability, and one tube for an emergency hematocrit and hemoglobin.

3. Start a saline infusion through a blood filter set.

4. Insert a nasogastric (NG) tube and completely aspirate the gastric contents by hand. Examine contents for pH and color of blood, if any (i.e., bright red, dark red, clots, coffee grounds). Rule out brownish acidic menstrumm of gastric retention (see Table 20.2).

5. Pass an Ewald tube if clots interfere with the evacuation of the stomach.

6. Continue the gastric lavage with tap water using 2–3 L over 20–30 minutes. Make estimate of rate of blood loss and its nature (arterial and/or venous).

7. Start a gastrointestinal bleed sheet. Record the patient's pulse, blood pressure, urine output, serial hematocrits as a function of time, and estimated blood losses recorded from the above. Clinical judgment will be needed to determine how often these data points should be obtained.

8. Give blood replacement early for arterial bleeding, decreased hematocrit or blood pressure, or increased pulse rate. Insert a central venous line and a urinary bladder catheter in patients in shock or with continued massive bleeding.

9. If the patient's vital signs are within an acceptable range, perform esophagoscopy and gastroduodenoscopy. If bleeding lesion is found, treat via the endoscope with bipolar coagulation or injection therapy. This should be done no later than 12 hours after admission.

10. If bleeding is from the rectum and the nasogastric tube aspirate is clear with bile, carry out colonoscopy. If the patient has stool and/or blood such that visualization of the colon is not possible, infuse 1–2 L of a nonabsorbable intestinal lavage solution through the NG tube. Repeat colonoscopy.

ml of blood should be withdrawn for hemoglobin/hematocrit determinations and blood typed and matched for 4–6 units initially. A saline infusion should be started through a blood filter set.

A tube should then be passed into the stomach and the gastric contents aspirated. The finding of a clear gastric aspirate containing bile in a patient with melena rules out bleeding from the upper gastrointestinal tract. (If the bleeding source is proximal to the second portion of the duodenum, blood will usually be found in the gastric aspirate along with bile.) Clots or bright red blood, or both, suggest an arterial source. It serves as a warning that abrupt, serious hemorrhage may ensue at any time. If the aspirate has a "coffee ground" appearance, it suggests past

or slow bleeding as the blood has had an opportunity to mix with acidic gastric contents. It is occasionally confused with gastric retention. Aids in the differential diagnosis of the gastric aspirate are shown in Table 20.2.

If blood is found, the tube should be aspirated continuously so that the rate of bleeding can be ascertained. If the stomach cannot be cleared by aspiration and irrigation with tap water lavage, a large bore orogastric tube (e.g., Ewald tube) should be inserted to remove remaining clots. Removal of all blood from the stomach is essential so that the rate of bleeding can be clearly gauged and endoscopy done. Furthermore, this maneuver will, on occasion, help reduce the likelihood of continued bleed, for example from erosive gastritis or tears in the mucosa at the cardioesophageal junction (Mallory-Weiss tears).

Use tap water for lavage because it is readily available. Iced water or saline is cumbersome and offers no advantage. Lavage should be performed with 2–3 L of water over a period of approximately 30 minutes. If no large clots are present, it is generally effective in clearing the stomach to allow endoscopic evaluation and to gauge the nature of the blood loss accurately.

Gastric retention is an important differential point in the examination of the gastric aspirate. As indicated in Table 20.2, several important features distinguish these two conditions. Obviously, it is important to tell them apart, since bleeding from duodenal ulcer may constitute an emergency, whereas bleeding associated with gastric outlet obstruction is not.

Bleeding from the upper gastrointestinal tract is strongly suggested by hematemesis. While hematemesis can be seen with bleeding from the nose, mouth, or pancreatic/biliary lesions, generally other clinical clues will suggest these sites.

Melena is strongly suggestive of bleeding from the upper gastrointestinal tract, but it can be seen with lesions of the small bowel or right colon. A gastric aspirate that is clear and that contains bile in a patient with melena is highly suggestive of bleeding from a more distal source than the duodenum. Hematochezia (obvious blood mixed with stool) not associated with hemodynamic instability is usually from a lower gastrointestinal site.

A brief physical examination is more important in determining the patient's clinical condition than in diagnosing the

TABLE 20.2 *Characteristics of gastric aspirate*

CHARACTERISTICS	ACUTE BLEEDING	GASTRIC RETENTION
Odor	None	Sour
pH	Neutral	Acid
Guaiac	Positive	Positive
Particles	Aggregate	Particulate
Menstruum	Watery	Mucoid

source of the bleed. The patient should be quickly examined for signs of chronic liver disease such as jaundice, ascites, splenomegaly, angiomata, tissue wasting, and gynecomastia. Skin lesions such as telangiectasia of Osler-Weber-Rendu or pigmentation in or about the oral buccal mucosa as seen in Peutz-Jeghers syndrome should be looked for.

Emergency endoscopy should be carried out in all patients who are determined to be bleeding from the upper gastrointestinal tract once the patient has been properly resuscitated. Its diagnostic accuracy and yield surpasses any other technique, and it can be done with great safety and speed. Some lesions can be treated through the endoscope, converting these emergency situations to less urgent ones.

Precise diagnosis through direct vision facilitates the proper treatment modality as discussed below. In addition, lesions associated with high risk of rebleeding (Table 20.3) can be identified with careful observation and consideration for other treatment can be made.

Endoscopic treatment should be considered in all patients with upper gastrointestinal tract bleeding as it reduces the bleeding and the need for emergency surgery. The bipolar electrocoagulation probe (BICAP) has proved the most generally available and practice instrument to treat these lesions. It is particularly useful in treating duodenal and gastric ulcers, specific superficial ulcers, hemorrhagic gastritis, Mallory-Weiss tears, and occasionally such lesions as polyps and angiomata.

Emergency esophagogastroduodenoscopy (EGD) depends on the skill of the endoscopist and on the condition of the patient. Patients in shock, those experiencing massive or exsanguinating bleeding, or those with concomitant myocardial ischemia or infarction may not safely undergo endoscopy. Upper gastrointestinal barium studies should only be done in patients in which the bleeding has stopped and their overall condition is good. Such studies are useful where anatomic considerations (e.g., previous unknown gastric operations or where gastrointestinal tract rearrangement, hiatal hernia are present.

TABLE 20.3 *Lesions with a high risk of rebleeding*

Upper
    Duodenal ulcer
        Visible vessel
        Clot in ulcer
        Active bleeding at endoscopy
    Gastric varices
    Cirsoid aneurysms
Lower
    Angiodysplasia
    Diverticulosis

Drug therapy for upper gastrointestinal bleeding using H_2 receptor antagonists is commonly employed but no benefit has been established. In the elderly, the antagonists may interact with other medications such as anticoagulants and aminophylline, β-blockers, and benzodiazepines. Once the bleeding has stopped, H_2 receptor antagonists plus liquid antacids may be given for selected conditions.

The more frequent causes of upper gastrointestinal tract bleeding are individual ulcer, gastritis, gastric ulcer, esophageal varices, and Mallory-Weiss tears in approximate descending order. Each is discussed briefly.

> **KEY POINTS**
>
> • Finding of clear gastric aspirate containing bile in patient with melena rules out bleeding from upper gastrointestinal tract
>
> • Emergency endoscopy should be done on all patients determined to be bleeding from upper gastrointestinal tract once patient properly resuscitated
>
> • Endoscopic treatment should be considered in all patients with upper gastrointestinal tract bleeding as it reduces the bleeding and the need for emergency surgery
>
> • Drug therapy for upper gastrointestinal bleeding using H_2 receptor antagonists commonly used but has no proven benefit

SPECIFIC UPPER GASTROINTESTINAL BLEEDING LESIONS

A previous history of epigastric distress of 1–2 hours, relieved by antacids, suggests ulcer disease. In particular, the use of nonsteroidal anti-inflammatory drugs (NSAIDs) in the elderly patient strongly suggests the presence of peptic ulcer disease or gastritis, or both, as these drugs are ulcerogenic. It is not generally appreciated that the incidence of bleeding peptic ulcer disease in the elderly is twice that seen in the younger patient. Bleeding is the most common complication of peptic ulcer disease in the elderly and accounts for almost one-half of deaths. The gastric aspirate will show hematemesis or bright red bleeding with clots, or both. Following initial cessation of the bleeding, the patient should be observed for signs of recurrent bleeding. Elderly patients (65 years or older) or patients who have had massive bleeding (>6 units), who have bled while in the hospital, or who are experiencing a second bleed, should be operated on.

Duodenal ulcers with a visible vessel, a clot overlying the ulcer, or with active bleeding at endoscopy are predictors for recurrent bleeding.

Operation includes a vagotomy and hemigastrectomy or proximal gastric vagotomy (highly selective vagotomy) plus suture ligation of the bleeding vessel. The latter has recently been shown to be equally effective and having lower operative risk and morbidity rate.

Idiopathic erosive gastritis or gastritis from ingestion of NSAIDs is best treated by vigorous nonoperative methods, as surgical treatment has a 70% or greater mortality rate. Nonoperative treatment includes the cessation of NSAIDs ingestion, use of triple antimicrobials, and mucosal protective agents containing sublimate of bismuth to control or eradicate *Helicobacter pylori* infection. The latter organism has been shown to influence, if not cause, the formation of gastritis. Bleeding in these cases is almost always controlled by these nonoperative measures. When operation is necessary because of uncontrollable bleeding, the most effective therapy is total gastrectomy to save the patient's life. Generally, these rare patients have no systemic predisposing factors, and the mortality rate is lower than those with systemic disease.

Unfortunately, the most severe forms of bleeding erosive gastritis have occurred in patients who are critically ill from systemic disease, such as sepsis. In a few patients gastritis develops following major operations (e.g., coronary artery bypass) in which bleeding occurs during the early postoperative period. In patients who are critically ill from other causes, or in whom bleeding gastritis is a complication and not a cause, the initial effort should be vigorous treatment of the infection or vigorous resuscitation and restoration of normal blood pH values and mesenteric perfusion in the postoperative patient. The operative mortality in these instances is exceedingly high; therefore, all efforts are directed as nonoperative management when possible.

Gastric ulcers are most commonly found on the lesser curvature of the stomach at the level of the incisura. The ulcers usually involve branches of the left gastric artery, producing severe bleeding.

Gastric ulcers greater than 3–4 cm in diameter respond less well to medical therapy and are more apt to rebleed. For these reasons, elderly patients or those who have had more than a 4-unit bleed should be considered for operation. The procedures of choice are excision of the ulcer with a distal portion of the stomach in the younger, healthier patient, or excision of the ulcer with gastric closure combined with vagotomy and pyloroplasty in the more elderly patient.

KEY POINTS

- Incidence of bleeding peptic ulcer disease in elderly twice that seen in younger patients, which is not generally appreciated

- Patients who are 65 years or older, have had massive bleeding (>6 units), have bled while in the hospital, or are experiencing a second bleed should undergo operation

- Predictors for recurrent bleeding are duodenal ulcers with a visible vessel, a clot overlying the ulcer, or with active bleeding at endoscopy

- Elderly patients or those who have had more than a 4-unit bleed should be considered for operation

SUGGESTED READINGS

Cook DJ, Fuller HD, Guyatt GH et al: Risk factors for gastrointestinal bleeding in critically ill patients. N Engl J Med 330: 377, 1994

Sugawa C, Steffel CP, Nakamura R et al: Upper GI bleeding in an urban hospital: etiology, recurrence and prognosis. Ann Surg 212:521, 1990

QUESTIONS

1. *The key steps in managing the patient with upper gastrointestinal bleeding?*
    A. Obtain a history, examine the patient, and start blood transfusion.
    B. Carry out emergency endoscopy and plan therapy around lesion found.
    C. Begin resuscitation, obtain a history, perform physical examination, then do endoscopy.
    D. Pass a nasogastric tube, evaluate the aspirate for arterial or venous bleeding, and carry out endoscopy.

2. *The primary reason for gastric intubation is?*
    A. To determine whether the bleeding is arterial or venous.
    B. To evacuate the stomach of clots to help stop continued bleeding.
    C. To prevent aspirations.
    D. To gauge the rate of bleeding.

3. *Upper gastrointestinal is considered more serious than lower gastrointestinal bleeding because?*
    A. It is more common.
    B. It is more apt to be associated with other diseases.
    C. The nature of the lesions can produce exsanguinating hemorrhage.
    D. The bleeding is less apt to stop spontaneously.

(See p. 603 for answers.)

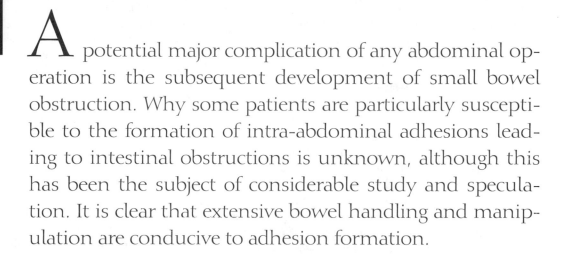

21

SMALL BOWEL

OBSTRUCTION

AND FISTULAS

EDWARD PASSARO, JR.

A potential major complication of any abdominal operation is the subsequent development of small bowel obstruction. Why some patients are particularly susceptible to the formation of intra-abdominal adhesions leading to intestinal obstructions is unknown, although this has been the subject of considerable study and speculation. It is clear that extensive bowel handling and manipulation are conducive to adhesion formation.

This chapter describes the principles underlying the development of small bowel obstruction and fistula formation. The goal is to provide the student with insight into this clinical problem that will aid both in its recognition and in its treatment.

CASE 1
FEMORAL HERNIA

A 55-year-old slightly obese male had rapid onset of nausea and vomiting over 6 hours. He had no previous operations. His last bowel movement was 12 hours earlier. His temperature was 38.6°C, WBC count 13,200. His abdomen was slightly distended and tender to deep palpation in the left lower quadrant. No groin hernias were felt. Plain abdominal films showed some dilated small bowel in the left lower quadrant without air-fluid levels. There was gas in the right colon and rectum. He was thought to have diverticulitis. He was started on a course of antibiotics and an NG tube was inserted. Four hours later, his abdominal

pain had increased and his temperature remained unchanged; operation was recommended.

At operation the descending and sigmoid colon was normal. Deep in the pelvis along the femoral vessels were several loops of dilated distal jejunum. During the process of retracting the small bowel into the field, the dilated jejunal loops were reduced from a femoral canal hernia. The incarcerated segment appeared reddish purple and slightly edematous and was sharply demarcated from the rest of the normal-appearing bowel. It was observed for the next 20 minutes and improved in color. The hernia defect was repaired and the abdomen closed. The patient was discharged on the fifth postoperative day.

CASE 2
POSTOPERATIVE ILEUS

A 47-year-old female had an abdominal hysterectomy for fibroids. An NG tube inserted during the operation was removed while she was awake in the recovery room. On the second postoperative day she consumed a liquid diet. The following day, she was started on solid foods. Her appetite was rather limited. The next day, while attempting to eat, she started to experience nausea. A few hours later, she had onset of vomiting. Her abdomen had become slightly distended, but she was without pain. She was made NPO and intravenous fluids were restarted. Because of increasing discomfort with abdominal distention, an NG tube was inserted and 800 ml of gastric contents withdrawn. She began to feel better. The following day she was being considered for an upper gastrointestinal contrast study when she began to pass flatus. The study was canceled and the NG tube withdrawn; the following day she was again started on a liquid diet. Over the next 48 hours she progressed to a regular diet and was discharged without incidence. Three months later on follow-up examination, she was found to be entirely asymptomatic.

CASE 3
POSTOPERATIVE ADHESIONS, FISTULA

A 37-year-old male presented with progressive nausea, vomiting, and crampy bilateral lower quadrant abdominal pain over the previous 48 hours. He had not had a bowel movement or flatus during this time. He had a perforated appendix at age 23 complicated by small bowel obstruction requiring reoperation on the 10th postappendectomy day. He had several prior similar episodes of crampy abdominal pain, successfully treated with NG tube decompression and IV fluids for 48–72 hours.

His abdomen was distended, tympanitic, and tender to palpation in both lower abdominal quadrants, with the right greater than the left. He was afebrile, his Hct was 50%, and the WBC count 10,600. Plain films of the abdomen showed many loops of small bowel with air-fluid levels in them. Only a few widely scattered patches of gas were found in the colon. An NG tube returned 1,200 ml of a brownish "feculent"-smelling fluid. He received more than 1,500 ml of saline infusion before he began to urinate. Over the next 12 hours, he felt much better, but his abdomen remained distended and he had passed no flatus. The NG tube had removed an additional 1,200 ml of bowel contents. His temperature was now 38°C and his WBC count 13,000. Both lower abdominal quadrants remained tender. Another set of plain films of the abdomen failed to show progression of gas into the colon. He was prepared for operation, as his obstruction had not resolved. Considerable difficulty was encountered in entering the abdominal cavity because of the dense adhesions, which were lysed by a combination of both sharp and blunt dissection. Several inadvertent enterotomies were made in the process, which were sewn closed. No clear point of obstruction (dilated bowel proximal and collapsed bowel distal) could be discerned.

On the seventh postoperative day he developed a temperature to 39°C and lower abdominal pain beneath the midline incision. The wound edges were gently spread apart, and bile-stained intestinal contents issued forth. Through a defect in the fascia, a sump drain was inserted, which promptly drained an additional 200 ml of enteric fluid. He was given antibiotics and 12 hours later was afebrile. He was started on TPN. Approximately 200 ml of fluid drained out daily. Five days later, he passed some flatus for the first time since operation and reported being hungry. Octreotide was started; 1 week later, catheter drainage was only 50 ml/day. The sump drain was removed, a small catheter inserted, and contrast injected by catheter ("fistulagram"). The contrast entered what appeared to be mid-small bowel and progressed into the colon. The catheter was removed and the fistula closed spontaneously 4 days later. He was maintained NPO on TPN for an additional 2 weeks before he was allowed to eat. He tolerated an oral diet and the TPN and octreotide were stopped. He remained asymptomatic during the next 2 years of follow-up.

GENERAL CONSIDERATIONS

Of the entire extent of the gastrointestinal (GI) tract only the duodenum and proximal 2 feet of the jejunum are essential for life. Seldom appreciated is that this meager portion of the bowel's length carries out most of its absorptive functions. The additional length of the bowel beyond this essential portion is thought to provide the great flexibility we enjoy in dietary habits.

Also not widely appreciated is the great variation in location and diameter of the small bowel. The duodenum is exclusively retroperitoneal and fixed in position. Portions of the hepatic flexure and transverse colon overlie it. Its diameter is 3–4 times greater than that of the distal ileum. Most of the small bowel comes to lie in the left lower quadrant of the abdomen, as its mesentery is fixed at the ligament of Treitz and the ileocecal valve. Based on this mesenteric plane, the bowel could flop into the right upper quadrant or left lower quadrant. The liver occupies the right upper quadrant so the small bowel is predominantly in the left lower quadrant.

From these anatomic considerations, we can deduce several important clinical considerations:

1. As the duodenum is large in diameter, retroperitoneal, and has portions of the colon as a shield, it is not the site of intestinal obstruction from adhesions or hernias, the two most common causes.

2. The distal ileum has the smallest diameter of the entire gastrointestinal tract and is therefore the easiest portion of the bowel to obstruct with adhesions. It is mobile in the lower abdomen and can be entrapped into hernias or be-

hind adhesive bands (internal hernias). Hernias are the second most common cause of obstruction.

3. Abdominal distention from intestinal obstruction will be primarily in the lower abdomen (the location of the small bowel).

4. As most obstruction occurs in the distal small bowel, the progressive symptoms of the obstruction (anorexia, nausea, abdominal distention, vomiting) take time (hours to days) to become manifest. Conversely, the more proximal the site of the obstruction the earlier and more prominent are the symptoms of the obstruction.

5. Plain abdominal films should show progressive loops of dilated small bowel proceeding from the ileocecal region to the ligament of Treitz (so-called stepladder pattern).

The other important consideration relates to the pathophysiology of obstruction. Recall that the intestinal tract has fluxes of 7–10 L of a salt solution every day. A slight shift of that equilibrium will cause several liters of fluid to accumulate quickly in either the bowel lumen or bowel wall or to transudate into the free peritoneal cavity quickly. We are exquisitely tuned to the condition of our bowels; anorexia is the first sign that something is wrong. With little or no intake and the shift of several liters of body fluids, a decrease in urine output and mild hypovolemia ensues. A few days of this and the patient is cool to touch, with slow, deep respirations and swollen abdomen. The patient is moribund and in a state of chronic shock. So insidious is its development that patient and physician alike are misled as to the seriousness of the condition. If these basic considerations relating to anatomy and physiology are understood and kept in mind, what follows relative to the diagnosis and treatment is both simple and logical.

KEY POINTS
- Extensive bowel handling and manipulation are conducive to adhesion formation
- Duodenum is large in diameter, retroperitoneal, and has portions of colon as shield; therefore is not site of intestinal obstruction from adhesions or hernias, the two most common causes
- Distal ileum has smallest diameter of entire gastrointestinal tract; therefore easiest portion of bowel to be obstructed by adhesions; in lower abdomen it is mobile and can be entrapped into hernias or behind adhesive bands (internal hernias); hernias second most common cause of obstruction
- Abdominal distention from intestinal obstruction primarily occurs in lower abdomen (location of small bowel)
- Most obstruction occurs in distal small bowel; thus, progressive symptoms of obstruction (anorexia, nausea, abdominal distention, vomiting) take time (hours to days) to manifest
- The more proximal site of obstruction, the earlier and more prominent the symptoms of obstruction

- Plain abdominal films should show progressive loops of dilated small bowel proceeding from the ileocecal region to the ligament of Treitz (so-called stepladder pattern)
- Intestinal tract has fluxes of 7–10 L/day of salt solution; a small shift of that equilibrium will cause several liters of fluid to accumulate quickly in either bowel lumen or bowel wall or to transudate into the free peritoneal cavity

DIAGNOSIS

Depending on the clinical information, the diagnosis can be relatively easy (Case 3) or nearly impossible (Case 1) or unsure (Case 2). The important clinical information from the history is previous operations or bouts of presumed obstructions (Case 3). Other features are the insidious and progressive development of anorexia, followed by nausea and finally vomiting. During this time the patient usually has not passed much or any flatus or stool.

Despite this understanding of the pathophysiology and progression of the symptoms, every study of this problem indicates that the clinical accuracy in arriving at a diagnosis based on history and physical findings alone is only fair. This is because many medical (e.g., pneumonia or surgical problems (Case 1) can mimic the findings.

Progression of the disease process (Cases 1 and 2) is the single best guide to determining what needs to be done (see Ch. 12). In Cases 1 and 2, this is how the clinicians arrived at the proper course of action. The progression, or lack of it, is assessed by repeated physical examination, looking for increasing abdominal distention, areas of focal pain or tenderness, and signs of peritonitis, and by observations that the patient has not had passage of flatus or stool. Plain films of the abdomen to monitor the progression of intraluminal gas down the gastrointestinal tract can be helpful. In selected instances, a contrast study using water-soluble contrast media inserted via a nasogastric (NG) tube may be useful. Delayed films will show accumulation of the contrast at the point of the obstruction. In some instances in which the obstruction is incomplete or the patient has an ileus (discussed below), the hypertonic contrast media can be therapeutic as well. Water-soluble contrast agents (hypertonic), draw fluid into the lumen. Additionally, these iodinated compounds are irritating to the bowel and therefore promote peristaltic activity. In patients with partial obstruction or ileus, this increased peristalsis may be sufficient to cause passage of gas and stool with considerable relief for the patient. Obviously, if the obstruction is complete, nothing will pass. The increased bowel activity may cause focal pain, pointing to the area of obstruction and aiding in diagnosis. However, the test would not be advisable in patients with longstanding obstruction or when compromise of the blood supply to the bowel is possible or likely.

Another approach to establish the diagnosis is through the use of long intestinal tubes. These tubes are particularly useful in very complicated patients who have undergone several abdominal operations previously. The Baker, Miller-Abbott, and Cantor tubes have the advantage of being therapeutic as well as diagnostic. Their disadvantage is that they require patience and some skill in getting them beyond the ligament of Treitz into the dilated proximal small bowel. If the obstruction is longstanding, peristalsis may be absent, preventing their advancement by bowel activity. When successful, however, the passage of a long tube evacuates the bowel of both gas and fluid, decompressing it. The long tube will advance to or near the point of obstruction. As the proximal bowel is decompressed, what was formerly an emergency is now a less emergent condition. When the progression of the tube has stopped, contrast media in limited quantities can be instilled and a selective study near the region made. This aids in locating the obstructed point which is difficult (Case 3) in many instances. Intraoperatively the intraluminal tube assists the surgeon in locating the obstruction among the many areas of adhesions and kinked bowel.

All in all, few conditions are as difficult to both diagnose and successfully manage as that of intestinal obstruction. Moreover, successful treatment in avoidance of major complications is absolutely dependent on the timely and proper management of this condition.

KEY POINTS

• Clinical accuracy is only fair in arriving at a diagnosis based on history and physical examination alone, despite understanding of pathophysiology and progression of symptoms

• Progression of disease process single best guide to determining what needs to be done

DIFFERENTIAL DIAGNOSIS

Any condition that can produce an ileus enters into the differential diagnosis of intestinal obstruction. Distinguishing an ileus from a presumed inflammatory process or from an obstruction is important. Ileus is a physiologic obstruction; that is, the bowel is patent but it lacks the force or peristaltic activity sufficient to propel bowel contents. Gas and fluid accumulate as in a mechanical obstruction where the lumen is blocked either partially or completely.

Postoperative ileus is often indistinguishable from postoperative intestinal obstruction due to adhesive bands (Case 2). Ileus does not require operation—in fact, operation only exacerbates the condition—whereas mechanical obstructions often do require operation for correction. Postoperative ileus that never resolves to the point that the patient can be started on oral feeds is most apt to be

due to mechanical obstruction and require reoperation in the postoperative period. Patients who appear to have resolved their postoperative ileus and who are started on diets, only to fail (Case 2) usually have ileus and not a mechanical problem. These cases typically resolve with additional supportive measures.

KEY POINTS

• Important to distinguish an ileus from a presumed inflammatory process (e.g., diverticulitis) from an obstruction

• Ileus does not require operation (which only exacerbates condition)

• Mechanical obstructions often do require operation for correction

TREATMENT

There are many oft-quoted statements regarding the treatment of intestinal obstruction ("the sun should never rise or set on a case of small bowel obstruction"). All convey a sense of urgency; that is, within a 12-hour period either the patient is better or should be operated on, or both, to make the diagnosis and treat it if correct. These aphorisms are misdirected, as there is universal agreement that if complete mechanical obstruction is present the patient will need operation for relief, and the more promptly this can be attended to, the less likely is the risk of complications such as bowel strangulation, infarction, or perforation. The problem therefore is not in treatment, it is in diagnosis. Does the patient have obstruction or ileus? Is the obstruction partial or complete? Where is the obstruction?

Insertion of an NG tube reduces the likelihood of aspiration, makes the patient feel better, and can aid in the diagnosis when combined with a period of observation (Cases 1, 2, and 3). In the first case, although the patient initially felt better, he did not improve with observation and underwent operation. In the second case, the patient improved following NG tube insertion and observation. In the last case, insertion of a nasogastric tube and observation led to successful resolution of his abdominal distention on two occasions in the past. On this admission he did not improve on observation and required operation.

The two most common causes of mechanical small bowel obstruction are postoperative adhesions and hernias of the abdominal wall. Obstructions resulting from adhesion formation is treated by dividing the adhesive bands producing the obstruction. Generally, many adhesive bands are found at operation, but only one is producing the obstruction. The rest need not be lysed. Hernias of the abdominal wall are repaired following a reduction of the obstructed bowel segment.

On occasion, the area of obstruction is either inaccessible because of scarring, or is too dangerous to remove because of an inflammatory process as in Crohn's disease. The obstruction can be relieved by bypass procedures, connecting proximal uninvolved bowel with bowel distal to the obstruction.

Small bowel obstruction due to tumor is a not infrequent complication of widespread metastatic tumors from the large bowel, pancreas, and stomach. Finding a discrete solitary point of obstruction in these patients is rarely possible. Unfortunately most of these patients cannot be aided by operation. When the tumor is localized to a segment of the bowel, it can either be resected or bypassed or an ostomy for decompression made proximal to it.

KEY POINTS

- Problem not in treatment but in diagnosis
- Two most common causes of mechanical small bowel obstruction are postoperative adhesions and hernias of abdominal wall

R FOLLOW-UP

Resumption of bowel activity with passage of gas and stool is the best measure of resolution of the obstruction. Patients with a discrete mechanical cause, as a solitary adhesive band, have an excellent prognosis on long term follow-up.

Patients with extensive intra-abdominal adhesions and previous bouts of obstruction require life-long follow-up for further bouts of obstruction.

Similarly, patients with obstruction from malignant tumors are at risk of additional episodes of obstruction before they succumb to the tumor. Many of these patients have small bowel obstruction as a terminal event.

A complication of small bowel obstruction seen during the immediate postoperative period, but more commonly on follow-up, is the development of small bowel fistula.

Small bowel fistulas arise because there is a recurrent obstruction (usually partial in nature) and a proximal weakened portion of the bowel that breaks down. The weakened area can be at a previous suture line or enterotomy closure (Case 3) or where the bowel was traumatized during the operation.

Fistulas are a connection between the bowel lumen and the skin surface. They are readily apparent as drainage or bowel contents issue forth on the skin usually at incisions or drain sites.

Infection, intra-abdominal as well as deep in the operative incision, are predisposing factors for fistula formation. Spontaneous fistulas can occur when an intra-abdominal infection, as from diverticulitis, erodes through the abdominal wall, draining externally.

Fistulas are categorized by their location and volume of drainage. In general, fistulas proximal in the gastrointestinal tract have a higher morbidity and mortality (approximately 40%) than those more distal such as colon fistula (2%). Similarly, fistulas draining large volumes are more hazardous than those draining smaller volumes. Duodenal fistulas have much higher volume outputs than ileal fistulas, for example.

The drainage contents are also important; bile, pancreatic juice, and other proteolytic juices from the duodenum are corrosive and extremely difficult to manage. Colonic fistulas draining fecal material are easier to control and can be managed similar to a colostomy.

Proximal fistulas require extensive drainage of the discharge. Not infrequently, the involved area needs to be excluded by operation from the remainder of the gastrointestinal tract. The voluminous discharge of a protein and salt rich fluid will rapidly deplete the patient. Thus patients require vigorous nutritional and fluid support via chronic intravenous catheters. By contrast, distal fistulas can be treated by a nutritional liquid diet that is absorbed proximal to the fistula site (elemental diet), total parenteral nutrition (TPN), NG intubation, and octreotide. These measures work by decreasing the volume of intestinal secretions passing through the fistula. As the bowel mucosa exhibits very high proliferative activity, it will grow and seal a collapsed fistulous tract but cannot do so if the fistula is actively discharging fluids.

Fistulas can close spontaneously when there is no diseased bowel involved and no obstruction distal to the fistula, and when the drainage through the fistula is minimal. Octreotide suppresses intestinal secretions of all kinds, reducing the volume of fluid passing through the fistula.

Conversely, fistulas will remain open if there is injured or diseased bowel or some degree of obstruction of the bowel distal to the fistula site. Foreign bodies (nonabsorbable sutures, retained sponges) at a fistula site, will promote infection and keep the fistula open.

KEY POINTS

- Resumption of bowel activity with passage of gas and stool best measure of resolution of obstruction
- Small bowel fistulas arise because of recurrent obstruction (usually partial in nature) and a proximal weakened portion of bowel that breaks down
- Fistulas are connection between bowel lumen and skin surface

SUGGESTED READINGS

Brolin RE: The role of gastrointestinal tube decompression in the treatment of mechanical intestinal obstruction. Am Surg 49: 131, 1983

Livingston EH, Passaro EP Jr: Postoperative ileus. Dig Dis Sci 35:121, 1990

QUESTIONS

1. The major difficulty in managing a patient with small bowel obstruction is?

    A. Determining whether the obstruction is complete or incomplete.

    B. Determining whether the obstruction is high in the gastrointestinal tract or lower.

    C. Determining the etiology of the obstruction as from tumor or an inflammatory process.

    D. Distinguishing between whether the patient has ileus or a mechanical obstruction.

2. In patient with suspected small bowel obstruction, the best course of action is?

    A. Immediate operation in all patients.

    B. Observe patient and carry out investigative test (e.g., plain films of abdomen, UGI series, CT) until the diagnosis is established.

    C. Initial resuscitation and observation followed by urgent operation in all patients who do not improve or in whom doubt remains.

    D. Passage of long gastrointestinal tubes to decompress the bowel and help establish the diagnosis.

(See p. 603 for answers.)

22

CIRRHOSIS

AND PORTAL

HYPERTENSION

FRED S. BONGARD

The causes of portal hypertension vary with geographic location. Worldwide, the most common cause is infection with schistosomiasis, which causes presinusoidal fibrosis of the liver. In the United States, alcohol intake with resultant cirrhosis is the most common etiology. In Asia, where infection with hepatitis B is endemic, postin-

fectious cirrhosis is prevalent. Common to all causes of portal hypertension is an obstruction to blood flow within the portal venous system. The effects of portal hypertension range from subclinical to massive hematemesis. This chapter discusses the pathophysiologic mechanisms of portal hypertension, the dependence on etiology of clinical presentation, a scoring system for the severity of the disease, and approaches to both surgical and nonsurgical management.

CASE 1
ALCOHOLIC CIRRHOSIS AND
PORTAL HYPERTENSION

A 54-year-old chronic alcoholic consumed at least 2 pints of whiskey a day for the past 13 years. On arising the morning of presentation, he began to feel nauseated and started to vomit dark red blood with clots shortly thereafter. On arrival at the hospital, he had a BP of 100/60 mmHg and an HR of 120 bpm. After several more bouts of bloody emesis, a nasogastric tube was inserted, which produced several hundred milliliters of dark blood. Lavage was begun with 2 L of fluid until the aspirate returned clear. Significant laboratory results were as follows: Hb, 9.2 g/dl: PT, 16.4 seconds (control = 12.0 seconds); K^+, 3.1 mEq/l; and BUN,

45 mg/L. A rapid infusion of saline was begun to correct hypotension, and blood was sent for type and cross-match. Emergent esophagogastroscopy found several large bleeding varices in the distal esophagus. An intravenous infusion of Pitressin was begun. Aspirate from the nasogastric tube cleared over the next 18 hours.

Further evaluation found the patient to have moderate ascites, no encephalopathy, a serum albumin concentration of 2.8 mg/L, and a bilirubin concentration of 3.2 mg/L. He was assigned a Child "B" classification. Evaluation for possible portasystemic shunting found that the splenic and portal veins were both patent. After several days of resuscitation and stabilization, he underwent a selective portasystemic shunt. Two years after the procedure he stopped drinking and experienced no further episodes of bleeding, but had a decreased attention span and was often confused.

CASE 2
HEPATITIS AND PORTAL
HYPERTENSION

A 36-year-old Chinese immigrant developed hepatitis B at age 13. Since that time, she has had chronic active disease with a fibrotic liver and signs of portal hypertension. Two previous hospitalizations have been required for hematemesis, which responded to nonoperative therapy. Her latest episode of bleeding was worse than those in the past. Her Hb had fallen to 7.2 g/dl from her usual value of 12.5 g/dl. Emergent esophagoscopy demonstrated multiple large bleeding varices. Significant laboratory values were as follows: albumin, 2.3 g/L; bilirubin, 4.1 g/L; PT, 15.3 seconds (control = 12.0 seconds). She was found to have moderate ascites, temporal wasting, and no encephalopathy. An NG tube was inserted and returned 750 ml of bloody fluid. A continuous infusion of vasopressin was begun, but the bloody aspirate persisted and her Hb continued to fall. Repeat esophagogastroscopy was done and the bleeding varices injected with a sclerosant solution. Despite three sessions of sclerotherapy over the next 36 hours, she continued to bleed and developed a profound coagulopathy. On the fourth hospital day, her urine output fell, despite adequate fluid resuscitation. In spite of dialysis and pressor support, she expired on the ninth hospital day.

GENERAL CONSIDERATIONS

The liver receives blood flow from the hepatic artery and from the portal vein. The hepatic artery arises from the celiac axis and terminates in the liver after branching into left and right tributaries. The portal vein begins at the confluence of the splenic and superior mesenteric veins behind the pancreas. It subsequently receives the inferior mesenteric vein before turning upward to enter the liver. Because of its position, it is susceptible to inflammatory processes in the pancreas that may cause portal vein thrombosis. Two-thirds of hepatic blood flow is from the portal vein, although most of the oxygen supply to the liver is through the hepatic artery. Hepatic arterial flow changes reciprocally with alterations in portal venous flow. However, acute changes in hepatic arterial flow do not produce significant increases in portal venous flow.

Portal hypertension occurs when there is an obstruction to blood flow through the portal venous (mesenteric) system. The location of the obstruction is related to the etiology of the disease. Mesenteric flow to the liver proceeds through the portal vein to the liver, through the portal sinusoids, into the hepatic veins, and finally into the inferior vena cava. Portal hypertension is divided into three broad categories, prehepatic, hepatic, and posthepatic. Rarely, it may be produced by increased portal blood flow, which occurs with splenomegaly, an arterioportal venous fistula, or with Banti's syndrome (primary splenic disease). Prehepatic causes are due to portal vein obstruction, which may follow congenital stenosis of the portal vein, thrombosis (following pancreatitis), or stenosis from extrinsic compression (e.g., tumor).

Schistosoma cruzii is a parasite, particularly common in the Middle East, that causes presinusoidal fibrosis. This prevents portal blood from flowing normally through the hepatic system. Even though portal hypertension is created, it occurs before blood reaches the sinusoids and liver function remains normal. Alcoholic cirrhosis and hepatitis, as well as a number of chemical agents, cause postsinusoidal fibrosis, which initially prevents blood from leaving the liver, but eventually causes such significant distortion that portal venous inflow is affected and portal hypertension results. Unlike the situation with presinusoidal disease, alcoholic cirrhosis causes profound hepatic dysfunction, which ultimately results in liver failure. An uncommon variant of postsinusoidal disease occurs in the Budd-Chiari syndrome, in which hepatic venous or vena caval outflow from the liver is limited, often by congenital stenosis, bands, or webs. This effectively constitutes a postsinusoidal obstruction and results in hepatic pathophysiology similar to alcoholic cirrhosis or viral hepatitis.

When portal venous pressure is increased, alternate pathways for mesenteric blood flow develop. Such *collateral* pathways are anatomic connections between the portal and systemic circuits, which normally have little or no flow through them. However, as portal pressure increases, these pathways enlarge and shunt blood away from the portal system to the lower resistance systemic veins (Fig. 22.1).

The portasystemic collaterals of greatest importance are in the esophagus, the pelvic circulation, the retroperitoneum, and the abdominal wall. The coronary (left gastric) vein connects the portal and systemic circuit through the veins of the esophagus and the azygos vein, which empties into the superior vena cava. When portal pressure increases, blood flows in a retrograde fashion (hepatofugal) through the esophagus to the low pressure systemic venous circuit. Veins that are usually very small, such as the esophageal submucosal veins, become engorged to carry the increased flow from the mesenteric circulation. The enlarged submucosal varices may erode through the mucosa and bleed into the lumen, resulting in severe hematemesis. Because of the increased pressure and flow within the collaterals, the hemorrhage tends not to stop once it has begun. Another important collateral pathway exists in the rectum between the superior hemorrhoidal veins of the portal system and the middle and inferior hemorrhoidal veins of the systemic circuit. Increased flow within these collaterals produces large hemorrhoidal veins that are easily damaged and may bleed profusely. In the retroperitoneum, in the veins of Retzius, which connect the mesenteric and peritoneal veins, hypertrophy occurs as flow increases. The abdominal wall contains communication between the superior and inferior epigastric veins and superficial systemic veins. The dilated veins produce a characteristic vascular pattern of radiating vessels around the umbilicus referred to as caput medusae.

In addition to the formation of varices and hemorrhoids, portal hypertension has other deterimental physiologic effects. Because mesenteric blood is shunted away from the liver, normal hepatocellular function cannot occur.

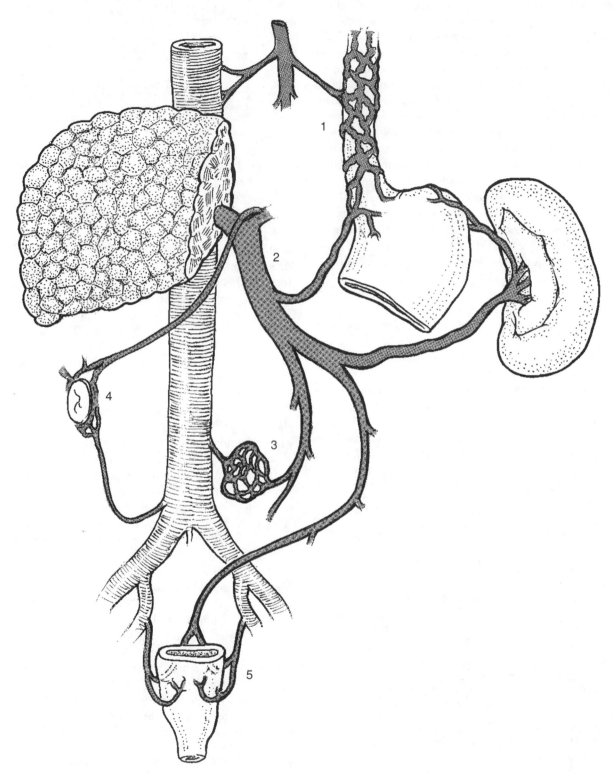

FIGURE 22.1 *Several pathways (portasystemic collaterals) develop so that blood can pass around the high pressure portal system into the systemic circuit. The major connections are between the (1) esophageal and azygos veins, (2) gastric veins and inferior vena cava, (3) retroperitoneal veins, (4) veins of the abdominal wall (caput medusae), and (5) hemorrhoidal veins.*

Hepatic encephalopathy is a reversible syndrome that occurs when toxins absorbed from the gut adversely affect the brain and central nervous system. The toxins arise from the action of bacteria on absorbed protein within the gut. Encephalopathy is particularly severe with increased protein intake, after episodes of esophageal variceal hemorrhage, infections, azotemia, and hypokalemic metabolic alkalosis. False neurotransmitters, formed in the gut, are thought to cross the blood-brain barrier and result in encephalopathy. The aromatic amino acids (tryptophan, tyrosine, and threonine) have increased access to the central nervous system where they serve as precursors of false transmitters. Additionally, γ-aminobutyric acid, which is formed by colonic bacteria, passes across the blood-brain barrier and serves as an inhibitory neurotransmitter. Ammonia is also formed by colonic bacteria and is normally converted to glutamine by the liver. When hepatofugal flow is present, increased ammonia concentrations are found in both arterial blood and cerebrospinal fluid.

When perisinusoidal pressure increases sufficiently, fluid transudation occurs. If production exceeds the reabsorptive capacity of hepatic lymphatics, ascites are produced. Protein rich ascites results in loss of volume from the intravascular space into the peritoneum. The physiologic response to this intravascular volume contraction includes salt and water retention due to the actions of aldosterone. The patient becomes hypokalemic, hypernatremic, and oliguric (Case 1). Ascites produces abdominal distention and may eventually result in spontaneous bacterial peritonitis if infection occurs.

KEY   POINTS

- In United States, alcohol intake with resultant cirrhosis is most common etiology

- Common to all causes of portal hypertension is an obstruction to blood flow within the portal venous system

- Two-thirds of hepatic blood flow is from the portal vein, although most of the oxygen supply to the liver is through the hepatic artery

- Three broad categories of portal hypertension: prehepatic, hepatic, and posthepatic

- Alcoholic cirrhosis and hepatitis, as well as a number of chemical agents, cause postsinusoidal fibrosis, which initially prevents blood from leaving the liver, but eventually causes such significant distortion that portal venous inflow is affected and portal hypertension results

- Unlike the situation with presinusoidal disease, alcoholic cirrhosis causes profound hepatic dysfunction, which ultimately results in liver failure

- Collateral pathways are anatomic connections between the portal and systemic circuits, which normally have little or no flow through them; however, as portal pressure increases, these pathways enlarge and shunt blood away from the portal system to the lower resistance systemic vascular resistance

- Portasystemic collaterals of greatest importance are in the esophagus, pelvic circulation, retroperitoneum, and abdominal wall

- Because mesenteric blood is shunted away from the liver, normal hepatocellular function cannot occur

- Hepatic encephalopathy is a reversible syndrome that occurs when toxins absorbed from the gut adversely affect the brain and central nervous system

DIAGNOSIS

Portal hypertension and variceal bleeding are sequelae of the underlying hepatic disease. Patients with cirrhosis will typically exhibit malnutrition, palmar erythema, encephalopathy, ascites, and jaundice. Splenomegaly is the most common physical finding, and is present in 80% of those with portal hypertension, regardless of the cause. Bleeding occurs in approximately 40% of those with cirrhosis. The first step in the treatment of presumed variceal hemorrhage is vigorous resuscitation. Fluid administration should consist of both balanced salt solution and red blood cells as required. Because the synthetic capacity of the liver may be severely impaired, prothrombin time (PT) should be checked and fresh frozen plasma administered as required to correct any coagulopathy. A nasogastric tube should be inserted for gavage and aspiration of clots, as well as to monitor continuing hemorrhage. A Foley catheter should be placed so that urine output can be used to guide further fluid resuscitation. If shock is present, or if the patient does not respond to initial resuscitative measures, central hemodynamic monitoring should be instituted.

Upper gastrointestinal endoscopy is the most useful procedure for the diagnosis of variceal hemorrhage. It should be performed as soon as possible after the patient is hemodynamically stable. Varices appear as large, bluish, submucosal vessels that run longitudinally along the length of the esophagus. Bleeding varices are easily identified, although fresh adherent clot may be present, indicating that hemorrhage was present recently. Occasionally gastric varices may be identified; this is particularly true when splenic vein thrombosis is the cause of portal hypertension.

Radiographic studies such as an upper gastrointestinal series are not helpful in identifying the source of hemorrhage, although they may confirm the presence of varices.

Laboratory studies including electrolytes, clotting parameters (PT and PTT [partial thromboplastin time]), blood type, platelet count, serum albumin, bilirubin, and liver and renal function tests should be obtained. The Child classification is a simple index of functional liver disease (Table 22.1) and should be calculated for all patients with portal hypertension. The Child-Pugh classification (Table 22.1) is the most recent modification. Earlier versions used nutritional status (good, fair, poor) instead of elevations in the PT. Mortality rate, both with and without surgery, is directly related to the Child classification.

> **KEY POINTS**
>
> • Splenomegaly most common physical finding; present in 80% of those with portal hypertension, regardless of cause
>
> • Bleeding occurs in approximately 40% of those with cirrhosis
>
> • Upper gastrointestinal endoscopy the most useful procedure for diagnosis of variceal hemorrhage; it should be performed as soon as possible after patient is hemodynamically stable
>
> • Radiographic studies such as an upper gastrointestinal series are not helpful in identifying the source of hemorrhage, although may confirm presence of varices
>
> • Mortality rate, with and without surgery, is directly related to Child classification

DIFFERENTIAL DIAGNOSIS

Upper gastrointestinal hemorrhage may be caused by a number of etiologies (see Ch. 20). Even when known portal hypertension and varices are present, one-half of those presenting with acute hemorrhage will be bleeding from a source other than their varices. Sources include gastritis and peptic ulcer disease. Therefore, it is imperative that the diagnosis of bleeding varices be confirmed by gastroesophagoscopy before any therapy is begun.

Other causes of hematemesis that are common among alcoholics and those with cirrhosis include: epistaxis, Mallory-Weiss syndrome, gastritis, and peptic ulcer disease.

TABLE 22.1 *Child-Pugh classification of functional status in liver disease*

	CLASS: A RISK: LOW	B MODERATE	C HIGH
Ascites	Absent	Slight to moderate	Tense
Encephalopathy	None	Grades I–II	Grades III–IV
Serum albumin (g/dl)	>3.5	3.0–3.5	<3.0
Serum bilirubin (mg/dl)	<2.0	2.0–3.0	>3.0
Prothrombin time (seconds above control)	<4.0	4.0–6.0	>6.0

(From Way L: Current Surgical Diagnosis and Treatment, 10th Ed. Appleton & Lange, E. Norwalk, CT, 1994, with permission.)

> **KEY POINTS**
>
> • Even when known portal hypertension and varices present, one-half of those presenting with acute hemorrhage will be bleeding from a source other than varices

TREATMENT

The goal of the acute management of variceal bleeding is to stop the hemorrhage as quickly as possible since the death rate increases quickly when more than 10 units of blood have been transfused. The mortality rate among those with acute variceal hemorrhage is 35%.

After fluid resuscitation and esophagogastroscopy have been completed, control of the hemorrhage should begin. Vasopressin and terlipressin (triglycyl lysine vasopressin) are compounds that lower portal blood flow and portal pressure by constricting splanchnic arterioles. When given intravenously (vasopressin 0.4 units/min), they control bleeding in 80% of patients. Because they are vasoconstrictors, they may produce myocardial and visceral ischemia. Concomitant administration of isoproterenol or nitroglycerin helps to ameliorate these side effects. Octreotide acetate (somatostatin) has similar effects on the splanchnic circulation as vasopressin, but without many of the side effects. It is given as an initial bolus of 100 μg followed by a continuous infusion of 25 μg/hr for 24 hours.

When vasopressin does not control the hemorrhage, mechanical tamponade with a balloon catheter is indicated. Several styles of balloons are available, but they all work on a similar principle. Most have two balloons, one gastric and one esophageal. After the tube has been inserted, the gastric balloon is inflated and pulled into position at the esophagogastric junction (the position must be confirmed radiographically). The balloon occludes the venous inflow from the stomach into the bleeding varices. If hemorrhage does not stop, the esophageal balloon should be inflated. A manometer must be used to ensure that the balloons are not overinflated, which might cause gastric or esophageal rupture. Balloon compression alone is successful 70% of the time. When used in combination with vasopressin, hemorrhage is controlled in 95% of patients. The balloons are deflated within 24 hours after bleeding stops. The esophageal balloon should always be deflated before the gastric balloon. In addition to the possibility of esophageal perforation, the other significant side effect is aspiration of saliva with subsequent pneumonia.

When small bleeding sites can be identified with the esophagogastroscope, injection of a sclerosing agent into the variceal lumen causes sclerosis and thrombosis of the vessel. Endoscopy should be repeated within 48 hours and for several weeks thereafter to treat residual varices. Sclerotherapy controls 80–95% of patients, although about one-half will rebleed during the same hospitalization.

A minimally invasive radiologic procedure is now available for emergency portasystemic decompression. The transjugular intrahepatic portasystemic shunt (TIPS) procedure involves fluoroscopic placement of a catheter in the liver substance (via the vena cava and hepatic veins), which is used to create a shunt between the two circulations. The shunt usually stays open for 1 year and is particularly useful in those being considered for liver transplantation.

Emergent surgery for acute variceal hemorrhage is required infrequently because of the success of sclerotherapy and vasopressin. Operative procedures fall into two groups: ligation and shunt. The Sugiura procedure consists of splenectomy, proximal gastric devascularization, vagotomy, pyloroplasty, esophageal devascularization, and esophageal transection and reanastomosis. Simple esophageal transection and reanastomosis with a mechanical stapler is used for variceal ligation in some centers.

Splenectomy is a nonshunting procedure performed when portal hypertension is due to splenic vein thrombosis, which may occur following pancreatitis or other inflammatory processes. Splenectomy, for this indication, lowers portal pressure, reduces gastric varices, and effectively prevents further hemorrhage.

Shunting procedures are usually performed on a semielective basis in good risk (Child A and B) patients whose acute bleeding has stopped. Operative shunt procedures are either selective or nonselective—that is, they either selectively decompress the esophageal varices or decompress the entire portal/mesenteric bed. Nonselective operations are far more common and consist primarily of end-to-side or side-to-side shunts. These terms are used to describe how the portal vein (or one of its tributaries) is connected to the inferior vena cava to create the shunt. In an end-to-side operation, the portal vein is transected before it enters the liver. The vein on the hepatic side is ligated. The end of the proximal portal vein is connected to the side of the inferior vena cava (Fig. 22.2A & B). Hence, all of the portal blood flow is shunted into the systemic circulation. Although this procedure acutely reduces portal pressure and may control ascites, it frequently worsens encephalopathy because all of the products of digestion bypass the liver and are routed into the systemic circulation.

A side-to-side (nonselective) portacaval shunt anastomosis connects the side of the portal vein to the side of the inferior vena cava (Fig. 22.2A & B). This procedure is differentiated from the end-to-side operation in that the liver is allowed to decompress while potentially maintaining some prograde (hepatopedal) flow through the portal vein. Like the end-to-side shunt, the major postoperative complication of the side-to-side shunt is worsened hepatic encephalopathy. The major variant is the mesocaval shunt in which the side of the superior mesenteric vein is connected to the side of the inferior vena cava (Fig. 22.2C). The advantage of the mesocaval shunt is that it is technically easier (does not require dis-

section at the porta hepatis) and can use a synthetic graft to connect the vessels. Its disadvantage is that the graft may clot quickly due to relatively low flows.

The distal splenorenal shunt is the only commonly performed selective shunt. In contradistinction to the end-to-side and end-to-end shunts, the distal (Warren) splenorenal shunt is selective because it "compartmentalizes" the portal flow, and shunts only that portion contributing to the bleeding varices (Fig. 22.3). By maintaining prograde flow through the liver, it is thought to have a lower incidence of encephalopathy than other operations. The increased portal flow may, however, produce ascites, and therefore should not be used in people with moderate or severe ascites before surgery.

Liver transplantation should be considered in young patients who have survived an episode of variceal bleeding. Candidates should have abstained from alcohol, or should have any systemic disease under control. If a patient under consideration for liver transplantation rebleeds, a TIPS procedure or a mesocaval shunt are the procedures of choice since they do not require dissection at the hepatic hilum, which would make subsequent transplantation more difficult technically.

KEY POINTS

- When given intravenously (vasopressin 0.4 units/min controls bleeding in 80% of patients

- When vasopressin does not control the hemorrhage, mechanical tamponade with a balloon catheter is indicated

- Balloon compression alone is successful 70% of the time; when used in combination with vasopressin, hemorrhage controlled in 95% of patients

- When small bleeding sites can be identified with the esophagogastroscope, injection of a slcerosing agent into the variceal lumen causes sclerosis and thrombosis of the vessel

- Sclerotherapy controls 80–95% of patients, although about one-half will rebleed during same hospitalization

- Emergent surgery for acute variceal hemorrhage required infrequently because of the success of sclerotherapy and vasopressin

- Operative shunt procedures are either selective or nonselective; that is, they either selectively decompress the esophageal varices or decompress the entire portal/mesenteric bed

- Liver transplantation should be considered in young patients who have survived an episode of variceal bleeding

---

FOLLOW-UP

Nonoperative therapy is now the standard treatment for patients acutely bleeding from varices. Hemorrhage can be controlled in 90%, although the early rebleeding rate is 30%. When medical and surgical treatment are compared, most trials have shown that surgical therapy is

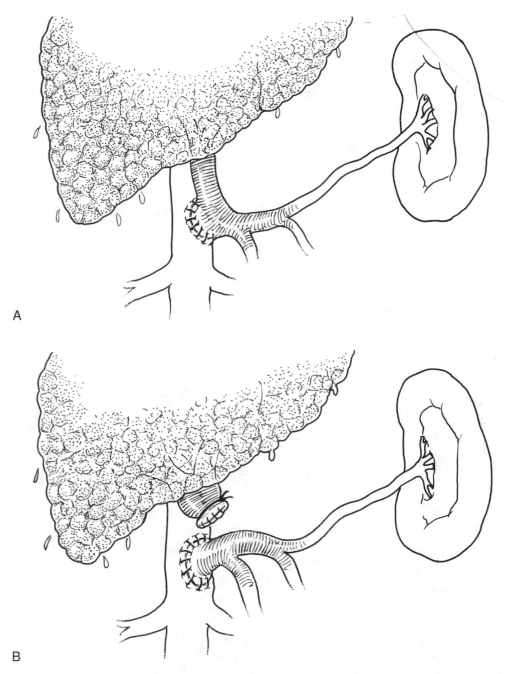

A

B

FIGURE 22.2 *(A)* *A side-to-side portasystemic shunt connects the side of the portal vein (shaded) to the side of the inferior vena cava. This allows the liver to decompress (retrograde) through the shunt while allowing prograde flow from the viscera into the inferior vena cava.* *(B)* *An end-to-side portasystemic shunt connects the proximal end of the portal vein (shaded) to the side of the inferior vena cava. Unlike a side-to-side shunt, the liver cannot decompress. (Figure continues.)*

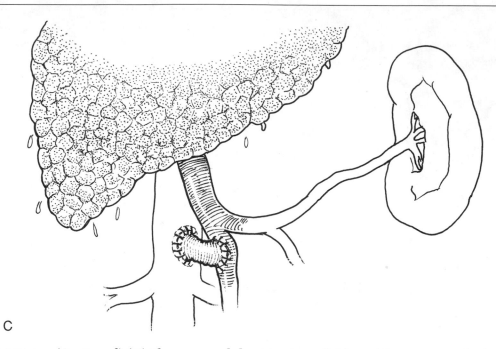

C

FIGURE 22.2   (Continued) *(**C**) The mesocaval shunt is a type of side-to-side portasystemic shunt. Rather than connecting the portal vein and inferior vena cava directly, a short graft is interposed between them. Either autogenous vein or prosthetic can be used. This operation is technically easier than a side-to-side shunt (Fig. A) and does not disturb the anatomy in the right upper quadrant, making a subsequent liver transplant easier.*

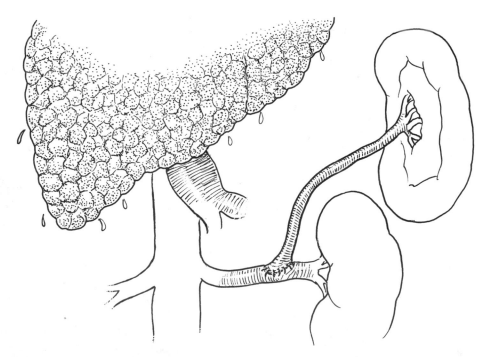

FIGURE 22.3   *The distal splenorenal ("Warren") shunt is created by disconnecting the distal splenic vein and turning it down to connect with the renal vein. This operation was thought to compartmentalize portal flow by returning blood from the high pressure esophageal veins into the renal vein and from there into the vena cava. This leaves undisturbed the portal flow from the superior and inferior mesenteric veins. In time, the shunt looses its selectivity. Increased ascites production is a common complication of the procedure.*

better at preventing subsequent bleeding than is medical treatment alone. Disturbingly, neither medical nor surgical therapy decrease the overall mortality rate from portal hypertension, which is directly related to the patient's Child classification. Furthermore, except for patients with extremely poor liver function (Child C), those treated by chronic sclerotherapy have a lower mortality rate than those treated with a portasystemic shunt. There is no proven benefit of prophylactic portasystemic shunting in patients with esophageal varices who have not experienced an episode of variceal bleeding.

Encephalopathy, ascites, and the hepatorenal syndrome are common complications of cirrhosis, portal hypertension, and shunt procedures. Encephalopathy is aggravated by increased amounts of intestinal protein, regardless of origin. It is worsened by intestinal hemorrhage, constipation, and continued alcoholism. It may be particularly problematic after an end-to-side portacaval shunt. Patients usually have increased arterial ammonia levels along with characteristic changes on electroencephalography. Acute treatment consists of stopping all dietary protein intake and cleansing the bowel using purgatives, enemas, and antibiotics. Lactulose, a minimally absorbed disaccharide, acidifies the colon and produces a catharsis thereby limiting protein absorption. Neomycin (2–4 g/day), a luminal antibiotic, may be helpful by reducing the endemic flora that convert protein to ammonia. Chronic encephalopathy is best treated by limitation of protein intake to less than 50 g/day and consumption of a high carbohydrate diet.

Ascites is treated with chronic diuretic administration aimed at reducing the response to aldosterone. When a patient's 24-hour urinary sodium is between 5 and 25 mEq, diuretic therapy is indicated. Spironolactone, an aldosterone inhibitor, is the drug of choice and is started at 25 mg three times a day, and advanced until ascites are controlled. The objective is to produce a weight loss of 0.5–0.75 kg/day until a stable weight is reached. Salt and water restriction is required only in the most difficult cases. Another diuretic, such as furosemide, may be used when a satisfactory diuresis is not achieved with spironolactone.

When diuretics (≤400 mg/day) are not effective in controlling or reducing ascites, a peritoneovenous shunt (LeVeen) may be performed. This procedure consists of placing a tube with a mechanical one-way valve between the peritoneal cavity and the jugular vein. The low hydrostatic pressure within the jugular vein allows ascites to flow from the peritoneum into the superior vena cava. Newer tubes have small pumps that allow patients to transfer fluid actively. Peritoneovenous shunts may also be used in those whose ascites are due to cancer. A functioning LeVeen shunt cannot completely eliminate ascites, but it makes the patient more responsive to diuretic therapy. The complications of shunt placement include peritonitis and disseminated intravascular coagulation (DIC). Post-shunt DIC occurs in up to 50% of patients and is evidenced by increased fibrin split products and decreased platelet count.

Bacterial peritonitis occurs commonly in patients with ascites and may produce a paucity of symptoms other than malaise and fever. It is diagnosed by aspirating a small amount of ascitic fluid. Typical findings include a white count greater than 250 cells/ml, and a protein concentration of less than 1 g/dl. The fluid should be sent for microbiologic culture and sensitivity testing. Most cases have only one infecting organism such as *Escherichia coli* or pneumococcus. Treatment is with intravenous antibiotics. Polymicrobial peritonitis suggests intestinal perforation or bowel ischemia.

Hepatorenal syndrome is one of the most feared complications of portal hypertension and operative shunting. It is characterized by oliguria, hyponatremia, and low urinary sodium concentration. Patients also exhibit evidence of liver failure such as hyperbilirubinemia and coagulopathy (due to reduced hepatic production of clotting factors). Other causes of renal failure, such as antibiotic induced failure, must be eliminated. Mortality rate approaches 100%, even with aggressive renal dialysis.

KEY POINTS

- Hemorrhage can be controlled in 90%, although the early rebleeding rate is 30%

- When medical and surgical treatment are compared, most trials have shown that surgical therapy is better at preventing subsequent bleeding than is medical treatment alone; neither medical or surgical therapy decrease overall mortality rate from portal hypertension, which is directly related to the patient's Child classification

- Except for patients with extremely poor liver function (Child C), patients treated by chronic sclerotherapy have a lower mortality rate than those treated with a portasystemic shunt

- Encephalopathy aggravated by increased amounts of intestinal protein, regardless of origin; it is worsened by intestinal hemorrhage, constipation, and continued alcoholism

- Chronic encephalopathy best treated by limitation of protein intake to less than 50 g/day and consumption of a high carbohydrate diet

- Ascites treated with chronic diuretic administration aimed at reducing the response to aldosterone

- Complications of shunt placement include peritonitis and DIC; postshunt DIC occurs in up to 50% of patients and evidenced by increased fibrin split products and decreased platelet count

- Hepatorenal syndrome one of the most feared complications of portal hypertension and operative shunting; characterized by oliguria, hyponatremia, and low urinary sodium concentration

- Patients also exhibit evidence of liver failure such as hyperbilirubinemia and coagulopathy (due to reduced hepatic production of clotting factors)

SUGGESTED READINGS

1. Cello JP et al: Endoscopic sclerotherapy versus portacaval shunt in patients with severe cirrhosis and acute variceal hemorrhage. N Engl J Med 316:11, 1987

   An important research study that helped establish sclerotherapy as the standard nonoperative treatment of acute variceal hemorrhage. Although almost 10 years old, it is a classic in the portal hypertension literature and merits close study.

2. Matloff DS: Treatment of acute variceal bleeding. Gastroenterol Clin North Am 21:103, 1992

   A good general review of the management of acute variceal hemorrhage.

3. Way LW: Portal hypertension. p. 520. In Way LW (ed): Current Surgical Diagnosis and Treatment. Appleton & Lange, E. Norwalk, CT, 1994

   A thorough review of the topic. Contains a very good summary of the surgical management of variceal hemorrhage. An excellent chapter by a world famous authority on the subject.

QUESTIONS

1. *The best diagnostic technique to establish the presence of variceal hemorrhage is?*

   A. Angiography.
   B. Esophagogastroscopy.
   C. Ultrasonography.
   D. Contrast radiography.

2. *The mortality rate among patients who present with acute variceal hemorrhage is?*

   A. 10%.
   B. 35%.
   C. 60%.
   D. 90%.

3. *The best initial measure to control variceal hemorrhage after diagnosis is?*

   A. Sclerotherapy.
   B. Balloon tamponade.
   C. Emergency surgery.
   D. LeVeen Shunt.

(See p. 603 for answers.)

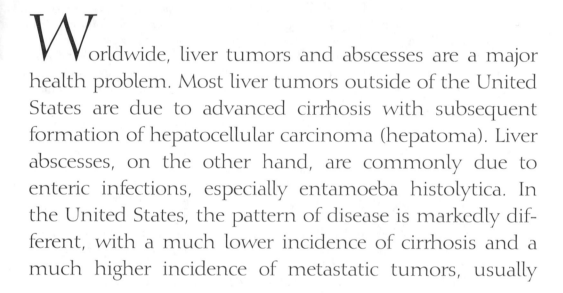

23

TUMORS AND
INFECTIONS
OF THE LIVER

MICHAEL J. STAMOS

Worldwide, liver tumors and abscesses are a major health problem. Most liver tumors outside of the United States are due to advanced cirrhosis with subsequent formation of hepatocellular carcinoma (hepatoma). Liver abscesses, on the other hand, are commonly due to enteric infections, especially entamoeba histolytica. In the United States, the pattern of disease is markedly different, with a much lower incidence of cirrhosis and a much higher incidence of metastatic tumors, usually from a primary gastrointestinal origin. Similarly, liver abscesses in the United States are typically pyogenic, with the most common source currently from the biliary tract. In certain areas there are high incidences of amoebic abscesses, primarily due to an immigrant population.

CASE 1
LIVER TUMOR

A 56-year-old male presented to the emergency room with complaints of right upper quadrant pain and a 40-lb weight loss. Upon questioning, he admitted to a feeling of malaise for the past 2 months with a generalized decreased level of energy. He denied any significant change in appetite or bowel movements. Initial physical examination was remarkable for a palpable nodular mass in the right upper quadrant apparently contiguous with the liver edge, and was otherwise unremarkable. Initial chest x-ray and abdominal films were within normal limits and labo-

ratory evaluation was significant for microcytic anemia with a Hb of 9.3 and an alkaline phosphatase of 187. A right upper quadrant ultrasound revealed a solid mass in the right lobe of the liver, contiguous with the gallbladder fossa, and measuring 8 cm in largest diameter. No other abnormalities were noted.

Due to the microcytic anemia, the patient underwent a colonoscopy, which showed a tumor in the ascending colon at the junction of the cecum. The patient underwent an uneventful right colectomy and intraoperative ultrasound. The liver tumor was noted to be lateral to the gallbladder fossa in segment 6 of the liver, and was left undisturbed. No other metastatic lesions were found in the peritoneal cavity or in the liver. The final pathology revealed a moderately well-differentiated adenocarcinoma of the colon with 0 of 14 lymph nodes involved with tumor. Vascular invasion was noted.

Six weeks later, the patient was brought back to the operating room and underwent a right hepatic lobectomy and cholecystectomy. His recovery was once again uneventful and 2 years postoperatively he had no evidence of disease.

CASE 2
ABSCESS OF THE LIVER

A 46-year-old white female presented to the emergency room with right upper quadrant pain, fever, nausea, and vomiting. On presentation, she was noted to have a blood pressure of 90/60 mmHg with a heart rate of 130 bpm and respiratory rate of 22 breaths/min. She was obviously jaundiced, and after obtaining intravenous access, resuscitation restored her blood pressure to 120/80 mmHg and her heart rate diminished to 108 bpm.

Physical examination failed to reveal any significant findings other than her jaundice and she was started on broad spectrum intravenous antibiotics for presumed cholangitis. A right upper quadrant ultrasound revealed stones within the gallbladder, a normal gallbladder wall, and a dilated common bile duct at 1.2 cm. The patient was admitted into the hospital and the following morning an ERCP was performed with the extraction of two common duct stones, the largest measuring 1.2 cm in size, following sphincterotomy.

The patient did well with normalization of her liver enzymes and bilirubin. After a 5-day course of intravenous antibiotics, she was afebrile with a normal WBC count. She was taken to the operating room for a laparoscopic cholecystectomy. Due to the prior ERCP, a cholangiogram was not performed. The patient's recovery was unremarkable and she was discharged the following day.

She returned 4 days later with complaints of right upper quadrant pain and fever. She was noted to be anicteric, but had a temperature of 39.7°C with a heart rate of 128 bpm and a WBC count of 22,000. She was admitted to the hospital and placed back on intravenous antibiotics, and an emergent right upper quadrant ultrasound showed a 10-cm cystic mass within the right lobe of the liver. Under ultrasound guidance, aspiration revealed 60 ml of purulent fluid. Following aspiration, the ultrasound showed near-complete resolution. Numerous WBCs and gram-negative rods were evident on Gram stain. The patient received antibiotics for an additional 10 days, at which time a repeat ultrasound showed complete resolution of the abscess. Klebsiella grew from cultures of the aspirate. The patient was discharged home for an additional 5-week course of oral antibiotics and had an uneventful recovery.

GENERAL CONSIDERATIONS

In the United States, liver abscesses are predominantly due to enteric bacteria, although certain areas of the country (California, Texas, Florida) see a reasonably high incidence of amoebic liver abscesses primarily due to a local immigrant population. The predominant cause of a pyogenic abscess is an ascending infection from the biliary tract (Case 2), while inflammatory conditions of the intestines (appendicitis and diverticulitis) continue to account for a distinct minority (Fig. 23.1). These cases of pylephlebitis or portal vein seeding of the liver were far more common before the advent of effective broad spectrum intravenous antibiotics.

The treatment of pyogenic abscess has similarly undergone a dramatic shift in the past two to three decades. Open surgical drainage is now rarely necessary or indicated and has largely been supplanted by radiologic guided percutaneous drainage procedures (Case 2). Additionally, more recent evidence suggests that antibiotics alone without percutaneous drainage will be effective in a significant number of cases, provided that the primary etiologic or causative process is resolved. Amoebic liver abscess should be suspected in a patient who has immigrated from a high risk area, or who has recently traveled in a high risk area. Importantly, however, a number of amoebic liver abscesses have been seen in patients without these risk factors, largely in inner city populations where high risk conditions may be reproduced. An antecedent history of a severe or protracted diarrheal episode may also raise suspicion, and amoebic serology will help confirm the diagnosis.

Liver tumors are typically classified as primary and secondary. Primary liver tumors are almost exclusively due to hepatocellular carcinoma (hepatomas), although primary neuroendocrine tumors can occur rarely in the liver. Hepatomas are seen in patients with cirrhosis and are particularly difficult to treat effectively because of the underlying liver disease. Secondary or metastatic liver tumors are most commonly of colorectal origin (Case 1). Gastric tumors, biliary tract tumors, and breast tumors may also metastasize to the liver, although with much less frequency. Neuroendocrine tumors of gastrointestinal origin, such as carcinoid and gastrinoma, also frequently metastasize to the liver, but their relative infrequency makes this presentation rare. Most liver tumors, whether primary or secondary, represent a grim prognosis. A small select number of patients (with both primary and secondary tumors) may be cured with surgical resection. Currently this treatment approach offers the only potential for cure, and a 5-year survival or cure can be seen in up to 40% of carefully selected patients (Case 1).

KEY POINTS

• In United States, liver abscesses predominantly due to enteric bacteria, although certain areas see high incidence due to amoeba, because of local immigrant population (California, Texas, Florida)

• Open surgical drainage is rarely indicated; supplanted by radiologic guided percutaneous drainage procedures

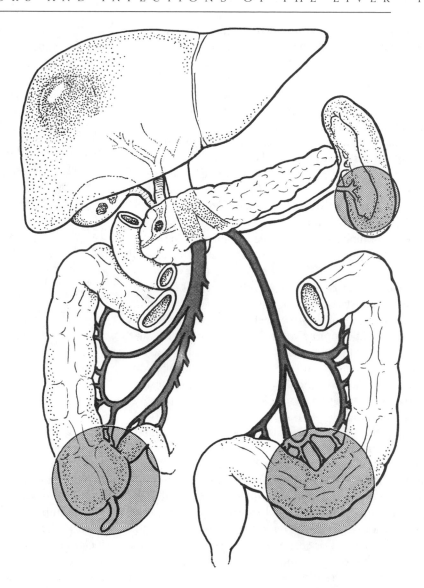

FIGURE 23.1 *The portal venous drainage system and biliary tract are responsible for most liver abscesses.*

• Hepatomas seen in patients with cirrhosis, and are particularly difficult to treat effectively because of underlying liver disease

• Most liver tumors, primary or secondary, present grim prognosis; small number cured with surgical resection

DIAGNOSIS

Most patients with liver abscess will present with fever and a variable amount of right upper quadrant pain. Importantly, however, the right upper quadrant pain is not experienced by a significant minority of patients, and evaluation for a fever of unknown origin with either ultrasound or computed tomography (CT) scanning will reveal the diagnosis. Most of these patients will have significant abnormalities of their liver enzymes, which should raise suspicion of the diagnosis.

The primary disease process (biliary tract, diverticulitis, etc.) will sometimes distract the examiner and indeed sometimes will precede the clinical or even radiographic evidence of the liver abscess (Case 2). In addition to elevation of the liver enzymes, an elevated white blood cell (WBC) count is usually seen and is sometimes quite dramatically elevated. Amoebic titers will be increased, not surprisingly, in 95% of patients with amoebic abscess. These titers should be measured, if suspicion exists, as the treatment protocol may be different. Ultrasonography and CT scanning have dramatically changed our diagnostic abilities and our therapy of liver abscesses (see Treatment section). They are essential tools in confirming the diagnosis, and ultrasound is also important in evaluating the biliary tract in a necessary search for the primary etiology.

Coincident with the diagnosis of a liver abscess or abscesses, a diligent search for the primary etiology is essential. In addition to biliary tract disease, appendicitis, diverticulitis, Crohn's disease, and colorectal cancer are all seen with some frequency. Further investigation should be guided by clinical presentation, specific patient factors (e.g., age, geographic location, prior complaints) as well as laboratory evaluation. Additional diagnostic evaluation may include contrast gastrointestinal studies, colonoscopy, nuclear medicine studies (WBC scan), and possibly laparoscopy.

Liver tumors are most commonly seen coincidentally during the preoperative staging or intraoperative treatment of patients with primary gastrointestinal malignancies (most commonly colon and rectal cancer). Up to 20% of patients initially evaluated for primary colon and rectal cancer will be found to have hepatic metastases at the time of diagnosis or treatment. An additional 20% will develop metastatic liver disease during the subsequent 5 years. The majority of these metachronous (occurring at a later time) hepatic tumors will be evident during the first 2 years (≤85%), therefore, efforts are frequently made in patients treated for primary colon and rectal cancer to detect these metastatic tumors early, with detailed history and physical examination as well as measurement of carcinoembryonic antigen (CEA).

Primary liver tumors (hepatoma) are most commonly found in cirrhotic patients and elevated α-fetoprotein (AFP) levels will typically be the first evidence of such a tumor in these high risk patients. Ultrasound and CT scanning are of less value due to the nodularity of the underlying liver and the decreased sensitivity of the radiologic evaluation as a result. Radiologic evaluation of the patient with a known or suspected metastatic liver tumor is of considerably greater value, both in the primary diagnosis as well as in the evaluation of patients with known liver tumors being considered for surgical resection. A necessary prerequisite to consideration of hepatic resection of metastatic liver tumors is effective treatment and control of the primary tumor sites. Additionally, there should be no other sites of metastatic disease outside of the liver. A thorough history and physical examination is essential, with an occasional patient found to have inguinal or supraclavicular adenopathy, or less commonly, a recurrence at prior incision sites.

Chest x-rays and CT scans of the chest, abdomen, and pelvis are important. CT portography is the most sensitive nonoperative test. This evaluation utilizes angiography of the mesenteric vessels followed in close sequence by CT scanning of the liver. The portal flow of contrast will highlight the normal liver parenchyma from the metastatic liver tumors, which are primarily supplied by the hepatic arterial circulation. Although this test has a high sensitivity, it suffers from a significant incidence of false-positive results (5–10%) and therefore should be used selectively. The best combination of tests currently available includes preoperative CT scanning followed by intraoperative hepatic ultrasonography and surgeon palpation of the liver. Other tests that are occasionally used but have unproven utility include laparoscopy and nuclear medicine scans.

KEY POINTS

• Ultrasonography and CT scanning are essential tools in confirming diagnosis, and ultrasound important in evaluating biliary tract in search for primary etiology

• Liver tumors most commonly seen coincidentally during preoperative staging or intraoperative treatment for primary gastrointestinal malignancies such as colon and rectal cancer

• Effective treatment and control of primary tumor sites necessary for hepatic resection of metastatic liver tumors; there should be no other sites of metastatic disease outside the liver

• Best combination of tests is preoperative CT scanning, intraoperative hepatic ultrasonography, and surgical palpation of the liver

---

DIFFERENTIAL DIAGNOSIS

Liver abscesses are conveniently classified as pyogenic and nonpyogenic, although some nonpyogenic abscesses can become secondarily bacterially infected. Most nonpyogenic abscesses are amoebic, although hydatid infections are occasionally seen in the United States. Immunocompromised patients, particularly hepatic transplant patients, may present with more unusual infections, including mycotic abscesses.

Occasionally, a simple liver cyst may be difficult to differentiate from a liver abscess. The clinical course will usually make the differential quite obvious, however. If doubt persists, simple aspiration of the fluid will confirm the diagnosis.

Liver tumors can be benign or malignant, and malignant tumors subdivided into primary and secondary. Benign liver tumors include adenomas, hemangiomas, and focal nodular hyperplasia (FNH). Adenomas and FNH are typically asymptomatic and are most commonly seen in female patients. They also may be hormonally influenced and contributed to by oral contraceptives. Magnetic resonance imaging (MRI) has greatly improved the ability to differentiate these tumors, particularly in the case of hemangioma and FNH. Serum tumor markers, including CEA (colorectal and breast) and CA-125 (ovarian) are frequently elevated in metastatic liver tumors, although poorly differentiated tumors may not produce these enzymes. If doubt persists, evaluation of likely primary sources should be conducted, particularly if the liver tumor is amenable to curative resection. If the pattern of liver tumor deems it unresectable or if doubt persists following extensive investigation, and hemangioma is unlikely by MRI scan, a percutaneous CT-guided liver biopsy may be indicated. Alternatively, a laparoscopic-guided liver biopsy may be safer and more sensitive.

TREATMENT

Most liver abscesses will respond to intravenous antibiotics, as long as the primary disease process is controlled. Larger abscesses (Case 2) or those that fail to respond to initial antibiotic treatment should be percutaneously drained. The primary disease process should be managed independently of the liver abscess, and with the exception of an incidentally discovered abscess in the peripheral liver at the time of operation, operative drainage is not indicated unless radiologic expertise is unavailable. The timing of the treatment of the primary process and the liver abscess is dependent on the nature of the primary disease process. Intravenous antibiotics are typically given for at least 7–10 days and, depending on the response and/or the bacteriologic evaluation, may be necessary for up to 6 weeks. Broad spectrum oral antibiotics may be used to replace intravenous antibiotics for a total of 6 weeks of therapy.

Liver tumors are most commonly untreatable for cure and signify a terminal prognosis. Palliative treatment of liver tumors is occasionally of value, although effective treatment modalities are limited. Systemic or regional chemotherapy can give a response in up to 40% of patients but with no proven survival benefit. Hepatic arterial embolization, with or without chemotherapy, hepatic arterial chemotherapy, cryotherapy, and percutaneous ethanol injections are currently available techniques that apply in select patients but remain unproven. Resection of liver tumors remains the only proven technique to elicit cure or prolong survival. Primary liver tumors are infrequently amenable to resection, primarily due to underlying cirrhosis making surgical resection hazardous. Secondary liver tumors are more commonly resected, particularly colorectal tumors. Tumors that arise from the breast or stomach are also seen with some frequency, but resection of these tumors is of no proven benefit.

Surgical resection of metastatic liver tumors requires extensive preoperative evaluation, including colonoscopy, detailed history and physical examination, laboratory evaluation (including CEA measurement), CT scanning of the abdomen and chest, and a thorough education and informed consent of the patient. Additionally, the tumors should be limited to no more than three and must be surgically resectable with adequate margins and adequate hepatic reserve. The patient must be otherwise in reasonable health to withstand a major hepatic resection. At the time of exploration and planned resection, a diligent search for extrahepatic metastasis must be conducted, and the find-

ing of any extrahepatic tumor should contraindict hepatic resection. If the above criteria are adhered to, and the tumor is resected with clear margins, a 30–40% cure rate or 5-year survival can be expected.

> ### KEY POINTS
> - Most liver abscesses will respond to intravenous antibiotics
> - Resection of liver tumors is the only technique proven to elicit cure or prolong survival

SUGGESTED READINGS

Lehert T, Otto G, Herfarth C: Therapeutic modalities and prognostic factors for primary and secondary liver tumors. World J Surg 19:252, 1995

A highly detailed analysis with an extensive reference list.

Machi J, Isomoto H, Yamashita Y et al: Intraoperative ultrasonography in screening for liver metastases from colorectal cancer: comparative accuracy with traditional procedures. Surgery 101:678, 1987

A nicely detailed work that points out the limitations of current staging and that should serve to highlight that most recurrent liver metastases actually represent residual disease.

Stain SC, Yellin AE, Donovan AJ, Brien HW: Pyogenic abscess: modern treatment. Arch Surg 126:991, 1991

This article describes an experience in the evolution of the treatment of liver abscesses.

QUESTIONS

1. *Appropriate treatment of liver abscesses may include?*
   - A. Surgical drainage.
   - B. Percutaneous drainage.
   - C. Intravenous antibiotics alone.
   - D. All of the above.

2. *Metastatic liver tumors may be cured by?*
   - A. Hepatic arterial chemotherapy.
   - B. Surgical resection.
   - C. Systemic chemotherapy.
   - D. Radiotherapy.
   - E. Percutaneous ethanol injections.

3. *Pyelephlebitis may arise from any of the following except?*
   - A. Appendicitis.
   - B. Diverticulitis.
   - C. Colon cancer.
   - D. Tubo-ovarian abscess.

(See p. 603 for answers.)

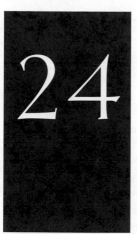

24

BILIARY

TRACT

DISEASE

BRUCE E. STABILE

Disease of the biliary tract is frequently encountered in clinical practice in Western society. Although the clinical manifestations of biliary tract disease are many and varied, in most instances the diagnosis is easily determined by history, and the treatment is fairly standardized. Other than gallstone disease, most other diseases affecting the gallbladder and bile ducts are uncommon or rare. Although clinical manifestations may be similar to those of gallstone disease, tumors, benign strictures, and

congenital cystic diseases of the biliary tree require treatments that are quite different. This chapter has several goals: (1) to define the different types of gallstones and their causes, (2) to enumerate the various complications of gallstones and their mechanisms of development, (3) to describe the clinical presentations and diagnostic evaluations pertinent to the complications of gallstones, (4) to describe the less common noncalculous lesions of the biliary tract and their associated clinical manifestations, and (5) to delineate the surgical and nonsurgical therapies available for treatment of biliary tract diseases.

CASE 1
RIGHT UPPER QUADRANT
ABDOMINAL PAIN AND FEVER

A 42-year-old overweight female had recurrent episodes of sharp, aching, right upper quadrant abdominal pain over the previous 3 months. Pain generally occurred

within 2 hours after eating and was particularly severe after fatty meals. Typically it lasted 30 minutes to 2 hours and then gradually subsided. She experienced associated nausea and occasional vomiting but no changes in bowel habits nor weight loss. Pain was not relieved by antacids or mild analgesics nor by vomiting or bowel movements. Both her mother and maternal aunt had undergone cholecystectomy. The patient was scheduled for an outpatient ultrasound examination of the gallbladder and was instructed to avoid fatty foods.

Three days later she experienced a severe episode of right upper quadrant pain that persisted over a 24-hour period with nausea, repeated episodes of vomiting, and, for the first time, fever. Because the pain was more severe, progressive, and prolonged than previously, she came to the emergency department. Her temperature was 38.3°C. Marked right upper quadrant abdominal tenderness was noted with voluntary guarding and arrest of inspiration on deep palpation (positive Murphy's sign). The WBC count was $13.1 \times 10^3/mm^3$, Hb 13 g/dl, Hct

40%, total bilirubin 0.9 g/dl, alkaline phosphatase 105 IU/L (normal <110), ALT 42 units/ml (normal <45), and AST 36 units/ml (normal <40). Serum amylase and lipase levels were normal. An ultrasound examination showed a dilated gallbladder containing multiple stones, with a thickened wall, and pericholecystic fluid. The common bile duct measured 0.6 cm in diameter; the liver, pancreas, and right kidney appeared normal.

She was admitted to the hospital, made NPO, and begun on intravenous fluids, broad spectrum antibiotics, and parenteral analgesics. Within 24 hours her pain and fever subsided and her WBC count returned to normal. Two days later, she underwent laparoscopic cholecystectomy. The gallbladder was noted to be distended, inflamed, and edematous. An intraoperative cholangiogram showed no abnormal findings. The gallbladder had acute and chronic cholecystitis with multiple 0.4–0.9-cm cholesterol gallstones contained within the lumen, including one stone that was impacted within the proximal cystic duct. Within 5 days she returned to her normal activities and experienced no subsequent bouts of abdominal pain or fever.

CASE 2
ABDOMINAL PAIN, FEVER, JAUNDICE, AND SEPTIC SHOCK

A 79-year-old demented male was brought by ambulance to the hospital emergency department. He was unable to give a history, but the supervising physician at his nursing home related a 2-day illness characterized by vague upper abdominal pain, anorexia, and fever. The illness had been attributed to gastroenteritis, and no specific diagnostic measures or therapy had been pursued. The patient had no other significant past medical history, and the family history was unobtainable. He appeared acutely ill with obvious jaundice and prostration. His temperature was 40°C, pulse 120 bpm, BP 90/60 mmHg, and respirations 24 breaths/min. He was moderately obtunded and had shaking chills. His abdomen was mildly distended but without guarding or rebound tenderness. The liver was slightly enlarged and tender.

Blood cultures were drawn from both antecubital veins, a urine culture was sent, and broad spectrum intravenous antibiotics immediately begun. After one hour of resuscitation, the pulse was 92 bpm, BP 124/76 mmHg, and respiration 18 breaths/min. Emergency abdominal ultrasound showed a gallbladder containing multiple large and small stones and a common bile duct measuring 1.2 cm in diameter. Twelve hours later, his confusion cleared somewhat, and he related that his abdominal pain had largely subsided. The total bilirubin was 9.8 g/dl with a direct bilirubin of 7.6 g/dl, and the alkaline phosphatase was 462 IU/L. ERCP was done with attempted extraction of

the obstructing common bile duct stone; multiple large and small common duct stones were detected, with a very large stone impacted just proximal to the ampulla of Vater. Despite multiple attempts, the stone could not be dislodged. At urgent open cholecystectomy, a chronically scarred gallbladder containing multiple stones was removed. A total of 11 common duct stones were retrieved, ranging in size from 0.3 to 1.1 cm, including the stone impacted just proximal to the ampulla of Vater. Flexible fiberoptic choledochoscopy was used to remove several additional small stones from within the intrahepatic biliary duct branches. Because of the presence of multiple stones and the concern that additional calculi might remain within the biliary tree, a side-to-side anastomosis between the distal common bile duct and proximal duodenum (choledochoduodenostomy) was created.

Postoperatively the patient recovered uneventfully, and by the sixth postoperative day his liver function tests were normal. On the eighth day he was transferred back to the nursing home tolerating a normal diet and ambulating with assistance. He had no further episodes of abdominal pain, fever, or jaundice.

GENERAL CONSIDERATIONS

Of all the diseases that affect the biliary tract, only calculus disease is common in the Western world. Gallstones are most often asymptomatic but are capable of causing both chronic symptoms and acute severe manifestations, both when confined to the gallbladder (Case 1) or when passed from the gallbladder into the common bile duct (Case 2). Benign strictures, malignant tumors, and congenital cystic dilatations are the other clinically important lesions of the biliary tract that can produce symptoms virtually identical to those of gallstone disease.

Gallstone disease is the most common reason for elective intra-abdominal operation in the United States, with approximately 500,000 cholecystectomies performed per year. It is not only an important clinical disease, but it is responsible for a large portion of total health care costs. Approximately 10% of the U.S. population has gallstones, but only a minority of affected individuals ever develop symptoms. Gallstones are particularly common among certain ethnic groups such as the Native Americans of the southwestern United States, Hispanics, and Asians harboring biliary parasites such as *Clonorchis sinensis*. Other risk factors for gallstone development include increasing age, female gender, obesity, pregnancy, hepatic cirrhosis, hemolytic anemia, and treatment with estrogens or total parenteral nutrition (TPN).

Gallstone disease is primarily a disease of hepatocellular origin, in that an abnormally lithogenic bile is secreted by the liver of affected individuals. The three principal constituents of bile are cholesterol, bile salts, and phospholipids, more than 90% of which is lecithin. As cholesterol is insoluble in aqueous solution, its solubility in bile is dependent on the formation of mixed micelles containing proper proportions and orientation of cholesterol, bile acid, and lecithin molecules and their aggregates. Approximately 75% of gallstones in the Western world are composed primarily of cholesterol. These stones are the result of hepatic synthesis of bile with supersaturated concentrations of cholesterol. Cholesterol stone nidation and growth occur in the gallbladder, where hepatic bile is concentrated and stored. Impaired gallbladder motility and stasis, along with other complex factors, also contribute to cholesterol gallstone formation.

Bile pigment stones form primarily in the gallbladder of patients with hepatic cirrhosis or chronic hemolytic diseases, such as sickle cell anemia and spherocytosis. Although most bile duct stones are present as the result of passage of gallbladder stones into the common duct (secondary bile duct stones), some are actually formed within the ducts and are typically composed of insoluble calcium bilirubinate (primary bile duct stones). These pigment stones most often form in the bile ducts of persons with biliary strictures or chronic bacterial infection of the biliary tree from any cause.

The clinical manifestations of gallstone disease are largely the consequence of obstruction of the gallbladder or bile duct. Stones within the gallbladder cause symptoms when they obstruct normal emptying as a result of impaction in the infundibulum or cystic duct. This obstruction leads to the intermittent pain of biliary colic and, when unrelieved, to the complication of acute cholecystitis (Case 1). Stones that pass from the gallbladder into the common bile duct or form within the bile duct may pass harmlessly into the duodenum or may obstruct the common duct, typically just proximal to the ampulla of Vater. Obstruction at this level causes jaundice, characterized by direct hyperbilirubinemia, and may be complicated by bacterial overgrowth, leading to ascending cholangitis and sepsis (Case 2). This contrast between the consequences of gallbladder versus common bile duct obstruction is crucial. While gallbladder obstruction can lead to acute cholecystitis, the infection is usually contained and leads to generalized sepsis only if appropriate treatment is delayed or unavailable. By contrast, obstruction of the common bile duct often leads to ascending cholangitis with translocation of bacteria into hepatic sinusoidal blood. This sequence leads to the rapid development of bacteremia and systemic sepsis (Case 2). Blood cultures are positive for the same organism infecting the bile in more than 90% of such cases. Failure to institute aggressive treatment of common duct obstruction causing acute cholangitis can result in septic shock and death with disturbing suddenness. Thus, gallstone obstruction of the common duct is a much more rapidly lethal complication than is obstruction of the gallbladder.

Gallstones cause several additional complications not directly associated with infection. Large stones (>2 cm) occasionally erode through the walls of both the gallbladder and the adjacent adherent duodenum and into the lumen of the small intestine. The resultant fistula between the gallbladder and duodenum rarely causes symptoms, but the large gallstone may fail to pass through the ileocecal valve, causing a distal small bowel obstruction. This unusual complication is known as gallstone ileus.

Transient or prolonged impaction of a common bile duct stone at, or just distal to, the entrance of the pancreatic duct is associated with development of acute gallstone pancreatitis. While the precise mechanism remains controversial, obstruction of the pancreatic duct by the gallstone is thought to be the primary inciting event. The pancreatitis is typically mild and transient, but in 5–10% of cases it progresses to severe necrotizing pancreatitis with associated complications such as peripancreatic fluid collections, pseudocyst formation, pancreatic sepsis, and multiple organ failure. In its most severe form, gallstone pancreatitis is associated with a mortality of 20–40%.

The other important complications of common bile duct stones are strictures associated with long-standing or repeated episodes of inflammation, infection, and scarring, and unrelieved biliary obstruction leading to secondary biliary cirrhosis. Advanced cirrhosis is manifested as hepatic insufficiency and ultimately failure with or without complications of portal hypertension.

Most benign biliary strictures follow injury of the common hepatic duct or its branches during cholecystectomy. In patients with chronic pancreatitis, particularly caused by alcoholism, chronic inflammatory fibrosis in the head of the gland causes stricture of the distal segment of the common bile duct.

Primary sclerosing cholangitis is a rare disease characterized by fibrous thickening and irregular narrowing of the bile ducts not attributable to stones, operative trauma, or malignant disease. One-third of patients have this condition in association with a history of ulcerative colitis. The strictures may be diffuse throughout the intrahepatic and extrahepatic biliary ductal system or may be segmental, involving only the intrahepatic or extrahepatic ducts. Although patients often tolerate the disease for a number of years without clinical deterioration, the onset of persistent jaundice or septic cholangitis indicates a poor prognosis.

Cystic disease of the biliary tree is quite rare and occurs as a spectrum of congenital dilatations and sacculations that affect the intrahepatic bile ducts (Caroli's disease), the common duct (choledochal cyst), or the intraduodenal terminal segment of the common bile duct (choledochocele). These cysts are associated with bile stasis, stone formation, and infection. Up to 15% of patients over age 20 years develop adenocarcinomas within the cyst wall.

Malignant tumors arising from the biliary tract are uncommon, with cancer of the gallbladder the most frequently encountered. Adenocarcinoma of the gallbladder accounts for less than 2% of all malignant tumors but is a highly lethal disease, with only a 5% 5-year survival. Approximately 80% of gallbladder cancers are associated with gallstones, but only 1% of patients who undergo biliary tract surgery have gallbladder cancer. There is an important association between gallbladder cancer and calcification within the wall of the organ. Approximately 40% of patients with a so-called porcelain gallbladder are found to have an adenocarcinoma.

Adenocarcinoma of the bile duct is referred to as cholangiocarcinoma; tumors arising from the extrahepatic ducts are quite rare. Conditions associated with these extrahepatic tumors include primary sclerosing cholangitis, familial adenomatous polyposis, choledochal cyst, gallstones, and *Clonorchis* infection. The most common variety of cholangiocarcinoma involves the proximal common hepatic duct or the confluence of the right and left hepatic ducts, or both, and is referred to as a Klatskin tumor. Cholangiocarcinomas are sometimes multicentric, particularly those involving the intrahepatic biliary tree. The prognosis is generally poor, with a 5-year survival of less than 20%. Cholangiocarcinomas, like carcinomas of the head of the pancreas, and unlike benign strictures, cause biliary obstruction manifested as jaundice without associated cholangitis.

KEY POINTS

- Of diseases that affect biliary tract, only calculus disease common in Western world

- Gallstones most often asymptomatic

- Benign strictures, malignant tumors, and congenital cystic dilatations are other clinically important lesions of biliary tract

- Approximately 500,000 cholecystectomies performed per year

- Gallstones particularly common among certain ethnic groups

- Other risk factors include increasing age, female gender, obesity, pregnancy, hepatic cirrhosis, hemolytic anemia, and treatment with estrogens or TPN

- Gallstone disease primarily disease of hepatocellular origin (an abnormally lithogenic bile is secreted by liver of affected persons)

- Three principal constituents of bile are cholesterol, bile salts, and phospholipids (>90% lecithin)

- Approximately 75% of gallstones in Western world composed primarily of cholesterol

- Cholesterol stone nidation and growth occur in gallbladder, where hepatic bile is concentrated and stored

- Bile pigment stones form primarily in gallbladder of patients with hepatic cirrhosis or chronic hemolytic disease (e.g., sickle cell anemia and spherocytosis)

- Most bile duct stones present as result of passage of gallbladder stones into common duct (secondary bile duct stones); some actuallly form within ducts, typically composed of insoluble calcium bilirubinate (primary duct stones)

- Clinical manifestations of gallstone disease largely consequence of obstruction of gallbladder or bile duct

- Stones within gallbladder cause symptoms when they obstruct normal emptying due to impaction in the infundibulum or cystic duct; this leads to intermittent pain of biliary colic and when unrelieved to acute cholecystitis

- Stones that pass from gallbladder into common bile duct or form within bile duct may pass harmlessly into duodenum or may obstruct common duct, typically just proximal to ampulla of Vater

- Obstruction at ampulla of Vater causes jaundice, characterized by direct hyperbilirubinemia; may be complicated by bacterial overgrowth, leading to ascending cholangitis and sepsis

- Difference between consequences of gallbladder versus common bile duct obstruction is crucial; gallbladder obstruction can lead to acute cholecystitis but is usually contained and leads to generalized sepsis only if treatment delayed or unavailable; obstruction of common bile duct often leads to ascending cholangitis with translocation of bacteria into hepatic sinusoidal blood, leading to rapid development of bacteremia and systemic sepsis

- Failure to institute aggressive treatment of common duct obstruction causing acute cholangitis can result in septic shock and death with disturbing suddenness

- Transient or prolonged impaction of a common bile duct stone at or just distal to the entrance of pancreatic duct associated with development of acute gallstone pancreatitis

- Most benign biliary strictures follow injury of common hepatic duct or its branches during cholecystectomy

- Primary sclerosing cholangitis is rare disease characterized by fibrous thickening and irregular narrowing of bile ducts not attributable to stones, operative trauma, or malignant disease

- Malignant tumors arising from the biliary tract are uncommon; gallbladder cancer most frequently encountered

- Adenocarcinoma of gallbladder accounts for less than 2% of malignant tumors but is highly lethal disease, with only a 5% 5-year survival

- Approximately 40% of patients with so-called porcelain gallbladder found to have an adenocarcinoma

- Adenocarcinoma of bile duct referred to as cholangiocarcinoma; tumors arising from extrahepatic ducts are quite rare

- Most common variety of cholangiocarcinoma (Klatskin tumor) involves proximal common hepatic duct or confluence of right and left hepatic ducts (or both)

- Cholangiocarcinomas, like carcinomas of pancreas head and unlike benign strictures, cause biliary obstruction manifested as jaundice without associated cholangitis

DIAGNOSIS

The diagnosis of biliary tract disease is generally not difficult. It is often strongly suggested by the history and physical examination. Blood tests are particularly useful when extrahepatic biliary obstruction is present. Imaging studies are extremely accurate in localizing the anatomic site of the lesion and also in pinpointing the precise etiology. Diagnosis of biliary tract conditions is very often a multidisciplinary effort that involves radiologist, gastroenterologist, and surgeon.

Patients with biliary tract disease generally present with right upper quadrant abdominal pain, jaundice, or sepsis. Although most patients with gallbladder stones are asymptomatic, those with symptoms typically complain of recurrent episodes of right upper quadrant postprandial abdominal pain, lasting minutes to hours. The pain is often particularly associated with fatty meals and may be accompanied by nausea and vomiting (Case 1). While the classic pain of transient gallbladder obstruction is referred to as biliary colic, the pain does not have the typical pattern of repetitive remissions and exacerbations commonly associated with other types of colic such as ureteral or small intestinal colic. When acute cholecystitis develops, the abdominal pain persists for days rather than hours and is usually associated with mild to moderate fever (Case 1). Common bile duct obstruction from any cause is classically manifested as jaundice. The patient may note scleral icterus, dark urine, or light colored stools before cutaneous jaundice is appreciated. If cholangitis accompanies biliary obstruction, the classic Charcot's triad consisting of right upper quadrant abdominal pain, jaundice, and high fever and chills may be present. In cases of advanced ascending or suppurative cholangitis, Reynold's pentad is sometimes observed and is defined by the addition of hypotension and mental confusion to Charcot's triad (Case 2).

Patients with primary biliary malignancies often present with jaundice uncomplicated by infection, but typically accompanied by chronic symptoms of pruritus, anorexia, and weight loss. Because the degree of obstruction is usually complete or near-complete, their jaundice is deep and obvious. Patients suffering from gallstone pancreatitis complain of mid-epigastric sharp pain penetrating directly through to the back. The pain generally lasts 1–3 days, is not localized to the right upper quadrant, and is accompanied by anorexia, nausea, and occasional vomiting. Fever is typically absent or low grade. The rare patient with gallstone ileus presents with a history typical of small bowel obstruction with hours to days of cramping abdominal pain, bloating, nausea, and repeated vomiting. Typically, constipation or obstipation is also present.

The physical examination of the patient with biliary tract disease very often confirms the suspicions raised by the history. Patients with biliary colic but with no other complication of gallstone disease may have only mild upper quadrant tenderness or a totally normal physical examination. By contrast, patients with acute cholecystitis have fever and moderate to marked right upper quadrant tenderness accompanied by voluntary guarding. A tender mass representing the distended and inflamed gallbladder may be appreciated. Deep palpation under the right costal margin causing sudden arrest of deep inspiration is referred to as Murphy's sign (Case 1). Biliary ductal obstruction manifested as jaundice is most readily appreciated by examination of the sclerae, the tympanic membranes, nail beds, and other nonpigmented tissues. Systemic sepsis accompanying biliary tract infection is manifested by high fever and shaking chills, or rigors. Tachycardia, hypotension, and obtundation may also be present (Case 2).

Laboratory examination of patients with biliary tract disease is intended to identify the presence of acute infection, biliary obstruction, or associated acute pancreatitis. An elevated white blood cell (WBC) count indicates inflammation and strongly suggests acute infection (Cases 1 and 2). Elevation of the serum amylase or lipase suggests pancreatitis and an amylase value of greater than 1,000 strongly supports the diagnosis of gallstone pancreatitis. An elevated serum bilirubin level, particularly with a predominantly direct component, supports ductal obstruction as the cause of jaundice (Case 2). Elevation of the serum alkaline phosphatase level is the most sensitive laboratory indicator of biliary obstruction and may be present in the absence of hyperbilirubinemia. Serum alanine aminotransferase (ALT) and aspartate aminotransferase (AST) levels may be elevated with biliary obstruction but less dramatically than the corresponding bilirubin and alkaline phosphatase levels (Case 2).

In patients with right upper quadrant abdominal pain or jaundice, abdominal ultrasound examination is the initial imaging procedure of choice. The sensitivity of ultrasonography in detecting gallbladder stones is greater than 95%. The characteristic finding is an intraluminal echogenic focus that casts a shadow (Fig. 24.1). In cases of acute cholecystitis, gallbladder wall thickening and pericholecystic fluid may also be demonstrated (Case 1). Furthermore, ultrasonography reliably demonstrates dilatation of the common bile duct or intrahepatic ducts characteristic of biliary tract obstruction.

While less accurate than ultrasonography in detecting gallstones, computed tomography (CT) scanning is at least as accurate in detecting biliary ductal dilatation (Fig. 24.2). CT with intravenous and oral contrast provides definition of anatomic structures and can precisely locate the level of the obstructing lesion in approximately 95% of jaundiced patients. Since it is highly accurate in identifying pancreatic, hepatic, and other mass lesions, CT is useful as the initial imaging study in patients with obstructive jaundice and a suspected or palpable tumor.

Hepatobiliary scintigraphy using intravenously administered iminodiacetic acid (IDA) derivatives is occasionally

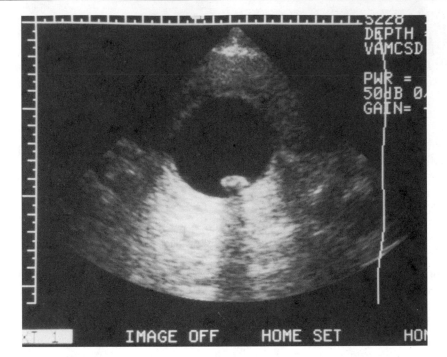

FIGURE 24.1 *Ultrasound of gallbladder showing a solitary stone with the characteristic sonolucent shadow.*

useful in cases of suspected acute cholecystitis. The isotope is excreted by the liver into the bile ducts. Failure to visualize the gallbladder implies cystic duct obstruction and acute cholecystitis.

Endoscopic retrograde cholangiopancreatography (ERCP) can detect gallstones within the gallbladder as well as the biliary ducts with great sensitivity. ERCP is also capable of accurately localizing other obstructing lesions, such as benign strictures, cholangiocarcinomas, and pancreatic and ampullary carcinomas (Fig. 24.3). After identification of the obstructing lesion, various endoscopic maneuvers can be performed to extract common bile duct stones (Case 2), to biopsy suspected tumors, or to decompress an obstructed duct with a stent.

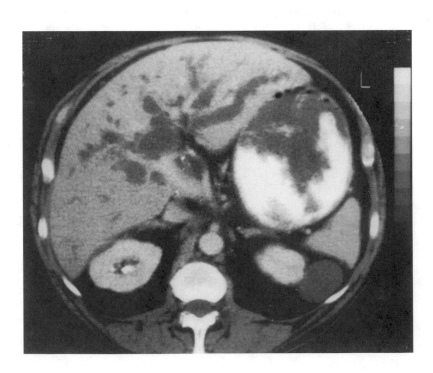

FIGURE 24.2 *CT scan showing markedly dilated intrahepatic biliary ducts due to a distal common bile duct cancer.*

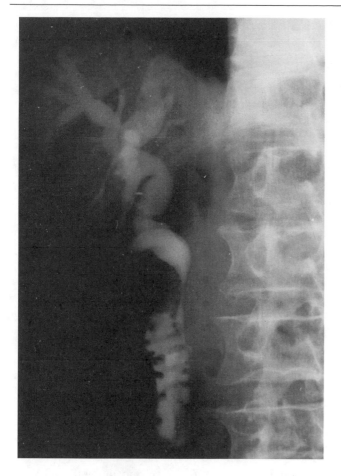

FIGURE 24.3 *ERCP showing dilated intrahepatic and extrahepatic bile ducts due to a distal common bile duct stricture from chronic pancreatitis.*

KEY POINTS

- Diagnosis of biliary tract disease not generally difficult; often strongly suggested by history and physical examination

- Patients with biliary tract disease usually present with right upper quadrant abdominal pain, jaundice, or sepsis

- Most patients with gallbladder stones asymptomatic but those with symptoms typically complain of recurrent episodes of right upper quadrant postprandial abdominal pain, lasting minutes to hours; pain often associated with fatty meals, may be accompanied by nausea and vomiting

- When acute cholecystitis develops, abdominal pain persists for days (not hours); usually associated with mild to moderate fever

- Common bile duct obstruction from any cause classically manifested as jaundice

- If cholangitis accompanies biliary obstruction, classic Charcot's triad (right upper quadrant abdominal pain, jaundice, and high fever and chills) may be present

- Reynold's pentad (hypotension and mental confusion in addition to Charcot's triad) sometimes observed in cases of advanced ascending or suppurative cholangitis

- Patients with primary biliary malignancies often present with jaundice uncomplicated by infection, but typically accompanied by chronic symptoms of pruritus, anorexia, and weight loss

- Patients with biliary colic but without other complications of gallstone disease may have only mild upper quadrant tenderness or a totally normal physical examination

- Patients with acute cholecystitis have fever and moderate to marked right upper quadrant tenderness accompanied by voluntary guarding

- Elevation of serum amylase or lipase suggest pancreatitis; an amylase value of greater than 1,000 strongly supports diagnosis of gallstone pancreatitis; an elevated serum bilirubin level, particularly with a predominately direct component, supports ductal obstruction as cause of jaundice

- Elevation of serum alkaline phosphatase level most sensitive laboratory indicator of biliary obstruction; may be present in absence of hyperbilirubinemia

- Abdominal ultrasound examination is initial imaging procedure of choice for patients with right upper quadrant abdominal pain or jaundice; sensitivity in detecting gallbladder stones is greater than 95%; characteristic finding is an intraluminal echogenic focus that casts a shadow (Fig. 24.1)

- Ultrasound reliably demonstrates dilatation of common bile duct or intrahepatic duct characteristic of biliary tract obstruction

- CT scanning is at least as accurate as ultrasound in detecting biliary ductal dilatation (Fig. 24.2) but less accurate in detecting gallstones

- CT useful as initial imaging study in patients with obstructive jaundice and a suspected or palpable tumor

- ERCP can detect gallstones within gallbladder as well as biliary ducts with great sensitivity; also capable of accurately localizing other obstructing lesions (e.g., benign strictures, cholangiocarcinomas, and pancreatic and ampullary carcinomas) (Fig. 24.3)

DIFFERENTIAL DIAGNOSIS

Since biliary tract disease without jaundice usually presents as abdominal pain with or without fever, the differential diagnosis may include a wide variety of inflammatory and neoplastic conditions within the abdomen. Afebrile patients complaining of "biliary colic" may have peptic ulcer disease, gastroesophageal reflux, esophageal motility disorders, nonulcer dyspepsia, irritable bowel syndrome, renal colic, or angina pectoris. When fever accompanies the abdominal pain, inflammatory conditions such as acute appendicitis, diverticulitis, colitis, acute pancreatitis, hepatitis, and pyelonephritis must also be considered. In most instances, ultrasound examination of the abdomen will identify stones within the gallbladder if gallstone disease is the etiology. Hepatobiliary scintigraphy is sometimes extremely helpful in differentiating acute acalculous cholecystitis from other inflammatory abdominal conditions that produce upper abdominal pain and fever.

When jaundice is the presenting symptom, the history, physical examination, and routine laboratory tests are most accurate and are highly cost effective in differentiating obstructive from nonobstructive jaundice. The accuracy of the basic clinical and laboratory assessment is 80–90%. With obstructive jaundice, an ultrasound examination should be performed to rule in or rule out gallstone disease (Case 2). In the absence of gallstones, chronic pancreatitis, or prior biliary surgery suggestive of a postoperative stricture, the chance of a malignant tumor is very high. The differential diagnosis includes carcinoma of the head of the pancreas, as well as cholangiocarcinoma, ampullary carcinoma, and hepatoma or metastatic tumor obstructing the major ducts at the porta hepatis. In most instances, malignant obstruction of the biliary tract is not associated with cholangitis. This clinical complication points to benign biliary obstruction due to calculus disease, strictures, or sclerosing cholangitis. CT scanning of the abdomen and ERCP are the diagnostic measures that best differentiate these clinical conditions.

KEY POINTS

- Afebrile patients complaining of "biliary colic" may have peptic ulcer disease, gastroesophageal reflux, esophageal motility disorders, nonulcer dyspepsia, irritable bowel syndrome, renal colic, or angina pectoris

- Acute appendicitis, diverticulitis, colitis, acute pancreatitis, hepatitis, and pyelonephritis must also be considered if fever accompanies abdominal pain

- Ultrasound examination should be done with obstructive jaundice to rule in or out gallstone disease

- In absence of gallstones, chronic pancreatitis or prior biliary surgery suggestive of a postoperative stricture, chance of malignant tumor very high; differential diagnosis includes carcinoma of pancreas head, cholangiocarcinoma, ampullary carcinoma, and hepatoma or metastatic tumor obstructing major ducts at the porta hepatis

TREATMENT

Once the diagnosis of biliary colic is confirmed by ultrasonography, initial treatment consists of pain management and avoidance of fatty meals, which are known to stimulate gallbladder contraction. In most instances, outpatient management is sufficient and oral analgesics appropriate. Once the diagnosis is firmly established, the patient should be scheduled for elective cholecystectomy unless concurrent medical conditions contraindicate general anes-

thesia. Laparoscopic cholecystotomy has replaced open operation for uncomplicated gallbladder disease. The operation is extremely safe and effective and, because of its minimally invasive nature, most patients are discharged within 1–2 days postoperatively. Approximately 10% of laparoscopic cholecystectomies must be converted to open procedures because of excessive inflammation, scarring, unusual anatomy, or complications such as bleeding or bile duct injuries requiring open repair. Mortality associated with the operation is almost nil and the bile duct injury rate is approximately 0.5%. An intraoperative cholangiogram is usually obtained, as 10–15% of patients will have clinically silent bile duct stones. With increasing experience, some surgeons are using laparoscopic techniques to manage common duct stones. Without this expertise, the surgeon has the option to convert to an open operation and perform a traditional common bile duct exploration or to refer the patient for postoperative ERCP and endoscopic stone extraction. When small stones are seen on intraoperative cholangiograms, a reasonable approach is simply to observe the patient postoperatively, with the expectation that the stones will be passed spontaneously harmlessly from the bile duct into the duodenum. The development of postoperative symptoms such as pain, jaundice, or sepsis is cause for concern for which ERCP is indicated.

Acute cholecystitis represents a potentially very dangerous complication of gallstone disease and in all instances patients should be hospitalized, made NPO, and begun on intravenous broad spectrum antibiotics (Case 1). The expectation is that the patient will improve within 24–48 hours and should then undergo cholecystectomy. If there is failure to improve or deterioration within this time, emergency operation should be undertaken. Although laparoscopic cholecystectomy can be undertaken in the setting of acute cholecystitis (Case 1), conversion to open operation is required in many instances. If a patient is suspected or known to have a complication of acute cholecystitis such as perforation or abscess, open operation is indicated. Immunocompromised patients, particularly those with diabetes mellitus or those treated with steroids or chemotherapy, are at great risk of severe cholecystitis that is unresponsive to medical therapy. These patients often require emergency open cholecystectomy for gangrenous cholecystitis (gallbladder necrosis), emphysematous cholecystitis (due to gas forming bacteria), or empyema of the gallbladder (gross pus within the gallbladder).

Acute septic cholangitis may progress rapidly to shock and to death if not promptly recognized and treated. Unfortunately, the classic Charcot's triad is present in fewer than 60% of patients with this condition. Intravenous broad spectrum antibiotics should be instituted as soon as the diagnosis is considered, regardless of whether a dilated biliary tree is visualized or a specific cause identified (Case 2). Common bile duct stones are the most common cause of septic cholangitis; the initial imaging procedure of choice is ultrasonography for its superior ability to identify calculi and its immediate availability and portability. Since the mortality for acute septic cholangitis is nearly 70% when managed without decompression of the common bile duct and less than 20% when treated by biliary decompression, the only real question is clearly the timing of the intervention to decompress the duct. When the patient in a state of septic shock fails to be resuscitated with volume expansion, cardiovascular support, and antibiotics, emergency decompression of the biliary tract is mandatory. This should be undertaken within the first 12–24 hours of hospitalization even in the absence of a precise cause. Open operation has been the traditional method of biliary decompression. However, the lower mortality and morbidity associated with ERCP make it the approach of choice, with endoscopic division of the sphincter of Oddi (sphincterotomy) and stone extraction or placement of a biliary stent for drainage. In some instances, percutaneous transhepatic placement of a drainage catheter into the intrahepatic biliary system serves as an effective alternative. This procedure is particularly applicable to patients with noncalculous obstructing lesions of the proximal biliary tree. If an operative decompression is undertaken, cholecystectomy, intraoperative cholangiography, and common bile duct exploration with placement of a decompressive T tube is the procedure of choice. Patients presenting with cholangitis due to noncalculous biliary tract obstruction require either dilatation and endoscopic stenting or surgical bypass of the biliary system proximal to the obstruction. Surgical procedures most commonly used to treat strictures involve anastomosis of the proximal bile duct to either the duodenum or a defunctionalized Roux-en-Y jejunal limb.

Acute pancreatitis caused by gallstones requires that the patient be hospitalized, maintained NPO, and treated with parenteral analgesics and intravenous fluids. In the vast majority of patients, the pancreatitis resolves within 1–3 days, after which laparoscopic cholecystectomy and intraoperative cholangiography are performed. For the very small proportion of patients who have severe or unrelenting pancreatitis due to gallstones, ERCP, endoscopic sphincterotomy, and stone extraction are recommended. No patient admitted with an acute complication of gallstone disease should be discharged without undergoing cholecystectomy. This is because of the high incidence of recurrence following discharge without removal of the gallbladder.

Malignant tumors obstructing the biliary tree are treated by surgical resection whenever possible. Unfortunately, most of these tumors are either locally unresectable because of invasion of adjacent critical structures or are widely metastatic, and therefore incurable. Carcinoma of the gallbladder is rarely resectable. When the tumor is confined to the gallbladder, cholecystectomy, wedge resection of the gallbladder fossa of the liver, and regional lymph node dissection are the optimal procedures. In the few patients who have resectable cancer of the distal bile duct, ampulla of Vater, duodenum, or pancreas, a Whipple pancreaticoduodenectomy is indicated. This resection includes the gallbladder, common bile duct, head and neck of the pancreas, and duodenum. The reconstruction is complex and involves multiple anastomoses to restore biliary, pancreatic, and gastrointestinal continuity. For malignant tumors involving the more proximal common duct or the confluence of the right and left hepatic ducts (Klatskin tumor), resection of the entire extrahepatic biliary tree is performed and biliary-enteric continuity restored by Roux-en-Y hepaticojejunostomy. When unresectable cancers obstructing the biliary tree are encountered, endoscopic biliary stent placement is the preferred procedure to provide palliation. If unresectability is not determined until operation, surgical decompression is provided whenever possible either by proximal biliary bypass or by stent placement without tumor resection. In all cases, the goal is to provide freedom from the intense itching associated with chronic biliary obstruction, as well as relief of jaundice itself.

Both pancreatic carcinoma and cholangiocarcinoma are generally unresponsive to chemotherapy or radiotherapy. Although transient tumor shrinkage may follow these therapies, significant prolongation of life is rarely achieved. Surgery and endoscopic stenting of malignant biliary obstruction are the only reliable means of palliation for these difficult tumors.

KEY POINTS

- Laparoscopic cholecystotomy has replaced open operation for uncomplicated gallbladder disease

- Mortality associated with operation almost nil; bile duct injury approximately 0.5%

- Intraoperative cholangiogram usually obtained as 10–15% of patients will have clinically silent bile duct stones

- Acute cholecystitis represents a potentially very dangerous complication of gallstone disease; in all cases, patients should be hospitalized, made NPO, and begun on intravenous broad spectrum antibiotics

- Conversion to open operation from laparoscopic cholecystectomy for acute cholecystitis required in many instances

- Acute septic cholangitis may progress rapidly to shock and to death if not promptly recognized and treated; classic Charcot's triad present in fewer than 60% of patients

- Intravenous broad spectrum antibiotics should be instituted as soon as diagnosis of acute septic cholangitis considered, regardless of whether dilated biliary tree visualized or specific cause identified

- Emergency decompression of biliary tract mandatory in patients in state of septic shock who cannot be resuscitated with volume expansion, cardiovascular support, and antibiotics

- Open operation traditional method of biliary decompression; however, ERCP with endoscopic division of sphincter of Oddi (sphincterotomy) and stone extraction or placement of biliary stent for drainage is approach of choice because of lower mortality and morbidity

- If operative decompression undertaken, cholecystectomy, intraoperative cholangiography, and common bile duct exploration with placement of decompressive T tube is procedure of choice

- No patient admitted with acute complication of gallstone disease should be discharged without undergoing cholecystectomy

- Malignant tumors obstructing biliary tree are treated by surgical resection whenever possible; most locally unresectable because of invasion of adjacent critical structures or widely metastatic and therefore incurable

- Endoscopic biliary stent placement is preferred palliative procedure for unresectable cancers that obstruct biliary tree

- Both pancreatic carcinoma and cholangiocarcinoma generally unresponsive to chemotherapy or radiotherapy

FOLLOW-UP

Patients treated for biliary calculus disease generally require no long-term follow-up. The vast majority are able to return to work within days or weeks of operation and experience no recurrence of symptoms. However, a small minority continue to experience pain, and such individuals should be re-evaluated with liver function tests, abdominal ultrasonography, and ERCP to rule out retained or recurrent bile duct stones. Since a small number of patients are capable of forming stones even in the absence of a gallbladder, aggressive evaluation is always indicated if recurrent pain or jaundice occur. Patients who undergo biliary reconstruction for benign strictures require several years of follow-up with monitoring of liver function tests, as anastomotic strictures may occur early or relatively late after surgery. Should a postanastomotic stricture occur, endoscopic balloon dilatation is an effective method of treatment and often provides a permanent cure for this complication. Occasionally a postoperative anastomotic stricture requires reoperation with reconstruction of the anastomosis. On rare occasion, benign strictures defy a surgical solution and liver transplantation becomes the only option for long-term survival.

In instances of malignant obstruction of the biliary tract, close follow-up for the duration of the patient's life is always required. Since cure is not achieved in most of these patients, even when tumor resection is accomplished, follow-up is intended mainly to provide symptomatic relief. There is no effective salvage therapy for residual or recurrent disease. Following resection, recurrent disease may be palliated by endoscopic stent placement across the tumor. Unfortunately, the recurrence of pain or jaundice after operation almost invariably signifies tumor recurrence and incurability.

KEY POINTS

- Patients treated for biliary calculus generally require no long-term follow-up; vast majority able to return to work within days or weeks of operation and experience no recurrence of symptoms

- Patients who undergo biliary reconstruction for benign strictures require several years of follow-up with monitoring of liver function tests, as anastomotic strictures may occur early or relatively late after surgery

- Patients treated for malignant obstruction of biliary tract always require close life-long follow-up

- Recurrence of pain or jaundice after operation almost invariably signifies tumor recurrence and incurability

SUGGESTED READINGS

Jacobson IM: Gallstones. p. 668. In Grendell JH, McQuaid KR, Friedman SL (eds): Current Diagnosis and Treatment in Gastroenterology. Appleton & Lange, E. Norwalk, CT, 1996

A comprehensive and current summary of the pathophysiology, clinical presentation, complications, and treatment of gallstone disease.

Pitt HA, Dooley WC, Yeo CJ, Cameron JL: Malignancies of the biliary tree. Curr Probl Surg 32:1, 1995

A comprehensive review of carcinoma of the gallbladder, cholangiocarcinoma, and metastatic tumors affecting the biliary tract.

Sharp KW: Acute cholangitis. p. 351. In Cameron JL (ed): Current Surgical Therapy. 5th Ed. Mosby–Year Book, St. Louis, MO, 1995

A concise review of the etiology, clinical presentation, evaluation, and treatment of acute bacterial cholangitis.

Soper MJ: Laparoscopic cholecystectomy. Curr Probl Surg 28: 581, 1991

A comprehensive review of the selection criteria, operative techniques, and clinical results related to laparoscopic cholecystectomy.

Yeo CJ, Venbrux AC, Thuluvath PJ: Cholangiocarcinoma. p. 305. In Pitt HA, Carr-Loche DL, Ferrucci JT (eds): Hepatobiliary and Pancreatic Disease: The Team Approach to Management. Little, Brown, Boston, 1995

An overview of the etiology, differential diagnoses, and multidisciplinary therapeutic approach to cholangiocarcinoma.

QUESTIONS

1. *Which of the following is not considered a principal constituent of bile?*
   A. Bile salts.
   B. Lecithin.
   C. Calcium bilirubinate.
   D. Cholesterol.

2. *The most immediately life-threatening complication of gallstone disease is?*
   A. Acute cholecystitis.
   B. Acute cholangitis.
   C. Gallstone pancreatitis.
   D. Gallstone ileus.

3. *Most benign bile duct strictures are the result of?*
   A. Gallstone disease.
   B. Chronic pancreatitis.
   C. Sclerosing cholangitis.
   D. Injury during cholecystectomy.

4. *The most useful initial imaging technique in the diagnosis of biliary tract disease is?*
   A. Ultrasonography.
   B. CT scan.
   C. Abdominal radiography.
   D. ERCP.

5. *The most important definitive treatment in the management of septic cholangitis is?*
   A. ERCP and endoscopic sphincterotomy.
   B. Removal of all common bile duct stones.
   C. Broad spectrum intravenous antibiotics.
   D. Biliary ductal decompression.

(See p. 603 for answers.)

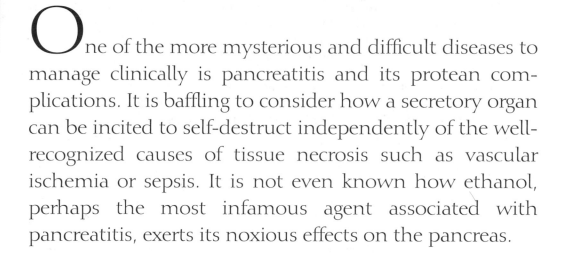

25 PANCREATITIS AND PSEUDOCYSTS

EDWARD PASSARO, JR.

One of the more mysterious and difficult diseases to manage clinically is pancreatitis and its protean complications. It is baffling to consider how a secretory organ can be incited to self-destruct independently of the well-recognized causes of tissue necrosis such as vascular ischemia or sepsis. It is not even known how ethanol, perhaps the most infamous agent associated with pancreatitis, exerts its noxious effects on the pancreas.

This chapter outlines the clinical and pathologic features of pancreatitis as well as some of the major complications. Among the latter, the focus is on pseudocysts and their management.

CASE 1
GALLSTONE PANCREATITIS

A 58-year-old female was seen because of fatty food intolerance, "excessive gas" or belching, and flatulence. Her gallbladder was found to contain multiple small stones on abdominal ultrasonography. The intrahepatic ductal structures were of normal size. She was scheduled for an elective laparoscopic cholecystectomy.

Two weeks before her scheduled operation she developed nausea and vomiting after a moderate size meal. She initially considered it to be a more pronounced form of her usual postprandial attack of excessive gas and bloating. Two hours later the distress did not abate but had progressed to epigastric distress and then pain. Five hours from onset, the pain had become unbearable, and she was aware of back pain, which she had not had previously. She was taken to the emergency room of a nearby hospital.

On arrival her temperature was 38°C and pulse 110 bpm. She appeared to be acutely ill and in severe pain.

She was diaphoretic and extremely restless in the bed but preferred to lie curled up about a pillow pulled close to her abdomen. Her Hct was 50, WBC 15,000, bilirubin 2.1, and amylase 800. Her abdomen was slightly distended, particularly in the epigastrium. It was tender to palpation throughout but more so in the epigastrium. An abdominal ultrasound was done promptly and showed the same findings as the previous one. A nasogastric tube was inserted as was a Foley catheter, and intravenous fluids and antibiotics were given. She was placed in the ICU. She improved over the next 72 hours; her serum amylase fell to 200, her upper gastric pain diminished, and her pulse was now 90 bpm. An ERCP was done. The ampulla of Vater was edematous. The common bile duct was cannulated and a cholangiogram showed the duct to be slightly dilated with several small (1–3 mm) filling defects in it. The pancreatic duct was not cannulated. Next, a sphincterotomy was done endoscopically. A large quantity of bile, seemingly under pressure, issued forth. Five small stones were expelled from the common duct. Following this, the patient became asymptomatic. Two days later her serum amylase was 90. The following day a laparoscopic cholecystectomy was done. The gallbladder specimen was slightly enlarged, edematous, and filled with many small stones similar to those found in the common bile duct. She was discharged the following day.

CASE 2
ALCOHOLIC PANCREATITIS
AND PSEUDOCYSTS

A 46-year-old male was hospitalized because of a 5-day history of epigastric pain that radiated straight through to his back. He had been hospitalized 3 years ago because of alcoholic pancreatitis. He had been drinking heavily (12 beers a day for 6–7 days) before the onset of the current abdominal pain. He had nausea but no vomiting over the 5 days. He had a watery bowel movement just before admission. He had a small bowel resection 24 years previously for an internal hernia producing intestinal obstruction.

His temperature was 38°C, and pulse 96 bpm. He appeared to be in mild distress from abdominal distention. He had no rebound tenderness but was tender to palpation in all quadrants. A stool guaiac was negative for blood.

Blood studies showed the following: Hct, 53%; WBC, 17,700; Ca, 8.1 mEq; total bilirubin, 1.0 mg/dl; amylase, 770 units; and lipase, 7,549.

He was started on intravenous fluids and given ampicillin, gentamycin, and metronidazole. A nasogastric tube was inserted. A CT scan showed an ill-defined pancreatic silhouette with peripancreatic fluid. On the fifth hospital day his temperature was 39.2°C and total parenteral nutrition was begun. On the seventh day, approximately 200 ml of a brownish turbid fluid high in amylase content was aspirated from the left upper quadrant and his abdomen became less distended. By the 12th day his abdomen became distended again. His temperature was 38.8°C. On CT scan there was a large peripancreatic fluid collection extending to below the liver. It was drained and examined for bacteria and fungi but none were found. A pigtail catheter was left in place. His abdomen was less distended and the following day his temperature was 38°C. On the 25th day he had mild abdominal tenderness and distention. Three pseudocysts were found on CT scan. Another pigtail catheter was placed in the larger collection and the other two were aspirated dry. Cultures showed coagulase negative staphylococci. He was given vancomycin and the intravenous catheters were changed. Two weeks later (40th hospital day) his temperature, which had been 38°–38.5°C rose to 39.5°C. A repeat abdominal CT scan showed no further fluid collections. He was given an antifungal agent. Over the following 2 weeks his temperature gradually came down to 37.7°C. On the 56th hospital day, two more pseudocysts were drained percutaneously under CT guidance and pigtail catheters placed. On the 60th day his temperature was below 37.5°C for the first time since his hospitalization. His remaining drains were removed, his antibiotics gradually stopped, and he was started on oral feeds. He was discharged on the 67th hospital day.

GENERAL CONSIDERATIONS

The two most common etiologies of pancreatitis are biliary tract disease and excessive alcohol ingestion. A few patients develop pancreatitis from hyperlipidemia, and some (10–15%) develop pancreatitis without any identifiable cause. Pancreatitis can also be a complication of an unrelated operation such as coronary artery bypass grafts (CABG), presumable because of the low blood flow state of the viscera, to which the pancreas is particularly sensitive.

Small- to moderate-size gallstones lodged in the ampulla of Vater (Case 1) are thought to produce pancreatitis by obstructing the outlet of the common bile duct, thereby allowing reflux of bile into the pancreatic duct. The theory is that bile refluxes into the main pancreatic duct because of a common junction between the common bile duct and the pancreatic duct just proximal to the ampulla of Vater (common channel theory of Opie). Even if this event initiates the process, it is not clear how the disease progresses to involve almost always the entire gland. However, the mechanical action of a stone impacted in the lower common bile duct as a cause of pancreatitis seems plausible because prompt removal of the stone is followed by the cessation of attacks of pancreatitis.

Alcoholic beverages taken in excess can cause pancreatitis in some individuals. Again, it is difficult to conceptualize how alcohol produces pancreatitis, either by direct or indirect mechanisms. In contrast to the pancreatitis associated with common bile duct stones, once pancreatitis is established in alcoholics it can progress or the patient may experience further attacks even when alcohol is no longer consumed. Again, just how and why this occurs is not known.

More baffling yet is idiopathic pancreatitis, which occurs without either biliary tract stone disease or alcohol ingestion (15%).

Whatever the cause, the chain of events is thought to be the interstitial release of the proteolytic enzymes of the acinar cells resulting in autolysis of the tissues. Large quantities of released enzymes can be found in the fluid that accumulates about the pancreas, in the peritoneal cavity, and in the blood. The most important of these are amylase and lipase, which can be readily measured and serve as markers of the autodigestive process. Amylase is found early in the process and then is rapidly cleared, whereas lipase concentrations increase slowly and are found later in the process.

Although fluid collections in and around the pancreas during an attack of pancreatitis is common (edematous pancreatitis) and can be detected by computed tomography (CT) scans, in most instances the fluid is reabsorbed. The fluid is thought to represent the direct leakage of pancreatic juices both from the injured parenchyma and the ductules, since a frank pancreatic fistula is occasionally the complication of an attack of pancreatitis.

When the fluid is excessive or becomes walled off from the peritoneal cavity by adjacent viscera it is called a pseudocyst (Fig. 25.1). Small pseudocysts may resolve spontaneously, while larger or multiple collections persist. Persistent collections may become infected or erode into adjacent vessels, producing bleeding. Thus, the complications of pancreatitis include sepsis (generally from infected collections), bleeding, and fistula formation, either from the pancreas or adjacent bowel. Long range complications include pancreatic exocrine insufficiency, diabetes, and malignancy.

The other form of pancreatitis is hemorrhagic pancreatitis. Whereas edematous pancreatitis has the escape of and transudation of large qualities of fluid (so-called internal burn) hemorrhagic pancreatitis is characterized by the extravasation of blood throughout the gland. The reasons for one form or the other occurring is not known, although hemorrhagic pancreatitis is more common among alcoholics.

KEY POINTS

• The two most common etiologies of pancreatitis are biliary tract disease and excessive alcohol ingestion

• Once pancreatitis is established in alcoholics, it can progress or the patient may experience further attacks even when alcohol no longer consumed—in contrast to pancreatitis associated with common bile duct stones

• The chain of events, whatever the cause of pancreatitis, is thought to be interstitial release of proteolytic enzymes of acinar cells resulting in autolysis of tissues

• When fluid is excessive or is walled off from the peritoneal cavity by adjacent viscera, it is called a pseudocyst (Fig. 25.1)

• Edematous pancreatitis has the escape of and transudation of large amounts of fluid ("internal burn"); hemorrhagic pancreatitis is characterized by extravasation of blood throughout gland

DIAGNOSIS

Ordinarily pancreatitis is not difficult to diagnose. It should always be considered in patients with the fairly rapid progression of upper abdominal pain, nausea, and vomiting. The character of the pain can be extremely variable. Classically, it is a deep-seated epigastric pain that radiates straight through to the back. Patients will often sit up and lean forward on a supporting table or chair back, or lie down over some support brought close to their abdomen (Case 1).

Obtaining a history of prior attacks of biliary colic from gallstone disease or excessive use of alcohol is very important as they are the prime etiologic factors. A history of either is present in about 80% of patients.

The patients least suspected of having pancreatitis and hence most difficult to diagnose are those in the hospital for other causes. For example, acute pancreatitis is a well-recognized complication of cardiac bypass procedures. It is thought to be due to inadequate perfusion of the pancreas during bypass. Similarly, patients with myocardial infarction and a low flow state from reduced cardiac output may develop pancreatitis.

Serial serum amylase determinations are an important aid in diagnosis, although the absolute level of amylase correlates poorly with the severity of the process. The

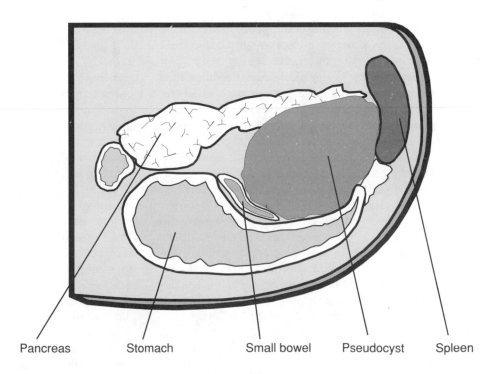

FIGURE 25.1 *Pancreatic pseudocyst.*

Pancreas   Stomach   Small bowel   Pseudocyst   Spleen serum amylase is elevated early and significantly in the disease and remains elevated during the acute phase. The determination can be made within a few hours and is extremely helpful in confirming the diagnosis. The finding of a normal serum amylase should lead to a reconsideration of the diagnosis.

A serum lipase determination is helpful when the patient is seen late in the clinical course. At that point the acute phase of inflammation and associated amylase release may be over and the excess amylase cleared by urinary excretion. As the lipase is released later and is slower to clear, it may serve as a marker for a resolving attack of pancreatitis.

Plain films of the abdomen and CT scans, while commonly obtained in the acute phase, provide little diagnostic assistance. They are more suited to evaluating the development of complications such as pseudocysts. Ultrasound may be helpful in confirming the presence of gallstones (the etiology) as well as pancreatic inflammation.

KEY POINTS

• It is important to obtain history of prior attacks of biliary colic from gallstone disease or excessive use of alcohol, because these are primary etiologic factors

• Serial serum amylase determinations important aid in diagnosis

DIFFERENTIAL DIAGNOSIS

Diseases producing the rather rapid progression of epigastric pain, nausea, and vomiting can mimic acute pancreatitis. These diseases include acute cholecystitis, perforated duodenal ulcer, and ruptured esophagus.

Acute cholecystitis is the most common differential diagnostic consideration. It shares a common history of prior attacks of biliary colic and the symptoms of nausea, vomiting, and epigastric distress. Aids in the differential diagnosis are that the pain is usually more prominent on the right and radiates around to the back rather than straight through to the back. Ultrasound and/or nuclear medicine scans (HIDA) may be useful as confirmation (see also Ch. 24).

Perforated duodenal ulcers or prepyloric ulcers also present as acute upper abdominal pain. On rare occasions duodenal contents high in amylase content leak into the peritoneal cavity, are absorbed, and transiently elevate the serum amylase, which can be misleading. Serial amylase determinations show the hyperamylasemia to be transient. Upright radiographs frequently show "free air" associated with a perforation.

Rupture of the esophagus at the cardioesophageal junction can occur as a result of forceful repetitive vomiting or retching. Such vomiting often accompanies bouts of alcohol abuse, which further compounds the problem. The patient experiences sudden epigastric pain that generally progresses in severity quickly. Experience has shown it to be a particularly difficult diagnosis to make early in the clinical course. Thus, many patients are considered to have acute pancreatitis because of the prominent features of alcohol abuse. Serial amylase determinations, follow-up CT scans, and water soluble contrast studies of the esophagus, are useful in making the differentiation.

Although the serum amylase is particularly useful in acute pacreatitis, it is not specific for this disease as is commonly assumed, nor is its concentration highest in the pancreas. Amylase is found in many tissues (its function there is not known), with the highest concentrations (severalfold over the pancreas) in the genital urinary tract. Ruptured ectopic pregnancies, for example, have had some of the highest values of serum amylase concentrations reported.

With the development of chronic pancreatitis, the pancreatic tissue levels are low. An acute attack in a chronic, diseased gland may cause only a very small increase in serum amylase concentrations.

KEY POINTS

• Acute cholecystitis most common differential diagnostic consideration

• Particularly difficult to diagnose in early clinical course; thus, many patients considered to have acute pancreatitis because of prominent features of alcohol abuse

TREATMENT

The treatment for acute pancreatitis is not specific and is supportive. Some aspects, such as the use of nasogastric tube decompression and antibiotics in mild cases, are controversial.

Critical elements in treatment are to correct the hypovolemic state and to detect and treat sepsis. Neither is simple in practice.

Large fluid shifts occur in acute pancreatitis, whether edematous or hemorrhagic, as explained above. Fluid requirements are further increased by the febrile response (Case 2), which can be marked and protracted. The best measure of adequate fluid replacement is a sustained urine output of 50 ml/hr or more. Complicating factors such as cardiac disease, sepsis, and diabetes may require that a central monitor of filling pressures and cardiac output (Swan-Ganz catheter) be inserted.

Antibiotic therapy may not be necessary in mild cases but is useful in severe forms of the disease and when infection of fluid collections is likely (Case 2). The continued use of antibiotics in these protracted cases may, however, make opportunistic infection from fungi more likely (Case 2). Antifungal agents are then required.

Serial CT scans are extremely useful in estimating the extent of the disease and in the recognition and treatment of pseudocysts. The clinical course of the patient in Case 2 points out the value of careful abdominal examination, noting the changes in abdominal distention, and the correlation with pseudocyst formation that were treated by repeated aspiration and catheter drainage.

Every attempt is made not to operate on these patients for either diagnosis or treatment. On occasion, particularly with hemorrhagic pancreatitis that becomes infected, nonoperative drainage techniques fail. In these circumstances, open debridement of some of the necrotic pancreatic tissue as well as wide drainage of the pancreatic bed is done. This treatment may be complicated either by pancreatic fistula formation or fistula from adjacent bowel.

KEY POINTS

• Critical elements in treatment are to correct hypovolemic state and to detect and treat sepsis

• Serial CT scans useful in estimating extent of disease and in recognition and treatment of pseudocysts

FOLLOW-UP

Recurrent attacks of pancreatitis are common, particularly after ethanol induced pancreatitis. Patients need help in refraining from alcohol consumption and in continued evaluation of any attack of abdominal pain for recurrent pancreatitis. Recurrent pancreatitis following elimination of biliary stone disease is uncommon and suggests either recurrent common bile duct stone formation or the development of a tumor in the periampullary region. Evaluation is best done by endoscopic retrograde cholangiopancreatography (ERCP) to both inspect the periampullary region for tumors and to look for common bile duct stones. If a stone is found it can usually be retrieved by repeat endoscopic sphincterotomy.

The end result of either an initial attack of severe pancreatitis or recurrent attacks of lesser severity is chronic pancreatitis. Chronic pancreatitis is characterized by the development of a nearly constant, dull, deep-seated epigastric or back pain. The pain is aggravated by eating, and patients lose weight. Additionally, with the progressive loss of acinar tissue, the pancreatic insufficiency leads to intestinal malabsorption. The patient's stools become frequent, foul, and float because of steatorrhea. Diabetes occurs in approximately one third of these patients. Hence, patients will need pancreatic enzyme supplements, vitamins, calcium, and correction of the hyperglycemia with either oral medication or insulin.

SUGGESTED READINGS

Schmitz-Moormann P, Schwerk W, Sinn P: Histological alterations of the preampullary common bile and pancreatic duct in acute biliary pancreatitis. Digestion 34:93, 1986

A good experimental examination of the pathologic events in gallstone pancreatitis.

Steer ML et al: Pancreatitis: the role of lysosomes. Dig Dis Sci 29:934, 1984

An excellent review of our current knowledge of the pathophysiology of acute pancreatitis.

QUESTIONS

1. Hemorrhagic pancreatitis rather than edematous pancreatitis is apt to result from?
   A. Gallstones disease.
   B. Alcohol abuse.
   C. Low perfusion state of the pancreas.
   D. Viral infections as mumps.

2. Major complications from acute pancreatitis include?
   A. Sepsis.
   B. Bleeding.
   C. Pseudocyst formation.
   D. All of the above.

3. CT scans are most useful to?
   A. Establish the diagnosis.
   B. Establish the extent of the pancreatic injury.
   C. To detect and treat complications such as pseudocysts.
   D. None of the above.

(See p. 603 for answers.)

26 TUMORS OF THE PANCREAS

MICHEAL RIDGEWAY

BRUCE E. STABILE

Carcinoma of the pancreas has the distinction of being one of the most lethal malignancies. With a widely quoted 5-year survival approaching 2%, it is easy to understand why most surgeons treat the typical patient with pancreatic cancer pessimistically. However, there are subgroups of patients with very early stage cancers or variant types of pancreatic cancer who can benefit from tumor excision. As nonpancreatic tumors in the region of the ampulla of Vater can produce identical signs and symptoms, it is especially important to identify them, as they are all more curable than carcinoma of the pancreas.

The goals of this chapter are to (1) describe the clinical presentations of pancreatic and periampullary tumors, (2) define the various diagnostic and staging techniques available, (3) outline the typical natural history, patterns of spread, and reasons for treatment failure, and (4) delineate the various treatments and palliative modalities available, their indications, and potential shortcomings.

CASE 1
PAINLESS JAUNDICE AND WEIGHT LOSS

A 61-year-old black male noted the recent onset of yellow sclerae. He had lost 10 lb over a 2-month period and had noted some deep-seated upper abdominal pain over the past several months. Although he had heavy alcohol use in the past, he denied any within the past 20 years. He was jaundiced and had an enlarged liver, mild epigastric tenderness, and a palpable gallbladder in the right upper quadrant. His Hct was 36%, WBC, 6.8; total bilirubin, 12.6 (direct 10.8); amylase, 68; alkaline phosphate, 656; GGT 442; AST, 36; ALT, 38; and PT, 11.8 seconds.

A CT scan of the abdomen showed a question of a "fullness" in the head of the pancreas, dilated intra- and extrahepatic bile ducts, an enlarged gallbladder without gallstones and no evidence of lymphadenopathy or intrahepatic disease. A CA 19-9 level was ordered. ERCP showed narrowed bile and pancreatic ducts within the pancreatic head. An endoscopic ultrasound demonstrated a 2 × 2-cm mass in the head of the pancreas and no evidence of regional adenopathy. Cytologic brushings taken of the biliary and pancreatic ducts along with ultrasound-guided FNA of the presumed pancreatic mass failed to show any evidence of tumor.

At operation, the liver was free of masses. An extensive search for regional lymphadenopathy was conducted in the hepatic hilum, celiac axis, transverse mesocolon, and greater omentum. A large periportal lymph node was sent to pathology for frozen section and revealed no evidence of tumor. The inferior vena cava and portal and superior mesenteric veins were found to be without evidence of tumor invasion. The decision was made to proceed with formal pancreaticoduodenectomy (Fig. 26.1). A mass was palapable in the head of the pancreas. The gastric antrum, gallbladder, common bile duct, duodenum, and head of the pancreas were all resected en bloc with pancreaticoje-junostomy and gastrojejunostomy performed for reconstruction (Fig. 26.2). The patient recovered uneventfully.

Pathologic examination of the resected specimen revealed a moderately differentiated ductal adenocarcinoma in the head of the pancreas. The surgical margins were clear of tumor and there was no tumor identified within the regional lymph nodes. The postoperative CA 19-9 level was within normal limits.

CASE 2
BACK PAIN AND GASTRIC OUTLET OBSTRUCTION

A 72-year-old white female developed severe mid-epigastric pain and mid-back pain, inability to take solid foods,

and weight loss. She had vomiting of solid foods within 1 hour and was unable to keep down anything but liquids. She reported a 40-lb weight loss over the past 6 months and was cachetic. A nonpulsatile mid-epigastric mass measuring approximately 6×6 cm was palpable. The stool was hemoccult positive. Her Hct was 29%, total bilirubin, 4.0 (direct 3.0); amylase, 45; alkaline phosphate, 422; GGT, 298; AST, 25; ALT, 26; PT, 12.2 seconds; albumin, 2.8; and serum glucose, 488. In the emergency room, a nasogastric tube was placed that initially drained 1 L of nonbilious material. Intravenous hydration was started and insulin given.

A CT scan of the abdomen showed a 5×5-cm mass in the head of the pancreas extending inferiorly into the transverse mesocolon. The mass impinged on the first and second portions of the duodenum. The stomach was distended. There were several enlarged lymph nodes noted in the periportal area and in the retroperitoneum surrounding the celiac axis. The liver was free of masses.

A large pancreatic head mass growing into the base of the transverse mesocolon was found at operation. Biopsy

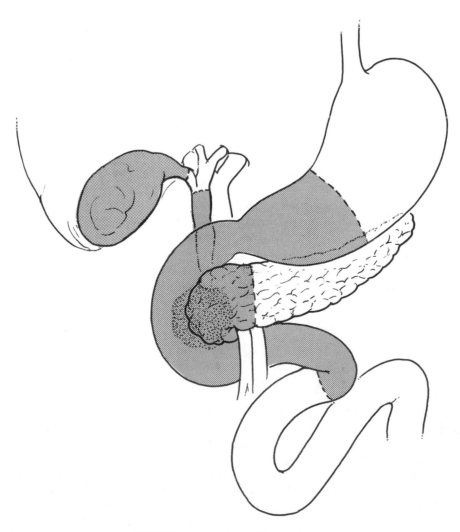

FIGURE 26.1 *Area of resection.*

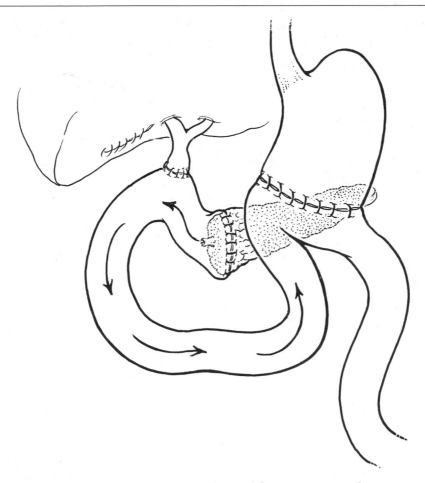

FIGURE 26.2 *Reconstruction of the gastrointestinal tract.*

showed ductal adenocarcinoma. The surface of the liver was studded with several suspicious lesions and a shave biopsy of one showed carcinoma. Cholecystojejunostomy and antecolic gastrojejunostomy were done. The gastrohepatic ligament was opened and a chemical splanchnicectomy was done by injecting 20 ml of 50% EtOH into the celiac plexus. The patient recovered uneventfully with improvement of her pain postoperatively. She died 3 months later from her tumor.

GENERAL CONSIDERATIONS

Pancreatic cancer is the fourth leading cause of cancer-related deaths in the United States. Approximately 28,000 new cases are diagnosed each year and almost as many patients die of advanced disease. Ductal adenocarcinoma accounts for 90% of all pancreatic malignancies, and 80% of these lesions are located in the head of the gland. Lesions located in the body or tail of the pancreas almost always produce symptoms late and therefore are almost always unresectable. Lesions located in the head of the gland are sometimes curable because they can produce obstructive jaundice when they are still small and without metastasis

(Case 1). Unfortunately, at the time of diagnosis, fewer than 10% of pancreatic tumors are confined to the head of the gland and most therefore are unresectable (Case 2). This fact has led to the generally nihilistic view of curative therapy held by many physicians today.

There are no universally acknowledged environmental risk factors for the development of pancreatic cancer. Several studies have suggested a slightly increased risk associated with coffee use, cigarette smoking, and increased levels of dietary fat, but other investigations have failed to confirm these findings. There is a twofold increase of pancreatic cancer in diabetics. In patients with inherited polyposis syndromes of the colon, there is an increase in incidence of periampullary tumors of 100–200 times that of the normal population.

The vast majority of pancreatic cancer patients, however, do not have an inherited syndrome. Most patients are elderly at the time of diagnosis, with 75% of patients older than 60 years of age. The overall survival is a dismal 2% at 5 years when all patients with the disease are considered. The median survival is 18–20 months after "curative" resection. A few high-volume centers have reported higher survival rates in the range of 20–40% following resection for cure. There are no reliable, cost-effective screening tests available to detect pancreatic cancer. A thorough history and physical examination, along with a high index of suspicion for the disease are required if the diagnosis is to be made early.

KEY POINTS

• Pancreatic cancer fourth leading cause of cancer-related deaths in the United States

• Ductal adenocarcinoma accounts for 90% of all pancreatic malignancies and 80% of these lesions are located in head of gland

• At time of diagnosis, less than 10% of pancreatic tumors confined to head of gland and, therefore are unresectable

• No universally acknowledged environmental risk factors for development of pancreatic cancer

• Most patients elderly at time of diagnosis, with 75% of patients older than 60

• Overall survival of 2% at 5 years, when all patients with disease considered

• No reliable, cost-effective screening tests are available to detect pancreatic cancer

---

DIAGNOSIS

The diagnosis of pancreatic cancer can be notoriously difficult. In rare cases, a small and curable lesion confined to the head of the gland is found, because the tumor produced obstructive jaundice early due to its strategic location (Case 1). In most cases, however, the diagnosis is much more elusive. The signs and symptoms may be subtle, leading to delays and the development of unresectable disease (Case 2). Pain, either deep-seated and subtle (Case 1) or boring and profound (Case 2), is the most common symptom associated with tumors of the pancreas, occurring in 80% of cases. When back pain occurs it is an ominous finding, implying retroperitoneal invasion by the tumor (Case 2). Other common presenting symptoms include jaundice, anorexia, and weight loss. Cholangitis is uncommon in patients with malignant bile duct obstruction. A palpable (Courvoisier's) gallbladder is seen in about 25% of patients (Case 1). The sudden onset of diabetes is noted in only about 20% of cases (Case 2). The finding of occult blood in the stool is related to tumor erosion into the duodenum (Case 2). Gastric outlet obstruction, usually a late finding, is associated with a worse prognosis (Case 2).

When a tumor of the pancreas is suspected, a computed tomography (CT) scan of the abdomen should be the first diagnostic test ordered. This test delineates the pancreas and surrounding structures and can be diagnostic for larger lesions (Case 2). Bile duct dilatation, lymphadenopathy, and evidence of hepatic metastases can be detected by this imaging technique, although it will often miss metastatic disease when the lesions are small (Case 2). When the diagnosis is in doubt after CT scanning (Case 1), endoscopic retrograde cholangiopancreatography (ERCP) is the next step in the evaluation of a patient with a suspected pancreatic head mass. ERCP suggests the diagnosis when the intrapancreatic common bile and pancreatic ducts are narrowed or obstructed and allows cytologic sampling of the pancreatic duct, which may reveal cancer in up to 80% of cases (Case 1). Endoscopic ultrasound is a new imaging modality that can detect smaller masses in the periampullary region, regional lymphadenopathy, and a safe means of biopsying lesions in the pancreatic head, (Case 1). Of the many serum markers that have been evaluated in pancreatic cancer, CA 19-9 is the most sensitive. Preoperative measurements can be useful when the diagnosis is in doubt and may be used to monitor the patient postoperatively for recurrence.

In many instances, despite the use of various preoperative imaging and diagnostic techniques, the diagnosis of pancreatic cancer cannot be made. In these cases, operative evaluation is indicated, with either laparoscopy or formal laparotomy, for both diagnostic and therapeutic reasons. At operation, biopsy of pancreatic head masses is done only for lesions that are considered to be unresectable. Symptomatic masses in the head of the pancreas that appear resectable are removed without biopsy because of the concern that biopsy can cause peritoneal seeding of the tumor.

KEY POINTS

• Pain, either deep-seated and subtle or boring and profound, is most common symptom associated with tumors of pancreas, occurring in 80% of cases

• When tumor of pancreas suspected, CT scan of abdomen should be first diagnostic test ordered

• When diagnosis in doubt after CT, ERCP is next step in a patient with suspected pancreatic head mass

• Of the many serum markers that have been evaluated in pancreatic cancer, CA 19-9 is most sensitive

---

DIFFERENTIAL DIAGNOSIS

Any mass lesion in the region of the ampulla of Vater can mimic carcinoma of the pancreas. Of the periampullary tumors, pancreatic cancer is by far the most common, accounting for 75% of all such lesions. Ampullary carcinoma is the next most commonly encountered periampullary tumor and is usually diagnosed or ruled out by endoscopy (Case 1). Its identification is important because the prognosis for patients with this tumor is vastly superior to that of pancreatic cancer. Other less common mass lesions in the region include bile duct carcinoma and duodenal carcinoma, which are usually excluded from consideration by endoscopy and ERCP. Very rarely, benign masses may be encountered in the region of the ampulla that can cause obstructive jaundice such as polyps or adenomas of the duodenum.

Chronic pancreatitis is always a consideration in patients with an abnormality of the head of the pancreas, especially if there is prior heavy alcohol use (Case 1). Scarring from chronic inflammation in the head of the gland can cause stricture of the distal common bile duct and painless jaundice. In the first case, the diagnosis is less likely because of the absence of an antecedent history of pancreatitis or gallstone disease, although this does not completely rule out the lesion. Often the differentiation between pancreatic cancer and chronic pancreatitis will be impossible, even at operation (Case 1). In these cases, if the lesion is deemed resectable, pancreaticoduodenectomy is performed.

Gallstone-related diseases must all be considered in the differential diagnosis of patients with jaundice or epigastric pain. The absence of fever, elevated white blood cell (WBC) count, and gallstones on ultrasound examination all help to rule out common bile duct stones in the jaundiced patient (Case 1). Cholangitis is rare in patients with obstructive jaundice from periampullary tumors, but more common in patients with choledocholithiasis. Any finding of a mass in the head of the pancreas eliminates the diagnosis of common bile duct stones, especially in the elderly patient (Case 2).

Gastric outlet obstruction from peptic ulcer disease should be considered in patients with epigastric pain and severe weight loss (Case 2). Absence of a history of ulcer disease makes this diagnosis unlikely, as do the findings of a large pancreatic mass. Peptic ulcer disease is best diagnosed by upper endoscopy.

KEY POINTS

• Any mass lesion in region of the ampulla of Vater can mimic carcinoma of pancreas

• Of periampullary tumors, pancreatic cancer most common, accounting for 75% of all such lesions

• Chronic pancreatitis always a consideration in patients with abnormality of head of pancreas, especially if history of prior heavy alcohol use

• Absence of fever, elevated WBC count, and gallstones on ultrasound all help to rule out common bile duct stones in jaundiced patient

---

TREATMENT

The principal goal of the care of patients with pancreatic cancer is to define the small subgroup who have a chance of being cured by resective therapy (approximately 10% of patients). Extensive preoperative evaluation is not necessary when the diagnosis is suggested and the patient is a good candidate for operation. A CT scan showing a pancreatic head mass in the jaundiced patient is enough to warrant operation if there are no contraindications. Often the diagnosis is less clear, and ERCP and endoscopic ultrasound are performed to determine the cause of jaundice (Case 1). Biopsy-proven diagnosis of pancreatic cancer is not required before planning operative intervention.

Curative resection of cancer of the pancreatic head (or any periampullary tumor, for that matter) is a pancreaticoduodenectomy or Whipple procedure. In this procedure, much of the dissection and time is spent determining resectability of the lesion. This is important since most patients undergoing "curative" resection do not live more than 2 years following surgery. The reason for treatment failure is obvious: unrecognized tumor spread at operation. A thorough search for tumor-positive lymph nodes is made. Direct extension of the tumor into the transverse mesocolon, celiac axis, superior mesenteric, or portal vein constitute absolute contraindications to resective therapy. In the standard Whipple procedure, the gastric antrum, gallbladder and common bile duct, head of the pancreas, and duodenum are all resected (Fig. 26.2). Reconstruction of the gastrointestinal tract following resection is complex, involving multiple anastomoses (Fig. 26.3). The procedure is fraught with potential complications, although most are not life-threatening. The most serious are brought on by the breakdown of the pancreaticoenteric anastomosis, which can lead to pancreatic fistula. The mortality of patients undergoing Whipple procedure ranges from 1–5% and is dependent on the experience of the operating surgeon.

When resective therapy is for possible, palliative measures are undertaken (Case 2). Palliation of pancreatic cancer usually involves three considerations: relief of pain, relief of jaundice, and relief of established or impending gastric outlet obstruction. If unresectable disease is found a palliative procedure can be performed (Case 2). This usually consists of a biliary bypass procedure, a gastrojejunostomy, and a chemical splanchnicectomy of the celiac ganglion to ameliorate the profound pain these patients often suffer in the end-stage of their disease. Nonoperative means of palliation include biliary stenting (either via an endoscopic or percutaneous transhepatic approach), percutaneous celiac block, and endoscopic stenting of the proximal duodenum to treat gastric outlet obstruction. However, when unresectable disease is found, operative palliation should be done then, since nonoperative measures all have appreciable failure rates.

Neither adjuvant chemotherapy nor radiotherapy has been found to alter the course or prolong life in patients with pancreatic cancer. Operation remains the only real hope for cure and the principal means of palliation for this lethal disease.

KEY POINTS

• Principal goal of care of patients with pancreatic cancer is to define subgroup who have chance of being cured by resective therapy (approximately 10%)

• Biopsy-proven diagnosis of pancreatic cancer not required before planning operative intervention

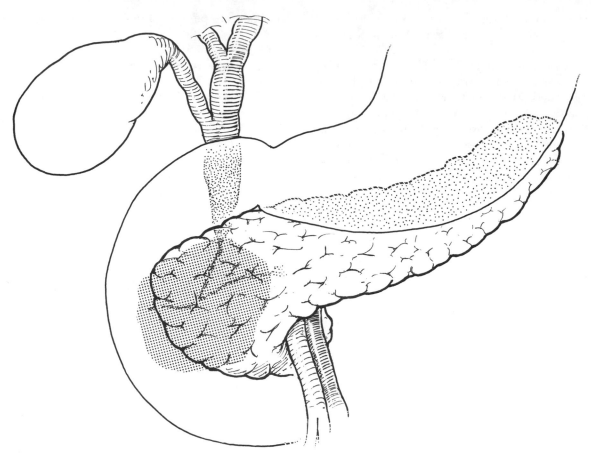

FIGURE 26.3   *Cancer of the head of the pancreas.*

• In this procedure, much of dissection and time spent determining resectability of lesion

• In standard Whipple procedure, gastric antrum, gallbladder, and common bile duct, head of pancreas, and duodenum all resected (Fig. 26.2)

• Palliation of pancreatic cancer usually involves relief of pain, relief of jaundice, and relief of established or impending gastric outlet obstruction

• Neither adjuvant chemotherapy nor radiotherapy has been found to alter the course or prolong life in patients with pancreatic cancer

check for symptoms that suggest recurrence (jaundice, gastric outlet obstruction, pain, or weight loss) and routine history and physical examination are performed at that time. Yearly CA 19-9 levels can be drawn to monitor for recurrence. A CT scan of the abdomen is the best test for detection of recurrent tumor or other treatable causes of the patient's symptoms.

KEY   POINTS

• For patients who successfully undergo resective therapy, follow-up is mainly syptomatic, since no good treatment for recurrence

FOLLOW-UP

Since long-term survival is the exception rather than the rule for patients with pancreatic cancer, no established guidelines exist regarding the follow-up management of these patients. Terminal patients are generally managed by medical oncologists and pain management specialists who attempt to control symptoms (principally pain) in the end-stage of the disease. For patients who successfully undergo resective therapy, follow-up is mainly symptomatic, since there is no good treatment for recurrence. Patients are seen at 6-month intervals to

SUGGESTED READINGS

Cameron JL, Crist DW, Sitzmann JV et al: Factors influencing survival following pancreaticoduodenectomy for pancreatic cancer. Am J Surg 161:120, 1991

An analysis of the most commonly performed curative operation for cancer of the pancreas from a high-volume center, delineating causes of treatment failure.

Lillemoe KD, Sauter P, Pitt HA et al: Current status of surgical palliation of periampullary carcinoma. Surg Gynecol Obstet 176:1, 1993

An overview of the various invasive and noninvasive means of palliating patients with unresectable pancreatic cancer.

Reber H: Tumors of the Pancreas. p. 1421. In Schwartz (ed): Principles of Surgery. 6th Ed. 1994

An excellent overview focusing on symptoms and signs of pancreatic cancer as well as algorithms for the work-up of tumors of the pancreas.

QUESTIONS

1. The findings of deep-seated, boring upper abdominal pain and jaundice can be associated with which of the following?

    A. Pancreatic cancer.

    B. Ampullary carcinoma.

    C. Duodenal carcinoma.

    D. Bile duct carcinoma.

    E. All of the above.

2. Surgical palliation of unresectable pancreatic cancer can include each of the following except?

    A. Gastric bypass.

    B. Biliary bypass.

    C. Chemical splanchnicectomy of the celiac axis ganglion.

    D. Pancreatic head biopsy for diagnostic purposes.

3. Adjuvant therapy for pancreatic cancer?

    A. Consists of well-established chemotherapy and radiotherapy regimens.

    B. Involves adjuvant adriamycin-based chemotherapy only.

    C. Involves adjuvant radiotherapy only.

    D. Has not been shown to improve survival.

    E. Should be offered to the patient as a means of palliation.

4. Which of the following findings at operation does not constitute a contraindication to pancreaticoduodenectomy?

    A. Periaortic lymph nodes positive for tumor on frozen section.

    B. Peritoneal implants of tumor.

    C. Direct tumor extension with the second portion of the duodenum.

    D. Liver metastases.

    E. Direct tumor extension into the rest of the mesentery.

(See p. 603 for answers.)

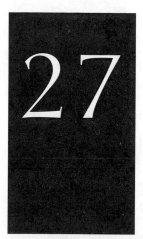

27

ITP AND

OTHER SPLENIC

DISORDERS

EDWARD PASSARO, JR.

The spleen occupies the attention of the surgeon because it is easily injured in trauma, whether external, internal, or as a complication of an intra-abdominal operation. In addition, a few diseases of the spleen produce hematologic disorders that require splenectomy. This chapter outlines the salient features of spleen disorders and the indication for splenectomy.

CASE 1
IDIOPATHIC
THROMBOCYTOPENIC PURPURA
(PRIMARY HYPERSPLENISM)

A 30-year-old female developed a cold over a 4-day period. A week later she noted for the first time purplish blotches over her lower torso and legs. She developed menorrhagia and easy bruisability. She was given steroids and her platelet count remained unchanged at 35,000. Her spleen was removed and appeared to be normal in size and consistency. Within 72 hours her platelet count had increased to 100,000. On follow-up 2 months later, her ecchymotic areas had cleared and her menses were normal.

CASE 2
SECONDARY HYPERSPLENISM
(MYELOPHTHISIC ANEMIA)

A 48-year-old female complained of lassitude and easy fatigability. Over the past 3 months she had noted progressive loss of energy to the point that she could no longer do her household chores.

She was pale, wan, with slight pedal edema. There was a large ecchymotic area over the right thigh laterally. A firm spleen could be palpated 6 cm below the left costal margin. It was not tender.

Her Hct was 22%, WBC count 8,000, and the platelet count 20,000. A BMA showed much of the marrow replaced by fibrosis. She was given blood, and a splenectomy, liver biopsy, and lymph node biopsy were done to look for myelogenous leukemia, which was not found. Four years later, however, she developed leukemia.

CASE 3
SPLENIC TRAUMA

A 23-year-old male's car jumped a curb and struck a glancing blow to a tree. When the paramedics arrived they found the driver sitting on a curb, bent forward and complaining of abdominal pain. He had grunting respirations. In the emergency department his vital signs were normal, as was an initial Hct. A chest film was reported as normal. He was very tender over the left 6th–10th ribs laterally and was thought to have rib fractures despite the chest films. He had abdominal guarding, particularly over a bruised area in the left upper quadrant. An IV catheter was started and he was observed over the next 2 hours. Serial Hct remained unchanged and he was discharged.

Approximately 36 hours later he returned because of the sudden onset of generalized abdominal pain. He was nauseated and slightly tachypneic. His abdomen was tender to palpation throughout and there was guarding. His Hct had fallen 20 points since he was last seen. He was rapidly given blood transfusions and an operation was performed. The posterior lateral aspect of his spleen had a large rent in the serosal covering. There was approximately 2,000 ml of unclotted blood with some clots free in the peritoneal cavity. A splenectomy was done and a large crack was found along the posterior lateral aspect that did not extend into the hilum.

Two months later his Hct was normal. He had been vaccinated against *Haemophilus influenzae*, *Streptococcus pneumoniae*, and *Neisseria meningitidis*.

GENERAL CONSIDERATIONS

The spleen has an unusually rich arterial blood supply and receives important collaterals from the stomach. It is useful to think of the spleen as a component of the hemopoietic system, as one of its major functions is to remove damaged or altered blood cellular components, store white blood cells (WBCs) and platelets, and occasionally, to produce these elements.

Splenic disorder can be grossly divided into primary and secondary types. The primary or intrinsic forms are identified by a normal sized spleen. These diseases can be accompanied by the inappropriate destruction of red blood cells (RBCs) as they pass through the spleen, as in hemolytic anemias, or the excess destruction of platelets, as in idiopathic thrombocytopenic purpura (Case 1). The causes of the increased breakdown of cellular components can be genetic defects in the production of cells (sickle cell anemia) or, more commonly, the development of autoimmune disease frequently related to viral infection.

Secondary splenic disorders are characterized by enlargement of the spleen—not infrequently to massive proportion—as well as the destruction of many blood cells. Thus, the spleen's disorder is a reflection of a systemic process, generally of the hemopoietic system, such as myelogenous leukemia (Case 2) or Hodgkin's disease.

The most common cause of splenic disorder relates to trauma. The spleen, being richly supplied with blood and nestled in the left upper quadrant beneath the rib cage, is frequently injured in both blunt as well as penetrating abdominal trauma. Because of its close proximity to both the stomach and the splenic flexure of the colon, the spleen can be readily injured during operations on either the stomach or the colon. It has a relatively thin fragile capsule, and minimal manipulation or traction on contiguous structures can produce a tear in the splenic capsule and bleeding.

KEY POINTS

- Splenic disorders are grossly divided into primary or secondary
- Primary splenic disorders identified by a normal size spleen
- Secondary splenic disorders characterized by enlargement of spleen—not infrequently to massive proportion—and destruction of blood cells
- The spleen, richly supplied with blood and nestled in the left upper quadrant beneath the rib cage, is frequently injured in both blunt and penetrating abdominal trauma

DIAGNOSIS

Primary and secondary splenic disorders are detected by the loss of RBCs, WBCs, and platelets in the blood from abnormal activity of the spleen. History and physical examination generally provide all of the necessary data, which can be confirmed by complete blood counts (CBCs) and occasionally a bone marrow aspiration (BMA). The finding of normal bone marrow indicates that the spleen is responsible for the loss of the blood cellular components. BMA determines whether the loss of the blood element is related to a systemic disorder that involves the spleen (Case 2).

Bleeding from the spleen, even when there is gross evidence of trauma (Case 3), is not always easy to detect. The patient in Case 3 had obvious signs of trauma in the left upper quadrant and clinical evidence of broken ribs on the left side despite a normal chest film—not an uncommon finding. He returned and was observed for several hours for bleeding and none was found. He returned some 36 hours later with obvious intra-abdominal bleeding. Thus, bleeding from a fractured spleen can be slow and occult, collecting beneath the splenic capsule until it breaks and releases blood into the peritoneal cavity. In addition to observing decreasing Hct, diagnostic aspiration of the peritoneal cavity (paracentesis) or peritoneal lavage for blood within the abdomen can be helpful. Computed tomography (CT) scanning frequently detects splenic injuries as well.

KEY POINTS

- Primary and secondary splenic disorders detected by loss of RBCs, WBCs, and platelets in the blood from abnormal splenic activity
- Normal bone marrow indicates that the spleen is responsible for the loss of blood cellular components

DIFFERENTIAL DIAGNOSIS

Splenic disorders can be divided in primary and secondary causes. The size of the spleen, normal in primary and enlarged in secondary, is a useful, practical method to distinguish between the two causes (with few exceptions). The importance of the differential is that primary splenic disorders can be readily treated, whereas secondary splenic disorders often identified as hypersplenism may or may not be ameliorated by splenectomy.

The specific hematologic defect found in primary splenic disorders, such as the loss of RBCs, WBCs, or platelets, is determined by appropriate laboratory studies. Practically, however, there is no great clinical difference between hemolytic anemia and thrombocytopenia produced by a primary splenic disorder.

The hematologic alterations produced by secondary splenic disorders are not limited to specific blood cell type. They are both more generic and more profound. The important differential in this group is between a more benign process and a malignant one. In Case 2 there was a concern that the patient had an occult myelogenous leukemia. Tissue biopsies were taken at operation. Biopsies are also useful to uncover extramedullary hemopoietic sites such as the liver or lymph nodes. Extramedullary hemopoietic sites are an indication that the patient's bone marrow has been replaced to a degree that these sites are needed to sustain the patient.

The differential diagnosis of splenic trauma is at times straightforward (Case 3), and other times is complex and confusing, such that laparotomy is necessary to determine whether the spleen is injured. This is particularly the case where extensive multiple injuries are involved (e.g., the thorax and extremities). Here, considerable experience and judgment is required to evaluate the patient for splenic injuries. CT scans are particularly useful in these instances and are almost always obtained, except where the rate of bleeding is such that the patient can only be saved by immediate exploration for the source of bleeding. CT scans reveal blood around the spleen and beneath the capsule, and also determine whether the tear is small and confined to the parenchyma or involves the hilum and thus the major vessels.

KEY POINTS

• Spleen size a useful, practical method to distinguish between the two causes (with exceptions)

• Differential important so that primary splenic disorders can be readily treated, and secondary splenic disorders identified as hypersplenism may be ameliorated by splenectomy

• Hematologic alterations produced by secondary splenic disorders are not limited to specific blood cell type, but are more generic and profound

• CT scans reveal blood around the spleen and beneath capsule, and determine if the tear is small and confined to parenchyma or involves the hilum and major vessels

TREATMENT

Primary splenic disorders are first treated by medical therapy. Idiopathic thrombocytopenic purpura, for example, is first treated with steroids. This is effective in more than one-half of patients. Only those who have failed medical management are referred for operative treatment.

The treatment of secondary splenic disorders is neither clear nor widely agreed on. The first criteria is to be sure that an occult malignancy is not present. The latter are not improved by splenectomy, which is usually contraindicated in these patients. The second criteria is to assess the potential for improvement of the patient's hematologic status or general health that can be expected by the splenectomy. Unfortunately, in many patients, such an assessment is either very difficult or impossible. The last criteria is symptomatic relief. Many patients develop huge spleens that are a source of discomfort in breathing, lying down, or bending over. Others have episodes of abdominal pain, nausea, vomiting, and fever because of infarcts in the spleen. Ascites and dependent peripheral edema may develop as a result of the spleen's pressure on the venous system and the increased intra-abdominal pressure.

In adults (beyond age 12) splenectomy is the best treatment for the injured spleen. The spleen injured from trauma is usually fragmented in multiple areas involving the arterial supply. Thus, continued bleeding is a serious threat to the patient's life. Under these circumstances, the prompt cessation of bleeding is of paramount concern. Attempting to repair such a spleen will cause even greater blood loss. Overwhelming sepsis is a rare but dreaded complication, so that patients are vaccinated against the organisms that commonly produce sepsis (Case 3). This is particularly important in pediatric patients undergoing splenectomy.

Patients found to have a tear of the spleen, not involving the hilum, and not actively bleeding after 48 hours of observation may be managed nonoperatively.

Similarly, patients found to have a subcapsular hematoma on a CT scan may be observed to see if the hematoma expands or not. Nonoperative management is indicated for those patients who demonstrate no further progression of the hematoma and no further evidence of bleeding.

On rare occasions, it is possible to save a portion of the injured spleen at operation. Judgment is required to ensure that blood loss will be no greater than that incurred by splenectomy. Splenorrhaphy or suture repair of splenic capsule tears is generally not suitable for splenic trauma as the tears or fractures are both deep and extensive.

Splenorrhaphy is effective when the splenic capsule is torn during the conduct of other surgical procedures such as resection of the splenic flexure of the colon. In these instances the tear is limited both in depth and length.

In pediatric patients it is possible and preferable to treat the injured or ruptured spleen nonoperatively. Considerable blood loss into the peritoneal cavity is replaced as needed with transfusion. In the pediatric patient, bleeding will stop, allowing sealing or healing of the injury, and reabsorption of the intra-abdominal blood without incident. The reason for this difference between children and adults is not fully understood, but it is thought to occur because children, in contrast to adults, have a lower systemic blood pressure; their arteries develop spasm more effectively and the intra-abdominal pressure increases more rapidly, thereby slowing bleeding.

KEY POINTS

- Primary splenic disorders first treated by medical therapy
- Treatment of secondary splenic disorders neither clear nor widely agreed on
- In adults (beyond age 12) splenectomy best treatment for injured spleen
- In pediatric patients it is possible and preferable to treat the injured or ruptured spleen nonoperatively

---

P FOLLOW-UP

Patients with splenic disorders are followed by hematologic studies postsplenectomy to monitor for correction of the defect. In addition, in the early postoperative period, they require close surveillance for signs of infection, which can develop and spread rapidly. Patients with secondary hypersplenism show only modest improvement in hematologic parameters but obtain considerable symptomatic relief. These patients need prolonged follow-up for the overt development of a malignant process (Case 2).

Postsplenectomy trauma patients are at risk of intra-abdominal abscess formation in the splenic bed or, rarely, pancreatitis or pancreatic fistula formation.

SUGGESTED READINGS

Coon WW: Splenectomy for splenomegaly and secondary hypersplenism. World J Surg 160:291, 1985

King DR, Lobe TE, Haase GM, Boles ET: Selective management of the injured spleen. Surgery 90:677, 1981

QUESTIONS

1. In instances of complex multiple trauma the best method of managing a possible splenic injury is?

    A. Obtain a CT scan at the earliest opportunity, and treat the patient based on the findings.

    B. Do a paracentesis. If blood is found operate on the patient for presumed ruptured spleen.

    C. Treat the other injuries (head, thorax, extremities) first and then, following transfusion, evaluate by a CT scan or operate.

    D. Resuscitate the patient initially. If the patient cannot be improved promptly an exploratory laparotomy should be done to find and control the bleeding. If the patient improves with resuscitation a CT scan may help determine if the spleen is injured.

2. Patients with primary splenic disorders should have?

    A. A trial of medical therapy. If that fails splenectomy is effective in treatment.

    B. Prompt splenectomy as medical therapy is not effective in their treatment.

    C. Vigorous treatment with steroids, as this is extremely effective in reversing these disorders.

    D. None of the above.

3. Patients with secondary splenic disorders (enlarged spleens)?

    A. May need splenectomy to alleviate symptoms.

    B. May have modest improvement in their hematologic parameters after splenectomy.

    C. Are subject to the development of malignant diseases such as myelogenous leukemia or Hodgkin's disease.

    D. All of the above.

(See p. 603 for answers.)

28

LOWER

GASTROINTESTINAL

HEMORRHAGE

MICHAEL J. STAMOS

Gastrointestinal hemorrhage encompasses a diverse spectrum of presentations and disease processes. Resuscitation and early establishment of the magnitude of the blood loss, as well as an accurate assessment of any ongoing blood loss, is critical to effective treatment and diagnosis. Accurate localization of the precise bleeding site and the etiology are frequently secondary concerns. Prompt triage, utilizing these criteria, will allow for appropriate utilization of resources and maximal patient benefit.

CASE 1
CECAL ANGIODYSPLASIA

A 73-year-old male presented to the emergency room with a 6-hour history of passing dark red blood and clots per rectum. His BP was 90/60 mmHg; pulse, 120 bpm; temperature, 36.7°C; and respiratory rate, 18 breaths/min. He denied any significant abdominal pain and his past medical history was significant only for hypertension controlled by diet alone. Resuscitation via two large bore (16 gauge) intravenous catheters with 2 L normal saline was started and the patient was administered supplemental oxygen via nasal cannula. On placement of the intravenous catheter, blood was obtained and sent for type and cross-match, coagulation profile, and CBC. A nasogastric tube that was placed shortly after arrival showed bile-stained gastric contents, and proctoscopy failed to reveal an anorectal source. The patient responded to initial hydration with heart rate decrease to 84 bpm and BP increasing to 140/80 mmHg. The patient again passed a moderate amount of dark red blood per rectum, but maintained his blood pressure. A tagged

RBC scan was obtained, with evidence of active bleeding in the cecum. He was then taken for SMA angiography. His initial Hct was 34% with MCV, 82. Selective SMA angiography failed to reveal any extravasation, but did show evidence of an angiodysplasia in the cecal region. On observation in the ICU, there was minimal further rectal bleeding and maintenance of his blood pressure and heart rate in the normal range. Two units of PRBC were required to maintain his Hct above 30%.

Colonoscopy after bowel preparation on hospital day 2 showed one large angiodysplastic lesion in the cecum. The patient subsequently underwent an elective right colectomy on the same admission and had an uneventful recovery.

CASE 2
DIVERTICULAR BLEEDING

A 57-year-old female presented to the emergency room with a complaint of passing a large amount of bright red blood and clots per rectum approximately 1 hour earlier.

She complained of crampy lower abdominal pain before passing the blood, but was currently asymptomatic. Her vital signs were BP, 110/80 mmHg; heart rate, 100 bpm; temperature, 37°C; and respiratory rate, 22 breaths/min. Her past medical history was significant for arthritis treated by Naprosyn and a hysterectomy 12 years earlier for fibroids.

While being initially evaluated and resuscitated, the patient again passed a large amount of bright red blood per rectum and her BP dropped to 80/50 mmHg and heart rate increased to 140 bpm. Resuscitation continued and a nasogastric tube aspirated only nonbloody gastric contents. Anoscopic examination was unremarkable and the patient was taken emergently for visceral angiography. SMA angiography was normal, while IMA injection showed extravasation from a sigmoid artery branch. The angiogram catheter was advanced selectively near to the site of extravasation and continuous infusion of vasopressin at 0.2 units/min was begun. Repeat angiographic contrast injection 15 minutes later confirmed cessation of bleeding, and the patient was transported to the ICU for continued vasopressin infusion and monitoring. The patient had minimal further bleeding and her vital signs and Hct remained stable over the next 24 hours; the infusion was then decreased to 0.1 units/min for 12 hours, then stopped. She continued to do well and on hospital day 4, colonoscopy was performed, revealing only scattered sigmoid diverticulosis. The patient was given dietary counseling and educated on the signs and symptoms of recurrent bleeding and discharged home.

GENERAL CONSIDERATIONS

Intestinal bleeding results when the mucosal barrier is broken down and the rich network of submucosal and intramural vessels are disrupted. The presentation of a patient suffering from intestinal bleeding varies greatly, depending on the site and nature of the bleeding and the inciting cause or etiology, as well as the severity and chronicity of the bleeding. Lower gastrointestinal bleeding encompasses all bleeding sites distal to the ligament of Treitz—a convenient and not entirely arbitrary distinction; anatomic distribution of the celiac trunk is responsible for upper gastrointestinal bleeding, and the superior mesenteric artery (SMA) and/or inferior mesenteric artery (IMA) for lower gastrointestinal hemorrhage.

Lower gastrointestinal bleeding, as defined, includes patients with blood loss of a variable degree emanating from between the ligament of Treitz and the anus. *Lower gastrointestinal hemorrhage* is descriptive of bleeding that threatens or causes hemodynamic compromise and/or requires transfusion of blood products (Cases 1 and 2). With notable exceptions, the problem primarily afflicts the elderly. Delay in appropriate diagnosis and/or therapy, coupled with frequent coexisting medical conditions, are responsible for the significant morbidity and mortality accompanying the diagnosis.

In the face of acute, life-threatening bleeding, an exact diagnosis is secondary to localizing the bleeding site and defining the severity and extent, if any, of continued bleeding. Crucial to the understanding and management of the problem is recognizing that at least 75% of acute bleeding episodes will cease spontaneously (Case 1). Recurrent bleeding may be encountered in up to 50% of cases, however, depending on the etiology and source of the bleeding.

KEY POINTS

• Resuscitation and early establishment of the magnitude of blood loss, as well as accurate assessment of ongoing blood loss, critical to effective treatment and diagnosis

• Delay in appropriate diagnosis and/or therapy, coupled with frequent coexisting medical conditions, responsible for the significant morbidity and mortality accompanying diagnosis

• In the face of acute, life-threatening bleeding, exact diagnosis secondary to localizing bleeding site and defining severity and extent of continued bleeding

• At least 75% of acute bleeding episodes will cease spontaneously

DIAGNOSIS

Although the diagnosis of lower gastrointestinal hemorrhage is usually obvious, there are several important initial diagnostic maneuvers crucial to appropriate patient care. A careful history documenting previous episodes and an attempt to quantify blood loss is initially indicated, although accurate assessment of the magnitude of bleeding can be difficult due to retrograde and prograde filling of the large and even small intestine. The nature of the bleeding (e.g., bright red, clots, melena) should be sought, preferably with the treating physician observing the blood that was passed. Hematemesis obviously is important in differentiating upper and lower gastrointestinal bleeding, as is a history of peptic ulcer disease, heavy alcohol ingestion, recent upper abdominal (epigastric) pain, and significant nonsteroidal anti-inflammatory drug (NSAID) intake. Intake of anticoagulants is obviously crucial information as well. Measurement of initial vital signs may show evidence of hypovolemia including tachycardia and/or hypotension. If these findings are absent, orthostatic changes should be evaluated (with close supervision) by sitting the patient up and looking for a decrease in blood pressure or increase in heart rate.

All patients presenting with major lower gastrointestinal hemorrhage should be considered to be possibly bleeding from a source proximal to the ligament of Treitz. Initially, a nasogastric tube should be utilized and should be considered incomplete (Case 2) unless a nonbloody bile-stained aspirate is obtained (Case 1) or upper gastrointestinal bleeding is confirmed. It is important to recognize that, even with a negative nasogastric aspirate, up to 10% of presumed lower gastrointestinal bleeding is actually arising from a proximal source. This confusion arises due to the intermittent nature of gastrointestinal bleeding and the sphincter effect of the pylorus. An approach to the diagnosis and management of patients with gastrointestinal bleeding is given in Table 20.1.

A hematocrit (Hct) and laboratory evaluation of coagulation should be done. Initial preresuscitation values are typically normal or even slightly elevated due to hemoconcentration, making early laboratory results deceptive. Serial values, however, are crucial to continued patient evaluation and therapeutic decisions.

A patient who shows any evidence of continued bleeding warrants prompt attention, with the specific goal of cessation of bleeding. Several diagnostic alternatives are available, including nuclear medicine bleeding scans (Case 1), mesenteric arteriograms (Case 2), endoscopy, and surgical exploration. Before consideration of these techniques, proctoscopy should be performed in the emergency room setting to rule out an anal canal source (hemorrhoids) and evaluate for evidence of distal colitis/proctitis.

Bleeding scans utilize a radioisotope injected intravenously (sulfur-colloid scan) or attached in vitro to red blood cells (RBCs) and reinjected (tagged RBC scans). The tagged RBC scan has the advantage of allowing delayed images ($\leq$24 hours), a significant advantage if the bleeding is episodic. Sulfur colloid scans are quicker and easier and potentially more sensitive. Bleeding scans are purported to be sensitive enough to detect blood loss as low as 0.1 ml/min, but great variability exists in their usefulness dependent on patient selection, timing of the study, and technical details.

Arteriography, with selective mesenteric arterial cannulation via a femoral artery (Cases 1 and 2), is an alternative in the diagnosis of suspected ongoing bleeding, or may be used following a positive bleeding scan. Angiography has the advantage of improved specificity of the bleeding site, and potential therapeutic benefit (see under Treatment). Disadvantages of angiography include nephrotoxicity of the intravenous contrast, as well as arterial injury, thrombosis, or embolism from the catheter.

Endoscopy plays a very important role in the management of the patient with gastrointestinal hemorrhage. Anoscopy or proctoscopy should be performed in every patient with a suspected lower gastrointestinal source. Additionally, upper endoscopy (esophagogastroduodenoscopy [EGD]) should be performed emergently on patients when the nasogastric output is bloody or nonrevealing or when suspicion of an upper gastrointestinal source remains. The colonoscope has potential benefit in localizing bleeding sites and in therapy, but its utility in the patient with lower gastrointestinal hemorrhage is severely limited. The subtlety of the source when viewed endoscopically, the temporary tamponade effect of the necessary insufflation and, most importantly, the great difficulty in visualization due to the intraluminal blood (obscuring the view and absorbing the light) conspire to diminish the potential of this technology. Colonoscopy is indicated and is the test of choice for the patient who ceases bleeding or who is bleeding slowly enough to allow bowel preparation (Cases 1 and 2). Surgical exploration for diagnosis has no role in the acutely bleeding patient and a limited role in therapeutic management (see under Treatment). Retrograde and prograde passage of blood make localization of the actual bleeding site difficult.

KEY POINTS

- All patients presenting with major lower gastrointestinal hemorrhage should be considered to be possibly bleeding from a source proximal to ligament of Treitz
- Colonoscopy indicated and test of choice for the patient who ceases bleeding or who is bleeding slowly enough to allow bowel preparation

DIFFERENTIAL DIAGNOSIS

The vast majority of major lower gastrointestinal bleeding episodes are due to diverticular disease or arteriovenous malformations (AVMs). Inflammatory bowel disease and Meckel's diverticula as sources of bleeding are significantly less common but should be considered in younger patients. AVMs, also referred to as angiodysplasia, are largely acquired lesions, typically found in the right colon of elderly patients (Case 1). These tortuous, thin-walled submucosal vessels may be more common in patients with aortic stenosis. Bleeding from AVMs typically will stop spontaneously, but recurrent bleeding is characteristic. Although endoscopic therapy with laser or heater probe treatment has been reported, elective surgical intervention (Case 1) should be considered in acceptable risk patients with a documented episode of hemorrhage from an AVM (i.e., angiographic extravasation).

Diverticula of the colon are also acquired lesions, with the exception of congenital diverticula of the cecum. These acquired diverticula originate at the site of penetration of the vasa recta through the seromuscular layer of the colon, and the anatomically weak areas allow outpouching of the mucosal and submucosal layers. The thinned out vasa recta (arteriole) overlying the diverticulum may rupture into the bowel lumen. Bleeding tends to be major due to the arterial source and may be accompanied by abdominal cramping (Case 2) due to rapid colonic filling and distention as well as the cathartic effect of the blood. Although most diverticular bleeding episodes can be expected to cease spontaneously, a significant minority (20–25%) may continue to bleed without intervention. Rebleeding from a diverticular source is relatively uncommon (<25%) and therefore surgical therapy is usually not indicated in patients who stop bleeding. Exceptions include patients with two or more episodes, in whom rebleeding can be expected in more than 50% of cases.

Colon cancer and/or polyps rarely present with gastrointestinal hemorrhage, although distal lesions commonly produce visible blood on or in the stool. Inflammatory bowel disease (Crohn's, ulcerative colitis), as well as other types of colitis (ischemic, infectious) may present with bloody diarrhea or even life threatening hemorrhage. Rigid sigmoidoscopy (proctoscopy) will reveal many of these by visualizing the abnormal mucosa, while also identifying the occasional hemorrhoidal source masquerading as a significant lower gastrointestinal bleed.

Meckel's diverticula, like all small bowel bleeding sites, are difficult to diagnose by a standard evaluation. Consideration of the diagnosis is crucial, as a Meckel's scan (nuclear scintigraphy ^{99}TC-pertechnate) will visually "light up" the ectopic gastric mucosa responsible for the adjacent ulceration and hemorrhage. Almost all bleeding from Meckel's diverticulum occurs in children and adolescents.

Other small bowel sources are fortunately uncommon and include angiodysplasia, varices, and tumors. Diagnosis of these lesions is usually delayed due to the relative inaccessibility of the small intestine. Potentially useful tests include small bowel contrast studies, arteriography, and enteroscopy.

TREATMENT

Following an assessment of the patient, intravenous resuscitation is mandatory for any patient with lower gastrointestinal hemorrhage. Early transfusion of blood and administration of supplemental oxygen should be considered to prevent cerebral and cardiac ischemia or hypoxia.

Following institution of these supportive measures, consideration should be given to halting the presumed ongoing blood loss. Although 75% or more of patients will cease bleeding spontaneously, there are no good initial indicators of continued hemorrhage. Therefore, an initial aggressive approach is warranted in all patients. Three disparate therapeutic approaches are available, and the selection of a particular therapy is made after consideration of patient factors and available expertise. Arteriography, as previously outlined, allows accurate localization of active bleeding. Administration of vasopressin may be conducted via the catheter (Case 2). Hepatic clearance via the portal system limits but does not eliminate the toxicity of the drug, which may include cardiac ischemia. Endoscopic therapy with laser, injection, or heater probe treatment has great attraction due to its relative safety. Unfortunately, difficulty in direct endoscopic localization of active bleeding and relatively high rebleeding rates have limited the application of these techniques. Surgical treatment entails resection of the segment of bowel from where the bleeding is emanating.

Accurate localization of an active bleeding site is mandatory before segmental bowel resection. "Blind" segmental colectomy performed for a presumed site based on clinical judgment is associated with an unacceptable postoperative rebleeding rate of 50%. A patient who shows evidence of ongoing bleeding and for whom localization studies are nondiagnostic or unavailable, or a patient who is hemodynamically unstable should be taken to the operating room for a planned total abdominal colectomy. At the time of exploration, a small intestinal source should be looked for and an upper endoscopy performed if not done earlier. Additionally, a careful proctoscopic examination should be repeated before resection of the entire colon. An ileorectal anastomosis can usually be performed and will lead to acceptable function in the majority of patients. Rebleeding rates of up to 10% can be expected in this situation.

FOLLOW-UP

Follow-up of the patient who ceases bleeding should include colonoscopy if not performed while hospitalized. The patient should be educated to present at the earliest sign of rebleeding, as diagnostic accuracy is very closely associated with the acuity of the bleed. Rebleeding rates of 20–100% can be anticipated depending on the actual etiology.

SUGGESTED READINGS

Baum S, Rosch J, Dotter CT et al: Selective mesenteric arterial infusions in the management of massive diverticular hemorrhage. N Engl J Med 288:1269, 1973

Landmark article detailing the use of selective vasopressors for therapy.

Richardson JD: Vascular lesions of the intestines. Am J Surg 161:284, 1991

A thorough description of the range of vascular lesions that contribute to gastrointestinal bleeding.

Ure T, Vernava AM, Longo WE: Diverticular bleeding. Seminars in Colon and Rectal Surgery 5:32, 1994

An overview on the pathogenesis, characteristics, and treatment of the most common source of lower gastrointestinal bleeding.

QUESTIONS

1. Initial approach to the patient with lower gastrointestinal bleeding and associated hypotension includes all of the following except?

A. Oxygen administration and fluid resuscitation.
B. Nasogastric aspirate and/or EGD.
C. Colonoscopy.
D. Bleeding scan and/or angiogram.

2. *Advantage of arteriography over bleeding scans include (choose all correct answers)?*

A. Increased specificity.
B. Therapeutic potential.
C. Increased sensitivity.
D. Increased safety profile.

3. *Bleeding from a colonic AVM?*

A. Is safely and reliably treated endoscopically.
B. Is characteristically episodic.
C. Is associated with atherosclerosis.
D. Is most frequently seen in the pediatric age group.

(See p. 603 for answers.)

29

LARGE BOWEL

OBSTRUCTION

AND VOLVULUS

MICHAEL J. STAMOS

Worldwide, large bowel obstruction (LBO) is a common problem, primarily due to the high incidence of colonic volvulus in developing countries. In the United States, LBO is a relatively uncommon admitting diagnosis, and is more frequently due to a malignancy (see Ch. 33).

CASE 1
SIGMOID VOLVULUS

An 85-year-old male was brought to the emergency room from his nursing home because of abdominal distention and discomfort. The patient had mild chronic dementia, but was awake and alert and able to answer most questions. He denied a similar problem in the past but did complain of chronic constipation. He reported no flatus or bowel movements for over 48 hours. He denied a history of blood per rectum. His family history was unknown. Physical examination was significant for a markedly distended abdomen and hyperactive bowel sounds with diffuse tympany. Moderate right lower quadrant abdominal tenderness existed. Rectal examination revealed an empty, collapsed rectal vault. After initial resuscitation, abdominal x-rays were obtained, demonstrating a massively distended large intestine with a cecal diameter of 14 cm and an apparent sigmoid volvulus. Small bowel distention was minimal.

Rigid sigmoidoscopy was performed with successful detorsion of the volvulus and decompression of the colon. A large red rubber catheter was passed above the site of torsion and secured in place. Three days later, after bowel

preparation, the patient underwent an uneventful sigmoid colectomy.

CASE 2
CARCINOMA

A 56-year-old white female was brought to the emergency room because of abdominal pain and progressive distention. The pain was colicky in nature and most severe in the lower abdomen. On questioning, she admitted to occasional dark red blood accompanying bowel movements for the past 3 months, as well as increased frequency of bowel movements. Family history was nonrevealing. On physical examination, moderate abdominal distention with tympany was noted, with high-pitched, hyperactive bowel sounds. No significant tenderness was appreciated, and no abdominal masses. On rectal examination, a firm, mobile intraluminal mass was felt at the tip of the examining finger. A proctoscopy performed to assess the mass better revealed a circumferential, exophytic tumor with no obvious lumen. The distal extent of the tumor was at 8 cm from the anal verge. On abdominal films a dilated colon with a cecal diameter of 12 cm and relative paucity of small intestinal gas was seen.

After fluid resuscitation, the patient was taken to the operating room and underwent a low anterior resection of the rectosigmoid colon encompassing the tumor. The proximal colon was lavaged clean and a primary anastomosis performed.

GENERAL CONSIDERATIONS

LBO accounts for only 10–20% of all cases of intestinal obstruction in the United States, but can present difficult diagnostic and management dilemmas due to the diversity of causes and the anatomic configuration of the colon and rectum. Carcinoma accounts for a clear majority of cases (Case 2), although diverticular disease (see Ch. 31) and colonic volvulus (Case 1) are also common causes of LBO. Other, less common etiologies include Crohn's colitis with stricturing, foreign bodies, hernias, anastomotic strictures, and fecal impaction. Carcinoma may obstruct any part of the colon or rectum, although most series show a preponderance of cases to involve the left colon, due to the smaller luminal diameter and more solid stool consistency. Similarly, colonic volvulus can involve virtually any segment of the colon, providing that a mobile mesentery is present. Since normal anatomy provides this prerequisite only in the sigmoid colon and in a minority of people with a congenital nonfixed right colon, sigmoid volvulus (60–70%) and cecal volvulus (30–35%) predominate.

Colonic volvulus is associated with chronic constipation and a sedentary lifestyle and, not surprisingly, many cases are encountered in nursing homes (Case 1).

Irrespective of the etiology of an LBO, important diagnostic and therapeutic decisions are predicated on the competency of the ileocecal valve. The small intestine will serve to "vent" a large bowel obstruction in the presence of an incompetent valve (Fig. 29.1). These patients, not surprisingly, will present and behave in a fashion indistinguishable from a distal small bowel obstruction (see Ch. 21).

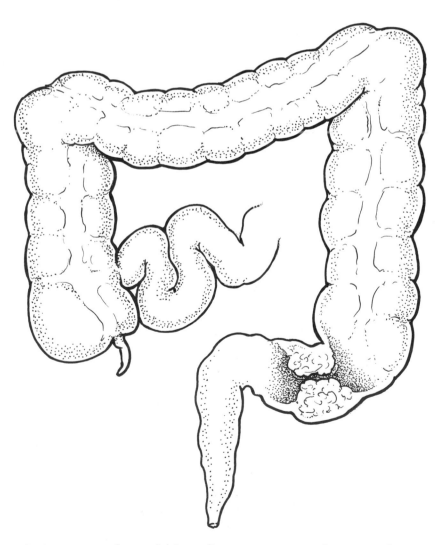

FIGURE 29.1   *An incompetent ileocecal valve will protect against perforation in the presence of a distal large bowel obstruction.*

A competent ileocecal valve, in the face of a complete distal obstruction, can quickly lead to vascular compromise and/or perforation (Fig. 29.2). A closed loop obstruction also exists with colonic volvulus.

> ### KEY POINTS
> • Irrespective of the etiology of LBO, important diagnostic and therapeutic decisions are predicated on competency of ileocecal valve

DIAGNOSIS

With the possible exception of acute volvulus, LBO presents in an insidious fashion. The most common presenting symptoms include abdominal distention, abdominal pain, and obstipation/constipation. Vomiting is an unusual and late symptom, although nausea and anorexia are common, nonspecific findings. Obstruction and constipation are typical, although partial LBO may allow continued flatus and even occasionally postobstructive diarrhea from mucous production and bacterial overgrowth.

Physical examination will reveal abdominal distention and tympany (Cases 1 and 2). Hyperactive bowel sounds are present unless bowel ischemia has developed. Tenderness on abdominal examination should be minimal in the absence of ischemia or impending perforation. Right lower quadrant tenderness and tympany should raise concern over cecal compromise in the face of a competent ileocecal valve, as this area of the large intestine is the most vulnerable due to its large diameter (Laplace's law). Rectal examination will reveal an empty rectal vault (Case 1) except for very distal tumors (Case 2). Plain radiographs of the abdomen are usually suggestive, and often diagnostic of LBO. An incompetent ileocecal valve will lead to extensive small bowel distention, which may be difficult to distinguish from large bowel loops. Colonic air fluid levels may be present, particularly on the right side. Minimal to no gas in the colon/rectum distal to the site of

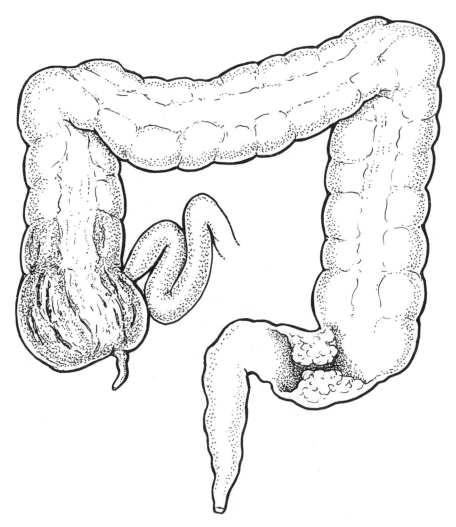

FIGURE 29.2 *A competent ileocecal valve, in the presence of a distal large bowel obstruction, produces a functional closed loop obstruction with a high risk of vascular compromise and perforation.*

obstruction is expected. Sigmoid volvulus appears as a large, single loop of intestine originating in the left lower quadrant and directed toward the right upper quadrant ("bent inner tube") (Fig. 29.3), while cecal volvulus reveals the cecum displaced from the right lower quadrant and a "kidney bean" appearance of the rotated segment in the upper abdomen.

Gastrointestinal contrast studies may be useful in confirming the diagnosis of an LBO, as well as localizing the site and suggesting the etiology. The latter issue is of minimal practical value in most cases. Although upper gastrointestinal contrast studies will occasionally demonstrate a proximal colonic obstruction, when LBO is suspected, a contrast enema is preferred. Water soluble contrast (Hypaque, Gastrografin) agents should be used in preference to barium, as the latter confers a prohibitive

morbidity and mortality in the event of perforation. The additional detail barium provides in defining the obstructive source is of little or no importance in the acutely obstructed patient.

Endoscopy has a limited role in the diagnosis of the patient with presumed/confirmed complete LBO. Flexible endoscopy is relatively contraindicated due to the risk that the insufflation required will worsen the obstruction or precipitate a perforation. Proctoscopy (rigid sigmoidoscopy) is initially preferred as it can be accomplished without insufflation and is useful in excluding a rectal obstruction, evaluating a rectosigmoid or rectal obstructing tumor, and confirming a sigmoid volvulus (see under Treatment). Occasionally the diagnosis is made intraoperatively, particularly in the presence of associated ischemia and/or perforation.

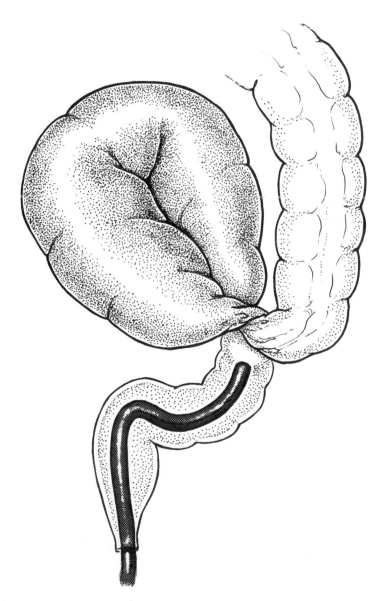

FIGURE 29.3   *The diagnosis of sigmoid volvulus may be confirmed by (rigid) proctosigmoidoscopy or flexible sigmoidoscopy.*

A DIFFERENTIAL DIAGNOSIS

Abdominal distention and abdominal radiographs demonstrating dilated loops of intestine are necessary for consideration of a bowel obstruction. These same findings are also seen in patients with colonic pseudo-obstruction (Ogilvie syndrome). Ogilvie syndrome, or colonic ileus, has a myriad of inciting factors and is felt to be due to a parasympathetic nerve dysfunction. It remains a diagnosis of exclusion and treatment should be directed at the identifiable cause (e.g., hypokalemia), with colonoscopic decompression or even cecostomy occasionally necessary.

A more specific form of colonic (and small intestinal) ileus may be seen with pancreatitis, due to the local effect of the proteolytic enzymes ("colon cutoff sign"). Serum amylase/lipase levels and selective abdominal imaging studies (computed tomography, contrast enema) along with a high index of suspicion may be helpful.

Perhaps the most difficult entity to distinguish from an LBO is a distal small bowel obstruction. In the setting of a complete obstruction, there is little to be gained by differentiation as both mandate early surgical intervention. With a partial obstruction, differentiating a distal small bowel source from a colonic source is often important, as a partial small bowel obstruction due to adhesions often responds to conservative treatment (Ch. 21), while a near obstructing colonic neoplasm requires surgery. Contrast enemas and or upper gastrointestinal contrast studies may be judiciously applied in this setting.

L TREATMENT

LBO invariably leads to significant intestinal edema and intraluminal fluid sequestration (third spacing). Intestinal ischemia, when superimposed, dramatically increases this fluid sequestration and may even lead to systemic fluid shifts when translocation and/or bacteremia result. It follows that volume resuscitation and electrolyte correction/replacement as necessary is an integral component of treatment. Nonoperative therapy (at least initially) is possible in only a minority of patients with complete or high grade LBO. These situations include sigmoid volvulus (Case 1) and distal rectal or rectosigmoid tumors. Proctoscopic (or occasionally flexible sigmoidoscopic) detorsion of sigmoid volvulus (Fig. 29.4) is successful in 80–90% of cases and allows an emergency situation to be converted into an elective condition. Most patients with sigmoid volvulus should undergo resective therapy following successful nonoperative detorsion of a single episode due to the high recurrence rate (75%). Exceptions would obviously include patients at prohibitive risk of complications from surgery. Initial nonoperative management of obstructing distal tumors is considerably more controversial, and should only be attempted by an experienced clinician. Options include passage of a well-lubricated tube through the visible lumen, or laser ab-

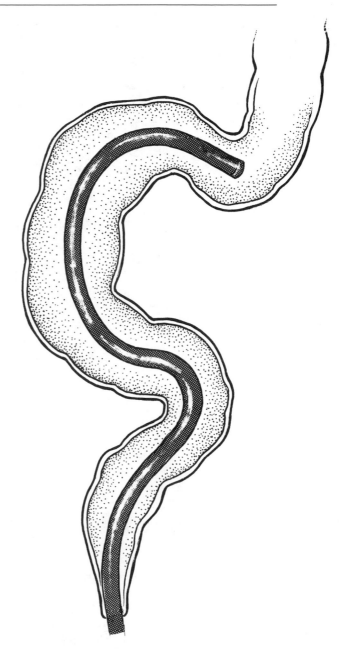

FIGURE 29.4 *Detorsion of a sigmoid volvulus with sigmoidoscopy is highly successful.*

lation (recanalization) (Fig. 29.5). The major advantage of these approaches are to allow conversion to an elective procedure and the attendant reduction in morbidity/mortality and avoidance of stoma formation.

Urgent operative intervention will be required in most patients with LBO (Case 2). Resection of the involved segment is usually indicated and the technical aspects should be dictated by the presumed etiologic factor (see Ch. 33). Resection of the entire colon proximal to the site of obstruction may be mandated by the operative findings (proximal ischemia, location of the obstruction) or may be an appropriate choice as an ileocolonic anastomosis is a safe and acceptable option. When extensive intestinal ischemia

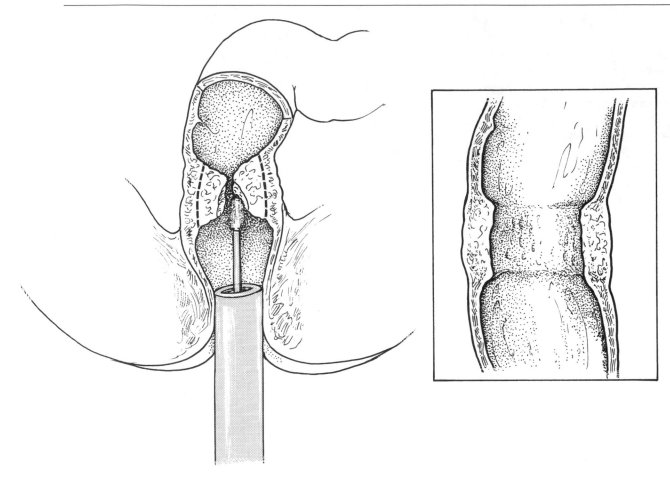

FIGURE 29.5 *Laser recanalization may be useful in carefully selected cases.*

and/or perforation is encountered, a colostomy or ileostomy is usually indicated as operative morbidity and mortality are considerable.

Distal colonic or rectal obstructions present the greatest management dilemmas. Resection, if straightforward, should be the primary treatment of choice. If the obstruction is due to a known or suspected neoplasm, however, consideration of a proximal diversion (i.e., loop colostomy) should be entertained if the tumor is adherent or fixed. Definitive treatment may then be conducted on an elective basis, with full bowel and patient preparation.

If resection is performed, a decision regarding restoration of intestinal continuity should be made. Appropriate options include the following:

1. Exteriorization of the proximal and distal segments of colon (end colostomy and mucous fistula)

2. Proximal end colostomy and oversewing of the distal rectal segment (Hartmann's procedure)

3. Primary anastomosis of the small intestine to the distal segment (as described above)

4. Intraoperative bowel preparation (on-table lavage) with primary colonic anastomosis or colorectal anastomosis (Case 2)

The last option should only be considered in a stable, relatively fit patient, and with an experienced surgeon. Benefits are obvious, including avoidance of a stoma and a second operative procedure.

If a volvulus is encountered intraoperatively, management is dictated by the condition of the involved intestine. If obvious irreversible ischemia is present, resection without detorsion is indicated. If the bowel is viable, detorsion is carefully performed and further options include resection and primary anastomosis (a good choice for cecal volvulus), resection with colostomy, and fixation of the bowel to the peritoneal surface (e.g., ceco"pexy").

KEY POINTS

• LBO invariably leads to significant intestinal edema and intraluminal fluid sequestration (third spacing)

• Proctoscopic or occasionally flexible sigmoidoscopic detorsion of sigmoid volvulus (Fig. 29.4) successful in 80–90% of cases and allows an emergency situation to be converted into an elective condition

• Distal colonic or rectal obstructions present the greatest management dilemmas

FOLLOW-UP

Further management of the patient with LBO will vary widely and is dictated by the underlying etiology. A patient with apparently localized large intestinal cancer should be followed as outlined in Chapter 33. Additionally, any preserved colon proximal to the obstructive site should be endoscoped in the early (1 6 weeks) postoperative period to eliminate a missed synchronous neoplasm (5–10%). Patients with volvulus treated by resection need no specific therapy or follow-up. Treatment of the underlying chronic constipation may improve their quality of life and prevent further problems.

SUGGESTED READINGS

Ballantyne GH, Brandner MD, Beart RW, Ilstrup DM: Volvulus of the colon. Ann Surg 202:83, 1985

A thorough review article based on a 20-year experience in the United States.

McGregor JR, O'Dwyer PJ: The surgical management of obstruction and perforation of the left colon. Surg Gynecol Obstet 177:203, 1993

An overview that covers collected experience with various options of management.

Stephenson BM, Shandall AA, Farouk R, Griffith G: Malignant left-sided large bowel obstruction managed by subtotal/total colectomy. Br J Surg 77:1098, 1990

Advocates one-stage operation and reports good functional results.

QUESTIONS

1. LBO is a common cause of intestinal obstruction worldwide and is most often due to?

    A. Cancer.

    B. Hernias.

    C. Adhesions.

    D. Volvulus.

    E. Foreign bodies.

2. Initial management of an obstructing rectal cancer may include?

    A. Passage of a catheter/stent through the area.

    B. Laser recanalization.

    C. Proximal colostomy.

    D. Resection, with proximal colostomy.

    E. All of the above.

(See p. 603 for answers.)

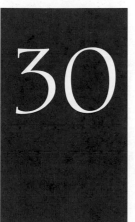

30 INFLAMMATORY BOWEL DISEASE

MICHAEL J. STAMOS

CHARLES N. HEADRICK

The term *inflammatory bowel disease* is nonspecific but is used in reference to two specific diseases: Crohn's disease and ulcerative colitis. The diagnosis of these entities is also often nonspecific and therefore it is important to evaluate for other more specific inflammatory diseases of the intestine, particularly infectious causes.

CASE 1
ULCERATIVE COLITIS

A 28-year-old male was referred to a gastroenterologist due to debilitating diarrhea for 2 months. Complete stool evaluation was nonrevealing and a flexible sigmoidoscopy showed moderately severe inflammation of the distal 60 cm of colon and rectum. The clinical, endoscopic, and histologic pattern were thought to be most consistent with ulcerative colitis and the patient was given steroids (prednisone) and Azulfidine. He noticed transient improvement but then suffered a relapse, requiring hospitalization for a brief period.

He responded to cyclosporine, and a surgical consultation was obtained. One week later he underwent proctocolectomy with sphincter preservation and an ileoanal pouch reconstruction. He was weaned off his steroids and other medication, and 3 months postoperatively was having six small bowel movements each day.

CASE 2
CROHN'S DISEASE

A 36-year-old female presented to the emergency room complaining of crampy abdominal pain and diarrhea. The pain was in the right lower quadrant and was similar but more severe than previous episodes. She had been diagnosed with Crohn's disease of the ileum 8 years earlier. Her current medications included prednisone and Azulfidine. She was noted to be febrile (T, 38.6°C), with a heart rate of 128 bpm. A tender mass in the right lower quadrant of the abdomen was noted. No peritoneal signs were present. CT scan of the abdomen showed a phlegmon in the region of the terminal ileum. Initial treatment was with broad spectrum intravenous antibiotics. Transient improvement in the clinical course was followed by worsening pain/tenderness and fever. The patient was operated on with findings of phlegmonous terminal ileal disease with fistula to the sigmoid colon. Resection of the

215

terminal ileum and local repair of the sigmoid colon was performed. Recovery was uncomplicated, steroids were stopped, and Pentasa prescribed.

GENERAL CONSIDERATIONS

Crohn's disease and ulcerative colitis are grouped together under the term *inflammatory bowel disease* (IBD) for a number of very important reasons. These reasons include their common predilection for a similar population, a lack of complete understanding regarding etiology and pathogenesis, a similar medical treatment regimen, an overlapping pattern of clinical presentation, and the common endoscopic and histologic appearances. These commonalities make up to 10% of all cases of IBD affecting the colon (colitis) impossible to differentiate, a situation termed *indeterminate colitis*. Despite these commonalities, significant differences exist between the two entities. These important differences include the pattern of intestinal involvement, recurrence rates following treatment, specific complications, and perhaps most important for the purpose of this textbook, surgical approaches. Crohn's disease is a transmural process, and the complications encountered (perforation/fistula, stricture) reflect that full thickness involvement (Case 2). Although Crohn's disease may involve any portion of the intestine, three patterns predominate: small intestine (usually ileum) only, colon/rectum only, and ileocolic disease. A small number of patients (<10%) will manifest anorectal disease as their first or only site. Ulcerative colitis is limited to the mucosa and submucosa and only involves the colon and rectum.

KEY POINTS

- Crohn's disease and ulcerative colitis are grouped together under the term IBD
- Crohn's disease is a transmural process, and complications encountered (perforation/fistula, stricture) reflect full thickness involvement
- Ulcerative colitis is limited to mucosa and submucosa and only involves colon and rectum

---

DIAGNOSIS

The diagnosis of IBD may be made at the time of acute presentation of a patient, or more commonly, in a patient who has had chronic symptoms. The acute presentation of a patient with IBD can vary from minor abdominal pain or minimal rectal bleeding to fulminant toxic colitis. Toxic colitis, most commonly seen with ulcerative colitis, is also known as toxic megacolon. Most commonly, the colon is indeed dilated and the patient is usually moderately to severely ill with systemic evidence of sepsis. Other complaints may include abdominal distention, abdominal pain, and diarrhea. Fortunately, this presentation is unusual, since most patients will have symptoms to suggest ulcerative colitis before this extreme presentation. A small subset of patients with Crohn's disease will also present acutely ill with signs and symptoms consistent with acute appendicitis. They may even progress to the operating room where the findings of acute terminal ileitis are discovered. Most patients with IBD, however, will present following weeks to months of symptoms. These symptoms will vary depending on the disease process and location.

More typically, ulcerative colitis presents with diarrhea (often with blood) and crampy abdominal pain that is partially relieved by bowel movements. Increased flatulence may also be noted and not infrequently the diarrhea may be grossly bloody.

Crohn's disease may present similarly, but commonly presents with abdominal pain as the predominant symptom (Case 2). Diarrhea is typically less than that seen with ulcerative colitis, and gross blood is relatively uncommon. Crohn's disease may also present with perianal complaints, including abscesses and fistulas. A family history of IBD should be sought, as up to 30% of patients with IBD may report such a history. Interestingly, there occasionally is crossover in patients with Crohn's disease having a family history of ulcerative colitis and vice versa.

Inspection of the perianal area may reveal unusual skin tags, fissures, and fistulas. If seen, these strongly suggest a diagnosis of Crohn's disease. These findings are distinctly unusual in ulcerative colitis and should raise serious doubts regarding that diagnosis. Evidence of weight loss may be apparent, and abdominal examination may reveal a phlegmon or indistinct mass in patients with Crohn's disease. Oral or aphthous ulcers are nonspecific, but can be seen in up to 20% of patients with IBD. Additionally, skin lesions are also nonspecific but may include pyoderma gangrenosum (a peculiar undermining skin ulceration) and erythema nodosum (tender subcutaneous nodules). Other extraintestinal manifestations include ocular diseases, arthritis, both central (ankylosing spondylitis and sacroiliitis) and peripheral joint synovitis, and liver disease (sclerosing cholangitis).

Crucial to the diagnosis of IBD is a negative stool evaluation for pathogens and endoscopic evaluation of the intestine. Stool studies should include ova and parasite examination as well as standard culture. Additionally, if any antibiotics have been taken by the patient within the last 6 months, *Clostridium difficile* toxin should be assessed to rule out pseudomembranous colitis. Flexible sigmoidoscopy may be the initial test performed. In the presence of ulcerative colitis, this test should reveal inflammatory changes beginning in the distal rectum and running without interruption proximally (Case 1). The extent of the inflammation may vary from a short segment (5–10 cm) to the entire colon. The finding of normal areas of mucosa between areas of inflammation should prompt a biopsy of the normal and abnormal areas. The finding of normal mucosa on histology eliminates ulcerative colitis as a diagnosis. If flexible sigmoidoscopy fails to reveal the extent of the disease, or if Crohn's disease is suspected and the flexible sigmoidoscopy is normal, colonoscopy may be indicated with an attempt at cannulation of the terminal ileum through the ileocecal valve for evaluation of this area, which is commonly involved with Crohn's disease. Alternatively, barium enema evaluation and/or small bowel follow-through studies may be helpful.

Typical endoscopic findings include loss of the normal vascular pattern, friability or easy bleeding, granularity of the mucosa, and ulcerations. Edema and erythema are universally seen. Pseudopolyp formation and mucosal bridging are usually seen in patients with more chronic manifestations. In addition to the skip areas typical of Crohn's disease, long linear or serpiginous ulcers are relatively characteristic and biopsies should always be obtained. If noncaseating granulomas are seen, the diagnosis of Crohn's disease is supported. Severe strictures, which may be seen on endoscopy or on barium studies, are more typical of Crohn's disease and are not seen in ulcerative colitis in the absence of a superimposed malignancy. Fistulas, most commonly between the terminal ileum and sigmoid colon (Case 2), may be seen on contrast studies and are also characteristic of Crohn's disease. If colonoscopy is performed, the terminal ileum should, as mentioned, be cannulated. Involvement of this area is highly characteristic of Crohn's disease. If the entire colon is involved with ulcerative colitis, a "backwash" ileitis may be seen, but this is a short segment of involvement and may be delineated from true IBD by biopsy. Small bowel radiographs may show loss of the normal mucosal pattern and a "string sign"—characteristically in the distal ileum—as a result of edema, bowel wall thickening, and/or fibrosis.

Blood tests are unfortunately nonspecific in the diagnosis of IBD although much attention has been paid to numerous potential serum markers, particularly for the value of differentiating Crohn's disease from ulcerative colitis. To date, none have proven sensitive or specific.

Pathologically, the disease can be easy to differentiate when a bowel resection has been performed, due to the transmural involvement characteristically seen in Crohn's disease, while ulcerative colitis is limited to the mucosa and submucosa. Unfortunately, we are often forced to make the diagnosis via mucosal biopsies, which are only obtained endoscopically. These, of course, do not allow evaluation of the deeper layers of the bowel wall and therefore a more difficult differentiation exists. The findings of noncaseating granulomas strongly suggest Crohn's disease as does narrow, deep ulcerations. Ulcerative colitis typically shows crypt abscesses and destruction of the normal goblet cell architecture, but these findings are nonspecific.

Ultimately, the diagnosis is often made on the basis of a combination of physical findings, clinical history, endoscopic and/or radiologic evaluation, and histologic appearance of biopsies (Case 1). Additionally, the behavior of the disease over time may allow differentiation. It is important that a premature, inaccurate diagnosis not be given to a patient solely to satisfy the physician's desire to label the disease and patient. Not infrequently, patients are classified as having indeterminate colitis.

KEY POINTS

- Acute presentation of a patient with IBD can vary from minor abdominal pain or minimal rectal bleeding to fulminant toxic colitis

- Most patients with IBD present following weeks to months of symptoms

- More commonly, ulcerative colitis presents with diarrhea (often with blood) and crampy abdominal pain that is partially relieved by bowel movements

- Crucial to diagnosis of IBD is negative stool evaluation for pathogens and endoscopic evaluation of intestine

- Severe strictures, which may be seen on endoscopy or barium studies, are more typical of Crohn's disease and are not seen in ulcerative colitis in the absence of a superimposed malignancy

- Diagnosis often made on the basis of a combination of physical findings, clinical history, endoscopic and/or radiologic evaluation, and histologic appearance of biopsies

DIFFERENTIAL DIAGNOSIS

The differential diagnosis of IBD is protean. Some of the more common entities to consider include infectious colitis (amebiasis, yersinia, giardia, *Clostridium difficile* colitis, salmonella or shigella infection, *Campylobacter* enteritis), irritable bowel syndrome and nonspecific or idiopathic colitis (microscopic colitis). Other diseases to consider in specific populations include unusual infectious organisms seen in immunosuppressed patients; radiation colitis or proctocolitis in patients who have had previous radiotherapy; and diversion colitis seen in patients who have proximal colostomies or ileostomies.

TREATMENT

The treatment of IBD is almost always medical treatment initially (Cases 1 and 2). It is important to recognize that many patients will eventually require operation. In the case of ulcerative colitis, this treatment is usually curative, although function and quality of life may be somewhat diminished. In Crohn's disease, the treatment is largely palliative, although some patients may be effectively "cured" by operation. It is also important to recognize that many of the medications used in the treatment of these diseases have significant and even life-threatening side effects and/or complications. Continued treatment of the patient with medication, despite the onset or predictable risk of complications, may have a greater morbidity and even mortality than a well-planned operation.

Initial medical therapy typically consists of anti-inflammatory medications. These medications may be delivered in a variety of ways, including orally, by suppository, or in enema form. For patients who are severely ill, intravenous therapy may even be necessary. The most common anti-inflammatory medications are steroids and 5-aminosalicylic acids (5-ASA). These 5-ASA derivatives (Azulfidine, Pentasa, Asacol, Rowasa) are particularly effective in allowing withdrawal of high dose steroids. High dose steroids, in addition to causing significant immunosuppression, can also lead to cataract formation, osteopenia, and even osteonecrosis. Antimicrobials have received a lot of attention in the treatment of IBD, and metronidazole can be extremely helpful in the management of patients with Crohn's disease, particularly in the presence of perianal complaints. Long-term use, however, has frequent, intolerable side effects, including nausea, metallic taste, glossitis, and peripheral neuropathy. Immunosuppressive drugs, including azathioprine and 6-mercaptopurine (6-MP) are frequently used medications for patients with Crohn's disease. They allow steroid tapering; 6-MP in particular may be helpful for patients with fistulas. More recently, cyclosporine (CsA), a drug best known for its use in transplantation, has been found to be of value in patients with fulminant or toxic colitis (Case 1). This short-term use seems to be well tolerated and efficacious. Use of cyclosporine in less ill patients is currently undergoing evaluation.

Operative intervention for IBD may be indicated for an acute, life threatening complication (toxic colitis, free perforation, hemorrhage); a nonemergent complication (fistula/abscess, cancer); or failure of medical therapy. The goals of an operation will vary depending on the indication. An acute abdominal catastrophe mandates both conservative resection of the grossly diseased intestine and diversion (stoma formation). Operation performed for a "chronic" complication will similarly require resection of the intestine but functional integrity of the intestine may often be restored (Cases 1 and 2). *Failure of medical therapy* is misleading terminology that has inappropriately led many patients and physicians to search for different pharmacologic solutions. A better term is *recalcitrant* or *unresponsive disease*. Operative intervention in this setting should offer the patient an improved quality of life and avoidance of or diminished requirement for potentially toxic drugs.

Operation for ulcerative colitis is relatively straightforward. Since the disease is limited to the colon and rectum, a total proctocolectomy is curative of the colitis, although any existing liver disease and/or central arthritis may persist. Most patients may be reconstructed by creation of a "neorectum" and preservation of the anal sphincters

(ileoanal pouch) (Case 1). Functional results are good in experienced centers, with patients averaging 5–7 bowel movements per day.

Operation for Crohn's disease is not truly curative since recurrence is common and any part of the intestinal tract may be involved. Operation may provide protracted relief in many patients, however, and will effectively "cure" a significant number. The guiding principle of surgery for Crohn's disease is bowel preservation, with conservative resection of the grossly involved intestine the most common procedure. Crohn's disease is a contraindication for complex continence-preserving procedures such as continent ileostomy (Koch pouch) or ileoanal pouch, due to the significant chance of complications (abscess/fistula) that will usually result in loss of the reservoir and a significant length of intestine.

IBD is a well-recognized risk factor for gastrointestinal cancer. This is particularly true for ulcerative colitis with total colonic involvement. This risk begins after 8–10 years of active disease. Current screening strategies in this population reflect that risk, and annual colonoscopy is recommended. Dysplasia, if seen on random biopsy, should warrant consideration for colectomy. Unfortunately, this screening strategy is far from perfect, with invasive cancer found in almost 20% of patients undergoing colectomy for this indication. Any patient with persistent pancolitis for more than 8 years should be counseled regarding cancer risk and should be offered "prophylactic" colectomy.

KEY POINTS

- Treatment of IBD almost always medical treatment initially

- Important to recognize that many patients will eventually require operation

- In cases of ulcerative colitis, operation usually curative

- In Crohn's disease, operation largely palliative; the guiding principle is bowel preservation

- Continued treatment of the patient with medication, despite onset or predictable risk of complications, may have greater morbidity and even mortality than a well-planned operation

FOLLOW-UP

Patients with IBD need follow-up as mandated by their disease activity initially. Patients with ulcerative colitis who undergo resection and ileoanal pouch reconstruction are followed closely for the first year to assist in restoration/stabilization of bowel function. Further follow-up is not necessary unless the patient develops a complication. These may include small bowel obstruction, "pouchitis" and liver disease. Pouchitis is a peculiar, poorly understood inflammation of the ileoanal pouch. The symptoms mimic ulcerative colitis with diarrhea, crampy abdominal pain, and malaise predominating. A short course of antibiotics (metronidazole) is "curative," and most patients remain free of further episodes. Liver disease is fortunately uncommon and includes sclerosing cholangitis, which may progress to liver failure and hepatic transplantation.

Patients with Crohn's disease who undergo operation should be followed long term due to the risk of recurrence and the efficacy of agents to prevent recurrence. In the past, operation for Crohn's disease was reputed to be risky, with enterocutaneous fistulas and other complications feared. Modern experience has disproven this "folklore"; appropriate, well-timed intervention is safe and efficacious. Medical treatment that is relatively safe and free of side effects (5-ASA derivatives, 6-MP) has recently been proved to prevent recurrent disease following resection.

SUGGESTED READINGS

Donowitz M, Kokke FT, Saidi R: Evaluation of patients with chronic diarrhea. N Engl J Med 332:725, 1995

An important article outlining the differential diagnosis and appropriate evaluation of patients with suspected inflammatory bowel disease.

Linn FV, Peppercorn MA: Drug therapy for inflammatory bowel disease: part I. Am J Surg 164:85, 1992

Current update for medical therapy of inflammatory bowel disease.

Werner SD, Jensen L, Rothenburger DA et al: Long-term functional analysis of the ileoanal reservoir. Dis Colon Rect 32: 275, 1989

An important article from an experienced center reporting on functional results of the ileoanal pouch.

Wolff BG: Crohn's disease: the role of surgical treatment. Mayo Clin Proc 61:292, 1986

An excellent overview of surgical indications and approaches for Crohn's disease.

QUESTIONS

1. Extraintestinal manifestations of inflammatory bowel disease may include?

    A. Skin lesions.

    B. Fistulas.

    C. Uveitis.

    D. Ankylosing spondylitis.

    E. All of the above.

2. Surgery for Crohn's disease is?

    A. Often disease complicated by fistula formation.

    B. Curative.

    C. Eventually necessary in the majority of patients.

    D. Guided by endoscopic and histologic findings.

    E. All of the above.

(See p. 603 for answers.)

31 DIVERTICULAR DISEASE

CHARLES N. HEADRICK

Diverticular diseases of the colon are extraordinarily common disorders among Americans. The actual incidence is unknown because most patients are asymptomatic or otherwise unaware of their symptoms. The aims of this chapter are to (1) define, precisely, the different diverticular diseases and their etiologies, and (2) review medical and surgical treatments for each.

CASE 1
ACUTE DIVERTICULITIS

A 40-year-old, moderately obese, white male presented to his physician with a 3-day history of increasing abdominal discomfort and fever. In the last 24 hours, he had been anorexic, nauseated, and his bowel movements had become irregular—looser, more frequent, and with increasing flatus. In the left lower quadrant there was a firm mass. On rectal examination, the rectal wall was tender and edematous. His temperature was 38.6°C and the WBC count $15.3 \times 10^3/mm^3$. The urine contained a few WBCs. Careful proctoscopy showed an erythematous upper rectum and lower sigmoid colon. The examination was limited to 15 cm because of pain.

He was admitted with a diagnosis of acute diverticulitis. Intravenous fluids were started and antibiotics given for gram-negative and anaerobic organisms. On CT scan, a thickened sigmoid colon with characteristics of a phlegmon and a distinct 5×4-cm abscess laterally was found. CT-guided drainage was done successfully.

He became afebrile and his WBC count returned to normal. Intravenous antibiotics were continued for approximately 5 days then discontinued. He was discharged on a low residue diet.

The patient was monitored with bimonthly office visits. Six weeks later, a colonoscopy showed moderate diverticulosis of the sigmoid and descending colon with mini-mal signs of residual sigmoid diverticulitis. At operation, a thickened sigmoid colon adherent to the dome of the bladder and laterally to the abdominal wall, with no residual abscess was resected. He was discharged 6 days later.

CASE 2
ACUTE DIVERTICULITIS
WITH ABSCESS

A 63-year-old female presented, having noted abdominal bloating and tenderness of several days duration. Her bowel habits were unchanged and she denied any urinary complaints. There was a tender, firm mass in the left lower quadrant without rebound tenderness. Her temperature was 38.8°C and the WBC count was 14,500/mm³. She was known to have sigmoid diverticulosis. She was admitted and intravenous antibiotics and hydration given. CT scan showed a thickened, phlegmonous colon without a fluid collection. Her tenderness and leukocytosis resolved. An attempt to feed her on the fifth hospital day produced a flare-up of abdominal pain and an increased WBC count. A repeat CT scan was unchanged. A gentle bowel preparation of laxatives and oral antibiotics was only partly successful. It was decided to operate because of continued sepsis. A thickened, boggy erythematous sigmoid colon was found, which on mobilization revealed a multiloculated abscess extending into the pelvis and adherent to the bladder. The diseased bowel was resected, leaving a rectal stump (Hartmann's pouch) and a proximal end colostomy in the left lower quadrant. The patient had an uneventful recovery and her colostomy was closed 3 months later.

CASE 3
DIVERTICULITIS WITH COLOVESICLE FISTULA

A 73-year-old female who had two previous hospitalizations for diverticulitis requiring intravenous antibiotics, presented to her internist for a routine visit. She had been treated for recent urinary tract infections and reported a new symptom of pneumaturia. She had a previous abdominal hysterectomy and a colonoscopy that showed only sigmoid diverticulosis. Urine cultures had grown *E. coli*, and large amounts of bacteria were seen in her urinary sediment. CT scan showed normal kidneys and ureters and a thickened sigmoid colon adherent to the bladder, with air in the dome of the bladder.

Following preparation, the patient underwent an elective sigmoid resection of a thickened, edematous sigmoid colon firmly adherent to the dome of the bladder. The fistula site was identified and bluntly separated from the bladder. A colorectal anastomosis was done. A single suture of chromic catgut was used to close the bladder fistula site and a Foley catheter was left in the bladder for 7 days. She was discharged on the eighth postoperative day after an uneventful recovery.

GENERAL CONSIDERATIONS

Diverticular diseases of the colon affect a large percentage of the American population. As much as 30% of the population over 60 years of age may be affected, and the incidence steadily climbs with age. Despite these large numbers, the population at risk is difficult to identify since the vast majority of people with diverticular disease of the colon are asymptomatic and/or unaware of their condition.

The term *diverticular disease* encompasses diverticulosis and diverticulitis. A diverticulum is a singular outpouching of the bowel wall. Diverticula may be located throughout the gastrointestinal tract, but this discussion is restricted to the large intestine. Diverticula of the colon are most commonly "pseudo" diverticula, rather than "true" diverticula, the distinction being that a true diverticulum contains all layers of the bowel wall. Common diverticula are "pseudo" because they contain only mucosal and submucosal elements of the bowel wall. The presence of more than one diverticulum constitutes a condition of diverticula or diverticulosis. An inflammation of a diverticulum is known as diverticulitis.

How are diverticula formed? To answer this question, the basic anatomy must be briefly reviewed. The large intestine is a hollow viscus with a large diameter proximally, which gradually narrows in diameter as it moves toward the rectum. There is a complete circular muscular layer and an incomplete longitudinal muscular layer known as the taenia coli. Cross-sectional anatomy (Fig. 31.1) demonstrates the vascular anatomy of the colon. As the blood leaves the mesentery, it passes around the colon, piercing the bowel wall along the mesenteric border of the taenia coli. It thus traverses the muscular wall supplying the mucosal and submucosal layers. It is at this site that most diverticula develop, as this anatomic weakness in the colonic wall allows herniation of the intestinal lining. It is a "pulsion"-type herniation—inner layers are extruded secondary to an increased luminal pressure. Most diverticula are located in the sigmoid colon, where the bowel has the smallest luminal diameter and thickest muscular wall, thereby generating the greatest pressures (Fig. 31.2). In the United States, where the advent of mass food processing has led to increasingly refined foodstuffs and lower dietary fiber intake, feces are smaller in volume. An additional increase in luminal pressure is therefore necessary to continue forward motion. The greater pressures generated create "pulsion" herniations (or diverticula) along the bowel wall at the anatomic sites of weakness. This process occurs over a considerable period.

The true incidence of diverticulosis is difficult to establish because the condition produces no symptoms, except bleeding in a minority of patients. The symptoms of diverticulitis are at times nondescript, making diagnosis difficult. Diverticulitis results from local inflammation and infection of a diverticulum. The disease can progress to perforation—from small, well-localized, pericolic abscesses to free feculent peritonitis (Fig. 31.3).

Medical treatment of the various forms of diverticular disease of the colon is directed at reducing the functional problems of colonic motility and resolving any infectious process. By providing a diet that is rich in fiber, bulk and volume are added to the fecal stream. Transit time is shortened and luminal pressures are decreased with a bulky stool. This requires a change in dietary practice and/or a dietary supplement (psyllium), a goal not always easy to achieve. Surgical treatment is reserved for complications of diverticular disease. In some instances, the decision to operate is easily made, such as the patient with an acute abdomen or life-threatening hemorrhage. In others, the decision is less clear cut. The option of operation is considered later in this chapter.

KEY POINTS

- Vast majority of people with diverticular disease of the colon are asymptomatic and/or unaware of their condition
- Most diverticula are located in sigmoid colon, where bowel has smallest luminal diameter and thickest muscular wall, thereby generating greatest pressures

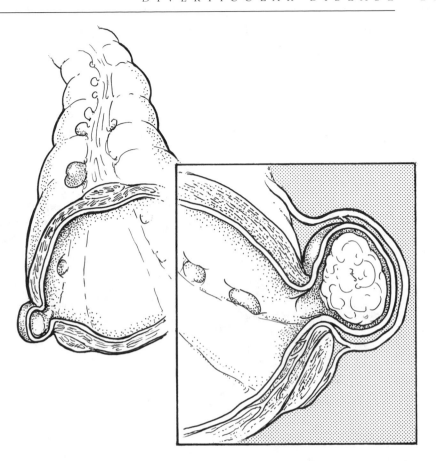

FIGURE 31.1 *Diverticula form at the site of muscular penetration of the vasa recta.*

• Diverticulitis results from local inflammation and infection of a diverticulum; the disease can progress to perforation—from small, well-localized, pericolic abscesses to free feculent peritonitis

DIAGNOSIS

Diverticula are frequently discovered during the course of routine examinations such as endoscopy and contrast enema. Active diverticular disease, however, may have no antecedent history or examination suggesting colonic disease. To be identified more easily, diverticular disease of the colon should be divided into diverticulosis and diverticulitis. Their presentations are quite different.

Diverticulosis is usually without symptoms. Some patients may describe occasional crampy abdominal pain, bloating, or gas, and intolerance of certain dietary items—complaints that are probably unrelated to the presence of diverticula. The most dangerous form of diverticulosis is massive hemorrhage. This typically occurs in the elderly patient without previous symptoms, and may present as a massive loss of bright red blood. Diagnosis utilizes nuclear scans (technectium-tagged red blood cells) and angiography with or without selective intervention. Once the hemorrhage is stabilized, complete evaluation of the entire colon by colonoscopy is indicated (see Ch. 28).

Diverticulitis has a much broader range of presentation. This diagnosis is most commonly made by physical examination, and usually by the primary care physician. Typically, tenderness in the left lower quadrant (Case 2) is accompanied by fever and leukocytosis. For mild presentations, no further workup other than history, physical examination, and laboratory analysis is necessary. At a later time, endoscopy or contrast enema will establish the diagnosis of diverticulosis, a necessary predisposing condition. For more severe cases, evaluation in the hospital is advisable. Imaging of the area can be accomplished by ultrasonography or computed tomography (CT) scanning. The advantage of CT over ultrasound is the more complete view of adjacent structures included in the image. In the patient with an acute abdomen, no studies are needed. Contrast studies using barium are contraindicated in the acute setting. If a perforation is suspected but not obvious, a gentle, water soluble contrast enema may be performed. Colonoscopy and barium enema are reserved until the inflammatory episode has resolved, which usually takes 6 weeks or longer. Rigid proctosigmoidoscopy with minimal insufflation is sometimes utilized in the initial workup of a patient, but great care should be taken, as the disease process could potentially be converted to a free perforation with too vigorous an examination.

Some patients present with evidence of a fistula (Case 3), most commonly to the bladder, although colovaginal and colocutaneous fistulas are not uncommon. Surpris-

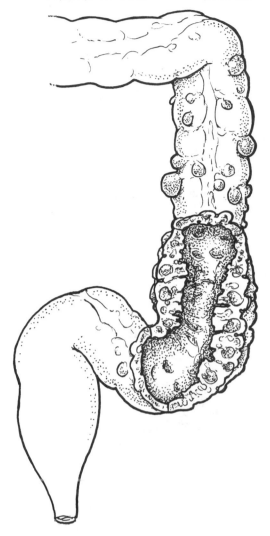

FIGURE 31.2 *Although diverticula often extend proximally to involve the descending colon, the inflammation is generally limited to the sigmoid colon.*

ingly, many of these patients will not recollect a history consistent with an episode of acute diverticulitis.

Unfortunately, the diagnosis is occasionally made at the time of surgery; this is discussed in the following section.

KEY POINTS

• Diverticulosis usually without symptoms; most dangerous form is massive hemorrhage

• Diverticulitis has broader range of presentation; diagnosis most often made by physical examination

DIFFERENTIAL DIAGNOSIS

As with any disease process, there is no substitute for a careful history and physical examination. A majority of patients with symptomatic diverticular disease can be

diagnosed on history alone. Factors such as general health of the patient, age, presentation of symptoms, and medical history are all helpful, although there may be no antecedent history of diverticular disease.

The most important diagnosis to exclude is the presence of carcinoma. Despite the many distinguishing characteristics of diverticulitis (an intact mucosa, fistula formation, longer segments of disease, and a gradual transition from abnormal to normal), carcinoma can often not be eliminated as a potential diagnosis. Endoscopy and radiologic studies are helpful after resolution of the acute episode.

Inflammatory bowel disease (ulcerative colitis, Crohn's disease) can mimic diverticulitis, as can appendicitis. Fistula formation is also common in Crohn's disease. Hemorrhage from colitis can also be confused with diverticular bleeding. Ischemic colitis may also present with a sudden onset of pain and change in bowel habit. Bloody diarrhea is characteristic of ischemic colitis and is distinctly unusual in diverticulitis. Small bowel obstruction, fecal impaction, gynecologic (pelvic inflammatory disease, endometriosis) and urologic diseases (ureteral colic, infections) should also be considered in a complete differential diagnosis.

Diverticulitis in the immunocompromised patient may be surprisingly asymptomatic. Transplant patients, patients with acquired immunodeficiency syndrome (AIDS), and patients on chemotherapy or steroids are groups that may not be able to manifest the classic signs and symptoms of diverticular infection. These patients are more likely to present with a free perforation or peritonitis and need urgent surgical treatment.

The differential diagnosis also includes irritable bowel syndrome. Although this is a functional ailment, it can mimic symptoms of diverticulitis. It most frequently affects female patients, and a long-standing history of symptoms with no real acute episodes helps differentiate it. Additionally, leukocytosis and fever are not expected with irritable bowel.

KEY POINTS

• Most important diagnosis to exclude is carcinoma; endoscopy and radiologic studies helpful after resolution of acute episode

• Differential diagnosis also includes irritable bowel syndrome; although a functional ailment, can mimic symptoms of diverticulitis; most frequently affects female patients—a long-standing history of symptoms with no real acute episodes helps differentiate it

TREATMENT

The diagnosis of diverticular disease does not always provide a clear-cut path to treatment. Symptoms can range from minimal to life-threatening. Much of diverticular disease is treatable medically, but there are distinct

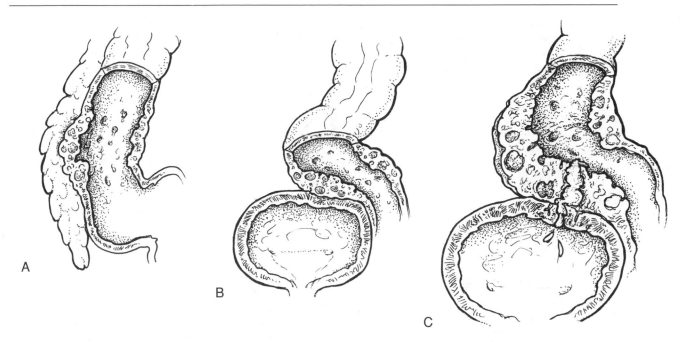

FIGURE 31.3 *Diverticular perforation is usually walled off by (A) the omentum or (B) an adjacent organ such as the bladder. (C) If the inflammation is severe and protracted, a fistula may develop.*

groups that require surgery. Roughly 20% of patients with diverticulosis will experience diverticulitis and perhaps 20% of that group will require surgery.

Diverticular hemorrhage is a topic covered more thoroughly in Chapter 28. Its treatment, however, is characterized by resuscitation and stabilization of the patient. In the majority of cases, the hemorrhage stops spontaneously. Workup with bleeding scans and/or colonoscopy are indicated unless surgery is required to halt the ongoing hemorrhage. Choice of operation is determined by radiologic findings and/or instability of the patient.

Diverticulitis can present with many variations, as noted. Most cases will be mild to moderate inflammatory episodes that can be treated medically as an outpatient. Physical examination and history, complemented by appropriate laboratory studies, will help the physician choose a treatment plan. Obstructive symptoms, fever and chills, peritoneal signs, elevated white blood cell count (WBC) or any signs of sepsis mandate admission to the hospital for more intensive evaluation and treatment. Milder forms can be treated with dietary restriction (liquids or low residue diet), oral antibiotics, and frequent reexamination and evaluation. When necessary, treatment in the hospital should include intravenous hydration, intravenous antibiotics, nothing by mouth, monitoring to include accurate intake and output, and serial laboratory and physical examinations. It should also include selective radiologic evaluation. Chest x-ray and plain abdominal films should be performed to look for free air and/or obstructive signs. Ultrasound and CT scanning should also be considered, particularly for patients who are not re-

sponding. Antibiotics should be chosen to provide broad coverage of gram-negative and anaerobic organisms.

Successful nonsurgical treatment of diverticulitis should always be followed by reliable examination of the colon. Colonoscopy or combination flexible sigmoidoscopy and air contrast barium enema should be performed after resolution of the inflammatory episode (usually at 6 weeks). This is to confirm the diagnosis and rule out any concurrent disease. Current standards advise elective operation following two episodes of uncomplicated diverticulitis. This is based on the success rate of medical therapy for recurrent diverticulitis, which drops rapidly after the first recurrence.

Operation entails sigmoid resection and primary anastomosis following bowel preparation. The proximal margin of resection is made on normal caliber, noninflamed, pliable bowel, while the distal margin is made at the rectum. The entire sigmoid colon is excised in this manner. There is a high rate of recurrent diverticulitis when distal sigmoid colon remains following surgery for diverticulitis.

In the patient presenting with more severe inflammation (Case 2) or even peritonitis, surgical treatment may be more urgent. Exploration may be required to control sepsis and establish adequate drainage of infection. Historically, a three-stage treatment plan was utilized: (1) exploration, drainage of abscess, and a proximally diverting stoma, (2) resection of disease, anastomosis, and a protective stoma, and (3) closure of stoma. Leaving the source of infection in stage 1 did not always cure the sepsis, however, and there is considerable morbidity and mortality with three operations. Currently, goals are to remove the diseased bowel if at all possible at the first operation, control sepsis, and then decide whether it is safe to perform an anastomosis. This removes the septic focus and gives the patient no more than two operations. Options include (1) Hartmann resection (Case 2), (2) resection and anastomosis with a proximal diverting stoma, and (3) single-stage operation with anastomosis (Cases 1 and 3).

Complications of diverticulitis do not always require urgent surgical treatment, although they usually mandate surgical treatment at some point in time (Case 3). These include abscesses, fistulas (colovesical, colocutaneous, coloenteric), obstruction/stricture, free perforation, and hemorrhage (rare).

Pericolic abscesses, as mentioned previously (Case 1), may be drained percutaneously, allowing a single stage surgical procedure after adequate bowel preparation. Incompletely drained abscesses or those not amenable to drainage will require exploration and are more likely to require a Hartmann resection with colostomy (Case 2).

After excluding other etiologies for fistula (irritable bowel disease, cancer, radiation) primary resection can usually be performed along with the repair of adjacent organs (Case 3). When faced with large bowel obstruction with diverticulitis, carcinoma should always be considered. Obstruction may need to be treated urgently with nasogastric decompression, rehydration, and even laparotomy (usually resection and stoma), or if decompression can be achieved, a one-stage procedure.

Free perforation is very uncommon but should be treated expeditiously after resuscitation. The procedure of choice would be segmental resection with colostomy. This complication carries a high mortality rate (6–35%).

In certain cases of diverticulitis, surgical treatment may be recommended early. Immunocompromise, as seen in transplant, AIDS, renal failure, and possibly neutropenic chemotherapy patients, carries a higher risk of free perforation. Medical treatment of these patients is also much less successful. Diverticulitis in a patient under 40 years of age is a more aggressive form of the disease, and resection after one documented episode should be strongly considered (Case 1).

> **KEY POINTS**
>
> • Diverticulitis can present with many variations; majority of cases will be mild to moderate inflammatory episodes that can be treated medically on outpatient basis
>
> • Obstructive symptoms, fever and chills, peritoneal signs, elevated WBC count, or any signs of sepsis mandate admission to hospital for more intensive evaluation and treatment
>
> • Successful nonsurgical treatment of diverticulitis should always be followed by reliable colon examination
>
> • In cases of severe inflammation, remove diseased bowel, if possible at first operation, control sepsis, and decide if safe to perform anastomosis

> • Pericolic abscesses may be drained percutaneously, allowing single stage surgical procedure after adequate bowel preparation

FOLLOW-UP

Follow-up of diverticular disease will vary, depending on the type of treatment utilized. Since most diverticular disease of the colon is treated medically, complete evaluation of the colon, with barium examination or colonoscopy, should be completed once the acute inflammatory episode has resolved. Following this, dietary counseling should be performed, either by the physician or a dietician. In more serious episodes of infection, surgery should be discussed in order to treat the disease electively rather than emergently.

For the postsurgical patient, follow-up includes routine postoperative care outside of the hospital. This should include sigmoidoscopy after 6–8 weeks of convalescence to examine the anastomosis. (Recall that this should be a colorectal anastomosis.) Dietary counseling will also be necessary as bowel habits frequently change after colonic resection. As a rule, high fiber foods are recommended. The patient should also receive yearly examinations for the first 3 years and as indicated thereafter. The American College of Surgeons recommends flexible sigmoidoscopy every 3–5 years in the individual who is asymptomatic or is not at increased risk of colon cancer. If all of the distal sigmoid colon has been resected, the likelihood of recurrent diverticulitis is very small, though still present (4–7%). In the final analysis, the best preventive medicine after an operative procedure will be regular visits with the patient's physician.

SUGGESTED READINGS

Gordon PH, Nivatvongs S: Principles and Practice of Surgery for the Colon, Rectum, and Anus. Quality Medical, St. Louis, MO, 1992

A good reference chapter encompassing the entire disease process and discussing specific surgical options.

Painter NS: Diverticular disease of the colon: the first of the western diseases shown to be due to a deficiency of dietary fiber. South Afr Med J 61:1016, 1982

Describes the dietary influence on diverticular formation.

Parks TG: Natural history of diverticular disease of the colon. Clin Gastroenterol 4:53, 1975

A classic look at the etiology and anatomy of diverticula.

Roberts P, Abel M, Rosen L et al: Practice parameters for sigmoid diverticulitis—supporting documentation. Dis Colon Rectum 38:126, 1995

A brief overview of treatment with an invaluable reference list.

QUESTIONS

1. Most patients with diverticulosis?
   A. Suffer from recurrent bleeding.
   B. Will eventually require surgery.
   C. Are asymptomatic.
   D. Have nightly fever and chills.

2. Diverticula are contributed to by?
   A. Aging.
   B. Inadequate fiber intake.
   C. High pressure peristaltic waves in the sigmoid colon.
   D. Anatomic weak areas in the sigmoid colon.
   E. All of the above.

3. An acute attack of diverticulitis may be appropriately treated with?
   A. Bowel rest, intravenous antibiotics.
   B. Emergent surgery.
   C. Oral antibiotics (bactrim and metronidazole).
   D. All of the above.

(See p. 603 for answers.)

32

POLYPS OF

THE COLON

HERNAN I. VARGAS

MICHAEL J. STAMOS

The normal colonic surface is smooth, except for the presence of mucosal folds. A polyp represents a discrete prominence seen in the mucosa as a consequence of alterations in the epithelial or stromal components. They may be found isolated or as part of a syndrome, morphologically pedunculated or sessile (Fig. 32.1). The aim of this chapter is to delineate the types of polyps commonly encountered and to outline a management strategy for patient care.

CASE 1
ADENOMATOUS POLYP

A 52-year-old male was referred by an insurance company physician after he was found to have a rectal mass on a routine physical examination. The patient was asymptomatic, in good health, and he denied any change in bowel habits, abdominal pain, or rectal bleeding. His past medical history was unremarkable. He was unaware of any relatives with cancer. His physical examination was remarkable for the presence of a 1-cm pedunculated mass in the anterior rectal wall.

A proctoscopic examination in the office confirmed the presence of this 1-cm polyp, pedunculated with a regular surface. This was snare excised at the time of evaluation and revealed a tubular adenoma. Subsequently, a colonoscopic examination showed a 4-mm adenomatous polyp in the sigmoid colon, a 5-mm hyperplastic polyp in the descending colon, and a 2-cm polyp in the descending colon that on pathologic examination showed a villous adenoma with carcinoma in situ. The patient was subsequently followed with yearly colonoscopy without any evidence of re-

current cancer. He has since developed two other benign polyps that have been excised. He has continued a routine surveillance protocol for the past 3 years and is doing well.

CASE 2
FAMILIAL ADENOMATOUS POLYPOSIS

A 39-year-old male presented with a 9-month history of bloody diarrhea, weight loss, and episodic abdominal distention for the past 4 weeks. He denied any other medical problems. His family history was significant for having a brother who died 2 months after having a colostomy for an obstructing colon cancer at age 34. A second brother, age 36, had developed bloody diarrhea but had not received medical attention. His father had died of an accident at age 28. He had two healthy sons, ages 17 and 18.

He had temporal wasting, weight loss, and a palpable, enlarged liver. On rectal examination, there were two palpable masses and guaiac positive stool. He had a hypochromic microcytic anemia, and elevated alkaline phos-

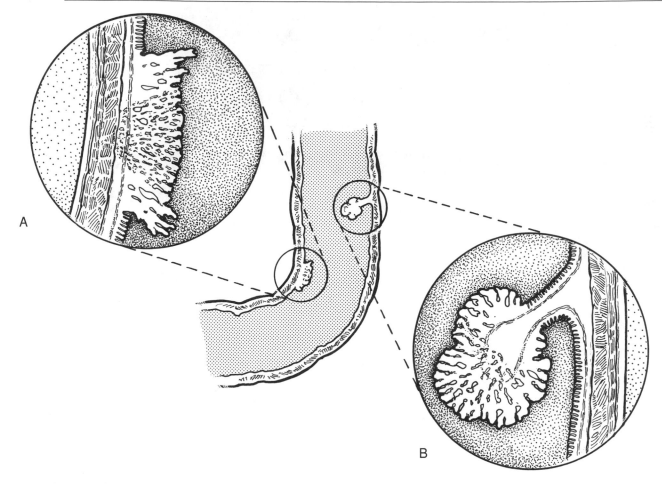

FIGURE 32.1 *(A) Sessile and (B) pedunculated colonic polyps.*

phatase and CEA level. A chest x-ray was normal and an abdominal CT scan showed several liver metastases in both lobes of the liver and a mass in the splenic flexure of the colon with a proximally dilated colon. On colonoscopy the rectum, sigmoid, and descending colon were carpeted with polyps, and a nearly obstructing mass was found in the proximal descending colon that did not allow the passage of the colonoscope; biopsies of this mass confirmed the presence of adenocarcinoma.

A palliative resection of the splenic flexure colon cancer was done and liver metastases confirmed intraoperatively. He was doing well but had continued to lose weight. His two sons were evaluated and did not have any colonic polyps; they were scheduled to undergo surveillance.

GENERAL CONSIDERATIONS

As is exemplified in both cases, the most significant fact about colonic polyps is that they represent a marker for high risk of developing colonic malignancies. Some polyps have precancerous potential, which is determined by the pathologic characteristics of the polyp. The histo-

logic classification of epithelial polyps is presented in Table 32.1. Hamartomatous polyps are essentially benign and represent disorganized growth of epithelial and stromal components. Juvenile polyps are more common in children and are also benign. Hyperplastic polyps are found most commonly in the elderly; they have been postulated by some to be a marker for adenomatous polyps. Inflammatory or pseudopolyps are seen most commonly with inflammatory bowel disease (see Ch. 30).

Adenomatous polyps are benign but premalignant epithelial neoplasms. They exhibit abnormal cell kinetics,

TABLE 32.1 *Colonic polyps*

HISTOLOGIC CLASSIFICATION OF COLONIC POLYPS
Neoplastic
Adenomatous carcinoma
Non-neoplastic
Hamartomatous polyps
Hyperplastic polyps
Inflammatory polyps (pseudopolyps)

showing unrestricted cell division and failure to differentiate. Adenomatous polyps can be tubular, tubulovillous, or villous; their relative frequencies are 75%, 20%, and 5%, respectively. Histology and size are the main determinants of their malignant potential. As many as 40% of villous adenomas have carcinomatous foci (Case 1). Among tubulovillous adenomas, 22% exhibit malignant transformation. Only 5% of tubular polyps are malignant. Polyps less than 1 cm in size rarely exhibit cancer, while polyps greater than 2 cm in size may contain cancerous elements more than 40% of the time.

ADENOMA-CARCINOMA SEQUENCE

It has now been accepted that colorectal carcinoma is preceded by adenoma formation in the vast majority of cases. This adenoma-carcinoma sequence theory is supported by the following evidence:

1. Adenomas are frequently seen in patients with colorectal cancer

2. Villous adenomas and large polyps frequently have areas of severe dysplasia or carcinoma (Case 1)

3. Residual adenomatous tissue is often seen in colorectal cancer

4. Adenomatous syndromes are strongly associated with colorectal cancer (Case 2)

5. De novo colorectal carcinoma is rarely seen

6. Anatomic distribution of adenomas and carcinomas is similar

7. Removal of polyps reduces the incidence of future carcinoma

8. Specific progressive changes in DNA have been described for each of these morphologic changes

KEY POINTS

• Adenomatous polyps are benign but premalignant epithelial neoplasms; they can be tubular, tubulovillous, or villous

• Histology and size main determinants of malignant potential

• Polyps less than 1 cm in size rarely exhibit cancer; polyps greater than 2 cm may contain cancerous elements more than 40% of the time

• Colorectal carcinoma preceded by adenoma formation in vast majority of cases

DIAGNOSIS

Most patients with colonic polyps do not represent a kindred of a polyposis syndrome. However, colonic polyps are seen more commonly in populations at higher risk of colon cancer. Polyps may be identified:

1. As part of a routine screening program with or without fecal occult blood (Case 1)

2. On radiologic or colonoscopic evaluation of a symptomatic patient with rectal bleeding, abdominal pain, or obstructive symptoms (Case 2)

3. In a patient with colon cancer subjected to colonoscopy to identify synchronous lesions

4. In a patient previously treated for colon cancer as part of routine follow-up surveillance

Once identified, removal and histologic evaluation of the polyp is essential to exclude the possibility of cancer and to identify the histologic type. This is done, in most cases, colonoscopically. Adenomatous polyps are multicentric and complete colonoscopy is therefore indicated.

DIFFERENTIAL DIAGNOSIS

Patients with familial adenomatous polyposis (FAP) (Case 2) have a genetic defect, traced to the long arm of chromosome 5, that leads to the development of adenomatous polyps. It has 100% penetrance and follows autosomal dominant transmission. Polyposis usually begins in early adolescence but may start as late as in the mid-30s. By age 35, 75% of patients have developed colon cancer. Eventually, 100% of patients develop colon cancer if untreated (Case 2). This defect is expressed in the foregut as well; these patients are at risk of polyps in the stomach, duodenum, and jejunoileum and of carcinoma of the stomach, duodenum, ampulla, bile duct, and small bowel.

Extraintestinal manifestations are noted in Table 32.2. Several variations of the genetic defect are grouped in different syndromes. Gardner syndrome includes colonic polyposis, desmoid tumors, dermoid cysts, and osteomas. Patients with colonic polyposis and brain tumors represent Turcot syndrome. Patients may have only colonic manifestations and are grouped as familial *Polyposis coli* (Case 2).

Peutz-Jeghers is a syndrome characterized by mucocutaneous pigmentation and hamartomatous polyps throughout the gastrointestinal tract. In decreasing fre-

TABLE 32.2 *Extraintestinal manifestations of familial polyposis syndromes*

Desmoid tumors
Osteomas
Epidermoid cysts
Retinal pigmentation
Adrenal adenomas and carcinoma
Congenital hypertrophy of the retinal pigment epithelium
Brain tumors

quency the jejunum, ileum, colon, and stomach are affected. Patients complain of gastrointestinal bleeding or abdominal pain due to intussusception, with the polyp as a lead point. Polypectomy is recommended in symptomatic patients or if a polyp larger than 1.5 cm is noted. In this situation, complete removal of all polyps is recommended to avoid the high symptomatic recurrence rate. These patients have a high incidence of extraintestinal malignancies, including ovarian, breast, thyroid, and cervical cancer. The risk of gastrointestinal malignancy is also higher than that of normal individuals.

Juvenile polyposis is characterized by the presence of multiple hamartomatous polyps. It is usually noted in children and it is the most common cause of major gastrointestinal bleeding in children. Treatment is directed at control of bleeding or intussusception but depends on the extent of disease. These patients have a 10% risk of cancer. In extensive colonic disease abdominal colectomy has been recommended.

Cronkhite-Canada syndrome consists of hyperpigmentation of the volar aspect of fingers and palms, pigmentation in the dorsum of the hands, alopecia, nail atrophy, and diffuse polyposis with juvenile polyps. Treatment is provided when intussusception or bleeding occur. There is no apparent increased risk of gastrointestinal malignancies.

In Cowden syndrome patients develop hamartomas of all three embryologic layers. It is characterized by mucocutaneous tricholemmomas and is also associated with thyroid and breast cancer. Three-fourths of patients have intestinal hamartomatous polyps.

Occasionally, hypertrophied anal papillae in the anal canal are confused with polyps. These papillae are often felt on rectal examination and may even prolapse out of the anus. They are a response to previous inflammation in the region (e.g., anal fissure) and are most readily distinguished by their location at the dentate line.

D TREATMENT

ue to the risk of harboring a malignancy as well as the malignant potential, colonic polyps should be removed. This can be done through proctosigmoidoscopy or through colonoscopy, depending on the location of the polyp. For smaller colonic polyps, a biopsy with endoscopic forceps is sufficient. Techniques for removal of larger colonic polyps include the following:

1. Snare polypectomy, most commonly applied to pedunculated polyps
2. Piecemeal polypectomy, which is used for large sessile polyps
3. Biopsy and fulguration
4. Surgical resection

Finding of an adenomatous polyp mandates complete colonic examination, as up to 40% of patients will harbor a synchronous polyp or cancer.

Approximately 5% of polyps have a carcinoma component ("malignant polyp"). These patients may require further treatment. When the risk of cancer recurrence is very small and considered less than the risk of surgery, polypectomy with a clear margin is sufficient treatment. Patients with carcinoma in situ, or a well-differentiated invasive carcinoma in a pedunculated polyp with a clear margin of resection are considered cured by a colonoscopic polypectomy.

Patients with invasive carcinoma in a sessile polyp, patients with a pedunculated polyp who do not meet the above criteria, or patients with polypoid carcinoma are better managed with a partial colectomy.

Management of patients with FAP and their family members is directed at

1. Identification of individuals at risk via proctosigmoidoscopic evaluation starting at age 10. Two-thirds of affected families develop congenital hypertrophy of the retinal pigment epithelium; fundoscopic examination may be a useful screening tool in these families

2. Once an individual at risk is identified, prophylactic colectomy is recommended to prevent the development of carcinoma. Several options are available, including total protocolectomy with ileostomy or Kock pouch, abdominal colectomy with ileorectal anastomosis, abdominal colectomy with rectal mucosectomy, and ileoanal pull-through

3. Patients who are identified after a malignancy has developed should receive the indicated treatment for their colon or rectal carcinoma and total colectomy

4. Upper endoscopy should be performed periodically in patients with familial adenomatous polyposis (FAP) to assess for gastric, duodenal, and ampullary polyps

5. Treatment for extracolonic manifestations should be provided as indicated by symptoms

KEY POINTS

• Due to risk of harboring malignancy as well as malignant potential, colonic polyps should be removed

• Management of patients with familial adenomatous polyposis directed at identification of individuals at risk via proctosigmoidoscopic evaluation starting at age 10; prophylactic colectomy to prevent development of carcinoma; patients identified after malignancy has developed should receive the indicated treatment for their colon or rectal carcinoma and total colectomy; upper endoscopy should be performed periodically in patients with FAP to assess for gastric, duodenal, and ampullary polyps; and treatment for extracolonic manifestations as indicated by symptoms

FOLLOW-UP

Follow-up in patients with colonic polyps is important due to the risk of recurrent polyps and the risk of developing colon cancer. They should be considered a group at high risk of development of colorectal malignancy. Follow-up colonoscopy should be done within 1 year for a benign adenomatous polyp. If a malignant polyp is completely excised with a clear margin and nonsurgical treatment is elected, a repeat endoscopy should be done within 3 months to exclude a local recurrence or incomplete excision.

Further endoscopy can usually be done at 3–5-year intervals due to the slow growth and progression of the adenoma-carcinoma sequence.

Follow-up of patients with familial adenomatous polyposis is directed at (1) identifying new polyps in any residual portion of colon, and (2) identifying polyps in the upper gastrointestinal tract, including the biliary tree and ampulla. Equally important is evaluation and follow-up of family members at risk of development of polyps and other manifestations of this genetic disorder.

SUGGESTED READINGS

Bapat BV, Parker JA, Berk T et al: Combined use of molecular and biomarkers for presymptomatic carrier risk assessment in familial adenomatous polyposis: implications for screening guidelines. Dis Colon Rectum 37:165, 1994

Cutting edge work on a disease (FAP) utilizing molecular diagnosis for primary prevention.

Desai DC, Neale KF, Talbot IC et al: Juvenile polyposis. Br J Surg 82:14, 1995

A review article that proposes a high rate of colorectal cancer with long-term follow-up.

Neugut AI, Jaconson JS, Ahsan H et al: Incidence and recurrence rates of colorectal adenomas: a prospective study. Gastroenterology 108:402, 1995

A prospective study providing important data regarding polyps to guide use of endoscopy.

Tierny RP, Ballantyne GH, Modlin IM: The adenoma to carcinoma sequence. Surg Gynecol Obstet 171:81, 1990

A good overview of the malignant potential of adenomatous polyps.

QUESTIONS

1. *Adenomatous polyps?*
   A. Usually progress to cancer.
   B. When larger than 2 cm, should be removed.
   C. Can occur anywhere in the colon or rectum.
   D. Usually warrant surgical resection.

2. *Familial adenomatous polyposis?*
   A. Is an autosomally dominant transmitted disease.
   B. May be associated with upper intestinal polyps or cancer.
   C. Is also known as Gardner syndrome.
   D. May be diagnosed in a presymptomatic stage by the finding of retinal pigmentation.
   E. All of the above.

(See p. 604 for answers.)

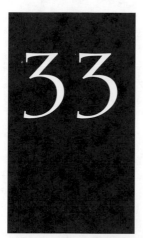

33

CANCER OF

THE COLON

AND RECTUM

MICHAEL J. STAMOS

Colon cancer is presented in many textbooks as a cut-and-dry issue. "This cancer is best treated by a left hemicolectomy"; "that cancer is cured by a right hemicolectomy," are prevailing attitudes. Often, the explanation for and even the rationale for a specific treatment are not given. The aims of this chapter are to (1) elucidate the risk factors for large bowel cancer, (2) produce an understanding of primary and secondary prevention, (3) help in the understanding of patterns of spread and reasons for treat-

ment failure, and (4) review the available therapies and their indications. Although the etiologic factors and therapeutic goals are similar when dealing with colon and rectal neoplasms, the treatment (both surgical and adjuvant) and patterns of failure are quite different.

CASE 1
ABDOMINAL PAIN AND
HEME-POSITIVE STOOL

A 56-year-old white male presented to his family physician with complaints of left-sided colicky abdominal pain for 2–3 weeks, worsening over that time. On further questioning, he admitted to a change in frequency of his bowel movements with recent use of laxatives. He denied fevers, chills, or weight loss. A detailed family history revealed breast cancer in his maternal grandmother but was otherwise unremarkable. Physical examination showed mild tenderness in the left lower quadrant with a possible mass

palpated, and heme-positive stool. Laboratory values at that time were WBC, $6.7 \times 10^3/mm^3$; Hb, 13 g/dl; Hct, 39%; MCV, 80.

Barium enema showed a lesion in the mid- to proximal sigmoid colon with irregular contours, completely obstructing retrograde flow. Additional laboratory evaluations (CEA, LFTs) were ordered and surgical consultation requested. Flexible sigmoidoscopy demonstrated an exophytic, annular mass at 40 cm (proximal sigmoid) that would not allow further passage of the scope. The distal sigmoid colon and rectal mucosa were normal. Biopsies of the lesion showed it to be a moderately differentiated adenocarcinoma. Additional laboratory evaluations included CEA, 14.0 ng/ml (NL <3.0); alkaline phosphatase, 140 IU/L (NL <110); ALT, 20 units/ml (NL <45); and AST, 32 (NL <40). The patient was counseled regarding options and operation planned. CT scan of the abdomen and pelvis showed a normal liver, normal kidneys and ureters, and an area of thickening of the bowel wall in the sigmoid colon region with encroachment of the lateral abdominal wall.

At operation, thorough exploration revealed a single 2-cm lesion in the left lateral lobe of the liver and a bulky tumor of the proximal sigmoid colon with adherence to the anterior lateral abdominal wall. A left hemicolectomy was performed with en bloc resection of adherent abdominal wall. Attention was then directed to the liver metastasis. Intraoperative liver ultrasonography found no other lesions, and excision of the isolated liver tumor was performed with a 1-cm margin. Pathology showed a moderately differentiated adenocarcinoma with full thickness invasion of bowel wall and invasion of the abdominal wall with clear margins. Three of 38 lymph nodes had metastatic deposits as did the liver mass (clear margins). The patient was again counseled and advised to receive adjuvant chemotherapy (5-FU and levamisole). Six weeks postoperatively, CEA had decreased to less than 2.0 and colonoscopy at that time found two ascending colon pedunculated polyps, approximately 1 cm in size, which were removed by snare polypectomy. Pathology revealed tubular adenomas.

CASE 2
IRON DEFICIENCY ANEMIA

A 38-year-old white female was referred for colonoscopy after discovery of an iron deficiency anemia and heme-positive stools. She denied any symptoms other than some easy fatiguability. She had not noted any abdominal pain or discomfort or change in her bowel pattern. Detailed family history revealed that her natural father (her parents were divorced during her infancy) had "intestinal cancer" and died before age 50. Her paternal grandmother died of "liver cancer" at the age of 42, before she was born. Physical examination was unremarkable, but her Hb was 8.2 g/dl; Hct, 24.5%; MCV, 76. After bowel preparation, colonoscopy showed a 5 × 6-cm friable, ulcerated tumor in the proximal ascending colon, which was biopsied. A small, flat 0.5-cm polyp in the sigmoid colon was also noted and treated by biopsy and fulguration. Additional laboratory tests (CEA, LFTs) were obtained. The ascending colon tumor was a poorly differentiated adenocarcinoma and the sigmoid polyp was a villous adenoma. CEA and LFTs were normal.

An exploratory laparotomy showed a normal liver and no evidence of other metastases. A total abdominal colectomy and bilateral oophorectomy was done. The specimen had a poorly differentiated adenocarcinoma with penetration to but not through the muscularis propria. None of the 56 lymph nodes found contained metastases. The patient's postoperative course was uneventful except for moderate diarrhea on regaining bowel function, which improved to 6–8 bowel movements per day at time of discharge on postoperative day 8. At 1-month follow-up, the patient was found to be doing well, with Hb, 11.2 g/dl; Hct, 34%; and having 2–3 well-formed stools per day.

GENERAL CONSIDERATIONS

Grouped together, colon and rectal cancers are the most common visceral malignancy in the United States, trailing only lung and skin cancer in overall incidence. Upward of 110,000 new cases of primary colon cancer and 40,000 new cases of rectal cancer are diagnosed in the United States each year. The incidence has remained relatively steady, increasing only in correlation with population size. Approximately 60–70% of cancers are distal to the splenic flexure and therefore potentially accesible to the standard 60-cm flexible sigmoidoscope (Fig. 33.1). Of significance, approximately 5% of patients will be found to have synchronous (occurring simultaneously) colon/rectal cancers and as many as 40% will harbor synchronous adenomatous polyps. In addition, 5% of patients will develop metachronous (occurring at a later time) colon cancers. These facts have obvious implications for patient management. All patients should have their entire colon examined preoperatively, by either colonoscopy or air-contrast barium enema. If this is not possible (Case 1) it should be done at an early postoperative time period. Also, annual postoperative surveillance of the remaining at-risk colonic and rectal mucosa is crucial. Historically, approximately 50% of colon cancer patients would succumb to the disease. With the relatively recent widespread use of effective adjuvant therapy there is cause for guarded optimism.

Greater advances can likely be achieved in the area of primary and secondary prevention, with the recognition of risk factors and liberal use of diagnostic and therapeutic endoscopy. Primary prevention is defined as "the prevention of development of disease in a susceptible population."

Is primary prevention of colon cancer possible? The answer is yes in many, if not all, cases. To examine this we must first define our "susceptible population." On one end of the spectrum is the familial adenomatous polyposis (FAP) patient, 100% of whom will develop colon cancer before age 40 if left untreated. Previously known as Gardner syndrome, this condition is caused by a genetic defect (chromosome 5) and is inherited in an autosomal dominant pattern (although up to 20% of cases are due to spontaneous mutations) (see Ch. 32). Primary prevention for these patients is prophylactic colectomy at the time of diagnosis. Other high risk groups include patients with longstanding ulcerative colitis and colonic Crohn's disease (to a lesser extent). An interesting and incompletely defined group are those with hereditary nonpolyposis colon cancer (HNPCC), or Lynch syndrome. Also an inherited syndrome (autosomal dominant), it is notable for affecting patients at a young age (mean, 46 years), a propensity for proximal colon involvement (69% proximal to the splenic flexure), and an increased incidence of synchronous (18%) and metachronous (≤40%) colon cancer. In addition, some families have specific extracolonic cancers (endometrium,

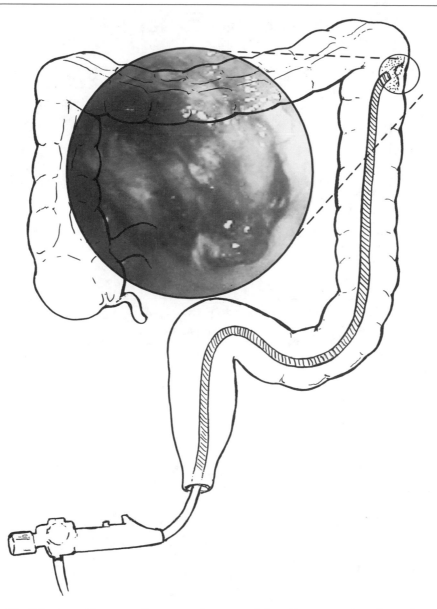

FIGURE 33.1   *Flexible sigmoidoscopy allows visualization of the colon up to the splenic flexure in most patients.*

ovary, etc.) as well (Lynch II). Lacking the characteristic features of FAP, one must rely on a detailed family history for its recognition. Case 2 represents a likely Lynch syndrome patient. The grandmother's liver cancer was likely metastatic from the colon, and the patient was appropriately treated by a total colectomy, given the high rate of metachronous cancer. Although lacking the numerous polyps of FAP patients, these cancers do seem to progress through the adenoma-carcinoma sequence as detailed in Chapter 32. Thus, primary prevention of colon cancer for any offsprings or siblings of the patient in Case 2 would consist of annual colonoscopy beginning at an early age (5–10 years less than the age of the youngest affected relative at time of diagnosis).

Most colon cancer patients, however, do not conform to an inherited syndrome or have a recognized inflammatory inciting factor. Are there any other recognized risks of adenomatous polyps or cancer? Environment is clearly implicated, primarily through dietary factors (Fig. 33.2). High fat, low fiber diets prevalent in Western industrialized countries are contributory. Increased fat intake leads to increased production of bile acids. These are deconjugated by colonic bacteria into secondary bile acids, which are known carcinogens. Fiber is thought to be protective by increasing fecal mass (dilutional) and by decreasing transit time through the colon, thus decreasing contact of colonic mucosa with fecal carcinogens. Other dietary factors (decreased vitamin D, decreased calcium intake) have also been implicated.

COLON CANCER RISK

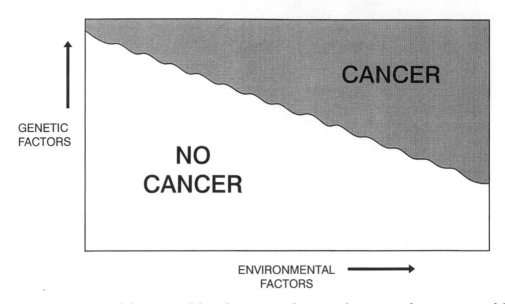

FIGURE 33.2 *A theoretical depiction of the relative contributions of genetic and environmental factors to cancer development.*

Evidence for environmental factors comes from epidemiologic studies. Native Africans have extremely low rates of colon cancer, while blacks in the United States have rates equal to whites. Further evidence comes from Japan, where native Japanese have a relatively low rate of colon cancer. After emigration to the United States, within two generations, the rate of colon cancer is nearly equal to the U.S. rate.

Age is perhaps the best recognized risk factor, with the incidence increasing significantly after 50 years, and peaking in the seventh decade. This trend is the basis for the American Cancer Society Screening Recommendations (Table 33.1).

Genetic factors are clearly contributory, even outside of an identifiable family syndrome. In fact, genetic alterations, primarily involving chromosomes 5, 17, and 18 have been identified in more than 75% of all colorectal cancers. The sequence of genetic changes in colorectal carcinogenesis is complex with multiple mutations and/or losses of genes apparently required for tumor development. The identification of these specific defects represents an exciting development in molecular biology with a myriad of po-

tential clinical applications, including targeting monoclonal antibodies for diagnostic and therapeutic benefits.

Family history is important. A first-degree relative with colon or rectal cancer imparts approximately 3 times the increased risk. Two such relatives impart up to 10 times increased risk (and raise the possibility of a familial syndrome). Personal history of breast and endometrial cancer may also be "markers" for increased risk (1.5–2 times).

Having identified high risk groups, what can we offer? Primary and secondary prevention are possible. Primary prevention options include dietary education and modification, and colonoscopy with identification and removal/destruction of premalignant lesions (adenomatous polyps).

Secondary prevention (early diagnosis and treatment to improve outcome) includes screening methods, colonoscopy, and surgery. In the absence of risk factors other than age, the 60-cm flexible sigmoidoscope is an appropriate screening tool. The finding of a cancer or adenomatous polyp mandates complete evaluation of the remaining colon. With the widespread availability and proven safety of colonoscopy, barium enema should be relegated to a lesser, complementary role. Even air-contrast barium enemas miss up to 30% of polyps and cancers, especially early tumors. Colonoscopy is more sensitive and is also potentially therapeutic or at least diagnostic.

TABLE 33.1 *American Cancer Society*

Colon and Rectal Cancer Screening Recommendations
After age 40
Annual digital rectal examination
After age 50
Fecal occult blood test and sigmoidoscopy

KEY POINTS

• When dealing with colon and rectal neoplasms, treatment and patterns of failure differ greatly

• Colon and rectal cancers most common visceral malignancy in the United States

- Approximately 60–70% of cancers are distal to splenic flexure and potentially accessible to standard 60-cm flexible sigmoidoscope (Fig. 33.1)
- Approximately 5% of patients will be found to have synchronous colon/rectal cancers
- 5% will develop metachronous colon cancers
- All patients should have entire colon examined preoperatively
- Primary prevention is defined as the prevention of development of disease in a susceptible population
- 100% of FAP patients will develop colon cancer before age 40 if untreated
- Primary prevention for FAP patients is prophylactic colectomy at time of diagnosis
- Also at high risk are patients with long-standing ulcerative colitis, colonic Crohn's disease, and HNPCC (Lynch syndrome), an inherited syndrome notable for affecting patients at mean age of 46, propensity for proximal colon involvement (69%), and increased incidence of synchronous (18%) and metachronous (40%) colon cancer
- High fat, low fiber diet also increases risk of adenomatous polyps or cancer; age perhaps best recognized risk factor
- Even air-contrast barium enemas miss up to 30% of polyps and cancers, especially early tumors
- Colonoscopy is more sensitive, and potentially therapeutic or at least diagnostic

DIAGNOSIS

The early diagnosis of colon/rectal cancer requires a high level of suspicion, with 1 of 20 Americans expected to develop colon or rectal cancer in their lifetime. Occasionally (Case 1) the diagnosis may be obvious, but more commonly the symptoms and signs are more subtle. It is critical to recognize that when diagnosed and treated before the appearance of symptoms, colon cancer is curable in more than 90% of cases. When diagnosed at a symptomatic stage, survival drops to approximately 50%. An attentive primary care physician can have more impact on patient survival than the greatest surgeon and latest adjuvant therapy!

Typically, right-sided colon cancers present with larger tumors, and a microcytic (iron deficiency) anemia (Case 2). Left-sided lesions, due to smaller lumenal diameter and increased stool consistency, present more commonly with obstructive symptoms (Case 1). Distal left-sided tumors may also exhibit obvious blood streaked stools, a symptom often attributed (by patients and even physicians) to hemorrhoids, leading to a delay in diagnosis. Blood per rectum (gross or occult) should never be attributed to hemorrhoids until proved otherwise. Conversely, current screening tests such as Hemoccult have a significant false-negative rate. A negative guaiac test in the face of an obvious risk factor or history of bleeding should never deter further investigation.

DIFFERENTIAL DIAGNOSIS

A sustained change in bowel habits, especially in a patient over age 50, should be viewed with suspicion and evaluated. Irritable bowel syndrome, a poorly understood functional intestinal disorder, will usually present with years of bowel habit irregularities. Gastrointestinal bleeding (occult or gross) is not part of this disease. A small number of patients in their fifth or sixth decade of life will present with new onset of inflammatory bowel disease (Crohn's or ulcerative colitis). Endoscopy will readily differentiate these as well as identify most infectious or other nonspecific colitis cases.

Diverticulitis is frequently encountered in the population at risk of colon cancer and is occasionally difficult to differentiate, particularly from a perforated cancer. Contrast enemas or endoscopy after resolution of the acute episode will definitively resolve most of these difficult dilemmas.

Symptomatic strictures from past diverticulitis or ischemic colitis often raise concern of a neoplasm and surgical resection may be needed for this suspicion. Endoscopy has limited this confusion and has even allowed therapeutic dilatation in selected cases.

Acute colonic ischemia often presents with left-sided abdominal pain, tenderness, and bloody diarrhea. The acute onset and rapid resolution in most cases aids in readily differentiating it from tumors, although obstructing or near obstructing lesions may cause proximal ischemia.

Iron deficiency anemia can occur from nutritional deficiency as well as from bleeding more proximally in the gastrointestinal tract (especially peptic ulcer disease). It may also result from excessive uterine bleeding in female patients.

KEY POINTS

- One of 20 Americans expected to develop colon or rectal cancer
- When diagnosed and treated before appearance of symptoms, colon cancer curable in more than 90% of cases
- Right-sided colon cancers present wth larger tumors and iron deficiency anemia; left-sided lesions, due to smaller lumenal diameter and increased stool consistency, present more often with obstructive symptoms
- Blood per rectum (gross or occult) should never be attributed to hemorrhoids until proved otherwise

TREATMENT

Having diagnosed a cancerous lesion of the colon or rectum, what further tests/studies are needed before therapy? As previously discussed, complete colonoscopy is mandatory when possible. If not possible due to an obstructing or near obstructing tumor (Case 1), at least two options exist. If intraoperative palpation of the proximal remaining colon is normal, early postoperative colonoscopy (Case 1) is acceptable, with only a slight chance of a missed synchronous cancer. A second option is to remove all of the colon proximal to the obstructing tumor with an ileocolonic or ileorectal anastomosis. This will increase the frequency of bowel movements but will be acceptable in all but very elderly patients and those with anal sphincter weakness or defects.

A combination of physical examination, carcinoembryonic antigen (CEA) levels, and liver function tests (LFTs) will identify most patients with liver metastases. Routine abdominal computed tomography (CT) scanning of patients with colon cancer has not been proven efficacious, yet is widely utilized. Possible indications include suspicion of hepatic metastases, either due to elevated CEA or LFTs (usually alkaline phosphatase) (Case 1) or the presence of hepatomegaly or ascites.

A large, possibly fixed abdominal mass may also warrant preoperative CT scanning to assess ureteral or other visceral involvement. Lastly, if laparoscopic resection is planned, CT scanning may supplant the deficiencies of laparoscopic exploration. Evaluation should also include a chest x-ray to assess for pulmonary metastases. Once we have made a diagnosis of cancer of the colon or rectum, what therapeutic options exists? On one end of the spectrum, a cancer detected in a polyp removed via colonoscopy may need no further therapy to enhance a cure. Conversely, a patient with a widely metastatic colon cancer who has minimal or no symptoms or side effects attributable to the primary tumor requires no surgical intervention. Most patients will fall between these two extremes, and will warrant surgical resection. How do we choose the extent of our surgery?

Knowledge of the patterns of tumor spread helps establish fundamental guidelines. Tumor growth begins on the mucosal surface and can spread to the wall of the bowel and/or "travel" via draining lympatics to regional lymp nodes. These lympatic channels parallel the blood supply (Fig. 33.3). Lymphatic channels only penetrate as superficially as the submucosal layer; cancers that have not penetrated to this level, therefore, have (for all practical purposes) no potential to metastasize. Less commonly, venous invasion by malignant cells occurs early, with subsequent embolization resulting in liver metastases. Cancers that have penetrated the full thickness of the colon wall can also invade adjacent structures/viscera or produce "drop" (gravitational) metastases.

These observations form the basis for our current staging systems and prognostic indices (Fig. 33.4). They also direct therapy. Outside of patients with obvious metastatic disease, preoperative staging of colon cancer is not possible with current technology. Most patients are staged at the time of surgery, with a thorough exploratory laparotomy, or by the pathologist postoperatively.

Before surgery, a cardiovascular evaluation is indicated. A mechanical bowel preparation is performed to decrease the bacterial and fecal load, utilizing purge laxatives or a large quantity of a balanced electrolyte solution. Oral and intravenous prophylactic antibiotics, effective against fecal flora, are given to decrease septic complications. At the time of initial exploration, as many as 20% of patients will have obvious hepatic metastases and between 10–20% of the remaining patients will be found to harbor occult metastases. Many of these can be detected by intraoperative ultrasound, which can detect lesions as small as 0.5 cm.

A complete and thorough examination of the remainder of the abdomen and pelvis should be conducted and the primary tumor assessed.

In the absence of evidence of incurable disease (peritoneal carcinomatosis, extensive hepatic involvement), a wide resection of the primarily involved bowel segment and its lymphatic drainage is the foundation of successful surgical therapy. If the tumor has an unpredictable lymphatic drainage pattern by the nature of its location (Fig. 33.3), a more extensive resection is indicated. This aggressive approach provides improved staging as well as a survival benefit. In palliative resections, a more limited segmental resection is justified. As previously discussed, a more extensive colon resection (i.e., total abdominal colectomy) is appropriate for patients at high risk of developing metachronous cancers as well as those with synchronous cancers (Case 2).

Rectal cancer treatment follows the same treatment principles as colon cancer, but presents the additional challenge of re-establishing intestinal continuity when possible. Before the turn of the century, treatment was primarily local (posterior approach), either transanal or parasacral. Improvements in perioperative care and technology have allowed an abdominal approach (anterior resection) with the advantage of lymphatic resection and wider tumor margins. Patients with low rectal tumors may undergo a low anterior resection, or may need a combined anterior and posterior approach to allow tumor resection (abdominal perineal resection [APR]). APR requires a permanent colostomy, as the sphincter muscles are excised along with the rectum and the cancer. Recent advances in the management of these patients include transrectal ultrasound for accurate preoperative staging and selection of appropriate candidates for sphincter salvage via a transanal (posterior) approach (limited to T1 and T2 tumors).

In the presence of apparent involvement of adjacent structures (Case 1), an en bloc resection without separation of organs is essential to preserve curability whenever possible. Separation of adherent adjacent structures dramatically increases recurrence and decreases survival (from 50–60% down to 15–20% at 5 years). Following re-establishment of bowel continuity (in most cases), any liver metastases should be addressed. Resection of liver metastases, in the setting of an otherwise negative meta-

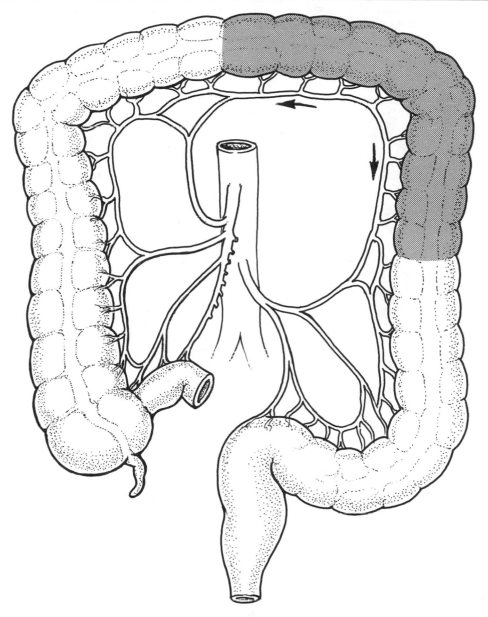

FIGURE 33.3   *The distal transverse colon and proximal descending colon (including splenic flexure) have an indeterminate blood supply and lymphatic drainage.*

static assessment, is an option. In selected populations, based largely on the stage of the primary tumor, up to 30% of these patients are cured by resection. The decision to proceed with hepatic resection at the time of colon resection or to return to the operating room at a delayed interval (usually 6–8 weeks) depends on the patient's physiologic tolerance, the extent of hepatic resection indicated, and ultimately, the surgeon's judgment. In female patients, oophorectomy may detect and treat occult ovarian metastases and prevent primary ovarian cancer (Case 2).

Following surgical treatment, as many as 30% of patients will have known incurable disease due to residual tumor burden. What is available for these patients? Adjuvant chemotherapy (5-fluorouracil and leucovorin) has been demonstrated to achieve tumor response (decreased or stable growth) but no consistent benefit in survival. Associated toxicity (nausea, vomiting, mucositis, neutropenia) can be severe and has limited its use in most centers to patients with disabling symptoms.

The remainder of the patients, with apparently curative resections, present a more promising outlook. Recent data has shown the benefit of adjuvant chemotherapy (5-fluorouracil and levamisole) for colon cancer in those patients with lymphatic involvement. Radiotherapy, usually combined with chemotherapy, is indicated (preoperatively or postoperatively) in patients with rectal cancer when the tumor is full thickness (T3) or involving local lymphatics (N1).

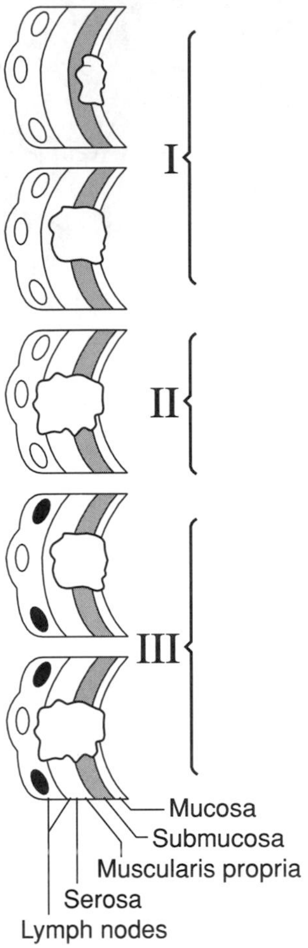

Stage	Dukes (Astler-Coller)	TNM	5-Year Survival (%)
I	A	T1N0M0	95
I	B1	T2N0M0	85
II	B2	T3N0M0	75
III	C1	T2N1M0	60[a]
III	C2	T3N1M0	55[a]

Mucosa
Submucosa
Muscularis propria
Serosa
Lymph nodes

FIGURE 33.4   *TNM staging system (with modified Dukes included for comparison) and modern prognosis.* [a]*With adjuvant chemotherapy.*

KEY POINTS

• Combination of physical examination, CEA levels, and LFTs identify most patients with liver metastases

• Evaluation should also include chest x-ray to assess for pulmonary metastases

• Tumor growth begins on mucosal surface and can spread through wall of bowel and/or travel via draining lymphatics to regional lymph nodes; these lymphatic channels parallel blood supply (Fig. 33.3)

• Outside of patients with obvious metastatic disease, preoperative staging of colon cancer is not possible with current technology

• Mechanical bowel preparation performed to decrease bacterial and fecal load, utilizing purge laxatives or large quantity of balanced electrolyte solution

• Oral and intravenous prophylactic antibiotics, effective against fecal flora, given to decrease septic complications

• At initial exploration, as many as 20% of patients will have obvious hepatic metastases and between 10–20% of remaining patients will be found to harbor occult metastases

• Wide resection of primarily involved bowel segment and lymphatic drainage is foundation of successful surgical therapy

• In presence of apparent involvement of adjacent structures, an en bloc resection without separation of organs is essential to preserve curability

• 30% of patients will have known incurable disease due to residual tumor burden

• Adjuvant chemotherapy (5-fluorouracil and leucovorin) has been demonstrated to achieve tumor response (decreased or stable growth) but no consistent benefit in survival for patients with incurable metastatic disease

• Patients with apparently curative resections have more promising outlook; recent data has shown the benefit of adjuvant chemotherapy (5-fluorouracil and levamisole) for colon cancer in patients with lymphatic involvement

FOLLOW-UP

Effective postoperative follow-up of these patients requires the recognition that any remaining colonic and rectal mucosa is at increased risk of developing neoplasia. Yearly colonoscopy with ablation/removal of any new polyps will likely prevent a second primary colonic malignancy. The primary benefit of CEA determinations is in postoperative follow-up and management. Keeping in mind the serum half-life of 7–10 days, levels can be obtained as frequently as every 6 weeks, although most clinicians follow levels every 3 months. An elevated level preoperatively that fails to return below normal (<3.0) suggests persistent (unresected) tumor. A level that is found to increase progressively postoperatively is suggestive of a recurrence and such a patient warrants an aggressive search for a potentially curative localized recurrence. It is important to note that other causes of an elevated CEA include cigarette smoking, cirrhosis, pancreatitis, inflammatory bowel disease, and renal failure. Also of importance is the observation that poorly differentiated tumors, which carry a worse prognosis, do not produce appreciable amounts of CEA and therefore do not yield elevated serum levels.

A yearly chest x-ray and frequent (possibly biannual) physical examinations and clinical history will detect a small number of early recurrences. Rectal cancer has a propensity for local recurrence, and physical examination should include digital rectal examination and/or palpation of the perineum. Recognition that only 5–7% of patients detected to have an "early recurrence" are resectable for cure, with only 25–30% of these surviving 5 years, is important to keep in mind. "Favorable" recurrence patterns include local (anastomotic) recurrence, isolated hepatic metastases, and isolated pulmonary metastases.

KEY POINTS

• Yearly colonoscopy with ablation/removal of any new polyps will likely prevent a second primary colonic malignancy

• Primary benefit of CEA determinations is in postoperative follow-up and management

• Only 5–7% of patients detected to have early recurrence are resectable for cure, with only 25–30% of these surviving 5 years

SUGGESTED READINGS

Ferguson E Jr: Operations of choice for cancers of the colon and rectum, an overview. Am Surg 50:121, 1984
A brief, to-the-point article highlighting surgical options, with decision-making points.

Jatzko G, Lisborg P, Wette V: Improving survival rates for patients with colorectal cancer. Br J Surg 79:588, 1992
Points out recent progress, cause for optimism, and directions for further improvement.

Ovaska J, Jarvinen H, Kujari H et al: Follow-up of patients operated on for colorectal carcinoma. Am J Surg 159:593, 1990
A pertinent and cogent article that looks at use and efficiency of follow-up studies on patients.

QUESTIONS

1. Characteristics of HNPCC (Lynch syndrome) include all of the following except?
   A. Proximal colon cancer involvement.
   B. Family history of colon cancer.
   C. Onset before age 40.
   D. Extracolonic cancers.

2. Hepatic metastases?
   A. Are considered as M1 disease in the TNM staging system.
   B. Are always incurable.
   C. Should always be resected if possible.
   D. Are most commonly detected on physical examination.

(See p. 604 for answers.)

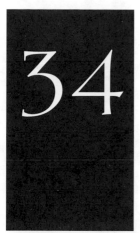

34

HEMORRHOIDS AND RECTAL PROLAPSE

CHARLES N. HEADRICK

MICHAEL J. STAMOS

Although disparate topics, these two different pathologic entities are commonly misdiagnosed by both layperson and physician alike. The inclusion of both topics in a single chapter allows us to examine their similarities and emphasize their differences. In the process, we hope to clarify common misconceptions regarding these anal/rectal disorders. We think you will see there is no one common profile particular to either diagnosis.

CASE 1
RECTAL PROLAPSE

A 33-year-old white female, who was gravida 0, para 0, presented with a chronic history of constipation and straining. She also gave a history of bright red blood per rectum and passage of mucus and "tissue" with each bowel movement. She denied any rectal pain. The prolapsed tissue reduced spontaneously at the completion of each bowel movement. She described these symptoms as lasting for the previous 4 months. She gave no history of any anal intercourse, trauma, or other significant past medical history. There had been no previous anorectal or abdominal surgery and she had no significant family history. Social history revealed that she did not smoke and was unmarried. Questions regarding her bowel habits revealed that she moved her bowels, at best, every other day, and occasionally every 3 days. There had been no history of laxative use in the past.

Physical examination revealed a healthy appearing young female. Her abdominal examination revealed a thin,

scaphoid abdomen. Examination of the perianus revealed some slight effacement of the anus. There was normal cutaneous sensation, somewhat diminished spinchter tone, and a good voluntary squeeze. There were no intra-anal masses. Anoscopy revealed prominent rectal mucosal folds with small internal hemorrhoids. These were moderately erythematous and with occasional superficial ulceration. Flexible sigmoidoscopy revealed a large rectal vault with moderate inflammation extending to the mid-rectum. She was also noted to have a redundant sigmoid colon. The remainder of her examination was normal.

The patient was asked to reproduce her symptoms by sitting on the toilet and straining. The result revealed a 3- to 5-cm circumferential prolapse that demonstrated circular, concentric folds consistent with rectal prolapse, or procidentia. The prolapse reduced spontaneously.

At the end of her consultation, the patient was counseled regarding her diagnosis. She was advised to increase the fiber in her diet and to take bulk fiber agents. A barium enema was ordered to evaluate the remainder of the colon. The air contrast enema revealed a normal mucosal outline without diverticula and a very redundant sigmoid colon. Subsequently, her bowel regimen improved to one bowel movement a day with only occasional straining during defecation. She continued to prolapse, however, with each bowel movement. Surgery was indicated because of her continued symptoms and the risk of sphincter damage. An abdominal approach was recommended as her best option. She underwent laparotomy, sigmoid resection, low rectal dissection, and rectopexy. Her postoperative recovery was uneventful.

CASE 2
RECTAL PROLAPSE
IN AN ELDERLY PATIENT

A 79-year-old white female who was gravida 4, para 4, presented with a history of constipation, stating that her rectum "falls out." She had a long history of taking laxative products (senna, herbal tea, cascara, and magnesium products). She was especially concerned because she sometimes moved her bowels without warning and soiled her undergarments. Other pertinent history revealed that she had coronary artery disease and medically controlled hypertension. She had previously undergone an abdominal hysterectomy and oophorectomy as well as an incidental appendectomy.

Physical examination revealed a moderately obese white female with lower midline abdominal scars. Rectal examination revealed both hemorrhoidal and rectal prolapse. The prolapse was easily reducible, but came back out with a moderate increase in intra-abdominal pressure. Digital examination revealed a diminished sphincter tone. Some soilage of stool and mucus was noted on her undergarments. Preoperative workup included contrast enema and flexible sigmoidoscopy. Anal manometry revealed a low-resting sphincter pressure.

The patient was deemed to be at high risk of an abdominal operation, and a perineal approach was recommended. The patient subsequently underwent perineal rectosigmoidectomy under spinal anesthesia. Postoperatively, the patient did well. Her prolapse was cured and she had perceptible improvement in her continence.

CASE 3
HEMORRHOIDAL PROLAPSE

A 43-year-old Hispanic male with a history of straining and constipation came in complaining of bright red blood per rectum. He denied pain. He was found to have prolapse revealing radial folds (hemorrhoidal prolapse) and anemia of 8 g Hb. Preoperative workup included a colonoscopy, which was normal, followed by surgical hemorrhoidectomy.

CASE 4
THROMBOSED EXTERNAL
HEMORRHOID

A 25-year-old male came in complaining of anal swelling and a sudden onset of pain. The patient recently had severe gastroenteritis with diarrhea. Physical examination revealed a thrombosed external hemorrhoid. Treatment consisted of excision in the office under local anesthesia.

GENERAL CONSIDERATIONS

Hemorrhoidal disease is very common. The number of over-the-counter remedies available is proof enough. Hemorrhoids are actually present in every person and have a normal physiologic function. They cushion the fecal bolus as it is expelled from the rectal reservoir and contribute to normal continence. Poor diet and hygiene, increases in intra-abdominal pressure, and family history may contribute to the development of abnormal hemorrhoids, which usually manifest as enlargement and/or inflammation. Hemorrhoids are classified as internal or external, based on their relationship to the dentate line. Distal to this junction of mucous membrane and anoderm there is normal somatic sensation. Proximal to this line, there is a transitional zone, measuring from 1 to 1.5 cm, in which sensation is lessened as the somatic sensory apparatus is diminished. It is in this zone, proximal to the dentate line, where internal hemorrhoids reside (Fig. 34.1). Symptomatic internal hemorrhoids may cause discomfort, prolapse, or even hemorrhage without pain to the individual (painless bleeding). External hemorrhoids rarely bleed, but may cause significant pain (Case 4) associated with thrombosis. Hemorrhoids may also bridge this anatomic boundary (mixed type) (Fig. 34.2).

Hemorrhoids have no sexual predilection, and span the range of ages. Certain conditions may predispose toward the formation of hemorrhoids: constipation, chronic diarrhea, and pregnancy. The most common causes of constipation are inadequate fluid intake, poor diet (low fiber intake), and infrequent exercise. There are also a number of medications that can cause constipation (calcium channel blockers, tricyclic antidepressants, diuretics).

Hemorrhoidal prolapse constitutes a special situation in hemorrhoidal disease. The tissue has enlarged enough to be partially expelled during defecation. A grading system is used to describe enlarged internal hemorrhoids: (1) grade I—enlarged hemorrhoidal tissue, (2) grade II—hemorrhoidal tissue that prolapses with straining but spontaneously reduces, (3) grade III—hemorrhoidal prolapse that requires manual replacement, and (4) grade IV—unreducible prolapse. Anatomic orientation is also helpful as one person may have coexisting grades of hemorrhoids. Left, right, anterior, posterior, and lateral are the

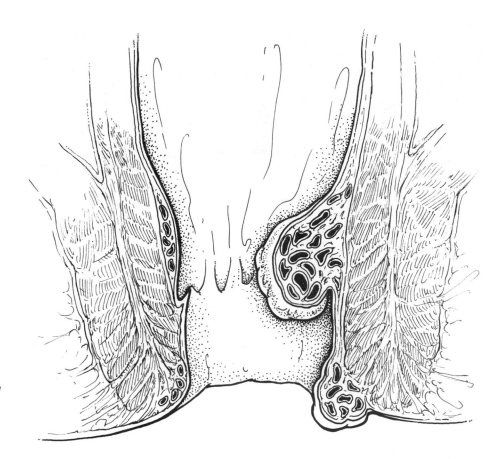

FIGURE 34.1 *Internal hemorrhoids, by definition, are lined by mucosa and rise above the dentate line. External hemorrhoids are lined by anoderm (skin).*

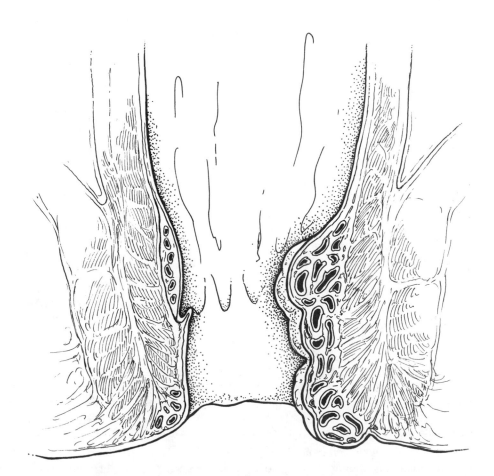

FIGURE 34.2 *The hemorrhoidal plexus may engorge and form collaterals to develop into a combined internal/external hemorrhoid.*

labels used to describe hemorrhoidal location. The typical distribution of hemorrhoids include left lateral, right anterior, and right posterior columns.

True rectal prolapse, or procidentia, can be confused with prolapse of hemorrhoids or mucosal prolapse. In true rectal prolapse, there is a full thickness prolapse. The rectum actually turns "inside out," similar to an intussusception. This situation connotes a loss of pelvic support and carries with it a risk of incontinence (Case 2)—either through stretching of the pudendal nerve or direct physical trauma to the sphincter complex.

Unlike hemorrhoidal disease, rectal prolapse is more common in women (Cases 1 and 2) (6:1 female/male) and can occur at any age (even in the newborn). Historically, it was thought to be associated with multiparous, elderly females, but may also occur in a young male or a nulliparous young female (Case 1). Doctors and patients alike may be confused by the symptoms and sensations of this ailment and frequently attribute them to hemorrhoids.

KEY POINTS

• Hemorrhoids present in every person and have a normal physiologic function

• Hemorrhoids classified as internal or external, based on relationship to dentate line

• Symptomatic internal hemorrhoids may cause discomfort, prolapse, or even hemorrhage without pain to the individual (painless bleeding)

• External hemorrhoids rarely bleed, but may cause significant pain associated with thrombosis

---

DIAGNOSIS

Diagnosis of these anorectal problems is based on a careful history and thorough physical examination. Ancillary tests such as air contrast barium enema and anal manometry may be helpful after the diagnosis is secure.

History taking for anal/rectal disorders can be very helpful in making a diagnosis. Particular attention should be directed toward the patient's diet, bowel habits, and description of any symptoms. This should include the average number of bowel movements per day or week, the presence of straining or any sensation or prolapse, the amount of time spent on the toilet, and the characteristics of any blood found during the movement. Associated abdominal complaints and concurrent usage of medication should also be discussed. Additionally, prior anorectal, abdominal, or pelvic surgery should be detailed, with particular attention given to vaginal childbirth, episiotomies, and/or tears.

As with any anal/rectal disorder, the following elements are essential to a good examination: (1) inspection of the perianus, including rudimentary sensory examination, (2)

digital examination to evaluate the canal for masses, tenderness, and sphincter tone, (3) anoscopy to examine the anal canal visually, (4) flexible sigmoidoscopy to visually examine the rectum and lower colon, and (5) when prolapse is suspected, visual examination of the anus and perineum during straining, preferably while sitting or squatting.

External hemorrhoids are visible on simple inspection, and in the noninflamed state simply may appear as fleshy skin covered protrusions (tags). They may become inflamed and edematous or may thrombose. Thrombosis (usually an acute event brought on by straining, constipation, or diarrhea), is typically very painful (Case 4). A firm tender mass is palpated adjacent to the anal canal. The mass may have a dark, bluish appearance. The overlying skin is usually normal although central ulceration is not uncommon due to pressure necrosis. The tenderness is localized to the thrombosis itself, unlike an abscess.

Internal hemorrhoids can only be appreciated adequately by visualization, either by inspection if prolapsed or by anoscopy. Palpation is unreliable in the diagnosis of internal hemorrhdoids.

Rectal prolapse can be difficult to diagnose. Even though the patient may report frequent prolapse, reproducing the event in the doctor's office may be difficult. Frequently, the experience can be embarrassing for the patient and even the physician. Often, the patient can only produce the prolapse while squatting and straining. A bathroom adjacent to the examination room is helpful for this part of the examination. When the prolapse is reproduced, it may protrude 1–2 cm or up to 15–20 cm. Rarely, a patient will present with an incarcerated prolapse, which should be treated as a surgical emergency.

Although flexible sigmoidoscopy is usually adequate, a more thorough colonic examination (colonoscopy, air contrast enema) may be helpful. Rarely, a tumor can act as a "bedpost" for intussusception or prolapse. Laboratory studies are not helpful in making the diagnosis, although the presence of anemia should mandate a full colonic evaluation.

KEY POINTS

• As with any anal/rectal disorder, the following elements are essential to good examination: inspection of perianus, digital examination, anoscopy, and flexible sigmoidoscopy

• Internal hemorrhoids can only be appreciated adequately by visualization, either by inspection if prolapsed or by anoscopy

---

DIFFERENTIAL DIAGNOSIS

The main difficulty in diagnosing these conditions is in distinguishing them from one another. True rectal prolapse produces circumferential mucosal folds while hemorrhoidal prolapse yields radial folds (Figs. 34.3 and

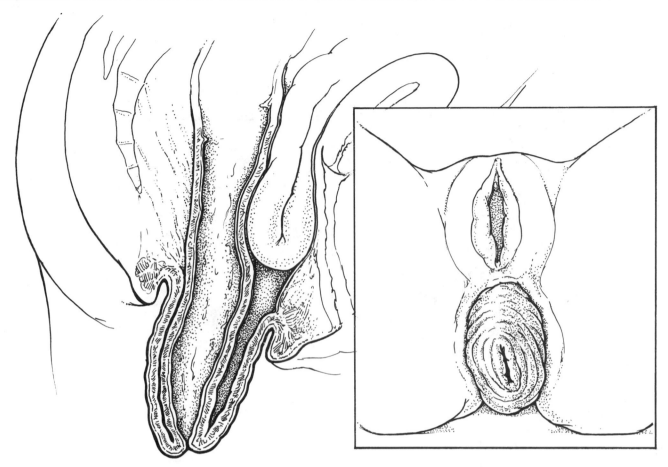

FIGURE 34.3 *True rectal prolapse. Note the circumferential mucosal folds and the sulcus outside the prolapse (fixation of the dentate line).*

34.4). Likewise, true rectal prolapse does not include the dentate line, leaving a deep sulcus outside of the prolapsed tissue.

Other tumors may also prolapse through the anal canal and be mistaken for hemorrhoids. Rectal polyps, tumors, and hypertrophied anal papillae are the most common. These are readily identified by anoscopy or proctosigmoidoscopy.

TREATMENT

Successful treatment of hemorrhoids requires an accurate diagnosis and elimination of other perianal disease as the cause of the patient's complaints. Since hemorrhoids are a normal part of human anatomy, they will invariably be present but may not be contributing to the patient's problems. Indeed, other pathology (e.g., anal fissures, proctitis) frequently will exacerbate existing hemorrhoids. Failure to appreciate and treat the primary disease process will likely lead to failure of therapy.

Internal hemorrhoids may be treated medically, with office treatments, or with surgery. The decision rests on the symptomatology and physical examination. For complaints of minor bleeding associated with bowel movements ("outlet bleeding"), dietary counseling and fiber supplementation (psyllium) may be adequate, although flexible sigmoidoscopy is mandatory to eliminate a distal colon or rectal cancer as the possible cause of the bleeding. For prolapse, or bleeding associated with prolapse, additional treatment is required. A variety of office treatments may be used, although sclerotherapy and rubber band ligation are the most commonly employed. All of these office based treatments are "fixation" techniques. They work primarily by creating scar tissue locally that "fixes" the mucosa overlying the hemorrhoid to the underlying internal sphincter muscle. Surgical treatment, including laser treatment, is reserved for more severe disease (Case 3) and for patients with associated external hemorrhoids that are not amenable to office treatment. Laser hemorrhoidectomy is identical to standard surgical hemorrhoidectomy in every parameter studied. Its only apparent advantage is in marketing. The disadvantage is solely in cost.

External hemorrhoids may also be treated medically or with surgery. Topically applied creams may help shrink

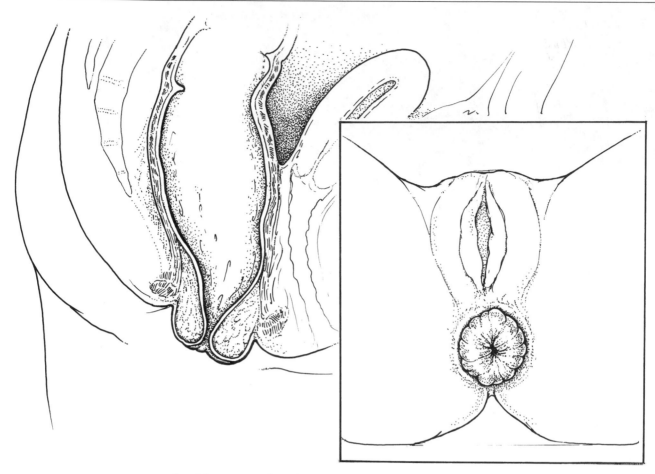

FIGURE 34.4 *Hemorrhoidal or mucosal prolapse. Note the radial folds and absence of rectal wall (muscle) within the prolapse.*

edematous and inflamed tissue, but office surgery is sometimes required to solve an acute painful process such as thrombosis (Case 4). On rare occasions, circumferential thrombosis is best treated in the operating room with anesthetic blockade.

As a rule of thumb, it should be remembered that most hemorrhoidal problems can be solved without surgical intervention.

Treatment for procidentia, unfortunately, does not enjoy the same success rate as hemorrhoidectomy. Once diagnosed, the solution is surgical, but the choices for repair are numerous. They fall into three basic categories: (1) anal encirclement procedures (Thiersch), (2) perineal approaches (Altmeier or Delorme), and (3) abdominal approaches.

Historically, the circlage, or Thiersch procedure, has been around the longest. The prolapse is reduced and maintained by reinforcing the external sphincter mechanism with a permanent material placed outside of the sphincter mechanism and underneath the skin. The recurrence and infection rates are high. It is now reserved for the very infirm.

Perineal solutions have enjoyed a resurgence in popularity, particularly among the elderly patient population, since the operation is performed under regional anesthesia. It involves resection or plication of the redundant bowel via the anal canal. Although this does not treat any underlying cause of the problem, the recurrence rate is somewhat lower than an encircling procedure and the operation is quite safe.

The abdominal approach has the lowest recurrence rate but also the greatest morbidity. Evaluation of the anatomy is more complete and the operation can be combined with a resection, rectopexy, or very low dissection. Most versions include a very low dissection in order to create a plane of scarring in the retrorectal space. The risks are the same as for low anterior resection. Choice of operation is based on an individual's activity, experience, and preference of the surgeon.

It should be noted that the pathophysiology of procidentia is not completely understood. A weakening of the pelvic floor leads to the intussusception or prolapse, but the role of bowel function and motility is not fully appreciated as a precursor to this event.

KEY POINTS

• Successful treatment of hemorrhoids requires accurate diagnosis and elimination of other perianal disease as the cause of patient complaint; since hemorrhoids are normal human anatomy, will invariably be present, but may not be contributing to patient's problem

• Rule of thumb: majority of hemorrhoidal problems can be solved without surgical intervention

FOLLOW-UP

Hemorrhoid disease and symptoms tend to recur in time if the inciting cause is not altered. The more conservative the therapy, the more likely the onset of recurrent symptoms. Follow-up should therefore emphasize avoidance of constipation and include dietary counseling.

Postoperative follow-up, however, should be done in a rigorous fashion to avoid the preventable complications—stenosis, prolonged pain, and constipative bowel habit. Counseling the patient on high fiber diet, hygiene, and pain control should be done both in the pre- and postoperative phase. Postoperative examinations should be done every 2 weeks until adequate healing has taken place to avoid postoperative stricture and stenosis. This may last up to 12 weeks. Additional informational exchanges can also take place on the telephone to eliminate anxiety and answer simple questions.

Rectal prolapse operations all carry a significant incidence of recurrence, perineal operations more so than abdominal operations. Although the exact cause of prolapse is unknown, avoidance of constipation and straining is felt to be important. Fecal incontinence is common in patients with prolapse (Case 2), and improvement is seen in approximately 50% of patients following operation. However, optimal function may take up to 6 months to achieve.

SUGGESTED READINGS

Corman ML: Rubber band ligation of hemorrhoids. Arch Surg 112:1257, 1977

Simplified technical description of the most common technique used for internal hemorrhoid treatment.

Huber FT, Stein H, Siewert JR: Functional results after treatment of rectal prolapse with rectopexy and sigmoid resection. World Surg 19:138, 1995.

Prospective study looking not just at anatomic but also functional results.

Loder KM, Kamm MA, Nicholls RJ, Phillips RKS: Hemorrhoids: pathology, pathophysiology and aetiology. Br J Surg 81:946, 1994

Comprehensive review focusing on pathophysiology.

Williams JG, Madoff RD: Perineal repair for rectal prolapse. Prob Gen Surg 9:732, 1992

Outlines perineal approach and options.

QUESTIONS

1. *Internal hemorrhoids?*
   A. Typically cause pain associated with bowel movements.
   B. Are universally present.
   C. Are most appropriately treated with the laser.
   D. Are readily diagnosed on digital examination.

2. *Rectal prolapse?*
   A. Can be difficult to differentiate from internal hemorrhoids.
   B. Is best treated surgically.
   C. Can lead to fecal incontinence.
   D. May be treated via an abdominal approach.
   E. All of the above.

(See p. 604 for answers.)

Case I. Declan Maguire.

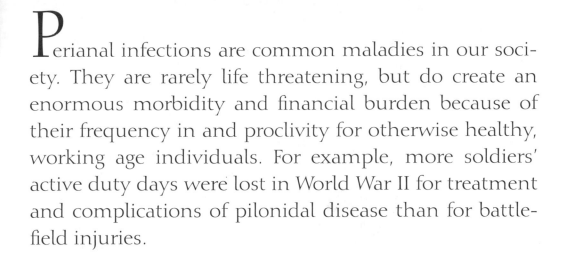

35

ANORECTAL ABSCESSES, FISTULAS, AND PILONIDAL DISEASE

MICHAEL J. STAMOS

Perianal infections are common maladies in our society. They are rarely life threatening, but do create an enormous morbidity and financial burden because of their frequency in and proclivity for otherwise healthy, working age individuals. For example, more soldiers' active duty days were lost in World War II for treatment and complications of pilonidal disease than for battlefield injuries.

CASE 1
PERIANAL ABSCESS

A 23-year-old male graduate student presented to the emergency room with a complaint of pain in the perianal area for the past 3 days. He was otherwise healthy. On examination, a 3-cm fluctuant mass was noted in the right posterolateral aspect of his perianal skin, approximately 2 cm from the anal opening (anal verge). No other abnormalities were noted. After infiltration with local anesthesia, a cruciate incision was made over the mass and 10 ml of purulent fluid drained under pressure. The patient was sent home with instructions and did well, but complained of persistent discharge from the region 2 months later.

CASE 2
ISCHIORECTAL ABSCESS

A 53-year-old female with a history of diabetes mellitus developed fevers, pelvic discomfort, and difficulty in controlling her glucose. Her primary care physician suspected a UTI but a spot urinalysis was normal. Due to discomfort on rectal examination, she was referred to a surgeon for suspicion of a anorectal abscess. She was noted to have a temperature of 38.6°C and a WBC count of 18,000. The surgeon evaluated her the same day and was unable to appreciate a definite abscess, but was concerned enough about infection in a diabetic to administer antibiotics and take her to the operating room for an examination under anesthesia.

At operation, a suspicious area in the left ischiorectal fossa was identified, and an incision through the overlying skin released a large (250 ml) foul smelling abscess. A drain was placed and the patient was treated with a 48-hour course of antibiotics and discharged home on the third hospital day with local wound care instructions. She was followed as an outpatient and eventually full healing was accomplished 6 weeks later.

A GENERAL CONSIDERATIONS

Anorectal abscess and fistulas (fistula-in-ano) represent different phases of a disease process that usually, in greater than 95% of cases, begins in the anal crypts and glands.

The crypts communicate with the anal canal at the level of the dentate line and function to lubricate the anal canal with secretions from the anal glands. The glands (and crypts) are of endodermal origin and therefore lie superficial to the external sphincter (mesoderm), either in the intersphincteric plane or within the internal sphincter or submucosa (Fig. 35.1). Obstruction of an anal crypt or gland causes an abscess to form (initially) at the location of the gland. This abscess will then grow locally and may

spread in any direction (Fig. 35.2). If the spread is through the adjacent external sphincter muscle, the ischiorectal fossa is involved (Case 2), an area prone to extensive infection due to its normal occupancy by poorly vascularized fatty tissue. Alternatively, the infection may spread caudally in the intersphincteric plane to the perianal region (perianal abscess), cranially to produce a supralevator abscess (rare), circumferentially to develop a so-called horseshoe abscess, or in some combination.

A fistula will develop in one-half to two-thirds of surgically drained abscesses due to persistence of the communication between the anal crypt and the location of the abscess. Anorectal fistulas are classified as intersphincteric, transsphincteric, suprasphincteric, or extrasphincteric. These differentiations simply describe the relationship between the fistula tract and the internal and external sphincter muscles. Occasionally, perianal fistulas are secondary to noncryptogenic sources, such as trauma (including iatrogenic), Crohn's disease (see Ch. 30) and intra-abdominal/pelvic infection (extrasphincteric).

Pilonidal disease is a poorly understood skin disease that occurs in the superior aspect of the midline gluteal cleft. Erroneously termed pilonidal cysts in the past, these problems arise as a result of the unique set of forces at work in the region. Due to the attachment and tethering of

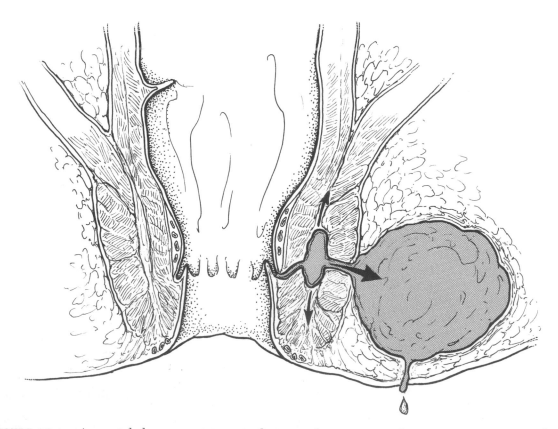

FIGURE 35.1   *Anorectal abscesses originate in the intersphincteric space but may progress across the external sphincter (transsphincteric) to develop an ischiorectal abscess.*

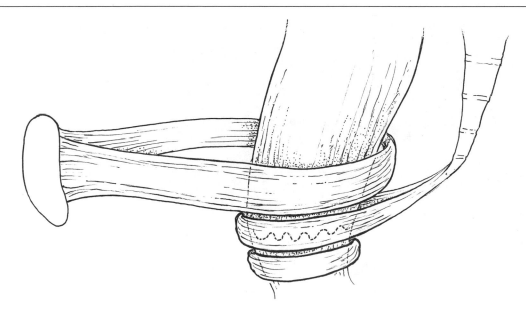

FIGURE 35.2 *The external sphincter is actually (somewhat arbitrarily) separated into three components. Anorectal abscesses develop in the intersphincteric plane and may spread in any direction.*

the skin in the midline to the underlying sacrum and coccyx, hair from the surrounding region is "drawn" into the midline cleft. Repetitive motion (e.g., riding on a bumpy road, horseback riding) may exacerbate this process. Hirsutism and obesity are recognized risk factors. The shaft of the hair will break down the skin, causing small sinuses to be produced in the cleft. Due to bacterial presence and growth, subcutaneous abscesses develop and smolder. The subsequent cavity is not epithelial-lined (and hence not a cyst), but is often full of hair (pilo-hair/nidal-nest).

KEY POINTS

- Anorectal abscess and fistulas (fistula-in-ano) represent different phases of disease process that, in more than 95% of cases, begins in anal crypts and glands

- Glands (and crypts) are of endodermal origin and therefore lie superficial to external sphincter (mesoderm), either in intersphincteric plane or within internal sphincter or submucosa (Fig. 35.1)

- Fistulas will develop in one-half to two-thirds of surgically drained abscesses due to persistence of communication between anal crypt and abscess location

- Anorectal fistulas are classified as intersphincteric, transsphincteric, suprasphincteric, or extrasphincteric

- Pilonidal disease is a poorly understood skin disease that occurs in the superior aspect of midline gluteal cleft

DIAGNOSIS

The diagnosis of an anorectal abscess is usually simple and straightforward. The patient, frequently a young male (Case 1), will complain of unremitting pain in or around the anus. Systemic signs of infection (fever, tachycardia) are uncommon except in immunocompromised patients (e.g., diabetics) (Case 2) or with delay in presentation/recognition. Laboratory evaluation contributes little or nothing to the diagnosis. Physical examination should be conducted in a well-lit area with appropriate attention to the patient's dignity. Accessory lights are essential, as is proper patient positioning. If a special examination table is available, the prone jackknife position gives optimal exposure, although the left lateral position (left side down, hips and knees fully flexed) will suffice. Inspection of the perianal region will often show an erythematous, swollen site of the abscess (Case 1). Gentle palpation will reveal fluctuance and tenderness as well as warmth. Crepitance is an ominous sign that signifies an advancing, necrotizing infection. If no abscess is seen, digital rectal examination and/or "bimanual" examination with careful palpation of the ischiorectal fossa should elicit point tenderness or "fullness." Particular attention should be directed to the presacral area (deep postanal space). When the clinical suspicion remains high despite an equivocal examination, an examination under anesthesia in the operating room is the appropriate option (Case 2). Computed tomography scans and other radiologic examination are of no value in the patient with an anorectal abscess.

Fistula-in-ano typically presents with a patient complaint of drainage from the anal area. Pain may be present, as may pruritus (itching). Importantly, the patient often has a history of a prior abscess that may have drained spontaneously. Examination should reveal the site of the external (secondary) opening where the drainage is noted by the patient. The fistula tract is usually palpable, coursing toward the anal canal and the internal (primary) opening at the dentate line. Goodsall's rule is helpful (Fig. 35.3) and states

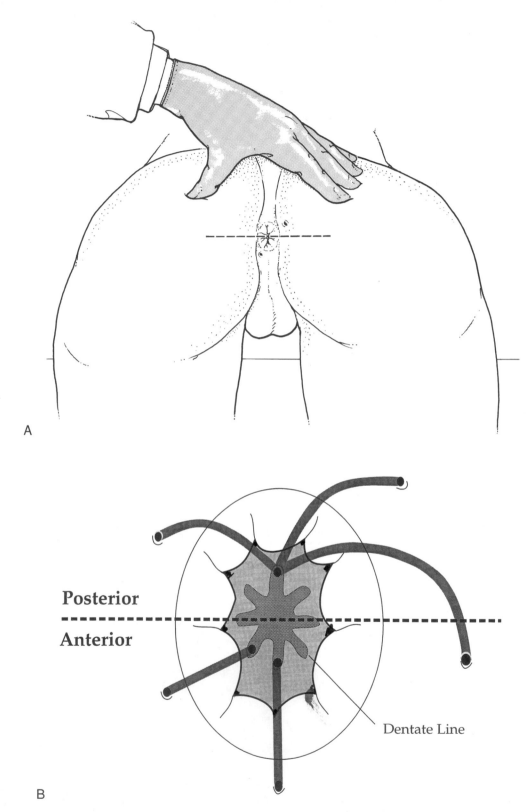

Posterior

Anterior

Dentate Line

A

B

FIGURE 35.3 *Goodsall's rule predicts the location of the internal opening of the fistula (see text for details).* **(A)** *Patient examination.* **(B)** *Diagram of Goodsall's rule.*

that secondary openings found in one of the posterior quadrants usually originate from the posterior midline, while secondary openings found in the anterior quadrants originate from a primary source at the dentate line oriented in a radial direction (i.e., straight tract).

Pilonidal disease may present as an acute abscess or as a chronic sinus. An abscess in this region is obvious, and the primary site of origin in the midline can usually be identified. Chronic pilonidal disease produces pain and drainage, and examination shows induration and scarring with one or more sinus tracts or openings. The key element in the diagnosis is the location of the process on and around the midline at the superior aspect of the gluteal cleft (Fig. 35.4).

> **K E Y   P O I N T S**
>
> • Crepitance is an ominous sign that signifies advancing, necrotizing infection

DIFFERENTIAL DIAGNOSIS

The most common diseases that may masquerade as an anorectal abscess are a thrombosed external hemorrhoid or an anal fissure, primarily due to their high prevalence. A thrombosed external hemorrhoid will typically have a bluish appearance, although the diagnosis may require incision/excision (see Ch. 34) (Fig. 35.4).

An anal fissure is a tear in the anoderm superficial to the dentate line. A common malady, it usually causes pain and minimal rectal bleeding and is aggravated by bowel movements. Confusion occasionally arises when severe pain/tenderness prevents adequate examination. In this situation, examination under anesthesia allows easy diagnosis.

Recurrent abscess and/or fistulas should raise the suspicion of Crohn's disease (see Ch. 30), especially if diarrhea and/or weight loss are present. Hidradenitis suppurativa is a disease of the apocrine glands that causes soft tissue infections, particularly in the perianal, groin, and axillary regions. These chronic, recurrent infections may be difficult to differentiate from complicated fistula-in-ano or even pilonidal disease. Involvement of other areas of the body is an important distinguishing feature.

TREATMENT

Most anorectal abscesses can be easily and safely drained in the emergency room or office. Local anesthesia followed by excision of an ellipse of skin is adequate. Packing of the wound should not be done except for the purpose of hemostasis, and probing with an instrument or finger is unnecessary and extremely painful. If the patient is immunocompromised or displays systemic signs of sepsis, pretreatment antibiotics should be administered, and treatment in the operating room is indicated. Post-treatment antibiotics are only indicated if evidence of cellulitis coexists. Antibiotics alone without surgical drainage are inadequate therapy. Hospital admission is required only for a small percentage of patients. At home, treatment consists of warm soaks (sitz baths) and avoidance of constipation, as well as local hygiene.

Before drainage of any anorectal abscess, the patient should be alerted to the possibility of progression to a fistula-in-ano. If treatment in the operating room is chosen, anoscopic examination should be done with an attempt at localization of the internal origin (offending crypt). Careful documentation of the site will make subsequent management easier if a fistula develops.

Successful fistula-in-ano treatment requires identification of the crypt of origin. Usually, palpation of the perianal region will reveal the location. Most fistulas are best treated by laying open the tract (fistulotomy). In the process, a variable amount of sphincter muscle is divided and defunctionalized. Caution should be observed, therefore, in patients at risk of incontinence. Anatomic factors are also important, as high transsphincteric fistulas and anterior fistulas (due to the normal anatomic weakness in this region) should be managed in alternative ways. These alternatives always include cryptectomy as part of the treatment. Options include anorectal advancement flaps and use of setons (see Suggested Readings). A seton is an elastic band or large suture that is passed through the fistula from the primary (internal) to the secondary (external) opening and the two free ends are joined tightly. Setons work by cutting through the muscle slowly (weeks) to effectively eradicate the tract, but also to bridge the resultant muscle gap with fibrosis (scar) and preserve some function.

Pilonidal disease should be treated like an abscess, with incision rather than excision. Attempts to keep the scar off the midline may lessen recurrence, and it is important to shave the adjacent area until healing is complete.

> **K E Y   P O I N T S**
>
> • Most anorectal abscess can be easily and safely drained in the emergency room or office; local anesthesia followed by excision of an ellipse of skin is adequate
>
> • Before drainage of any anorectal abscess, the patient should be alerted to the possibility of progression to fistula-in-ano
>
> • Successful fistula-in-ano treatment requires identification of crypt of origin
>
> • Most fistulas are best treated by laying open the tract (fistulotomy); in the process, a variable amount of sphincter muscle is divided and defunctionalized
>
> • Pilonidal disease should be treated like an abscess, with incision rather than excision

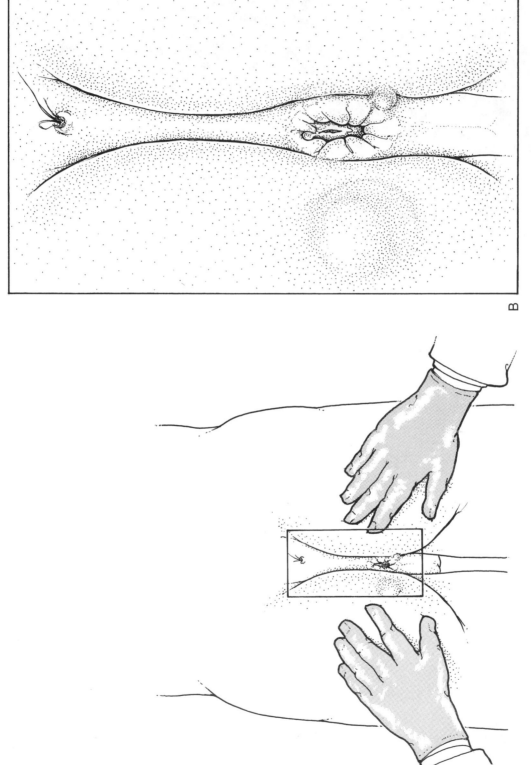

FIGURE 35.4 (**A** & **B**) A variety of maladies commonly occur in a limited anatomic area, including pilonidal disease, anal fissures, perirectal abscesses, and perianal abscesses.

FOLLOW-UP

Following drainage of an anorectal abscess, patients should be seen in 1–2 weeks to ensure adequate drainage. Following this, persistence of drainage beyond 4–6 weeks usually signifies formation of a fistula (Case 1). After complete healing of an abscess drainage site or fistulotomy site, no follow-up is necessary. Dietary fiber supplements may prevent recurrence. Follow-up after pilonidal treatment must be diligent until healing is complete. Education of the patient to the signs/symptoms of early recurrence may allow easier treatment.

SUGGESTED READINGS

Parks AG, Gordon PH, Hardcastle JD: A classification of fistula-in-ano. Br J Surg 63:1, 1976

A classic treatise with exceptional anatomic descriptions.

Seow Choen F, Nicholls RJ: Anal fistula. Br J Surg 79:197, 1992

Excellent review of pathogenesis and treatment options.

McCourtney JS, Finlay IG: Setons in the surgical management of fistula-in-ano. Br J Surg 82:448, 1995

Shemesh EI, Kodney IJ, Fry RD, Neufeld DM: Endorectal sliding flap repair of complicated anterior anoperineal fistulas. Dis Colon Rect 31:22, 1988

The above articles outline the management options for complex, high-risk fistulas.

QUESTIONS

1. *Anorectal abscesses?*
   A. Should be treated initially with broad spectrum antibiotics.
   B. Should always be drained in the operating room.
   C. Are usually due to viral infections.
   D. May evolve into a fistula following simple drainage.
   E. All of the above.

2. *Effective treatment of anal fistulas requires?*
   A. Identification of the internal opening (offending crypt).
   B. Understanding of local sphincter anatomy.
   C. Adequate drainage of any associated abscess.
   D. All of the above.

3. *Pilonidal disease?*
   A. Is a cystic process originating from the neuroenteric canal.
   B. Should be treated by excision.
   C. Is a soft tissue infection.
   D. Is best treated with antibiotics.

(See p. 604 for answers.)

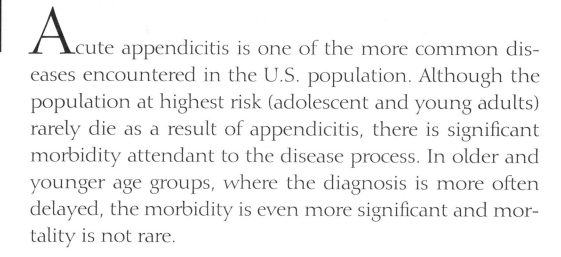

36

ACUTE

APPENDICITIS

MICHAEL J. STAMOS

Acute appendicitis is one of the more common diseases encountered in the U.S. population. Although the population at highest risk (adolescent and young adults) rarely die as a result of appendicitis, there is significant morbidity attendant to the disease process. In older and younger age groups, where the diagnosis is more often delayed, the morbidity is even more significant and mortality is not rare.

CASE 1
ACUTE APPENDICITIS

A 17-year-old white female presented to the emergency room with a 36-hour history of abdominal pain, originating in the periumbilical region and now localized to the right lower quadrant. She also reported anorexia with one episode of minimal nonbilius emesis. She reported feeling febrile, but had not measured her temperature. She denied any previous episodes and reported that she was sexually active with one steady partner. She also denied any history of sexually transmitted diseases and had never been pregnant. Her menstrual history was noncontributory and her last menstrual period was 10 days earlier.

On physical examination, she was noted to have a mildly distended abdomen with normal to slightly hypoactive bowel sounds. No scars were noted and she was tender to moderate palpation in both lower quandrants, right slightly greater than left. There was no rebound tenderness, negative psoas sign, and negative Rovsing's sign. Pelvic examination showed mild to moderate cervical motion tenderness and rectal examination was normal except for moderate tenderness on the right side in the supralevator region. Her WBC count was 11,000/mm³ with a left shift, normal Hb and Hct, and a urinalysis with small

amount of ketones and otherwise normal. An abdominal x-ray showed a nonspecific bowel gas pattern.

She was admitted for observation, was resuscitated with intravenous fluids, and 6 hours later, upon re-examination, was noted to be persistently tender and was taken to the operating room where laparoscopy confirmed acute nonperforated appendicitis. A laparoscopic appendectomy was performed. The patient was discharged home 48 hours later.

CASE 2
PERFORATED APPENDICITIS

A 28-year-old black male presented to the emergency room with a 24-hour history of right flank pain and fever to 38.8°C. The patient reported feeling fine the day prior and noted that the onset of the pain was gradual and was currently only moderate in severity. He also reported watery bowel movements for the past 48 hours, occurring five to six times a day. He denied any previous similar episodes, denied any recent travel outside of the United States, and also reported that no other family members or friends were currently ill. He otherwise felt well and had a normal appetite and denied nausea and vomiting. He did admit to increased frequency of urination in the past 3 days but denied nocturia or dysuria.

On physical examination, the patient was noted to be a healthy appearing young black male in apparent mild distress. His temperature was 38.7°C, HR, 118 bpm; and respiratory rate, 14 breaths/min. His heart and lung examination were normal and he had only mild tenderness deep in the right lower abdominal quadrant and iliac fossa. He had moderate CVA tenderness on the right side, a strongly positive psoas sign on the right, and a negative obturator and Rovsing's sign. Laboratory evaluation included a WBC count of 18,000/mm^3 with a left shift and a normal Hb and Hct. A urinalysis showed two to five WBC per high power field, and no bacteria, and a KUB demonstrated a nonspecific bowel gas pattern with an absent psoas shadow on the right side. An ultrasound showed a complex periappendiceal mass consistent with perforated appendicitis. He was given intravenous fluids and broad spectrum antibiotics. At laparotomy, on exploration, a phlegmonous mass was noted. With some difficulty the appendix was located and removed and the base of the appendix oversewn. A small amount of purulent fluid was present and drains were placed in the area. The fascia was closed and the skin left open to heal by secondary intention. He was continued on intravenous antibiotics for 5 days. The drains were advanced and after a 7-day hospitalization the patient was discharged home with wound care instructions.

GENERAL CONSIDERATIONS

The vermiform appendix is a largely vestigial organ in humans. In its normal position in the right lower quadrant, as an extension of the cecum, it is lined with normal colonic epithelium, but its wall is rich in lymphatic tissue. This abundance of lymphatic tissue gives support to the theory that the appendix once played an important role in the immune system, a role that has been diminished with evolution. Appendicitis denotes inflammation of the appendix, usually involving the distal portion of the appendix for a variable length, and usually caused by obstruction of its lumen at some point along its length. In the pediatric population, this obstruction is often caused by inflammation and engorgement of the lymphatic tissue; in adults it is more commonly due to a fecalith or foreign body (vegetable matter). Once started, this inflammation will rapidly progress to a transmural process and lead eventually to necrosis and at least localized peritonitis (Case 2).

Appendicitis is exceedingly common and its manifestations are diverse, although most cases are relatively easy to recognize. Most of the morbidity and occasional mortality of this disease is related to complications of transmural necrosis and perforation. It follows, therefore, that delay in diagnosis and therapy is in large part responsible for the morbidity and mortality.

Two overriding factors contribute to a continued, steady incidence of 10–15% of clinically perforated appendicitis. The first is the lack of a noninvasive, sensitive, and specific means of making or confirming the diagnosis of acute appendicitis. The second is the considerable expense and definable morbidity associated with a negative appendectomy, which leads physicians to wait until the diagnosis is obvious because of the advanced disease.

Acute appendicitis is most commonly seen in the second and third decades of life, but can occur at any age. Indeed, the extremes of age account for morbidity out of proportion to the percentage of the population who are treated for the disease. The reasons for this are clear and include (1) failure to consider the diagnosis due to the atypical patient population and presentation, (2) the difficulty in obtaining a history from many patients in the pediatric and geriatric populations, and (3) the comorbid conditions encountered in the geriatric population.

KEY POINTS

• Most of the morbidiy and occasional mortality of this disease is related to complications of transmural necrosis and perforation; therefore, delay in diagnosis and therapy is in large part responsible for morbidity and mortality

DIAGNOSIS

Acute appendicitis remains a clinical diagnosis. Numerous tests have been advocated and are often useful in evaluating a patient with suspected appendicitis. The singular fact remains that the best reported results of the currently available tests show a diagnostic sensitivity of approximately 90% and will therefore miss at least 10% of cases of acute appendicitis if relied on. The obvious conclusion, therefore, is that a heightened clinical acumen is essential and no test should be used to rule out appendicitis.

The diagnosis starts with a thorough history. The typical patient will be in the second or third decade of life. The onset of pain will be gradual and in the periumbilical region. Over the ensuing 24–36 hours, the pain will typically radiate to the right lower quadrant and be associated with anorexia. Nausea and vomiting are also common and low grade fever may be noted.

In the pediatric population, a prior upper respiratory infection is a helpful clue to the diagnosis, as this may incite the local lymphatic response leading to obstruction of the appendiceal lumen and appendicitis. In the adult population, the lymphatic tissue is diminished and the lumen large. A history of a prior upper respiratory infection is generally not helpful.

Although cases of recurrent appendicitis undoubtedly occur, they are rare and a prior history of similar pain should raise the suspicion of an alternative diagnosis. Similarly, urinary symptoms, at least early in the course of acute appendicitis, are uncommon and should lead to suspicion of urinary tract pathology as an alternative diagnosis. Diarrhea may be seen (Case 2) but is usually found in late or advanced cases when an inflammatory reaction creates an irritant affect on the adjacent colon with subsequent secretory diarrhea.

Anorexia, or loss of appetite, is an early and almost invariable consequence of acute appendicitis (Case 1). Nausea is also common, although vomiting is an infrequent complaint. Urinary symptoms are not normally seen although frequency may be noted, usually with a low-lying appendix directly irritating the bladder dome (Case 2).

Physical examination should start with observation of the patient. General assessment will reveal a patient not moving around much, and gentle nudging of the bed or a "heel tap" will often elicit pain due to peritoneal irritation. Vital signs may reveal mild tachycardia and low grade fever; a temperature greater than 39°C should raise suspicion of perforation. Examination should include auscultation of breath sounds and gentle percussion of the costovertebral angle (CVA) for tenderness over the kidney, primarily to evaluate for alternative diagnoses (Table 36.1). Abdominal examination will reveal mild to moderate distention, while bowel sounds are usually hypoactive to absent. Gentle palpation with warm hands should begin away from the right lower quadrant to improve the patient's comfort. Distracting the patient with conversation while continuing gentle palpation toward the right lower quadrant will improve the clinical acumen. Focal tenderness will usually be elicited by mild to moderate palpation in the region; occasionally a mass (phlegmon)

will be palpable. Guarding, involuntary or voluntary, may also be present. Rebound tenderness can be assessed by gentle percussion of the abdomen, not by deep palpation and release.

Psoas muscle irritation (Case 2), usually from a retrocecal appendicitis, can be assessed best with the patient on the left side; the hip is then hyperextended with the knee slightly bent (Fig. 36.1). An obturator sign is evaluated by flexing the hip and knee and then internally rotating the hip. Pain on this motion signifies irritation of the obturator nerve by a pelvic inflammatory process (such as a low-lying appendicitis). Rectal (and pelvic in female patients) examination is mandatory in assessing lower abdominal complaints. Performing these examinations with the patients in slightly reverse Trendelenburg's position or on the left side may improve diagnostic acumen by allowing the appendix to "fall" into the low pelvis (Fig. 36.2). Tenderness and/or a mass can frequently be appreciated on the right side in the supralevator region when the examination is properly performed.

Laboratory evaluation for suspicion of acute appendicitis is best described as supportive, not diagnostic. Leukocytosis is usually seen (Cases 1 and 2), although a normal white blood cell count does not rule out appendicitis, particularly in the elderly population. Urinalysis is nonspecific, often showing evidence of dehydration (high specific gravity) or starvation (ketones) (Case 1). Not infrequently, a few white blood cells (Case 2) or red blood cells are seen due to irritation of the ureter and/or bladder from the adjacent inflamed appendix. Radiologic examinations (plain abdominal films) are most frequently nonspecific, although the visualization of an appendicolith in the setting of right lower quadrant pain is suggestive. Visualization of a ureteral stone may suggest an alternative diagnosis. Computed tomography (CT) scans and ultrasound scans may infrequently be useful, although the sensitivity of these examinations is not great. They may have value in advanced cases (see under Treatment). Laparoscopy has an important role in diagnosis and treatment, especially in female patients in whom clinical diagnostic accuracy is relatively low.

TABLE 36.1 *Differential diagnosis*

Mesenteric adenitis

Meckel's diverticulitis

Gastroenteritis

Crohn's disease (acute ileocolitis)

Cholecystitis

Nephrolithiasis/urinary tract infection

Endometriosis

Mittleschmertz (pain of ovulation)

Torsion of ovary/ovarian cyst

Pelvic inflammatory disease

Perforated peptic ulcer

Cecal diverticulitis

Sigmoid diverticulitis

Perforated colon cancer

Hernia (incarcerated)

Torsion of testicle

KEY POINTS

- Acute appendicitis remains a clinical diagnosis
- Anorexia, or loss of appetite, is early and almost invariable consequence of acute appendicitis

DIFFERENTIAL DIAGNOSIS

The list of possible causes of right lower quadrant pain and tenderness are legion (Table 36.1). One can, however, narrow the list down considerably based on the

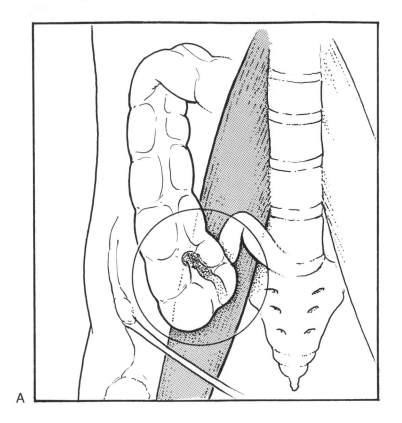

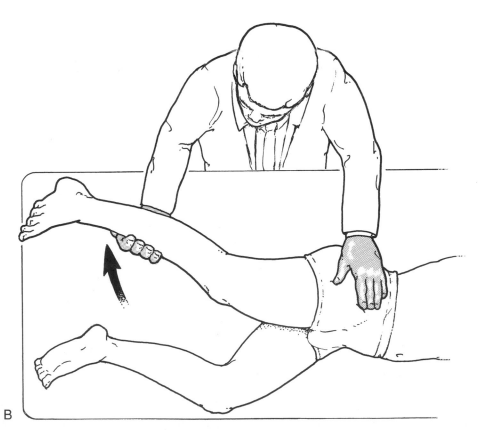

FIGURE 36.1 *The iliopsoas muscle is vulnerable to irritation by* **(A)** *a retrocecal appendicitis and* **(B)** *can be evaluated for by hyperextension of the hip.*

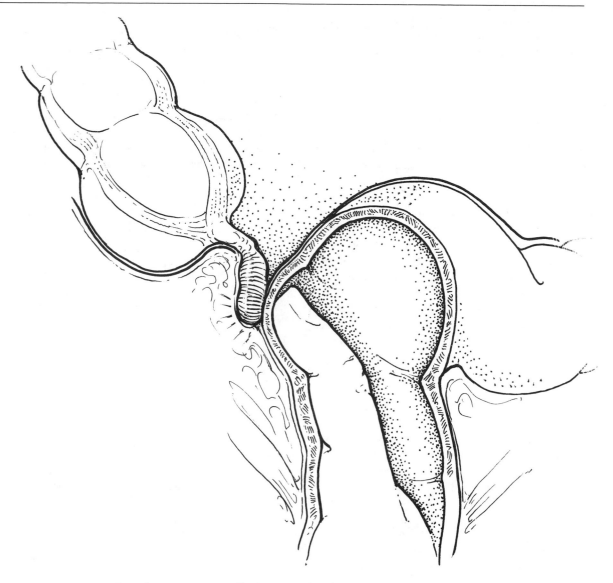

FIGURE 36.2   *Rectal examination will often reveal right-sided supralevator tenderness and/or a mass.*

patient's presentation, age, and sex. A preoperative diagnosis of acute appendicitis will be correct in 90–95% of young male patients, while in older and female patients clinical acumen is much less reliable, with up to 20–25% inaccurate diagnoses. The most common alternative diagnoses in female patients, not surprisingly, involves gynecologic disease and conditions, including symptomatic ovarian cysts, ovarian torsion, and pelvic inflammatory disease. In older patients, where acute appendicitis is much less common, other diseases may clinically mimic acute appendicitis, including diverticulitis.

Children present an additional dilemma contributed to by the larger number of alternative diagnoses and their difficulty in communicating an accurate history. Common causes of right lower quadrant pain in children include mesenteric adenitis and gastroenteritis. Since these are self-limited diseases, close and frequent observation over 12–14 hours will usually demonstrate improvement. Less

common or infrequently seen diseases include Meckel's diverticulitis and even Crohn's disease. These are usually intraoperative diagnoses, although CT scans obtained in confusing cases may be suggestive.

KEY POINTS

• Preoperative diagnosis of acute appendicitis will be correct in 90–95% of young male patients

• In older and female patients, clinical acumen much less reliable, with up to 20–25% inaccurate diagnoses

TREATMENT

Most patients with acute appendicitis will require minimal resuscitation before operative intervention. However, some patients will present late in the clinical course, occasionally with vomiting. They may require a brief period of intravenous fluid replacement and electrolyte correction. Typically, this resuscitation is guided by urine output. Once the diagnosis and the decision to operate has been securely established, intravenous antibiotics should be administered. They should be directed towards enteric flora and include coverage for gram-negative rods, enterococci, and anaerobes.

Controversy exists regarding the optimal surgical management of acute appendicitis, with the options including open appendectomy through a right lower quadrant muscle-splitting incision or, alternatively, a laparoscopic approach utilizing minimally invasive techniques. A laparoscopic approach appears to cause less pain, and in particular patient subgroups, including older and female patients, improves diagnostic accuracy. Obese patients may also benefit from the laparoscopic approach as the wounds are considerably smaller in this subgroup and access to the appendix improved. For the thin male patient, laparoscopy clearly increases the expense and offers little, if any, advantage.

If a normal appendix is found, a diligent search for an alternative cause of the pain is undertaken and the normal appendix is removed to prevent any future diagnostic dilemma. If acute appendicitis is encountered, an appendectomy is performed and antibiotics are continued for a brief period. If a perforated appendicitis is found, the local area is irrigated after removal of the appendix and antibiotics may be continued for 72 hours. If a large pelvic or periappendiceal abscess is found, drains are typically left to prevent reaccumulation and antibiotics are again continued for 3–5 days. Occasionally, a patient will present late with a large appendiceal phlegmon and/or abscess. If this is appreciated on physical examination by palpation of a large mass or by clinical suspicion, preoperative imaging studies, including ultrasound and/or CT scan, may be useful. Although not a widely utilized strategy, these patients can be initially managed nonoperatively with intravenous antibiotics and drainage of any associated large abscesses. The success rate with such an approach is upward of 90% and allows a rather difficult, complex operation and dissection to be converted into an elective situation. Following successful resolution of this appendiceal phlegmon, an interval appendectomy can be performed 6–8 weeks later, possibly utilizing a laparoscopic approach. Failure to perform an interval appendectomy will put the patient at moderate risk of recurrent appendicitis.

KEY POINTS

• Controversy exists regarding the optimal surgical management of acute appendicitis

• If a normal appendix is found, a diligent search for alternative cause of pain is undertaken and normal appendix is removed to prevent any future diagnostic dilemma

FOLLOW-UP

No particular follow-up is required in most patients with acute appendicitis beyond the immediate postoperative period, although patients with wound infections or open, granulating wounds will require longer convalescence (Case 2). Occasionally, a patient will present after discharge with an intra-abdominal abscess. Long-term risks include adhesive small bowel obstruction and, rarely, recurrent appendicitis if the stump of the appendix is inadvertently left too long. Patients who have negative explorations and no alternative diagnosis discovered may warrant close follow-up and attention to recurrent symptomatology, and further investigations may be necessary.

SUGGESTED READINGS

Franz MG, Norman J, Fabri PJ: Increased morbidity of appendicitis with advancing age. Am Surg 61:40, 1995

An interesting article that shows a dramatic increase in septic morbidity and mortality in elderly patients mostly due to delays in diagnosis and treatment.

Ford RD, Passinault WJ, Morse ME: Diagnostic ultrasound for suspected appendicitis: does the added cost produce a better outcome? Am Surg 60:895, 1994

Study failed to show benefit for ultrasound in acute appendicitis.

Frazee RC, Roberts JW, Symmonds RE, Snyder SK et al: A prospective randomized trial comparing open versus laparoscopic appendectomy. Ann Surg 219:725, 1994

Well performed study showing less pain and earlier return to full activity in the laparoscopy group.

Levine JS, Gomez GA, Dove DB: Negative appendix with suspected appendicitis: an update. South Med J 79:177, 1986

Retrospective study highlighting value and importance of clinical judgment.

QUESTIONS

1. Acute appendicitis may result in?
   A. Leukocytosis.
   B. Cervical motion tenderness.
   C. A tender mass on rectal examination.
   D. Infertility in female patients.
   E. All of the above.

2. Laparoscopic appendectomy may provide an advantage for the following patient groups?
   A. Obese patients.
   B. Male patients.
   C. Pediatric patients.
   D. Thin patients.
   E. Patients with a palpable abdominal mass.

(See p. 604 for answers.)

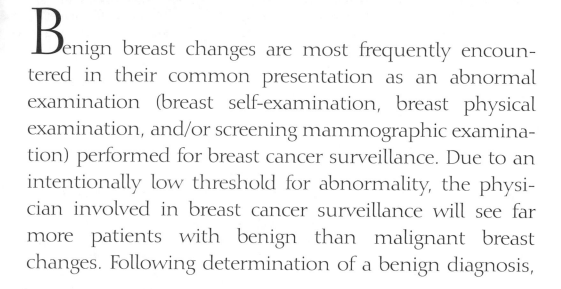

37

BENIGN

BREAST

DISEASE

GERALD MOSS

STANLEY R. KLEIN

Benign breast changes are most frequently encountered in their common presentation as an abnormal examination (breast self-examination, breast physical examination, and/or screening mammographic examination) performed for breast cancer surveillance. Due to an intentionally low threshold for abnormality, the physician involved in breast cancer surveillance will see far more patients with benign than malignant breast changes. Following determination of a benign diagnosis,

clinical interest is lost in most patients. Less commonly, symptomatic benign breast disease requires therapeutic intervention. The aims of this chapter are to identify and categorize (1) benign changes within the breast, (2) their relevance to breast cancer surveillance, (3) the workup to exclude a malignancy, and (4) associated etiologies, symptoms, and therapeutic interventions.

CASE 1
BENIGN BREAST CYST

A 38-year-old white female presented to her primary care physician with a 6-month history of a left breast mass. Uncomfortable with his knowledge of breast pathology, he referred her for surgical consultation. Before consultation he requested a mammogram since he was sure that his consultant would require it. The screening mam-

mogram reported a left breast density that was smooth walled and coincided in location with the palpable finding. Ultrasound was recommended to differentiate cystic from solid nature. The primary care physician ordered left breast ultrasound, which was performed the day before her surgical appointment. Ultrasound revealed a cystic lesion. Follow-up left mammography was advised in 4 months to exclude any change in size that would indicate an intracystic neoplasm and require a tissue diagnosis.

At her surgical evaluation, further questioning confirmed a 6-month history with slight enlargement and pain the week before menstrual flow. A history of local trauma, prior breast biopsy (demonstrating atypical lobular/ductal hyperplasia), mother or sister with breast cancer, and previous screening mammogram were denied. FNA was performed, revealing 5 ml of straw-colored fluid. At the completion of FNA the dominant left breast mass had disappeared. The patient was advised to return in 1 month for re-evaluation, at which time the left breast mass was absent. She was discharged from further surgical follow-up and advised to perform monthly breast self-examination, to undergo yearly breast physical examination by her primary care physician, and to have her next screening mammogram at age 40.

CASE 2
BREAST CYST

A 62-year-old Hispanic female, having had her annual screening mammogram, presented to her primary care physician for her annual breast physical examination and report of her mammogram. It was reported to her that her breast physical examination was without change but that her mammogram demonstrated a new smooth walled density in the left breast. Ultrasound was advised for further workup of the mammographic finding. A cystic lesion was reported with recommendation to repeat unilateral mammography in 4 months. The patient was advised of the ultrasound findings upon her follow-up appointment. She expressed concern regarding the 4-month wait until follow-up unilateral mammography and requested a second opinion.

Referral to a surgeon was obtained. The history revealed a mother and one of three sisters with the diagnosis of breast cancer. Both remained alive following treatment after 5 and 3 years, respectively. A history of local trauma and prior breast biopsy (demonstrating atypical lobular/ductal hyperplasia) were denied. Physical examination was free of any dominant masses. Review of the mammograms confirmed the presence of a new upper outer quadrant left breast density with smooth borders, consistent with a cyst. A phone call confirmed the sonographic diagnosis of a cyst and the feasibility of ultrasound guided FNA.

Ultrasound guided FNA demonstrated a 3-ml cyst. After aspirating the fluid, 3 ml of air was injected into the cyst in preparation for performing pneumocystography. A unilateral mammogram followed, which demonstrated a smooth inner wall. The patient was advised that the findings were diagnostic of a benign cyst and excluded malignancy. She was advised to continue annual breast physical and screening mammography examinations with her primary care physician.

B GENERAL CONSIDERATIONS

Benign breast changes are common. As many as one-third of all women have benign changes of the breast diagnosed through symptoms, physical examination, or mammographic findings. To some degree there exists a commonality with breast cancer of proliferative breast tissue. However, atypical ductal/lobular hyperplasia are the only benign breast changes associated with a significant (five times the baseline) risk of breast cancer development.

Although the histologic diagnosis of benign breast changes has little bearing on breast cancer development, the overlap in abnormal breast cancer surveillance studies is formidable (Cases 1 and 2). Proliferative disease without atypia, fibrocystic changes, sclerosing adenosis, and fibroadenoma commonly present with a palpable mass on breast physical examination. Proliferative disease without atypia, fibrocystic changes, sclerosing adenosis, fibroadenoma, and complex sclerosing lesion/radial scar are often associated with focal mammographic abnormalities detected by screening mammography. Less often, infectious and noninfectious inflammatory breast processes are associated with abnormal breast cancer surveillance studies.

The symptomatology of benign breast changes includes focal or diffuse breast pain, recognition of a lumpy breast by breast self-examination, and nipple discharge. Breast pain may be either cyclical, with premenstrual or midcycle discomfort being most common, or noncyclical. Cyclical pain may respond to hormonal therapy and disappears with menopause. Noncyclical pain occurs in a slightly older age group and shows no response to hormonal therapy, making management more difficult. The role of caffeine consumption in symptomatic fibrocystic changes is somewhat controversial. Caffeine abstinence has been reported to reduce cyclical breast pain in patients who consume caffeine.

Infectious (viral, bacterial, fungal, and parasitic) and noninfectious inflammatory (puerperal mastitis, breast thrombophlebitis, and sarcoid) breast abnormalities present with constant local or diffuse pain and associated skin changes. In addition, associated dominant/nondominant mass, fistulas, mastitis, or constitutional symptomatology may be present. All breast physical changes may demonstrate an associated abnormality when imaged by mammography.

Breast lumpiness is most evident in women around the time of menopause. Increasing fat replacement augments the physical presentation of benign breast lumps. Lumpiness may be quite varied, from diffuse small irregularities to discrete masses. Changes related to the menstrual cycle are most evident in the week preceding menses. Interestingly, patients who are symptomatically responsive to caffeine abstinence often demonstrate no associated change in breast physical examination.

The majority of nipple discharges are nonbloody in character. Nonbloody nipple discharges are physiologic and not associated with breast cancer. Bloody nipple discharges originate from pathology within the individual duct, with benign intraductal papillomas responsible for most cases. Papillomas may be associated with a dominant palpable mass or a dominant mammographic density; abnormal studies warrant a tissue diagnosis. Galactography (contrast radiography of the duct) may be performed when bloody nipple discharges are not associated with a dominant palpable mass or a dominant mammographic density. However, galactography cannot distinguish papilloma from cancer, thus warranting a tissue diagnosis of associated focal galactogram abnormalities (obstructed duct and/or filling defect).

K E Y P O I N T S

- Due to an intentionally low threshold for abnormality, physicians will see far more patients with benign than malignant breast changes

- One-third of all women have benign breast changes diagnosed through symptoms, physical examination, or mammography

- Symptomatology of benign breast changes includes focal or diffuse breast pain, recognition of a lumpy breast by self-examination, and nipple discharge

- Cyclical breast pain responds to hormonal therapy and disappears with menopause; noncyclical breast pain occurs in an older age group and does not respond to hormonal therapy

- Infectious and noninfectious inflammatory breast abnormalities present with constant local or diffuse pain and associated skin changes

- All breast physical changes may demonstrate an abnormality on mammography

- Breast lumpiness is most evident in women around time of menopause

- Most nipple discharges are nonbloody

- Bloody nipple discharges originate from pathology within the individual duct, with benign intraductal papillomas responsible for most cases

---

DIAGNOSIS

The diagnosis of benign breast changes can only be definitely made through a tissue diagnosis. This is a fundamental principle. Most often, patients are diagnosed with benign breast changes through history and physical examination and in the absence of a tissue diagnosis. This is an acceptable practice, provided that benign breast changes are not associated with an abnormal breast cancer surveillance study (new or increasing dominant breast mass, new or old nondominant breast mass with recent increasing size, or new abnormal mammogram). With the presence of an abnormal breast cancer surveillance study, a tissue diagnosis is mandated (Fig. 37.1). In the absence of a tissue diagnosis or confirmatory microbiology, biochemical, or immunohistochemical studies, the diagnosis of benign breast disease is a diagnosis consistent with but not confirmatory of benign breast changes.

Fine needle aspiration (FNA) can reliably diagnose some benign neoplastic changes, the most common of which is fibroadenoma. However, FNA cytopathology in benign disease (the most common of which are fibrocystic changes) is most commonly regarded as nondiagnostic, requiring tissue for histopathology.

In guarding against a false-negative diagnosis, both benign neoplastic and non-neoplastic FNA diagnoses require further evaluation within the context of the "triple test" (FNA, physical examination, and mammography). A single abnormality on any of the three tests constitutes a positive triple test. Low probability (risk of breast cancer) physical examination and low probability mammography findings do not qualify as abnormal results within the context of the triple test. A positive (abnormal) triple test warrants an actual tissue diagnosis, obtained through the performance of an open biopsy.

When FNA of a dominant mass, or ultrasound of a new smooth walled mammographic density, reveals a cyst (Cases 1 and 2), two subsequent courses may be followed. First, the mass that resolves through aspiration is re-evaluated in 1 month (Case 1), and the mass that has not resolved undergoes open biopsy. Any mammographic density is remammogrammed within 4–6 months. Alternatively, the dominant mass/mammographic density undergoes pneumocystograpy (Case 2), any inner wall pathology that is found mandates open biopsy. Negative results allow discharge from care.

Nipple discharge cytology has insufficient predictive value to qualify as a useful screening/diagnostic test. A significant correlation between tissue and nipple discharge exists for atypical hyperplasia only. Associated focal breast physical and mammographic findings warrant a tissue diagnosis. Diagnostic intervention proceeds relative to the abnormal finding. In the absence of an associated focal finding, galactography is performed (Case 2). Galactography demonstrating ductal ectasia represents a definitive benign diagnosis without the need for a tissue diagnosis. Demonstration of an obstructed duct or filling defect warrants a tissue diagnosis through excision of the specific duct.

K E Y P O I N T S

- Diagnosis of benign breast changes only made definitively through tissue diagnosis

- Tissue diagnosis mandated with abnormal breast cancer surveillance study

- In guarding against a false-negative diagnosis, both benign neoplastic and non-neoplastic FNA diagnoses require further evaluation within the context of the "triple test" (FNA, physical examination, and mammography); a single abnormality on any of the tests constitutes a positive triple test, warranting a biopsy

- When FNA reveals a cyst, the mass that resolves through aspiration is re-evaluated in 1 month and the dominant mass/mammographic density undergoes pneumocystography

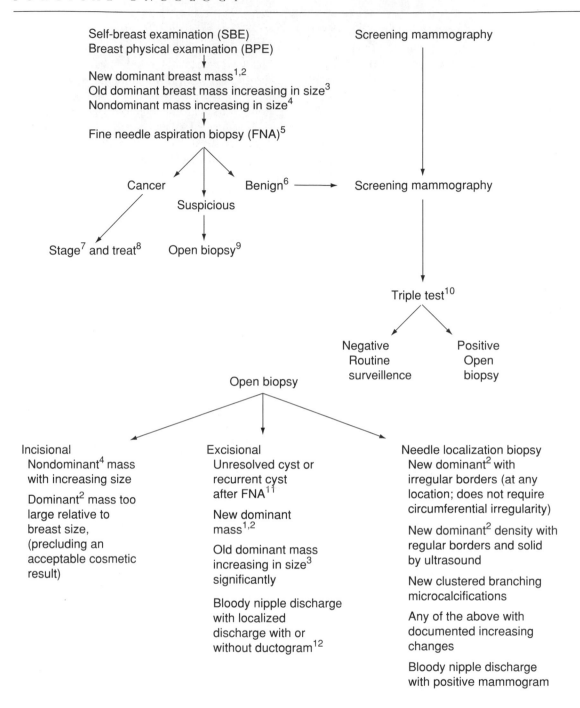

Self-breast examination (SBE)
Breast physical examination (BPE)
↓
New dominant breast mass[1,2]
Old dominant breast mass increasing in size[3]
Nondominant mass increasing in size[4]
↓
Fine needle aspiration biopsy (FNA)[5]

Screening mammography

Cancer   Benign[6] ————→ Screening mammography
     Suspicious

Stage[7] and treat[8]   Open biopsy[9]

Triple test[10]

Negative   Positive
Routine   Open
surveillence   biopsy

Open biopsy

Incisional
Nondominant[4] mass
with increasing size

Dominant[2] mass too
large relative to
breast size,
(precluding an
acceptable cosmetic
result)

Excisional
Unresolved cyst or
recurrent cyst
after FNA[11]

New dominant
mass[1,2]

Old dominant mass
increasing in size[3]
significantly

Bloody nipple discharge
with localized
discharge with or
without ductogram[12]

Needle localization biopsy
New dominant[2] with
irregular borders (at any
location; does not require
circumferential irregularity)

New dominant[2] density with
regular borders and solid
by ultrasound

New clustered branching
microcalcifications

Any of the above with
documented increasing
changes

Bloody nipple discharge
with positive mammogram

DIFFERENTIAL DIAGNOSIS

Asymptomatic breast changes do not require a specific benign pathologic diagnosis. In the absence of symptoms, the sole purpose in seeking a pathologic diagnosis is to exclude the diagnosis of breast cancer. The exclusion of breast cancer is necessary when these patients present with an abnormal breast cancer surveillance study. However, symptomatic benign breast changes may benefit from a specific benign pathologic diagnosis that dictates selection of therapy.

Symptomatic fibrocystic changes that are cyclical in nature exhibit the best response to therapeutic intervention. Symptomatic infectious changes require appropriate therapy to combat the infection. Selection of drug therapy may require microbiology studies. The presence of an underlying abscess can be determined by FNA or ultrasound. Noninfectious inflammatory breast changes may involve skin alone or in combination with underlying parenchyma. When only skin is involved, therapy selection may be determined based on physical findings alone. If the changes remain unresponsive to initial topical

FIGURE 37.1   *Surveillance study workup for breast cancer.*
[1]*New (within 2 years)*
[2]*Dominant (discretely separated from surrounding breast parenchyma)*
[3]*Increasing in size (greater than or equal to twice the previous size)*
[4]*Nondominant (not discretely separated from the surrounding parenchyma)*
[5]*FNA should be performed on initial examination*
[6]*Benign is a cytologic diagnosis that can be neoplastic (i.e., fibroadenoma) or non-neoplastic (fibrocystic change). This is not the practice of most institutions. Therefore, there must be quality assurance review of cytopathologic results specific to the institution and/or cytopathologist*
[7]*Routine staging includes chest x-ray mammography, liver function tests. Bone scan for stage III lesions, increased alkaline phosphatase, new bone pain*
[8]*See treatment guidelines*
[9]*Tru-cut biopsy may be performed as an open incisional biopsy. Biopsy should be scheduled within the month*
[10]*"Triple test" is FNA, physical examination, and mammography*
[11]*Residual dominant mass (immediately following aspiration) and/or recurrent (at 1 month follow-up) dominant mass*
[12]*Focal findings by breast physical examination, mammography, or ductogram (obstructed duct and/or filling defect. Appearance of ductal ectasia representative of definitive nonmalignant diagnosis, obviating open biopsy)*

agent therapy, skin biopsy with immunohistochemical studies should be performed.

KEY POINTS
• Without symptoms, the sole purpose of a pathologic diagnosis is to exclude breast cancer

TREATMENT

Puerperal (lactational) mastitis is treated by emptying the breast of milk while instituting properly selected antibiotic coverage. Nonpuerperal/noninfectious inflammation/mastitis is more common in women whose age places them at risk of breast cancer. Therefore, mammography is required to exclude breast cancer, which may also present in this manner.

Symptomatic (focal or diffuse breast pain) fibrocystic changes are treated with nonsteroidal anti-inflammatory agents. Refractory cases can be treated with oil of primrose, bromocriptine, and/or danazol. Bromocriptine and Donacrine usage have associated unpleasant side effects that, in most cases, cause women to lose interest in pursuing a therapeutic course. In fact, once women are assured that this symptomatology has little to no relation to breast cancer (provided there are no associated abnormal breast cancer surveillance studies), the pursuit of symptom palliation is greatly reduced.

Granulomatous (tuberculous) mastitis also warrants mammography to exclude cancer. Pathology results, sometimes combined with microbiology and immunohis-

tochemistry, determine the need for systemic therapy. Mammillary fistula can be effectively treated by either laying open or excising the fistula tract.

Infectious mastitis (viral, bacterial, fungal, parasitic) warrants mammography for patients of screening mammography age. An abnormal study requires a tissue diagnosis to exclude breast cancer. In the absence of any focal mammographic finding, properly selected antibiotic coverage is initiated. Evidence of an abscess, by either FNA or ultrasound, should lead to incision and drainage within 24 hours. At the time of incision and drainage, an incisional biopsy of the abscess wall must be performed to exclude the presence of cancer. Appropriate drug therapy may be selected on the basis of clinical and/or microbiologic findings.

Localized thrombophlebitis is treated with salicylates and warm compresses. When abnormal breast cancer surveillance studies are present a tissue diagnosis is warranted to exclude breast cancer.

Asymptomatic nonproliferative lesions, proliferative lesions, localizing sclerosing lesions, duct ectasia, fat necrosis, fibroadenoma/phyllodes tumor, and papillomas are all benign diagnoses that may present as a mass or abnormal mammogram. When presenting with an abnormal breast cancer surveillance study, a tissue diagnosis is required to exclude the diagnosis of breast cancer. Patients with pathologically proven atypical ductal/lobular hyperplasia may require modification of the standard breast cancer surveillance program (see Ch. 38) based on an increased risk of developing future invasive breast cancer. Modifications never narrow the time interval to less than 1 year. Therefore, patients over age 50 require no modification; between age 40 to 50, screening mammography is modified to annual testing; and under age 40, screening mammography is initiated earlier (at intervals of 1–2 years) and breast physical examination is performed yearly.

Phyllodes tumors present as an abnormal breast cancer surveillance study and mandate tissue diagnosis. Once the diagnosis is established, the pathologic distinction of malignancy (10% incidence) is paramount. Rapidly growing benign phyllodes tumors require complete excision. Malignant phyllodes tumors of the breast (breast sarcoma) require treatment that is similar to that associated with breast carcinoma (see Ch. 39).

KEY POINTS

- Puerperal mastitis is treated by emptying the breast of milk while instituting antibiotics

- Symptomatic fibrocystic changes are treated with NSAIDs, oil of primrose, bromocriptine, and/or danazol

- Mammillary fistula can be effectively treated by either laying open or excising the fistula tract

- In absence of focal mammographic finding, infectious mastitis is treated with antibiotics; abscesses should be incised and drained and a biopsy performed of the abscess wall

- Localized thrombophlebitis is treated with salicylates and warm compresses

---

FOLLOW-UP

Patients with infectious benign breast changes require observation during their therapeutic course, until complete resolution of the infection as well as the associated physical breast changes. Systemic spread should be considered and treated if present. Patients with noninfectious benign breast changes also require observation until complete resolution and/or stability of associated physical breast changes.

Following the open biopsy method for obtaining a tissue diagnosis (not FNA or core needle biopsy), patients require routine wound observation. In addition, for patients of screening mammography age, a new baseline unilateral mammogram is required within 4–6 months. The purpose of the new baseline mammogram is to record the image associated with breast healing following breast intervention. In the absence of a new baseline study, the subsequent routine screening mammograms of the area of breast healing cannot be temporally distinguished from an interval malignant neoplasm. Therefore, an additional biopsy may be necessary to exclude an interval malignancy.

SUGGESTED READINGS

Bland KI, Copeland EM: The Breast: Comprehensive Management of Benign and Malignant Diseases. WB Saunders, Philadelphia, 1991

Extensive coverage of benign diseases of the breast.

Grant CS, Goellner JR, Welch JS, Martin JK: Fine needle aspiration of the breast. Mayo Clin Proc 61:377, 1986

An overview of the role of FNA in breast disease and the potential pitfalls.

Haagensen CD: Diseases of the Breast. 3rd Ed. WB Saunders, Philadelphia, 1986

Extensive coverage of benign diseases of the breast.

Powell DE, Stelling CB: The Diagnosis and Detection of Breast Disease. CV Mosby, St. Louis, 1994

Multidisciplinary approach to breast imaging and disease.

QUESTIONS

1. *Bloody nipple discharge?*
    A. Is usually due to a malignancy.
    B. Can be studied conclusively with mammography.
    C. Should be evaluated with galactography first.
    D. Is an indication for excisional biopsy when associated with an abnormal mammogram.

2. *The "triple test" refers to?*
    A. Three sequential breast examinations 1 month apart.
    B. Breast examination, FNA, and mammography.
    C. FNA, core needle biopsy, and excisional biopsy.
    D. Breast examination, axillae examination, and mammography.

(See p. 604 for answers.)

38 BREAST CANCER

GERALD MOSS

STANLEY R. KLEIN

Traditionally, medical students and residents have described difficulty in mastering the topic of breast cancer. This is likely the result of an unwarranted emphasis on various aspects of breast cancer therapy. An acquired knowledge in pretreatment aspects of breast cancer—epidemiology, pathophysiology, surveillance, and diagnosis—would actually find greater utility. With the majority of medical students and residents completing their training and practicing in nononcologic fields, their greatest

contribution will be in encouraging screening and subsequent early detection and in providing early referral to a definitive medical specialist (radiation, medical, or surgical oncologist). As medical resources become increasingly scarce, surveillance for recurrence of breast cancer patients may be added to these responsibilities. Thus, this chapter is directed toward the elucidation of (1) the natural history of breast cancer, (2) breast cancer surveillance, (3) risk factors for the development of breast cancer and their effect on surveillance guidelines, (4) abnormal breast cancer surveillance criteria, (5) diagnostic management of abnormal breast cancer surveillance results, and (6) breast cancer risk factors and recurrence sites.

CASE 1
BREAST MASS

A 49-year-old white female with new onset of a right breast mass was referred for evaluation. Further questioning identified a 2-month history without change in size of the mass. A history of local trauma, prior breast biopsy

(demonstrating atypical lobular/ductal hyperplasia), mother or sister with breast cancer, and previous screening mammogram were denied. Physical examination revealed a mobile 2 × 2-cm dominant upper outer quadrant right breast mass without associated skin changes. FNA cytology was performed and initial screening mammography requested. Having had the requested screening mammogram, the patient returned for her follow-up appointment 1 week later. The FNA showed infiltrating ductal carcinoma. The mammogram demonstrated a right upper outer quadrant stellate density, suspicious for malignancy, that correlated with the position of the physical finding.

The patient was advised of the diagnosis of breast cancer along with treatment options for early breast cancer. Metastatic workup was requested, which was negative. The patient elected breast preservation and underwent surgical lumpectomy with axillary lymphadenectomy. Final pathology confirmed infiltrating ductal carcinoma with negative margins on the lumpectomy and 1 of 21 axillary lymph nodes involved with cancer (T1, NI, M0, stage IIA). Following hospital discharge and wound healing, medical and radiation oncology consultations were arranged. Adjuvant chemotherapy and breast irradiation were planned and completed within 6 months. Recurrence surveillance was outlined and initiated.

CASE 2
OCCULT LESION

A 64-year-old black female had a new mammographic lesion identified on her most recent annual screening mammogram. Her primary care physician referred her for surgical oncology consultation. She had undergone annual screening mammography since age 50. All prior mammograms were reported to be normal. A history of local trauma, prior breast biopsy (demonstrating atypical lobular/ductal hyperplasia), and mother or sister with breast cancer were denied. Physical examination revealed no dominant mass, nipple discharge, or skin changes. Review of the recent mammogram, with comparison to prior mammograms, was performed by both surgical oncologist and dedicated mammographer. The mammographic lesion was confirmed as new, highly suspicious for malignancy (new density with irregular borders), and warranting a tissue diagnosis through needle localization biopsy.

The patient was advised of the findings and recommendations. Needle localization biopsy revealed benign fibrocystic changes without evidence of neoplasm. One week later she was seen in order to evaluate wound healing, advise her of the final diagnosis, and schedule a 1-month wound check and new baseline unilateral mammogram (to be performed between 1 and 3 months postbiopsy). The next screening breast physical and mammographic examinations were scheduled for 1 year.

B GENERAL CONSIDERATIONS

reast cancer is the number one malignancy in women. It ranks second to lung cancer in cancer-related deaths. Currently, one out of every eight women will be diagnosed with breast cancer within her lifetime. The incidence continues to rise at a rapid pace, and it is estimated that 183,400 new cases of breast cancer will be diagnosed in 1995 (182,000 in women and 1,400 in men) in the United States.

A well-defined etiology is present in less than 10% of all patients diagnosed with breast cancer. A genetic etiology (hereditary breast cancer) may be demonstrated by a family history of breast cancer in one or more first-degree relatives (mother or sister). A positive family history increases the risk of breast cancer fivefold relative to the baseline female population. A similar increase in risk is associated with a history of a prior breast biopsy demonstrating atypical ductal/lobular hyperplasia. (The proliferative cellular pattern found in atypical ductal/lobular hyperpla-

sia may indicate a common proliferative etiology for the development of breast cancer.) However, reported associations between breast cancer development and cigarette smoking, fat intake, alcohol consumption, early menarche, late menopause, and delayed first pregnancy (after age 30) fail to define an etiology or significant association with the development of breast cancer (sporadic breast cancer) in an individual patient, although epidemiologic data suggest their influence.

The relevance of grading risk of breast cancer development is to guide breast cancer surveillance (Table 38.1 and Fig. 37.1). Documentation of a positive family history and/or prior pathologically proven atypical ductal/lobular hyperplasia may require modification of the standard breast cancer surveillance program, although the time interval will not be less than 1 year. Therefore, patients over age 50 require no modification; between age 40 to 50, screening mammography is modified to annual testing; and under age 40, screening mammography is initiated earlier (at intervals of 1–2 years) and breast physical examination performed yearly.

Breast cancer most commonly arises from either ductal or lobular epithelium. Breast sarcomas and lymphomas arise from mesenchymal cells in the supporting structure of the breast. The most common histologic type of breast cancer is infiltrating (invasive) ductal carcinoma. There exist numerous other histologic types; the only value of their recognition is to identify an altered prognosis (e.g., improved prognosis associated with medullary and colloid carcinoma). Noninvasive ductal/lobular carcinoma in situ (DCIS/LCIS) represent cancers that have not invaded the basement membrane.

Carcinoma of the breast spreads by lymphatic and vascular channel permeation and embolization. Common regional lymphatic sites of spread include the axillary, supraclavicular, and internal mammary nodes. The axillary nodal basin is most commonly involved. Although defined as regional lymphatic metastasis, patients without spread beyond this level are referred to as early breast cancer and may be cured of their disease through proper treatment.

TABLE 38.1 *American Cancer Society breast cancer surveillance recommendations*

Test or Procedure	Age (yr)	Frequency
BSE	≥20	Every month
BPE	20–40	Every 3 years
BPE	≥40	Every year
Screening mammography	40	Baseline
	40–49	Every 2 years
	≥50	Every year

Abbreviations: BSE, breast self-examination; BPE, breast physical examination.

The exception is supraclavicular nodal involvement, which is tantamount to distant metastasis. This is supported by the recent inclusion of supraclavicular nodal involvement in M1 disease, as specified by the Tumor, Node, and Metastasis (TNM) staging classification (Table 38.2). Less information regarding internal mammary nodal involvement and prognosis is available. Nevertheless, it would be reasonable to conclude that the addition of internal mammary nodal involvement would bear a worse prognosis, yet still be amenable to cure in the absence of distant metastatic disease.

DCIS/LCIS, by definition, represents noninvasive cancer of the breast ductules and lobules. In the absence of invasion, there exists the risk of local recurrence but not metastasis, with its associated risk to survival. Nevertheless, poorly or untreated DCIS/LCIS may lead to invasive disease, with all the attendant risks of metastatic disease and loss of life.

TABLE 38.2 *Breast cancer staging*

Stage I	T1 N0 M0		T2 N2 M0
Stage IIA	T1 N1 M0		T3 N1 M0
	T2 N0 M0		T3 N2 M0
Stage IIB	T2 N1 M0	Stage IIIB	T4 Any N M0
	T3 N0 M0		Any T N3 M0
Stage IIIA	T0 N2 M0	Stage IV	Any T Any N M1
	T1 N2 M0		

T	Primary tumors
TX	Primary tumor cannot be assessed
T0	No evidence of primary tumor
Tis	Carcinoma in situ: intraductalcarcinoma, lobular carcinoma, or Paget's disease with no tumor
T1	Tumor >2 cm or less in its greatest dimension
T2	Tumor >2 cm but not more than 5 cm in its greatest dimension
T3	Tumor >5 cm in its greatest dimension
T4	Tumor of any size with direct extension to the chest wall or to skin[a]
N	Regional lymph nodes
NX	Regional lymph nodes cannot be assessed
N0	No regional lymph node metastases
N1	Metastasis to movable ipsilateral axillary node(s)
N2	Metastasis to ipsilateral axillary nodes, fixed to one another or to other structures
N3	Metastasis to ipsilateral internal mammary lymph node(s)
M	Distant metastasis
M0	No evidence of distant metastasis
M1	Distant metastases (including metastases to ipsilateral supraclavicular lymph nodes)

[a]Chest wall includes ribs, intercostal muscles, and serratus anterior muscle, but not pectoral muscle.

Mammary sarcomas may be classified by histology (liposarcoma, leiomyosarcoma, fibrosarcoma, angiosarcoma, malignant fibrous histiocytoma, and malignant cystosarcoma phyllodes). However, their incidence is rare and biologic behavior so similar that they may be grouped as a whole for consideration of diagnostic and therapeutic intervention. Lymphatic spread is exceedingly rare, obviating the need for diagnostic axillary node dissection. Metastasis occurs by vascular spread with the lungs being the most common distant site of spread.

Primary breast lymphoma is extremely rare. It tends to be larger than mammary carcinoma at the time of diagnosis. There is a high incidence of axillary nodal involvement, which may make it difficult to ascertain whether the tumor is primary or secondary within the breast.

KEY POINTS

• Breast cancer number one malignancy in women, second to lung cancer in cancer-related deaths

• One of every eight women will be diagnosed with breast cancer within her lifetime

• Risk increases with a history of prior breast biopsy demonstrating atypical ductal/lobular hyperplasia

• Grading breast cancer development guides surveillance

• Most common histologic type of breast cancer is infiltrating (invasive) ductal carcinoma

• In DCIS/LCIS, noninvasive cancer of breast ductules and lobules, there exists risk of local recurrence but not metastasis

---

DIAGNOSIS

In general, patients with breast cancer present in one of three manners. These include a new (within 2 years) dominant (discrete borders relative to surrounding parenchyma) breast mass identified by the patient (Case 1); a dominant breast mass identified by a physician at breast physical examination; and a dominant density and/or clustered microcalcifications identified at screening mammography (Case 2). Smooth-walled lesions may be examined by ultrasound to differentiate solid from cystic, with solid lesions suspicious for cancer. Densities with irregular borders are suspicious for malignancy and do not warrant ultrasound. Clustered microcalcifications are those greater than five in number. Suspicious microcalcifications are linear and branch-like, not punctate. A less common presentation is that of symptomatic metastatic breast cancer (most common sites for metastatic spread are lung, liver, and bone).

Breast cancer surveillance guidelines have been developed as a result of our knowledge of presentation. As recommended by the American Cancer Society, they include first screening mammogram at age 40; screening mammogram every 2 years through age 50 and yearly thereafter;

breast physical examination by a physician every 3 years between ages 20 to 40 and yearly thereafter; and monthly breast self-examination (Table 38.1) initiated at age 20.

Abnormal surveillance studies warrant a tissue diagnosis (see Fig. 37.1). The preferred method for obtaining a tissue diagnosis is a cytologic diagnosis furnished through fine needle aspiration (FNA). For palpable masses this may be performed on the initial surgical consultation (Case 1). For occult lesions (nonpalpable, identified by mammography only), FNA is only available to select centers that possess a stereotactic mammographic unit. The accuracy of breast FNA is cytopathologist dependent. In the hands of skilled cytopathologists, accurate diagnosis can be rendered for malignant breast neoplasms (cancer more so than sarcoma/lymphoma) and benign neoplasms (fibroadenoma). Less common and somewhat controversial, a benign non-neoplastic (fibrocystic changes) diagnosis can be rendered through FNA alone.

When reliable FNA is unavailable, or insufficient to establish a diagnosis, actual tissue must be retrieved. This can be achieved through either excisional (removal of entire palpable mass or occult lesion) or incisional biopsy (partial removal of a palpable mass when removal would cosmetically alter the breast). A form of incisional biopsy is the core needle biopsy. This can be performed under local anesthesia in the office/clinic at the same time that FNA results (nondiagnostic) are rendered. In centers performing stereotactic breast FNA, concomitant core needle biopsy may be performed.

KEY POINTS

• Patients with breast cancer present with a new, dominant breast mass identified by the patient; a dominant breast mass identified at examination; or a dominant density and/or clustered microcalcifications identified at mammography

• Breast cancer surveillance guidelines recommended by the American Cancer Society, include first mammogram at age 40; mammogram every 2 years through age 50 and annual breast examination by a physician every 3 years between ages 20 to 40 and yearly thereafter; and monthly self-examination, initiated at age 20

B DIFFERENTIAL DIAGNOSIS

Breast cancer surveillance studies are evaluated with an intentionally low threshold to increase their sensitivity. The greater the sensitivity, the greater the biopsy/cancer ratio. A good example of this process is seen in the comparison of biopsy/cancer ratios in Europe and the United States. The biopsy/cancer ratio in the United States is double that seen in Europe. This difference is likely accounted for by this country's current malpractice climate. The Euro-

pean practice of observing low probability mammographic lesions is considered to be prohibitive in the United States.

Breast trauma (with resultant fat necrosis), locally thrombosed veins, benign neoplasms (most commonly fibroadenomas), fibrocystic changes (Case 2), and non-neoplastic inflammation/infection all may mimic breast cancer and present as an abnormal surveillance study. Fortunately, most methods for achieving a tissue diagnosis are minimally invasive without significant risk of disability and/or impaired cosmesis, and allowing for tissue diagnosis and avoidance of potentially delayed diagnosis (associated with a higher threshold).

KEY POINTS

• Breast cancer surveillance studies are evaluated with an intentionally low threshold to increase sensitivity

• The greater the sensitivity, the greater the biopsy/cancer ratio

---

H TREATMENT

Having established the diagnosis of breast cancer, the extent of disease (stage) must be determined (Case 1). Accurate staging of a patient's breast cancer is necessary for treatment selection and prognosis, as well as outcome comparisons. The TNM classification is the universally accepted staging system currently in use (Table 38.2). TNM permutations are divided into four staging groups (I–IV). Further diagnostic intervention (metastatic workup) is required to complete this process. Diagnostic study selection is based upon the knowledge of common metastatic organ sites (lung-chest x-ray, liver-liver function tests, bone-serum alkaline phosphatase).

Not all stages of breast cancer are curable. Metastatic breast cancer (stage IV) is incurable. All other stages are treatable for cure, yet all are at risk of recurrence/progression with advancement to metastatic disease and ultimate loss of life. Therapeutic intervention is subdivided into local, regional, and systemic therapy. Multimodality therapy (combination of surgery, radiotherapy, chemotherapy, and/or hormonal therapy) is customary. Nevertheless, surgical removal of the local tumor remains common to all therapeutic options performed for cure.

Surgery is a local/regional therapy applied to the primary tumor within the breast and axillary lymph nodes, respectively. Lumpectomy (removal of the breast tumor while preserving the natural cosmetic appearance of the breast) and mastectomy are the two local surgical therapeutic options. Patients with breast cancer are candidates for lumpectomy (breast preservation) as long as the tumor mass can be grossly removed without an unacceptable cosmetic effect. When lumpectomy is followed by breast irradiation, local control and survival are equivalent to mastectomy. With rare exception, both surgical procedures are associated with an axillary lymph node dissection to identify nodal involvement for TNM classification. (Axillary lymph node dissection is a diagnostic, not therapeutic intervention.)

Radiotherapy is routinely used in association with lumpectomy (Case 1). Adjuvant, postoperative chest wall (in patients who have undergone mastectomy) and supraclavicular fossa irradiation are advised by some when risk of local and regional recurrence is increased (tumor greater than 5 cm in diameter, positive deep margin of breast tumor removal through mastectomy, and/or greater than four axillary lymph nodes involved with tumor). The intention is to reduce the problematic chest wall/regional recurrence, which may be painful, difficult to control when present, and may compromise upper extremity function.

Chemotherapy and hormonal therapy affect systemic disease. Following local/regional treatment of early breast cancer (removal of all gross disease), the patient remains at risk of recurrent local/regional as well as systemic disease. Systemic recurrence occurs secondary to progressive growth at metastatic sites that were present at the initial patient presentation, yet not identifiable through routine metastatic workup. Systemic treatment at this stage is referred to as adjuvant systemic treatment. The earliest role for adjuvant systemic treatment was in treating patients with axillary nodal involvement. Adjuvant systemic treatment of node-positive breast cancer resulted in improved survival. More recently, adjuvant systemic treatment of node-negative breast cancer has similarly demonstrated improved survival. Thus, it is common practice to advise systemic treatment in patients with node-negative as well as node-positive breast cancer (Table 38.3).

Although metastatic breast cancer is incurable, therapeutic intervention for palliation may have significant clinical relevance. Pain is the most common symptom warranting palliative intervention, usually local irradiation. This may be augmented through systemic therapy (chemotherapy or hormonal therapy) when bony/visceral metastases are present. Less commonly, prophylactic therapeutic intervention may be advised in the absence of symptoms. The best example of this recommendation is the asymptomatic weight bearing skeletal metastasis. In an effort to prevent a future pathologic fracture, with its attendant effect on quality of life, it is wise to treat such metastases prophylactically.

TABLE 38.3 *Breast cancer management guidelines*

TNM	SURGERY	RADIATION	CHEMOTHERAPY/HORMONAL THERAPY			
			RECEPTORS[a] ABSENT		RECEPTORS[b] PRESENT	
			PRE	POST	PRE	POST
Tis N0 M0	Lump vs TM	Breast (for diameter between 2 and 5 cm)	/	/	/	/
T1 N0 M0	Lump/Ax vs MRM	Breast for Lump/Ax	+/	+/+	+/+	/+
T0 N1 M0	AX vs MRM	Breast, SCF, CW	+/	+/+	+/+	+/+
T1 N1 M0	Lump/Ax vs MRM	Breast, SCF, CW	+/	+/+	+/+	+/+
T2 N0 M0	Lump/Ax vs MRM	Breast	+/	+/+	+/+	+/+
T2 N1 M0	Lump/Ax vs MRM	Breast, SCF, CW	+/	+/+	+/+	+/+
T3 N0 M0	Lump/Ax vs MRM	Breast, SCF, CW	+/	+/+	+/+	+/+
T0 N2 M0	Lump/Ax vs MRM	Breast, SCF, CW	+/	+/+	+/+	+/+
T1 N2 M0	Lump/Ax vs MRM	Breast, SCF, CW	+/	+/+	+/+	+/+
T2 N2 M0	Lump/Ax vs MRM	Breast, SCF, CW	+/	+/+	+/+	+/+
T3 N1 M0	Lump[b]/Ax vs MRM	Breast, SCF, CW	+/	+/+	+/+	+/+
T3 N2 M0	Lump/Ax vs MRM	Breast, SCF, CW	+/	+/+	+/+	+/+
T4 Any N M0	Lump/Ax vs MRM	Breast, SCF, CW	+/	+/+	+/+	+/+
Any T N3 M0	Lump vs TM	Breast, AX, SCF, CW, IMN	+/	+/+	+/+	+/+
Any T Any N M1 (SCF)	Lump vs TM	Breast, AX, SCF, CW, IMN	+/	+/+	+/+	+/+
Any T Any N M2 (all other)	Lump vs TM	Symptomatic site (any) and/or asymptomatic weight bearing bone	+/	+/+	+/+	+/+

Abbreviations: Pre, premenopausal; Post, postmenopausal; Lump, lumpectomy; TM, total mastectomy for tumor diameter >5 cm; Lump/Ax, lumpectomy and axillary lymph node dissection; AX, axillary nodes; MRM, modified radical mastectomy; SCF, supraclavicular fossa (for T3 or T4 lesions and/or >4 axillary nodes involved; CW, chest wall when >4 axillary nodes involved; IMN, internal mammary nodes.
[a]Estrogen and progesterone receptors (+, present; –, absent).
[b]Provided primary tumor mass can be excised with clear margins and without disturbing the cosmetic appearance of the breast.

Having established a sarcoma diagnosis through open biopsy (FNA is unreliable in sarcomas), the local tumor undergoes wide excision that may require total mastectomy when wide excision would cosmetically alter the breast. Since lymphatic spread is unusual, axillary lymph node dissection is performed for clinical axillary lymph node involvement only. When total mastectomy is not required, the remaining breast should be irradiated in the early postoperative period. Chemotherapy remains investigational at this time. For established pulmonary metastasis, pulmonary metastectomy is advised, as up to 20% of patients with resectable metastases can be cured.

Total mastectomy and axillary lymph node dissection is advocated for large primary lymphomas of the breast. Recurrent local disease and accessible regional disease should be managed with radiotherapy, and systemic or multiregional disease with chemotherapy using current regimens for non-Hodgkin's lymphoma.

KEY POINTS

• Having established diagnosis of breast cancer, accurate staging is necessary for treatment selection, prognosis, and outcome comparisons

• When lumpectomy is followed by breast irradiation, local control and survival are equivalent to mastectomy

• It is common practice to advise adjuvant systemic treatment, which has improved survival in patients with node-negative and node-positive breast cancer

FOLLOW-UP

Similar to breast cancer surveillance and metastatic evaluation (at initial diagnosis), breast cancer recurrence surveillance requires the knowledge of body sites at risk of recurrent/progressive disease. The frequency of surveillance follows our knowledge of time interval to recurrence. As previously discussed, lung, bone, and liver are the more common sites of systemic disease. Axillary and supraclavicular fossa lymph nodes are the more common sites of regional disease. The breast (in patients locally treated with breast preservation) and chest wall (in patients locally treated with mastectomy) are common sites of local recurrence. Therefore, anatomic sites of recur-

PATIENT _____   Hospital # _____

	PREOP	3MO	6MO	9MO	1YR	15MO	18MO	21MO	2YR	2.5YR	3YR	3.5YR	4YR	4.5YR	5YR[2]
PHYS EXAM															
MAMMO															
CXR															
LFTs & CBC															
BONE SCAN[1]															
OTHER															

[1]For T3 lesions, new bone pain, elevated alkaline phoshatase @ pre-op or recent elevation during follow-up.
[2]Annual follow-up, only, beyond five years. Continue annual follow-up for life of patient.

STAGE	THERAPY	RECURRENCE
T _____ N _____ M _____ If Node Positive, ?/? nodes are +. ___ / ___ SITE _____	OPERATION _____ DATE _____	SITE _____ DATE _____
HISTOLOGY:	RADIATION: (circle one) YES NO	RESTAGING:
RECEPTORS: (circle one) ER positive negative PR positive negative	CHEMOTHERAPY: (circle one) YES NO	TREATMENT:
	HORMONAL THERAPY: (circle one) YES NO	

FIGURE 38.1   *Harbor/University of California at Los Angeles, follow-up regimen for breast cancer patients.*

rence surveillance include bilateral supraclavicular fossa, breast/chest wall, bilateral axillae, bone, and liver. The modalities for surveillance include history/alkaline phosphatase (bone), palpation (supraclavicular fossa), auscultation/chest x-ray (chest), palpation (axilla), palpation/mammography (breast, chest wall), and palpation/liver function tests (liver). Recurrence risk is greatest within the initial 5 years and continues for as long as 20 years, reflected in the frequency of recurrence surveillance (Fig. 38.1).

Recurrence sites for mammary sarcomas and lymphomas are pulmonary (local) and multiple bony and visceral sites, including bone marrow (local/regional) respectively. With one exception, these body sites should be surveyed in a manner similar to that of mammary carcinoma. In the presence of a diagnosis of mammary sarcoma, compared tomography (CT) scans of the chest should be performed when radiography is negative and mastectomy is planned.

SUGGESTED READINGS

Devita VT, Hellman S, Rosenberg SA: Cancer: Principles and Practice Oncology. Lippincott-Raven, Philadelphia, 1993

Comprehensive multidisciplined oncology text (weakest discipline is surgery).

Donegan WL, Spratt JS: Cancer of the Breast. WB Saunders, Philadelphia, 1995

Comprehensive breast cancer text (strong surgical presence).

Early Breast Cancer Trialist Collaborative Group: Systemic treatment of early breast cancer by hormonal, cytotoxic, or immune therapy. Lancet 39:8784, 1992

Overview analysis of systemic breast cancer treatment. Highly technical process yet simplified end product (treatment algorithm).

QUESTIONS

1. Breast cancer screening includes?
   A. Breast self-examination.
   B. Breast ultrasonography.
   C. FNA of a suspicious breast mass.
   D. Mammography obtained in a 35-year-old patient with a self-discovered lump.

2. Staging of breast cancer may include?
   A. Physical examination.
   B. CT scan of the liver.
   C. Axillary node dissection.
   D. Serum alkaline phosphatase.
   E. All of the above.

(See p. 604 for answers.)

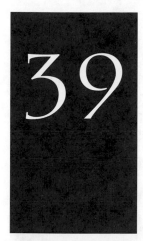

39

SKIN AND
SOFT TISSUE
TUMORS

GERALD MOSS

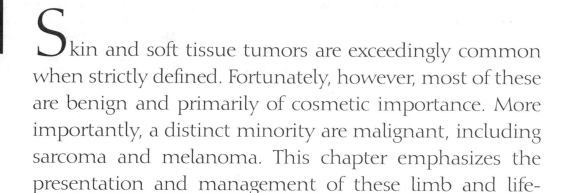

Skin and soft tissue tumors are exceedingly common when strictly defined. Fortunately, however, most of these are benign and primarily of cosmetic importance. More importantly, a distinct minority are malignant, including sarcoma and melanoma. This chapter emphasizes the presentation and management of these limb and life-threatening neoplasms.

CASE 1
SOFT TISSUE SARCOMA

An 18-year-old black male was recruited to the University of Michigan with a full scholarship to play football. Like all freshman athletes he was required to have a recent physical examination. This was performed at the student health clinic by a family practitioner who noticed a 3 × 4-cm soft tissue mass present in the right anterior thigh. The mass was soft, with discreet borders and was consistent with a lipoma. Further questioning revealed an 11-month history without much appreciation for changing size. The patient was fairly sure of this history because he first noticed the mass after he had sustained a bruised right thigh during his last high school game. The doctor informed him of the lipoma diagnosis with the advice for no further workup for this benign lesion. The doctor described his comfort with this diagnosis, explaining that a malignancy in an 18-year-old would be quite rare.

Approximately 1 month into the freshman football season the patient pulled a right hamstring muscle and required attention from the team trainer, a physical therapist in his third year of medical school. While attending to

the injury, the right thigh mass was noted and the prior history recounted. The trainer's suspicion for malignancy led to a second opinion obtained through the university medical center's surgical clinic. The concern for malignancy was echoed by the surgical oncologist, who advised and performed an FNA and core needle biopsy the very same day. The FNA result was consistent with a sarcoma but a specific classification was only revealed with the core needle biopsy—malignant fibrous histiocytoma. Subsequently, definitive therapeutic intervention was planned with surgical extirpation followed by external beam irradiation to the tumor bed.

CASE 2
MELANOMA

A 20-year-old white male presented to his primary care physician describing a 1-month history of a nontender, right groin bulge. The primary care physician appreciated some transmission of intra-abdominal pressure, which led him to consider this an incarcerated femoral hernia. Alarmed with the possibility that an incarcerated hernia may progress to strangulation, he requested an immediate surgical evaluation.

The general surgeon was not impressed with the transmission of intra-abdominal pressure and found the right groin mass to be indurated and nontender. Furthermore, there was no associated rubor, erythema, and/or edema to be suspicious of an underlying infectious etiology. Although the patient offered no prior malignant history or associated constitutional symptomatology, the surgeon was suspicious of an underlying malignancy. He performed an FNA, which confirmed a solid consistency.

The following day the FNA results revealed a diagnosis of melanoma. Further questioning revealed a history of a prior pigmented right thigh nevus that had spontaneously disappeared 2 years earlier. Metastatic workup revealed no evidence of further disease spread. A right groin dissection was advised and performed. Postoperatively, no further therapy was recommended.

GENERAL CONSIDERATIONS

Soft tissue sarcomas are uncommon malignant neoplasms, accounting for less than 1% of all cancers. A relative clustering seen in a younger population increases the prominence of this diagnosis, and soft tissue sarcomas rank fifth in cancer-related incidence and death in children under the age of 15.

Although the classification of most malignant tumors relies upon the tissue of origin (connective tissue—sarcoma, epithelial tissue—carcinoma), soft tissue sarcomas represent a large variety of malignant tumors for which distinction for the tissue of origin alone does not best classify these tumors. Instead, similarities in pathologic appearance, clinical presentation, and behavior have led to their grouping.

Little is known about epidemiologic or etiologic factors of importance in patients who develop a soft tissue sarcoma, although a 15% incidence of neurofibrosarcoma development is found in patients with the genetic abnormality that leads to von Recklinghausen's disease.

With the ubiquitous presence of connective tissue, soft tissue sarcomas may arise anywhere in the body. A somatic site of origin is far more common than a visceral site, with extremity tumors predominating. The lower extremity is the most commonly affected with the majority occurring at or above the knee. Other sites include the head and neck region and trunk, which is subdivided into retroperitoneum, abdominal wall, chest wall, mediastinum, and breast.

The pathologic classification of soft tissue sarcomas is as varied as that for connective tissue itself. Pathologic distinction by cell of origin is pathologist dependent, and it is fortunate that cell of origin is of minimal value for prognostication and treatment selection, thus compelling the treatment of soft tissue sarcomas as a group.

Melanoma represents a highly lethal form of cancer, and is by far the most deadly form of skin cancer. The incidence continues to rise, and is rising more rapidly than other solid malignant neoplasms. In the absence of a clear cause and effect relationship, this phenomenon is best explained by the combined effects of increased recreational exposure to sunlight, increased amounts of ultraviolet B irradiation reaching the earth's surface, and efforts toward early detection.

The more common nonmelanoma skin cancers include squamous cell carcinoma (SCC) and basal cell carcinoma (BCC). Other nonmelanoma skin cancers include apocrine, eccrine, sebaceous, and nonmammary Paget's disease. Relative to melanoma, SCC and BCC represent the more prevalent cutaneous malignancies, while ranking a distant second and even more distant third in site-related mortality, respectively.

Melanoma is a disease primarily confined to whites (as are SCC and BCC). The typical patient has a fair complexion and a tendency to sunburn rather than tan (both due to a decreased content of melanin). Geographic clustering reflects the level of sunlight and associated ultraviolet exposure. Similarly, prevalence by anatomic site reflects the relationship between gender specific fashion and exposure (prevalence for truncal sites in men versus lower extremity sites in women). Most melanomas arise from a pre-existing benign nevus, although the vast majority of nevi will not undergo neoplastic changes. The exception is the congenital giant hairy nevus. Up to 30% of these will develop into a malignant melanoma.

The four major growth patterns of melanoma are superficial spreading, nodular, lentigo maligna, and acral lentiginous melanoma. Each variable growth pattern is associated with distinct clinical features that depict divergent prognoses. Such clinical and prognostic variability make it imperative that these distinctions be recognized by the physician.

KEY POINTS

• Soft tissue sarcomas may arise anywhere in the body; somatic site more common than visceral, with extremity tumors predominant

• Most melanomas arise from a pre-existing benign nevus, although vast majority of nevi will not undergo neoplastic changes

DIAGNOSIS

The typical presentation of a soft tissue sarcoma is of a large tumor that is relatively asymptomatic. A location among compressible tissues, often far from vital organs, leads to a delay in symptomatic presentation. The absence of reliable clinical signs to aid in distinguishing between benign and malignant soft tissue neoplasms (Case 1) requires a lower threshold for the performance of a biopsy in order to seek early identification. Indications for biopsy include a growing soft tissue mass or any persistent soft tissue mass in which lack of growth cannot be ensured through a reliable history.

Having made the decision to biopsy a soft tissue mass, the nature of the biopsy plays an important role in the overall management of patients with a soft tissue sarcoma. Although fine needle aspiration (FNA) biopsy has found increasing use in the diagnosis of solid neoplasms, the subtle distinctions necessary to distinguish benign from malignant variants are often not available within the small sample size and cytologic characteristics available with FNA (Case 1). By contrast, core needle biopsy offers the availability of tissue for a histologic evaluation, and may be considered as a form of incisional biopsy indicated for larger soft tissue masses (>3 cm).

Excisional biopsy (removal of the entire tumor) is an appropriate technique only for small tumors (<3 cm) in which adequate margins can be obtained without compromising cosmetic outcome. Incomplete excisional biopsy (with positive or inadequate margins) will mandate re-excision, including excision of previously created scar. In addition, wide excision performed at the time of initial biopsy may result in adverse cosmetic consequences for what may be a benign lesion. Incisional biopsy (see Ch. 11) is a more appropriate choice for larger tumors when the suspicion of sarcoma exists.

Regardless of the choice of biopsy technique, the placement of the incision or Tru-cut (core needle) biopsy tract needs to be well thought out. Improper placement may preclude proper radical resection of the lesion and may lead to large increases in the radiation fields necessary to encompass areas of possible spread. Incisions on the extremities should be placed longitudinally, so as not to compromise subsequent muscle group excision. At other sites, the incision should be parallel to the long axis of the underlying principal muscle. Biopsies of lesions in the buttocks should be placed as inferior as possible to allow for subsequent development of skin flaps if hemipelvectomy is necessary.

Although melanomas may have a variety of clinical appearances, the common denominator is their changing nature. Any pigmented skin nevi that ulcerate, bleed, or undergo a change in size, configuration, color, or even (rarely) spontaneous resolution (Case 2) should be considered a melanoma and considered for biopsy. Nonpigmented skin nevi with progressive nodular growth, unresponsive associated inflammatory changes, signs of underlying fixation, or prominent regional lymph nodes should also undergo biopsy.

Biopsies performed for the consideration of melanoma require full thickness tissue in order to properly stage the local disease. Shave or curette biopsies may be useful in nonmelanoma skin cancers but, due to the inability to properly assess the full thickness of the local disease, are contraindicated for pigmented skin nevi. Similarly, FNA biopsy serves no useful role in evaluating primary melanoma. However, FNA may be useful in evaluating spread of disease (regional lymphatic and/or systemic organ sites) once the initial diagnosis has been made.

Excisional biopsies may be performed for skin nevi that are less than 1.5 cm in diameter and are located in areas where the amount of skin is not critical for functional or cosmetic needs (i.e., trunk). An elliptical incision is made, while considering the orientation and effect of re-excision should the lesion prove to be malignant. For lesions larger than 1.5 cm, or in sites where skin loss may have formidable consequences, an incisional biopsy is advised. Initially, this should be performed using a punch biopsy technique.

Local assessment of melanoma and nonmelanoma skin cancers are evaluated within the context of the tumor criteria (T) of the Tumor Node Metastasis (TNM) classification (Tables 39.1 and 39.2). Centrally important for prognostication and treatment selection, and unique to melanoma, is the need to microstage local disease. Historically, two systems (Clark and Breslow classifications) have been developed to determine the microstage of melanoma. More recently, studies have found that Breslow's depth of invasion represents the more accurate classification. Additional prognostic factors specific to melanoma include anatomic site, sex, the presence of ulceration, growth pattern, and age.

Melanoma is remarkable for its ability to spread to any organ site. The most common area of spread, which may or may not precede that of systemic organ sites, is the regional lymphatic basin. By contrast, systemic spread is far less common to nonmelanoma skin cancers, the greatest risk occurring with SCC found in areas of chronic

TABLE 39.1 *AJCC staging system for melanoma*

STAGE	CRITERIA
IA	Localized melanoma ≤0.75 mm (T1N0M0)
IB	Localized melanoma 0.76–1.5 mm (T2N0M0)
IIA	Localized melanoma 1.5–4 mm (T3N0M0)
IIB	Localized melanoma >4 mm (T4N0M0)
III	Limited nodal metastases involving only one regional lymph node basin, or <5 in-transit metastases but without nodal metastases (any T, N1M0)
IV	Advanced regional metastases (any T, N2M0) or any patient with distant metastases (any T, any N, M1 or M2)

Abbreviation: AJCC, American Joint Committee on Cancer.

TABLE 39.2 *TNM Classification for squamous and basal cell carcinoma*

Primary tumor (T)

Tx   Minimum requirements to assess the primary tumor cannot be met

Tis   Carcinoma in situ

T0   No primary tumor present

T1   Tumor 2 cm or less in its largest dimension, strictly superficial or exophytic

T2   Tumor > 2 cm but ≤5 cm in its largest dimension or with minimal infiltration of the dermis, irrespective of size

T3   Tumor > 5 cm in its largest dimension or with deep infiltration of the dermis, irrespective of size

T4   Tumor involving other structures such as cartilage, muscle, or bone

Nodal involvement (N)

The nodal involvement for cervical nodes is identical to that of the head and neck cancers, this can also be applied to other nodal regions

Nx   Minimum requirements to assess the regional nodes cannot be met

N0   No evidence of regional lymph node involvement

N1   Evidence of involvement of movable contralateral or bilateral regional lymph nodes

N3   Evidence of involvement of fixed regional lymph nodes

Distant metastasis (M)

Mx   Minimum requirements to assess distant metastasis cannot be met

M0   No (known) distant metastasis

M1   Distant metastasis present (specify site: pulmonary, osseous, hepatic, brain, lymph nodes, bone marrow, pleura, skin, eye, other)

Staging

I   Localized T1

II   Regional nodal involvement (first chain of drainage)

III   Distant metastases

Tumor grade

G1   Well differentiated

G2   Moderately well differentiated

G3–G4   Poorly to very poorly differentiated

KEY POINTS

• Indications for biopsy include growing soft tissue mass, or any persistent soft tissue mass in which lack of growth cannot be ensured through reliable history

• Nature of biopsy plays important role in the overall management of patients with soft tissue sarcoma

• Excisional biopsy, removal of entire tumor, appropriate technique only for small tumors (<3 cm)

• Regardless of choice of biopsy technique, placement of incision or Tru-cut (core needle) biopsy tract needs to be well thought out

• Although melanomas may have variety of clinical appearances, the common denominator is changing nature

• Biopsies performed for consideration of melanoma require full thickness tissue in order to properly stage local disease

• Microstaging local disease is centrally important for prognostication and treatment selection, and is unique to melanoma; Breslow's depth of invasion represents most accurate classification

---

DIFFERENTIAL DIAGNOSIS

With their potential for large growth, benign soft tissue tumors, especially lipomas, represent the most common entity from which a soft tissue sarcoma must be distinguished. Similar to soft tissue sarcomas, there exists little or no reason to distinguish the cell of origin for a benign soft tissue tumor. Of greater importance is the ability to distinguish nonmetastasizing soft tissue tumors that behave in a malignant manner, exhibiting locally aggressive growth (i.e., desmoid tumors or dermatofibrosarcoma protuberans). Such otherwise benign growths will require specific therapeutic decision making.

Injury may also provoke localized proliferative soft tissue growth from which a soft tissue sarcoma must be distinguished. Due to a high mitotic rate, these growths may be difficult to distinguish from a soft tissue sarcoma. Such an example is exhibited by the entity of myositis ossificans.

Virtually any skin lesion may be considered suspicious for a melanoma. The most common lesions considered include pigmented nevi, actinic keratoses, seborrheic keratoses, and BCCs. A low threshold for excision or biopsy should be maintained.

TREATMENT

Once the diagnosis of a soft tissue sarcoma is established, the extent of disease (stage) must be determined. Accurate tumor staging is necessary for appropriate treatment selection, prognostication, as well as outcome comparisons. The TNM classification, with slight modification for the addition of a tumor grade classi-

---

inflammation and bum scar (10–30%). Metastatic disease confined to the regional lymphatics may be cured, placing great emphasis on both initial as well as follow-up surveillance. As previously stated, tissue diagnosis confirmation of nodal involvement may be quickly and easily accomplished through FNA (Case 2). Less often, an open biopsy (incision versus excision) may be warranted.

fication (TGNM), is the accepted tumor staging system (Table 39.3).

Further diagnostic evaluation (metastatic workup) is required to complete the tumor staging process. Diagnostic study selection is based on the knowledge of local growth as well as the common metastatic organ sites (computed tomography [CT] of the chest to check the lungs when chest x-ray is negative; palpation, alkaline phosphatase, and CT of the abdomen to check the liver; history, alkaline phosphatase, and bone scan to check the bones; and palpation of the regional lymphatic basin for rhabdomyo, alveolar, and/or synovial sarcoma cell types).

Therapy of soft tissue sarcomas must bear in mind the formidable site related morbidity/mortality that is associated with inadequate local control. This concept is relevant for patients with or without systemic metastases at the time of initial diagnosis. To this end, surgical resection represents the primary therapeutic intervention, with all other therapeutic options acting in an adjuvant role.

The essential ingredient in the surgical approach to a soft tissue sarcoma is the achievement of adequate margins. Against the historical background of major amputations performed for most extremity soft tissue sarcomas, a more recent practice of wide excision followed by adjuvant irradiation of the tumor bed has resulted in the achievement of limb sparing without compromise in survival (Case 1). (Unlike osteosarcomas, a solid therapeutic role for adjuvant chemotherapy has yet to be established.) In the rare occurrence of regional lymphatic spread, regional lymphadenectomy is advised.

Patients with systemic disease (pulmonary site only) may also be candidates for surgical resection. Isolated pulmonary metastases may be cured by complete surgical excision. Similar survival benefits may be achieved when recurrent isolated pulmonary disease can be completely removed.

Patients with nonresectable pulmonary and/or nonpulmonary systemic disease are candidates for palliative therapy only. Standard therapy includes a doxorubicin-based chemotheraphy regimen. Although newer agents have exhibited promising preliminary results, their role will likely continue to be relegated to salvage (recurrence/progression during treatment) regimens.

Local control of cutaneous malignancies, as well as survival, may suffer as a result of the timing and choice of biopsy technique. Acknowledging the historical background of routine wide (>5 cm circumferential margins) local excision, recent data demonstrating the importance of tumor thickness have led to a policy of surgical margin width reflecting the level of invasion of the primary tumor.

Noninvasive melanomas (<0.76 mm depth of invasion) have a minimal local recurrence rate, and survival appears unaffected by resection margin width. Minimally invasive melanomas (0.76–1 mm depth of invasion) are well controlled with 1-cm margins. Although additional data are available to support the safety of 1-cm margins for depth of invasion up to 2 mm, many surgeons prefer to extend the margin to 2 cm. Similarly, data exist to support the use of 2-cm margins for 2–4 mm depths of invasion but most surgeons prefer a 3-cm margin. Primary lesions having a 4 mm or greater depth of invasion exhibit a significantly increased risk of local recurrence as well as systemic disease, thus warranting the widest margin of resection (3 cm).

Special anatomic sites require unique guidelines for the local resection of melanoma. Upper or lower extremity dig-

TABLE 39.3 *AJC staging system for soft tissue sarcomas*

Primary tumor (T)

 T1 Tumor <5 cm

 T2 Tumor ≥5 cm

Histologic grade of malignancy (G)

 G1 Low

 G2 Moderate

 G3 High

Regional lymph nodes (N)

 N0 No histologically verified metastases to regional lymph nodes

 N1 Histologically verified regional lymph node metastasis

Distant metastasis (M)

 M0 No distant metastasis

 M1 Distant metastasis

Stage I

 Stage IA

  G1T1N0M0

 Stage IB

  G1T2N0M0

Stage II

 Stage IIA

  G2T1N0M0

 Stage IIB

  G2T2N0M0

Stage III

 Stage IIIA

  G3T2N0M0

 Stage IIIB

  G3T2N0M0

Stage IV

 Stage IVA

  G13T12N1M0

 Stage IVB

  G13T12N01M1

its require amputation to achieve optimal local control. Facial melanomas are often treated with smaller margins due to the functional and cosmetic consequences. Melanomas of the ear are treated with wedge excision when possible.

Local resection for nonmelanoma skin cancers require less variability in margin width. BCC may be treated with 3–5-mm margins; SCC and other nonmelanoma skin cancers require 1-cm margin widths to achieve adequate local control. Similar to the consideration for melanoma, special body sites will require special considerations, including narrower margins with or without radiation. Less commonly utilized local techniques include cryosurgery, chemotherapy, and immunotherapy.

Surgical excision of involved regional nodes is the only effective treatment for regional control or cure. With respect to melanoma, the decision to excise clinically negative nodes (elective or prophylactic lymphadenectomy) has been debated most when the regional lymphatic basin of concern is the ilioinguinal region (additional common regional areas include the cervical and axillary region). The decision to perform elective ilioinguinal lymphadenectomy must be weighed against the incidence of associated wound and extremity lymphedema complications. To date, the best available studies have not shown a survival advantage to patients undergoing elective lymphadenectomy. Nevertheless, the low complication rate associated with axillary lymphadenectomy has led many surgeons to lower their threshold for the performance of elective axillary lymphadenectomy.

Additional therapeutic modalities that require expanded reading include isolated limb perfusion, radiotherapy, intralesional immunotherapy, and systemic chemotherapy and/or hormonal therapy.

KEY POINTS

• The essential ingredient in the surgical approach to soft tissue sarcoma is the achievement of adequate margins

• Recent data demonstrate the importance of tumor thickness, leading to a policy of surgical margin width reflecting the level of invasion of the primary tumor

• Surgical excision of involved regional nodes is the only effective treatment for regional control or cure

---

FOLLOW-UP

The principles of recurrence surveillance are quite similar to those involved in tumor staging of newly diagnosed patients. An understanding of the sites at risk of recurrent/residual disease as well as the time interval to recurrence is required. The local tumor bed and the pulmonary parenchyma represent the most common sites for recurrence. Additional metastatic sites to consider on a selected basis include the liver (retroperitoneum/intra-peritoneal viscera primary sites) and regional lymphatic basin (synovial/rhabdomyo/alveolar sarcoma histologic cell types).

Recurrence surveillance techniques include history and physical examination, chest x-ray, selective use of CT scans (chest/abdomen), and bone scans. An understanding of the time frame related to recurrence (major risk occurring within the initial 2–3 years) should be reflected in the frequency of surveillance.

The principles of recurrence surveillance for skin cancer are quite similar to those involved in defining the appropriate metastatic workup for newly diagnosed patients. An understanding of the sites at risk of recurrence as well as the time interval to recurrence is required. The local tumor bed as well as the complete mucocutaneous surface area (including the oral and anal verge, and the vaginal introitus mucosa for patients with melanoma) are at risk of local recurrence or the development of a second primary tumor.

The regional lymphatic basin is at risk of melanoma recurrence regardless of the performance of a prior prophylactic or therapeutic lymphadenectomy. Although melanoma demonstrates one of the broadest patterns of systemic organ site involvement, the more frequent sites that should be reflected in a recurrence surveillance program include lung, liver, bone, and brain.

Recurrence surveillance techniques should be utilized only with recognition of the current limitations in altering the outcome. Assessment should include a thorough history and physical examination with emphasis on the local tumor site and regional lymphatic basin. Local and regional recurrence risk is greatest within the first 5 years, but second primary and systemic risk may exceed this time frame, which should be reflected in the determination of the frequency of surveillance.

SUGGESTED READINGS

Brennan MF, Casper ES, Harrison LB et al: The role of multimodality therapy in soft-tissue sarcoma. Ann Surg 214:328, 1991

A large prospectively gathered experience reported from a single institution, highlighting the use of adjuvant treatment.

Drepper H, Kohler CO, Bastian B et al: Benefit of elective lymph node dissection in subgroups of melanoma patients. Cancer 72:741, 1993

A large retrospective study evaluating the potential benefit of "prophylactic" lymph node dissection.

Evans GR: Review and current perspectives of cutaneous malignant melanoma. J Am Coll Surg 178:523, 1994

An excellent overview article with an extensive reference list.

Yang JC, Rosenberg SA: Surgery for adult patients with soft tissue sarcomas. Seminars in Oncology 16:289, 1989

A good review article that covers "all the bases."

QUESTIONS

1. A 28-year-old male with a 12-cm soft tissue sarcoma of the posterior thigh may be appropriately treated by?

    A. Amputation.
    B. Wide local excision.
    C. Local excision followed by radiotherapy.
    D. Wide local excision and inguinal lymphadenectomy.
    E. All of the above.

2. A melanoma on the calf of a 48-year-old white female is found to be 0.74 mm thick by punch biopsy. The most appropriate definitive management of this case would be?

    A. Excision with 2-cm margins.
    B. Excision with 5-cm margins.
    C. Excision with 2-cm margins and inguinal lymphadenectomy.
    D. Shave biopsy and curettage.

(See p. 604 for answers.)

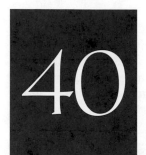

40

THYROID

TUMORS

HERNAN I. VARGAS

STANLEY R. KLEIN

T he surgeon is commonly asked to see a patient with a thyroid nodule or diffuse enlargement of the gland, a goiter. Occasionally, a patient with hyperthyroidism will be considered for surgical therapy.

The aims of this chapter are to (1) emphasize the evaluation and treatment of a patient with a thyroid nodule or goiter, (2) identify patients at risk of thyroid cancer, and (3) explain the alternatives for treatment of a patient with a thyroid nodule and/or thyroid cancer.

CASE 1
FOLLICULAR CARCINOMA

A 22-year-old female recently noted a low anterior neck mass. She did not have weight change, feelings of hot or cold, or change in bowel habits. She had no known exposure to radiation. There was no familial history of thyroid or other endocrine disease. She had a firm 2 × 2-cm mass below the cricoid ring, to the right of the midline, that moved with deglutition. There was no cervical or supraclavicular adenopathy. Serum TSH and T_4 levels were normal.

An FNA showed a follicular lesion of the thyroid. A right thyroid lobectomy was done. Intraoperative microscopic examination (frozen section) showed vascular and capsular invasion, consistent with follicular carcinoma. A completion total thyroidectomy was then done. A postoperative iodine scan did not show any thyroid remnant or other areas of uptake. She did well, taking 200 μg of levothyroxine daily.

CASE 2
GOITER WITH HYPERTHYROIDISM

A 50-year-old female who had a goiter for 30 years noted insomnia, nervousness, irritability, weight loss, and palpitations for the past 3 months. Her symptoms started 2 weeks after she had a complete evaluation for a lower abdominal mass, which on CT scan of the abdomen and pelvis (with intravenous iodine contrast), was consistent with a uterine fibroid. She elected not to have a hysterectomy. On presentation she was tachycardic (heart rate, 108 bpm). Other findings were a 15 × 10-cm low anterior neck mass consistent with a goiter, and a palpable and enlarged fibroid uterus. She also had evidence of hyperreflexia.

The serum TSH was less than 0.01 μU/ml and T_4 was 16 μg/dl (normal, 5–12 μg/dl). A thyroid scan showed a "hot" nodule in the right lobe. She was initially treated with propylthiouracil and propranolol. During the following 4 weeks her symptoms resolved and she became clinically euthyroid. A total thyroidectomy was done for cosmetic benefit. She was asymptomatic and taking 100 μg of levothyroxine daily.

GENERAL CONSIDERATIONS

Goiter is an enlargement of the thyroid gland as a consequence of elevated levels of thyroid stimulating hormone (TSH). The most significant cause worldwide is iodine deficiency. Goiter can also occur in persons with intrinsic thyroid dysfunction in spite of adequate amounts of iodine. The most common complaint is a growth in the neck. When the thyroid reaches a significant size, it may cause symptoms in the aerodigestive tract and complaints of dysphagia, dyspnea, or hoarseness are not uncommon.

Some patients will develop a defined thyroid nodule. This occurs in approximately 4–7% of the population. The main significance of a thyroid nodule is a 5–10% risk of malignancy. In populations exposed to ionizing radiation, the incidence of thyroid nodules is higher (20–30%), and of these, 30–50% are malignant. Solitary nodules in patients younger than 25 or older than 60 are more likely to be malignant (Case 1).

There are approximately 10,000 new cases of thyroid cancer in the United States yearly, although only 10% of these patients die as a consequence of thyroid carcinoma. Perhaps the most fascinating characteristic of thyroid cancer is its unique biologic behavior. It ranges from being a dormant, poorly understood, occult neoplasm found incidentally in thyroid specimens or at autopsy, to being a very aggressive malignancy, such as in anaplastic carcinoma, with nearly a 100% mortality.

Risk factors for the development of thyroid carcinoma include (1) head and neck irradiation in childhood, (2) multiple endocrine neoplasia syndrome IIa, IIb, (3) familial medullary thyroid carcinoma, and (4) poor iodine intake.

KEY POINTS

• Main significance of thyroid nodule is a 5–10% risk of malignancy; in populations exposed to ionizing radiation, the incidence is 20–30%, and of these, 30–50% are malignant

DIAGNOSIS

The diagnosis of goiter is made on clinical examination. It is important to note the presence of multinodular goiter and to search for any dominant nodules that may represent cancer. Although most patients are euthyroid, thyroxine (T_4) and TSH studies are important in determination of thyroid function.

Indirect laryngoscopy is essential in the patient who complains of hoarseness or stridor, to assess vocal cord function. In the absence of prior surgery, vocal cord paralysis is almost always due to malignancy involving the recurrent laryngeal nerve. In the patient with dysphagia, an esophagogram or upper endoscopy is prudent to exclude other causes.

The most important task is to determine whether a thyroid nodule is malignant or benign. The history may provide some clues, like recent change in size (rapid growth). Hoarseness, although nonspecific, occurs more commonly in malignant disease. The presence of a nodule of long duration (even years) does not exclude the possibility of malignancy due to the slow growth of most thyroid tumors. A history of radiation exposure or a familial history is most relevant. Examination for cervical adenopathy must be complete.

The diagnosis rests on sound clinical judgment and interpretation of ancillary tests. Laboratory evaluation is not helpful in the initial assessment of most patients with a thyroid nodule. In patients with a history suggestive of medullary carcinoma, calcitonin levels should be drawn.

The role of thyroid scintigraphy is controversial. Malignant thyroid nodules concentrate less iodine than the surrounding thyroid parenchyma ("cold" nodules), but so do thyroid cysts, colloid nodules, and adenomas. A cold lesion is likely benign; only 16% of cold nodules are malignant. A "hot" lesion represents an area of increased uptake and clinically corresponds to a hyperfunctioning benign nodule; still, 4% of hot nodules are malignant.

Ultrasound has a limited role in evaluating thyroid nodules. It is very sensitive for cystic lesions and detecting additional occult nodules, but has a very low specificity for solid nodules.

Thyroid suppression is advocated by some as a means of not only treating benign thyroid nodules but also as part of the diagnostic algorithm. The size of the nodule is followed at 6-month intervals; if it diminishes in size it can be followed, but if there is no change or an increase in size, a biopsy is required.

Thyroid lobectomy was once the standard method of diagnosis and treatment of thyroid nodules. Since the advent of fine needle aspiration (FNA), thyroid lobectomy has been limited. FNA is the first and most important diagnostic study in the evaluation of a thyroid nodule (Case 1). It provides valuable material in more than 90% of cases; however, false-negative results may be noted in up to 25% of cases. Some of the caveats of this technique are (1) sampling is operator dependent, (2) interpretation is highly dependent on the experience of the cytopathologist, (3) small lesions (<2 cm) are difficult to biopsy, and (4) large lesions (>4 cm) may lead to sampling error. Core needle biopsy is as accurate as FNA but the discomfort and complication rate are higher.

DIFFERENTIAL DIAGNOSIS

Goiter can be a manifestation of several processes. In the hyperthyroid patient, Graves disease is the most likely cause; this should be differentiated from iodine induced hyperthyroidism in multinodular goiter (Case 2) and from a hyperfunctioning autonomous thyroid nodule. In the euthyroid or hypothyroid patient, chronic thyroiditis, iodine deficiency, use of antithyroid drugs (propylthiouracil, methimazole) or some plants (casaba meal, rutabaga) can cause goiter.

In the patient with a goiter who complains of hoarseness, vocal cord paralysis by a thyroid malignancy should be excluded. Other causes of hoarseness are a laryngeal tumor or inflammatory process, or recurrent laryngeal nerve involvement by a mediastinal mass. Esophageal obstruction by tumor or stricture, esophageal motility dysfunction, or diverticula may present as dysphagia.

Differential diagnosis of a thyroid nodule includes the following:

1. *Infectious diseases*: viral, pyogenic, or granulomatous
2. *Inflammatory processes*: Hashimoto's thyroiditis, subacute thyroiditis
3. *Congenital anomalies*: cystic hygroma, dermoid cyst, teratoma, thyroglossal duct cyst
4. *Neoplastic disorders*: adenoma, carcinoma, lymphoma
5. *Miscellaneous*: thyroid cyst

TREATMENT

The main goal of therapy in patients with goiter is to suppress the TSH stimulus that incites thyroid growth and hyperplasia. Levothyroxine (100–200 µg daily) is the treatment of choice for patients who are euthyroid or hypothyroid. It is not effective in patients with autonomous hyperfunctioning nodules; they are best identified with a thyrotropin hormone (TRH) stimulation test and treated with radioactive iodine.

Thyroidectomy for goiter is indicated in (1) failure of or contraindication to medical therapy, (2) tracheal or esophageal compression, (3) sudden change in a goiter, (4) suspicion of cancer, (5) appearance (Case 2), and (6) autonomous hyperfunctioning nodule.

The management of thyroid nodules is based on the clinical history and on cytologic and histologic diagnosis, as presented in Table 40.1.

A benign diagnosis on FNA should be interpreted cautiously and the patient followed at 6–12-month intervals; if any growth is observed, thyroid lobectomy with intraoperative frozen section is indicated to exclude the presence of cancer. In the case of follicular lesions, cytology (FNA) is inadequate to detect capsular or vascular invasions that are markers of malignancy. Therefore a thyroidectomy is indicated in patients with a cytologic diagnosis of a follicular lesion.

Therapy of patients with thyroid carcinoma is planned according to the known biology of the tumor. The different histologic types are listed in Table 40.1. Histologic classification is important because it correlates closely with the biologic behavior of thyroid cancer (Case 1).

Papillary carcinoma is a well differentiated malignancy and is the most common type of thyroid carcinoma. Age is the most significant prognostic indicator, followed by size and extent of the tumor. Patients younger than 50 years or with small (<1.5 cm) tumors have an excellent prognosis, having less than 2% mortality after 25 years of follow-up. Older patients, patients with tumors larger than 4 cm, or with extrathyroidal extension have more aggressive disease.

Controversy exists regarding the extent of operation. The accepted modalities of therapy are (1) total thyroidectomy, (2) subtotal thyroidectomy, or (3) thyroid lobectomy with isthmusectomy. Total thyroidectomy is advocated on the basis of multicentricity of thyroid cancer and the incidence of recurrence in the preserved thyroid tissue. Other advantages are that follow-up and treatment with iodine 131 (^{131}I) and monitoring of thyroglobulin levels is feasible. Proponents of less than total thyroidectomy emphasize the lack of clinical significance of multicentricity and

TABLE 40.1 *Histologic classification of carcinoma of the thyroid*

Papillary carcinoma

Follicular carcinoma

Hürthle cell carcinoma

Medullary carcinoma

Anaplastic carcinoma

Lymphoma

Sarcoma

Metastasis

the increased risk of complications (hypoparathyroidsm, injury to the recurrent laryngeal nerve).

The presence of lymph node metastases is common, reported as high as 40–90%. This has no major prognostic significance and if the nodal metastases are clinically palpable, node removal is the treatment of choice. A modified neck dissection is only done if necessary to include all palpable disease. The presence of distant metastases is rare and denotes an unfavorable prognosis; patients are treated with total thyroidectomy and radioactive iodine. Subsequently, regardless of the type of operation, patients require lifelong suppression of TSH with thyroid hormone. This is directed to inhibit the growth of any foci of tumor in the thyroid remnant or in metastases, as well as to render the patient clinically euthyroid.

Follicular carcinoma is also a well differentiated malignancy. Older age, size of the lesion, and evidence of invasion are poor prognostic indicators. It may metastasize to lung and bone, significantly worsening the prognosis. Treatment is similar to papillary carcinoma of the thyroid.

Hürthle cell carcinomas are thought to be more aggressive than follicular and papillary thyroid carcinoma, having a higher local recurrence rate. They frequently metastasize. Age of the patient or size of the tumor are not considered as significant prognosis factors. Due to the aggressive behavior, total thyroidectomy is recommended. These tumors do not concentrate iodine, and thus patients do not benefit from radioactive iodine therapy.

Medullary thyroid carcinoma is a tumor of the C-cells (parafollicular cells) of the thyroid. It is commonly associated with multiple endocrine neoplasia (MEN syndrome) IIa and IIb, and screening for pheochromocytoma and hyperparathyroidism should be done preoperatively (Table 40.2). It can occur as a familial or sporadic presentation.

TABLE 40.2 *Multiple endocrine neoplasia (MEN) syndromes*

MEN I

   Parathyroid hyperplasia

   Pituitary adenomas (prolactinoma)

   Pancreatic islet cell tumors (gastrinoma/insulinoma)

MEN IIa

   Medullary carcinoma of the thyroid

   Parathyroid hyperplasia

   Pheochromocytoma

MEN IIb

   Medullary carcinoma of the thyroid

   Pheochromocytoma

   Ganglioneuromatosis

   Marfinoid habitus

The C-cells produce calcitonin, and thus calcitonin levels should be checked in patients with a thyroid mass and a significant family history. Total thyroidectomy with lymph node dissection is done because of the 50% incidence of lymphatic metastases. Radioactive iodine is not effective.

Anaplastic carcinoma is the most aggressive thyroid neoplasm. At the time of presentation, it commonly invades vital structures and is not resectable. Recent rapid growth of a thyroid nodule or nodular goiter should increase the suspicion of this entity. Therapy for these tumors includes chemotherapy and radiotherapy. Prognosis is dismal.

KEY POINTS

• In cases of follicular lesions, cytology (FNA) inadequate to detect capsular or vascular invasions that are markers of malignancy; therefore, thyroidectomy indicated in patients with cytologic diagnosis of follicular lesion

• Papillary carcinoma well differentiated malignancy and most common type of thyroid carcinoma; age most significant prognostic indicator

FOLLOW-UP

Thyroid hormone replacement for life is required in patients who are subjected to total or subtotal thyroidectomy (Cases 1 and 2), patients with thyroid cancer, and patients with goiter. Patients subjected to thyroid lobectomy for benign adenoma may not require hormonal replacement. TSH levels are followed in patients receiving hormonal replacement and in patients after lobectomy to ensure proper thyroid function.

Follow-up of patients with thyroid cancer should include

1. Physical examination: searching for recurrence in the thyroid bed, residual lobe, or cervical lymph nodes
2. Thyroglobulin level: elevation of the serum level indicates recurrence. It is only useful in patients subjected to total thyroidectomy or subtotal thyroidectomy with iodine ablation
3. Radioactive iodine scanning: to detect systemic metastases or locoregional recurrence in patients who have undergone total thyroidectomy or ablation
4. Chest x-ray: to evaluate for pulmonary metastases

SUGGESTED READINGS

Kramer JB: Thyroid carcinoma. Adv Surg 22:195, 1989

   Discusses options and controversies in the management of thyroid carcinoma.

Mazzaferri EL: Management of a solitary thyroid nodule. N Engl J Med 328:553, 1993

Review article with in-depth analysis and extensive references.

Woeber KA: Cost-effective evaluation of the patient with a thyroid nodule. Surg Clin North Am 75:357, 1995

Particularly useful in the current socioeconomic climate.

QUESTIONS

1. The following are risk factors for the development of thyroid carcinoma, except?

    A. A family history of papillary thyroid carcinoma.

    B. A family history of medullary thyroid carcinoma.

    C. Exposure to ionizing radiation.

    D. History of low iodine intake.

2. Which of the following is true regarding FNA of a thyroid nodule?

    A. It is not a very useful study in the evaluation of a thyroid nodule.

    B. The best results are obtained with a skilled and experienced cytopathologist.

    C. The size of the lesion does not influence the accuracy of the study.

    D. If a benign diagnosis is obtained, no further evaluation and follow-up is required.

3. The differential diagnosis of a thyroid nodule includes?

    A. Viral, bacterial, or granulomatous infections.

    B. Inflammatory process (thyroiditis).

    C. Benign tumors (adenoma).

    D. Cancer of the thyroid.

    E. All of the above.

4. The following are indications for surgery?

    A. Suspicion of cancer.

    B. Airway compromise.

    C. Failure of medical therapy.

    D. Cosmetic reasons.

    E. All of the above.

5. The following is false regarding thyroid cancer?

    A. Age is an important predictor of outcome in well differentiated carcinoma of the thyroid.

    B. Total thyroidectomy, subtotal thyroidectomy, and thyroid lobectomy with isthmusectomy are accepted modes of therapy for patients with well differentiated thyroid cancer.

    C. Risk of thyroidectomy includes recurrent laryngeal nerve injury and hypocalcemia.

    D. Radioactive iodine is effective in metastatic medullary carcinoma of the thyroid.

    E. Anaplastic carcinoma of the thyroid is an aggressive malignancy and is usually fatal.

(See p. 604 for answers.)

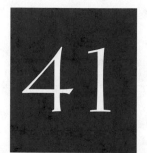

41 HYPERPARATHYROIDISM

HERNAN I. VARGAS

STANLEY R. KLEIN

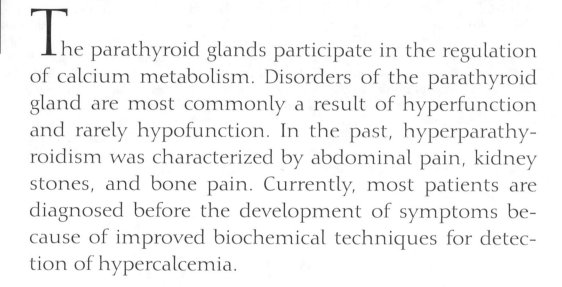

The parathyroid glands participate in the regulation of calcium metabolism. Disorders of the parathyroid gland are most commonly a result of hyperfunction and rarely hypofunction. In the past, hyperparathyroidism was characterized by abdominal pain, kidney stones, and bone pain. Currently, most patients are diagnosed before the development of symptoms because of improved biochemical techniques for detection of hypercalcemia.

Hypofunction of the parathyroid glands is primarily iatrogenic, as a complication of thyroid or parathyroid surgery, and only rarely of congenital origin.

CASE 1
ASYMPTOMATIC
HYPERPARATHYROIDISM

A 42-year-old female patient was seen for elective cholecystectomy. A calcium level obtained the day of admission was elevated. She denied any history of malignancy, weight loss, bone pain, renal stones, ulcers, or pancreatitis.

Her calcium level was 12.8 mg/dl and serum phosphorus level 2.8 mg/dl. A 24-hour urinary collection for calcium was 280 mg/24 hr. A serum PTH level was elevated at 600 pg/ml. The patient underwent a neck exploration and removal of a left superior parathyroid adenoma, with frozen section confirmation of a normal left inferior parathyroid gland.

CASE 2
SYMPTOMATIC
HYPERPARATHYROIDISM

A 60-year-old female presented with a second episode of back pain, hematuria, and passage of a renal stone. She again became asymptomatic with a calcium level of 13.6 mg/dl. She had an episode of pancreatitis 5 years previous attributed to cholelithiasis. She also admitted a history of peptic ulcer, treated with H$_2$ blockers.

In addition to the calcium elevation, her serum phosphorus was 3.1 mg/dl and a 24-hour urinary calcium excretion was 300 mg/24 hr. The PTH level was 550 pg/dl. A chest x-ray showed diffuse osteopenia.

The patient underwent neck exploration with findings of four diffusely enlarged parathyroid glands. All four glands were removed and one gland was minced. One-half of the tissue was placed into the muscles of the forearm through a small incision, and the remaining tissue was preserved.

GENERAL CONSIDERATIONS

Hyperparathyroidism is a metabolic disorder characterized by increased production of parathormone (PTH). It is the most common cause of hypercalcemia in nonhospitalized patients; however, patients with hyperparathyroidism may have low, normal, or high serum calcium levels, mostly depending on renal function. It occurs in 1 of 1,200 adults, more commonly in women.

The most common cause is a parathyroid adenoma (Case 1) (Fig. 41.1). It accounts for approximately 85% of cases. It is a benign, encapsulated neoplasm involving only one parathyroid gland. The tumor is composed of closely packed cells, predominantly chief cells. The diagnosis is safely confirmed when normal or suppressed parathyroid tissue is seen in a second gland (Case 1) or in a remnant of normal tissue in the diseased gland.

Primary parathyroid hyperplasia is the cause of hyperparathyroidism in approximately 12% of patients (Case 2). It consists of proliferation of parathyroid cells in the absence of a known stimulus for PTH hypersecretion. Typically, all parathyroid glands are enlarged; however, there may be a significant difference among the glands due to variation in the extent of enlargement. On light microscopy there is an increased parenchymal cell mass with predominance of chief cells or clear cells. Stromal fat cells are markedly decreased.

Of particular interest is the association of chief cell hyperplasia and multiple endocrine neoplasia (MEN) syndromes. The different components of the MEN syndrome and subtypes are noted in Table 41.1.

Rarely, a parathyroid carcinoma is responsible for hyperparathyroidism. Characteristically, patients have higher calcium levels than patients with adenoma or hyperplasia, and most patients have metabolic alterations. On physical examination a palpable nodule in the neck may be noted. The parathyroid gland is markedly enlarged, ill-defined, and densely adherent to the surrounding tissues. Microscopically, vascular and capsular invasion may be seen.

In patients with chronic renal failure or malabsorption syndromes there is an increase in secretion of PTH as a consequence of chronically low serum calcium levels. This is called secondary hyperparathyroidism. Patients develop bone pain or pathologic fractures that are secondary to bone resorption, decalcification, cysts, and brown tumor formation. In renal failure patients this is complicated by hyperphosphatemia and the inability to hydroxylate vitamin D_2.

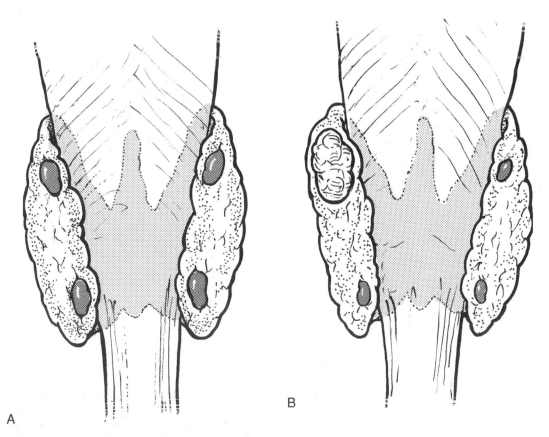

A

B

FIGURE 41.1 *(A) The normal parathyroid glands are in close proximity to the thyroid gland. (B) A parathyroid adenoma will lead to feedback inhibition and atrophy of the normal glands.*

TABLE 41.1 *Multiple endocrine neoplasia (MEN) syndromes*

MEN I (Werner)
    Parathyroid hyperplasia
    Pituitary adenoma
    Pancreatic islet cell tumors

MEN IIA
    Parathyroid hyperplasia
    Medullary thyroid carcinoma
    Pheochromocytoma

MEN IIB
    Parathyroid hyperplasia
    Medullary thyroid carcinoma
    Pheochromocytoma
    Ganglioneuromatosis
    Marfanoid habitus

In some patients with secondary hyperparathyroidism the parathyroid glands function autonomously and patients develop hypercalcemia, paralleling rising levels of PTH. This is called tertiary hyperparathyroidism.

KEY POINTS

• Some patients with secondary hyperparathyroidism develop tertiary hyperparathyroidism; parathyroid glands function autonomously and patients develop hypercalcemia, paralleling rising PTH levels

DIAGNOSIS

The classic description of a patient with "painful bones, renal stones, abdominal groans, and psychic moans" is infrequently seen nowadays. Clinical manifestations related to hypercalcemia are listed in Table 41.2, and include peptic ulcer disease, kidney stones, and pancreatitis (Case 2). Demineralization of the skeleton, pathologic fractures, bone cysts, and brown tumors are a direct consequence of elevated PTH.

TABLE 41.2 *Symptoms and complications of hypercalcemia*

Peptic ulcer, pancreatitis, anorexia

Muscle weakness

Inability to concentrate, depression, delirium, coma

Polyuria, polydipsia

Renal stones, nephrocalcinosis

With the advent of the blood biochemical analyzers, the measurement of calcium levels has become part of routine evaluation and over 50% of patients are identified by an elevated calcium level while they are asymptomatic (Case 1).

The triad of hypercalcemia, hypercalciuria, and hypophosphatemia is suggestive of primary hyperparathyroidism. If these findings are coupled with an elevated PTH level, the biochemical diagnosis of primary hyperparathyroidism is very accurate, particularly since the introduction of the immunochemiluminiscence methodology for measurement of the intact hormone (Case 1).

KEY POINTS

• Triad of hypercalcemia, hypercalciuria, and hypophosphatemia is suggestive of primary hyperparathyroidism

DIFFERENTIAL DIAGNOSIS

Causes of hypercalcemia are noted in Table 41.3. A careful history may reveal vitamin D or thiazide diuretic intake. A thorough physical examination may disclose a breast, abdominal, or prostatic mass responsible for hypercalcemia as a consequence of a paraneoplastic syndrome (usually due to ectopic production of PTH). Evaluation should include a chest x-ray as a survey for lung cancer or pulmonary metastases with the added benefit of an assessment of bone density (Case 2). A mammogram or a bone scan may be necessary if malignancy is strongly suspected, often on the basis of a depressed PTH level or associated hyperphosphatemia.

TABLE 41.3 *Differential diagnosis of hypercalcemia*

Primary hyperparathyroidism

Humoral hypercalcemia of malignancy

Multiple myeloma

Metastatic bone disease

Sarcoidosis

Thyrotoxicosis

Thiazide diuretics

Vitamin D toxicity

Familial hypocalciuric hypercalcemia

Prolonged immobilization

KEY POINTS

• Careful history may reveal vitamin D or thiazide diuretic intake

• Thorough physical examination may disclose breast, abdominal, or prostatic mass responsible for hypercalcemia as consequence of paraneoplastic syndrome (usually due to ectopic production of PTH)

• Evaluation should include chest x-ray as survey for lung cancer or pulmonary metastases with added benefit of assessment of bone density

• Mammogram or bone scan may be necessary if malignancy is strongly suspected, often on basis of depressed PTH level or associated hyperphosphatemia

TREATMENT

Classically, hyperparathyroidism has been treated by excision of the adenoma. The goal is to remove the hyperfunctioning parathyroid gland or glands with preservation of sufficient parathyroid tissue to maintain normal calcium homeostasis.

The decision to operate is more difficult in asymptomatic patients (Case 1). Approximately 30–50% of asymptomatic patients will progress to develop a metabolic complication. Neck exploration is recommended for those who develop increasing hypercalcemia, evidence of loss of bone mass, or for those patients with impairment of renal function.

At operation, the parathyroid glands are carefully examined and frozen sections are obtained as needed for confirmation of the clinical diagnosis (Case 1). A diagnosis of parathyroid adenoma is made if only one parathyroid gland is enlarged and the rest of the glands are normal or small.

All parathyroid glands are enlarged in hyperplasia. On occasion, a minimally enlarged gland may be confused on gross examination with a normal gland. Hyperplasia is confirmed by hypercellularity in more than one gland on frozen section. Three and one-half glands are removed, leaving the equivalent of one normal gland as a functioning organ.

Due to the chance of recurrent hyperparathyroidism from the remnant gland, some advocate total parathyroidectomy with autologous transplantation into the forearm in cases of parathyroid hyperplasia (Case 2). If recurrent hyperparathyroidism develops, re-excision of the extra parathyroid tissue is carried out under local anesthesia, avoiding the hazards of re-exploration of the neck.

When the diagnosis of parathyroid carcinoma is made, wide excision with clear margins including the ipsilateral thyroid lobe and frequently the ipsilateral recurrent laryngeal nerve is necessary. The tumor must not be violated or recurrence in the soft tissues of the neck is likely.

Many modalities are available for preoperative localization of the enlarged parathyroid glands; none are uniformly successful. These are listed in Table 41.4. When primary exploration of the neck is being performed by an experienced surgeon, these localizing techniques are not necessary. Radiologic studies are valuable and cost-effective in the patient with recurrent hyperparathyroidism or

TABLE 41.4 *Accuracy of localization studies*

	SENSITIVITY (%)	FALSE-POSITIVE RATE (%)
Noninvasive techniques		
Barium swallow	Historical interest	
Ultrasound	75	20
Differential thallium technitium scan	74	25
Computed tomography	70	30
Magnetic resonance imaging	80	20
Invasive techniques		
Aspiration biopsy	80	0
Arteriography	85	5
Venous sampling	80	0
Intraoperative ultrasound	80	2

in a patient in whom the diseased parathyroid gland was not identified on the first neck exploration.

A parathyroid gland may be localized in the mediastinum and it may be the cause of failure of the neck exploration. Ectopic parathyroid glands may also be located in the carotid sheath or retropharyngeal space, or may even be intrathyroidal. Ectopic location is the result of embryologic migration.

Autopsy studies have revealed four parathyroid glands in only 80% of patients. Thirteen percent of patients have five glands and 3% of patients have only three glands. This may cause difficulty at the time of surgery for obvious reasons.

Postoperatively, bleeding and hematoma formation can be hazardous due to compression of the airway; meticulous attention to hemostasis is critical. Damage to the recurrent laryngeal nerve occurs in approximately 1–2% of cases. Hypoparathyroidism can occur but is usually transient unless all four parathyroid glands have been removed or devascularized. It is chronically treated with oral calcium and vitamin D_3.

KEY POINTS

• Classically, hyperparathyroidism has been treated by excision of adenoma; goal is to remove hyperfunctioning parathyroid gland or glands with preservation of sufficient parathyroid tissue to maintain normal calcium homeostasis

FOLLOW-UP

Patients with parathyroid adenoma have the best prognosis. Postoperatively, the calcium level decreases and normalizes over the course of hours or days. Transient (hours to days) hypocalcemia is common as the remaining glands have been chronically suppressed. Patients with parathyroid hyperplasia are more likely to experience recurrent hypercalcemia and long-term follow-up is therefore recommended.

If hypercalcemia persists or recurs postoperatively, a thorough assessment should question the previous diagnosis of primary hyperparathyroidism. Review of the operative report and pathology specimen may help clarify an erroneous diagnosis of hyperplasia versus adenoma. Persistent hypercalcemia is defined as an elevated calcium level within 6 months of surgery. It is most commonly due to a missed adenoma. A localization study is indicated to help direct the reoperation to the most likely location of the gland. If recurrent hypercalcemia develops 6 months after surgery, it is called recurrent hypercalcemia and usually indicates hyperplasia.

SUGGESTED READINGS

Clark OH: Surgical treatment of primary hyperparathyroidism. Adv Endocrinol Metab 6:1, 1995

A nice review of surgical management.

Kaye TB: Hypercalcemia. How to pinpoint the cause and customize treatment. Postgrad Med 97:153, 1995

A straightforward approach to diagnosis.

Kaplan EL, Yashiro T, Salti G: Primary hyperparathyroidism in the 1990s. Ann Surg 215:300, 1992

Current views on the diagnosis and management of hyperparathdroidism.

Cope O: The story of hyperparathyroidism at the Massachusetts General Hospital. N Engl J Med 274:1174, 1966

Historical perspective on parathyroid disease, including the natural history of untreated hyperparathyroidism.

QUESTIONS

1. The following are complications of hypercalcemia, except for?

   A. Renal stones.
   B. Gallstones.
   C. Pancreatitis.
   D. Inability to concentrate, depression, delirium, coma.

2. The following are causes of hypercalcemia, except for?

   A. Hyperparathyroidism.
   B. Cancer metastatic to bone.
   C. Use of thiazide diuretics or vitamin D toxicity.
   D. Prolonged immobilization.
   E. Renal failure.

3. Which of the following laboratory examinations is characteristic of primary hyperparathyroidism?

   A. Elevated serum calcium.
   B. Low serum phosphate.
   C. Elevated PTH.
   D. Chloride/phosphate ratio greater than 33.
   E. All of the above.

4. Which of the following statements is false regarding hyperparathyroidism?

   A. The most common cause is a parathyroid adenoma.
   B. Parathyroid hyperplasia is seen in patients with renal failure or MEN syndrome.
   C. Parathyroid carcinoma is a common cause of hyperparathyroidism.
   D. Removal of the abnormal parathyroid tissue is the treatment of choice.

(See p. 604 for answers.)

42 ADRENAL
DYSFUNCTION

HERNAN I. VARGAS
STANLEY R. KLEIN

The embryologic origin of the adrenal gland is dual: the adrenal cortex as well as the gonads arise from the urogenital portion of the celomic mesoderm, while the adrenal medulla arises from a portion of the neuroectoderm. In conformity with the different embryologic origin, the two parts serve different functions. Patients with disorders of the adrenal gland may present with functional disorders or with an adrenal mass. The surgeon in particular is asked to see patients with syndromes of hyperfunction, or patients who have an adrenal mass.

CASE 1
CUSHING SYNDROME

A 42-year-old female presented with a large ecchymotic painful area in the lateral aspect of the right thigh that rapidly developed after she bumped into a coffee table. She admitted that she bruised easily and had had "coagulation tests" on many occasions with no abnormality noted. She denied any fevers or constitutional symptoms, but admitted to a 40-lb weight gain during the previous 4 or 5 years. On further questioning, she had noted the growth of excessive hair on her face, arms, and legs during the past 3 years. She denied taking any medication regularly. She had an uneventful appendectomy 15 years ago. She had had dental extractions in the past without any complications. She had no family history for hematologic or endocrine disorders. Her physical examination was significant for a temperature of 37°C; HR, 72 bpm; respiratory rate, 16 breaths/min; BP, 160/85 mmHg. She was awake, alert, and cooperative. She had central obesity and very thin extremities. Examination of her skin revealed hirsutism and striae along the shoulder girdle and anterior and lateral abdominal wall. A large ecchymotic area in the lateral aspect of the right thigh was noted, with no evidence of skin abrasion. The proximal musculature of her thighs and upper extremities was diminished and proximal motor weakness was apparent. The rest of her examination was normal.

Coagulation tests and electrolytes were normal. The chest and femur x-rays were unremarkable. An endocrine evaluation was requested to exclude Cushing syndrome. Initial testing included a morning cortisol level that was elevated at 49 μg/dl. A 24-hour urine collection of free cortisol was elevated at 250 μg/24 hr; 17 hydroxycortisol and 17 ketosteroids were also elevated at 31 and 26 mg/24 hr, respectively. A single dose dexamethasone suppression test was significant for a persistently elevated plasma cortisol. The diagnosis of Cushing syndrome was confirmed with a low dose dexamethasone suppression test that revealed 32 mg of 17 hydroxycortisol in a 24-hour urine collection, consistent with autonomous secretion of cortisol and lack of suppression.

The 17 hydroxycortisol level in the urine during a high dose dexamethasone suppression test was 29 mg/24 hr, again without evidence of suppression. This suggested an adrenal source. This was confirmed by an abdominal CT that showed a 2-cm right adrenal mass. An iodocholesterol scan to confirm the functional status of this mass revealed uptake of the isotope in the right adrenal gland without any uptake in the left adrenal gland, confirming the diagnosis of Cushing syndrome arising from a right adrenal adenoma.

The patient was subsequently hospitalized and received preoperative preparation with stress doses of hydrocortisone and underwent a right adrenalectomy and recovered uneventfully. She required steroid replacement for a period of approximately 2 months. She was doing well, 3 years after surgery. She lost approximately 30 lb and regained her strength.

CASE 2
PHEOCHROMOCYTOMA

A 28-year-old female presented with a 2-month history of headaches; some episodes were associated with sweating, palpitations, nausea, and sensations of anxiety. These episodes occurred almost every day and lasted from 30 minutes to 2 hours. She had had a normal first pregnancy 3 years prior, but developed severe toxemia during her second pregnancy 1 year later, requiring a cesarean section. Since then, she had been told that her blood pressure was high and she was being treated with nifedipine and a thiazide diuretic. She denied the use of any other medication or street drugs. Her past medical history was only significant for having an aunt with breast cancer. On physical examination, her BP was 195/120 mmHg; HR, 100 bpm; and respiratory rate, 24 breaths/min. She looked chronically ill, anxious, and had a tremor in both hands. Cardiopulmonary evaluation revealed a II/VI systolic ejection murmur. Fundoscopy revealed changes consistent with severe hypertension. The rest of the physical examination was unremarkable.

Laboratory evaluation was significant for an Hb of 16 g/dl and an Hct of 48% with no leukocytosis. Electrolytes and liver panel were within normal limits. A chest x-ray revealed mild cardiomegaly and an ECG showed mild left ventricular hypertrophy consistent with the history of hypertension.

A pheochromocytoma was suspected due to the presence of uncontrolled hypertension and paroxysms of hyperadrenergic symptoms consistent with her complicated obstetric history of hypertension and toxemia. Urinary VMA, normetanephrine, and metanephrine were 15 mg, 2.5 mg, and 6 mg, respectively, in a 24-hour urine col-

tion. Total urinary catecholamines were 72 μg in 24-hour urine sample. All these levels were elevated, consistent with hypersecretion of catecholamines, confirming the diagnosis of pheochromocytoma.

She was started on phenoxybenzamine, 10 mg twice daily for 2 days, and the dose was subsequently increased to 20 mg twice daily. She experienced some improvement of her headaches and on follow-up her BP was 165/95 mmHg. The phenoxybenzamine dose was progressively increased to 60 mg twice daily. Due to continued complaints of palpitations, propranolol was started, but not until α-blockade had been obtained. She felt a bit dizzy upon getting up quickly and had gained 12 lb since the α-blockade was started. Her Hb and Hct were 12 g/dl and 38%, respectively.

An MRI showed a 4-cm mass in the right adrenal gland. It was very bright on T_2 images and was isodense to the liver on T_1 images. No evidence of invasion into adjacent structures or vena cava thrombus was noted. The left adrenal was normal. An uneventful right adrenalectomy was performed. Her blood pressure, urinary catecholamines, VMA, and metanephrines were normal 2 years later.

GENERAL CONSIDERATIONS

Excess production of adrenal hormones may be caused by a diffuse enlargement of the adrenal gland, called hyperplasia, or by a tumor. When the pathologic process is located in the adrenal cortex, the consequence is excess production of corticosteroids (cortisol, aldosterone, testosterone).

Cushing syndrome is characterized by an excess production of glucocorticoids. Glucocorticoids are adrenal steroids that play a major role in the regulation of intermediary metabolism of protein, lipids, carbohydrates, and nucleic acids. The effects of these steroids are predominantly catabolic and are grossly exaggerated when hypercortisolism ensues. These patients suffer from excess protein breakdown and mobilization of fatty acids. Glucose metabolism and gluconeogenesis are also impaired. The anti-inflammatory characteristics of glucocorticoids are also exaggerated when there is increased production, causing disturbances in leukocyte- and cell-mediated immune function. Regulation of glucocorticoid secretion is dependent on adrenocorticotropin (ACTH) and corticotropin release factor (CRF). CRF and ACTH secretion is dependent on the circadian cycle, plasma cortisol levels, and stress (i.e., infections, trauma, emotional trauma, exercise, hypoglycemia). A servocontrol mechanism decreases ACTH release when cortisol levels are elevated by decreasing the sensitivity of pituitary cells to CRF. Glucocorticoids are metabolized in the liver and the products of catabolism, 17 hydroxycortisol and 17 ketosteroids, are excreted in the urine.

Primary hyperaldosteronism, also known as Conn syndrome, is the cause of hypertension in less than 1% of patients with hypertension. Hyperaldosteronism is more commonly secondary, due to excessive renin production in the presence of cardiac, renal, or liver disease. Conn syndrome can be caused by an adenoma (80%) or by idiopathic adrenal hyperplasia (20%). The role of aldosterone and other mineralocorticoids is to regulate the extracellular fluid volume and to control potassium homeostasis. Aldosterone acts on the distal convoluted tubule in the kidney, causing reabsorption of sodium and water in exchange for potassium. Hyperaldosteronism causes increased reabsorption of sodium and excessive excretion of potassium, leading to hypokalemia. Expansion of the intravascular space occurs through reabsorption of sodium and water but subsequently natriuresis develops, preventing the formation of edema ("escape" phenomenon). The regulatory mechanisms of aldosterone secretion include the renin-angiotensin-aldosterone axis, potassium concentration, and ACTH. These are impaired when the adrenal gland becomes autonomous as a consequence of a tumor or hyperplasia of the gland.

Pheochromocytoma is a tumor of the adrenal medulla or sympathetic ganglia. Nonfunctional tumors of the same embryologic origin and histology are known as paraganglioma. Pheochromocytoma is the cause of hypertension in only 0.2% of patients with hypertension. However, it constitutes an important, underdiagnosed cause of surgically correctable hypertension.

Pheochromocytoma occurs as a sporadic disease in 90% of cases. The remaining 10% of cases occur in the setting of a familial syndrome with genetic transmission. The more common familial syndrome is MEN II; other cases with a strong familial component are associated with von Recklinghausen's disease, Sturge-Weber syndrome, tuberous sclerosis, and von Hippel-Lindau disease. Ten percent of patients have bilateral disease and 10% of tumors occur in an extra-adrenal location, along the sympathetic chain, at the bifurcation of the aorta in the organ of Zuckerkandle, and at the root of the neck or carotid bifurcation (chemodectoma). Pheochromocytomas are malignant only 10% of the time.

A functional pheochromocytoma synthesizes catecholamines through pathways similar to normal adrenal medulla. The fraction of norepinephrine is disproportionally more elevated, and extra-adrenal pheochromocytomas produce norepinephrine exclusively. Clinical presentation is due to an expression of elevated catecholamines.

Benign lesions of the adrenal gland are far more common than primary malignant tumors. The vast majority of tumors are nonfunctional, benign adrenocortical adenomas or other benign solid tumors or cysts. A rare event is the identification of a malignant neoplasm of the adrenal cortex. It represents less than 0.05% of all cancers.

Adrenocortical carcinoma is a rare form of cancer with a high mortality. Mean age at presentation is in the early to mid-fifth decade; 75% of tumors are functional, with clinical evidence of secretion of glucocorticoids, estrogens, androgens, or aldosterone in order of frequency. Patients with clinically nonfunctional adrenocortical carcinomas present with symptoms of local progression, commonly flank pain, and may be found on examination to have a palpable abdominal mass. Pain is usually due to rapid growth, bleeding, or invasion to adjacent structures.

An adrenal mass fortuitously discovered on an imaging study is known as an incidentaloma. As a consequence of wider application of computed tomography (CT) scanning, increasing numbers of patients with an incidentally discovered adrenal mass have been identified. Incidentally discovered masses occur in approximately 0.6% of CT scans. Characteristically, these are patients that have a chest or upper abdominal CT for an unrelated problem.

KEY POINTS

- Primary hyperaldosteronism (Conn syndrome), is the cause of hypertension in less than 1% of patients with hypertension
- Clinical presentation of a pheochromocytoma is due to expression of elevated catecholamines

DIAGNOSIS

The diagnosis of adrenal pathology requires a thorough and detailed history and physical examination and a high index of suspicion. Once an adrenal cortex endocrine syndrome is suspected, a stepwise approach is essential, as noted in Figure 42.1. Biochemical testing is of paramount importance in making the diagnosis and in establishing the cause of impaired adrenal function; it provides documentation of elevated hormonal levels and of the regulatory pathways that participate in hormonal control. Finally, localization is completed via radiologic and nuclear medicine techniques.

Cushing syndrome usually occurs in the fourth decade of life and more commonly in women (Case 1). If untreated, it has a mortality of approximately 50% at 5 years. The clinical characteristics of Cushing syndrome are due to the effects of altered intermediate metabolism (Fig. 42.2). The patient described in Case 1 presented primarily with symptoms and signs of decreased protein synthesis and protein catabolism, characterized by striae, easy bruisability due to capillary fragility, muscle wasting, and proximal muscle weakness. Her weight gain, central obesity, and moon facies are attributed to deposition of adipose tissue in characteristic sites. The elevated blood pressure is attributed to a mineralocorticoid effect of excess glucocorticoids.

The biochemical diagnosis of Cushing syndrome is based on the following criteria: (1) increased cortisol production, (2) loss of circadian rhythm, and (3) inability to suppress cortisol secretion by the administration of dexa-

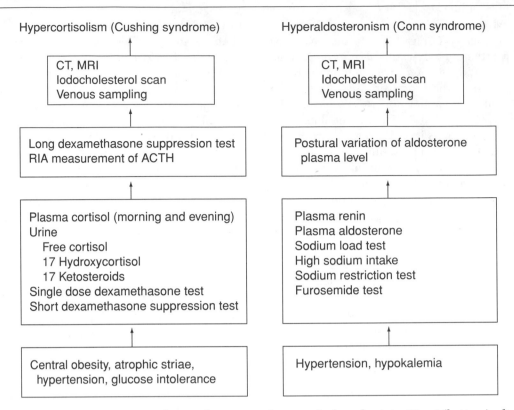

FIGURE 42.1   *Diagnostic approach to endocrine syndromes of adrenal origin. Tier I (bottom), clinical characteristics; tier II, biochemical confirmation; tier III, biochemical identification of the source; tier IV, radiologic localization.*

methasone (Case 1). Initial laboratory evaluation is directed toward documentation of abnormal cortisol production. A morning plasma cortisol level is a sensitive test, but lacks specificity and can be falsely elevated with other conditions such as obesity, alcoholism, and stress. Measurement of free cortisol in a 24-hour urinary collection is a reliable method to estimate elevated total cortisol production. It is highly sensitive and specific. Collection of urine for the metabolites 17 hydroxycortisol and 17 ketosteroids is also sensitive but not very specific. A loss of the normal circadian rhythm may be documented with an evening plasma cortisol level. Loss of regulation and feedback is a significant component of Cushing syndrome. A single dose dexamethasone suppression test is performed as part of the initial evaluation by giving a 1-mg dose of dexamethasone the night before and drawing a morning plasma cortisol level. In Case 1 it was elevated, suggesting loss of regulation and thus Cushing syndrome. A more reliable test is a low dose dexamethasone suppression test. In this test, the patient is given 0.5 mg of dexamethasone every 6 hours for 48 hours; during the last 24 hours, urine is collected for 17 hydroxycortisol. If elevated, it is diagnostic of Cushing syndrome (Case 1).

The loss of feedback is more severe in patients with Cushing syndrome of adrenal origin than in patients with Cushing's disease (pituitary origin). This concept is used to identify the source of hypercortisolism. A high dose dexam-

ethasone suppression test is used to define the source of excess hormonal production by measuring loss of regulation. Two milligrams of dexamethasone are given orally every 6 hours for 2 days. During the last 24 hours, urine is collected for 1 hydroxycortisol. A suppression to less than 40% of baseline indicates pituitary origin. In patients with primary adrenal pathology, no suppression is evident (Case 1). Patients with ectopic ACTH production exhibit a mixed response, but occasionally evidence of suppression is noted. The lack of suppression with this test (Case 1) directs our attention to the adrenal gland as the origin of a patient's problem.

The ACTH plasma level may be measured by radioimmunoassay (RIA) and is also helpful in defining the source of hypercortisolism. ACTH levels are markedly elevated in ectopic ACTH producing tumors; it is normal or elevated in pituitary disease and is low in Cushing syndrome of adrenal origin.

Once the source of hypercortisolism has been defined, imaging studies are used to localize the pathologic process that will likely require surgical resection. This discussion focuses on adrenal imaging studies. The resolution of CT and magnetic resonance imaging (MRI) is very good and lesions larger than 1 cm are easily visualized. Iodocholesterol is a radionuclide concentrated in hyperfunctioning adrenal cortex and is used as an anatomic as well as a functional nuclear medicine study. Possible results are (1) bilateral up-

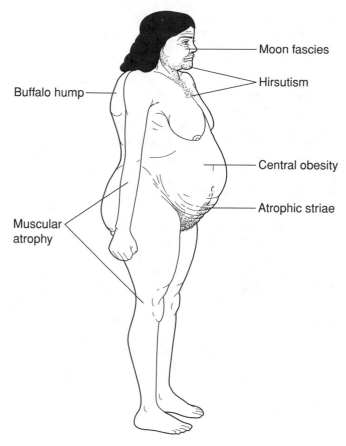

FIGURE 42.2 *Clinical, metabolic, and physiologic changes in patients with Cushing syndrome (see also Table 42.1).*

take that is associated with processes that stimulate the adrenal cortex diffusely, like Cushing's disease or ectopic ACTH production, (2) lateralized uptake that is pathognomonic of an adenoma (Case 1), or (3) bilateral nonvisualization, when an adrenal carcinoma should be considered.

The classic description of paroxysms of severe headache, sweating, tachycardia, severe hypertension, and anxiety (Case 2) occur in approximately one-third of patients with a pheochromocytoma. Paroxysms may be triggered by a variety of stimuli, such as exercise, trauma, parturition, induction of anesthesia, radiologic procedures with use of intravenous contrast, change in position, micturition, and defecation. Sustained hypertension is common, and sudden death, arrhythmia, and cardiac arrest can be the first manifestation of disease. Other common forms of presentation are anxiety, nervousness, and tremulousness.

A high index of suspicion is necessary to identify patients with pheochromocytoma. Patients to be considered are those with hypertension refractory to medical therapy (Case 2) and patients with paroxysms. Initial evaluation should include 24-hour urine collection for vanillylmandelic acid (VMA), metanephrine, and normetanephrine or free catecholamine levels. These tests in combination are very sensitive and specific for the diagnosis of pheochromocytoma. On the rare occasion when these tests are not conclusive, a clonidine suppression test may be necessary. Clonidine normally reduces sympathetic tone and plasma catecholamine levels in patients with essential hypertension. Due to autonomous, nonregulated production, a persistent elevation of catecholamines in patients with pheochromocytoma is noted.

Once a diagnosis of pheochromocytoma has been made, localization of the tumor is essential to provide adequate therapy. MRI and CT are the most useful tests. Most lesions are easily identified because they are larger than 3 cm at the time of diagnosis and are characteristically bright on T_2-weighted images (Case 2). MRI is also helpful in defining vascular invasion of the vena cava, evaluation for liver metastases, and to assess the contralateral adrenal gland. Imaging with CT before α-blockade should be approached with caution, due to the risk of hypertensive crisis precipitated by intravenous contrast. A metaiodobenzyl-

TABLE 42.1 *Clinical, metabolic, and physiologic changes in patients with Cushing syndrome*

	METABOLIC CHANGES	CLINICAL EXPRESSION
Protein metabolism	Increased protein breakdown and nitrogen excretion	Muscle weakness Striae
	Mobilization of glycogenic amino acid precursors from muscle, bone, skin, connective tissue	Osteoporosis Bruises easily
Carbohydrate metabolism	Gluconeogenesis	Glucosuria
	Inhibited glucose uptake by peripheral tissues	Glucose intolerance
Lipid metabolism	Lipolysis, redistribution of fat	Central obesity, "buffalo hump," "moon facies"
Immunologic changes	Inhibited macrophage and neutrophil chemotaxis	Poor wound healing
	Decreased complement levels	Susceptibility to and inability to fight infections
	Suppressed natural killer cell activity	
Miscellaneous changes	Mineralocorticoid action	Hypertension, hypokalemia
	Androgen effect	Hirsutism

The labels on the figure read: Moon fascies, Hirsutism, Buffalo hump, Central obesity, Muscular atrophy, Atrophic striae.

guanidine (MIBG) nuclear medicine scan may be useful in identifying the primary tumor, bilateral tumors, extra-adrenal tumors, and metastases. Rarely, venous sampling may be necessary to define the location of the pheochromo-cytoma; this technique should only be attempted after appropriate blockade has been achieved.

Conn syndrome should be suspected in patients who develop hypertension and have unexplained hypokalemia. Hypertension is due to retention of sodium and water; it is usually moderate but malignant hypertension is not uncommon. When hypokalemia is severe, muscle cramps, proximal muscular weakness, and fatigue may ensue. Metabolic alkalosis is usually asymptomatic but, when severe, patients may develop tetany and muscle paralysis.

Initial laboratory evaluation is directed to documenting retention of sodium and excretion of potassium by the kidneys and to verify the increase in aldosterone production (Table 42.2). It should include a 24-hour collection of urine for sodium, potassium, and aldosterone levels. Plasma renin level, aldosterone, and serum electrolytes should be checked. It is important to stop all diuretics and spirono-lactone, as well as most antihypertensive medication before functional evaluation of these patients. Hypokalemia should be corrected as well. Patients with autonomous production of aldosterone exhibit a persistent elevation and loss of regulation of aldosterone secretion. This concept is tested by administering a large sodium load either intravenously or orally, followed by measurement of the aldosterone urinary excretion. The normal response is to experience a marked decrease in aldosterone secretion and excretion after a large sodium load. If the urinary levels of aldosterone are persistently elevated (>17 μg/24 hr) it indicates lack of suppression, supporting the diagnosis of an autonomous source of aldosterone production.

In patients with primary hyperaldosteronism, renin is suppressed due to the persistent autonomous elevation of aldosterone. With the loss of physiologic regulation of the renin-aldosterone-angiotensin axis, the normal renin elevation following sodium depletion is absent. Two methods to accomplish sodium depletion are (1) sodium restriction of 10 mEq/day for 3 days (2) administration of furosemide in the evening before sampling of blood. Renin levels are measured the following morning, after the patient has been in the upright position for 2 hours. Normally the renin level rises to more than 3 μg/ml. In patients with primary hyperaldosteronism the renin level fails to rise.

Postural studies are most valuable in differentiating an aldosterone producing adenoma from hyperplasia. This test is performed by maintaining the patient on a 12 mEq sodium/day diet for 3 days. The patient should be recumbent the night before the test. The morning of the test, after 4 hours in the upright position, levels of plasma

TABLE 42.2 *Renin-angiotensin-aldosterone axis in different pathologic conditions*

	Normal Sodium Recumbence	Normal Sodium Upright Position	High Sodium Load	Sodium Restriction
	Test performed in the morning after overnight recumbence	Test performed after 4 hours in the upright position and ambulating	1. Oral: 250 mEq/day 2. IV: 2 L of NS	1. Oral: 10 mEq/day 2. Furosemide the evening prior
Normal				
Renin	N	⇑	⇓	⇑
Angiotensin I	N	⇑	⇓	⇑
Angiotensin II	N	⇑	⇓	⇑
Aldosterone	N	⇑	⇓	⇑
Aldosterone producing adenoma				
Renin	⇓⇓	⇓⇓	⇓⇓	⇓⇓
Angiotensin I	⇓⇓	⇓⇓	⇓⇓	⇓⇓
Angiotensin II	⇓⇓	⇓⇓	⇓⇓	⇓⇓
Aldosterone	⇑⇑⇑⇑⇑	⇑⇑⇑	⇑⇑⇑⇑⇑	⇑⇑⇑⇑⇑
Idiopathic hyperplasia				
Renin	⇓⇓	⇓	⇓⇓	⇓⇓
Angiotensin I	⇓⇓⇃	⇓	⇓⇓	⇓⇓
Angiotensin II	⇓⇓	⇓	⇓⇓	⇓⇓
Aldosterone	⇑⇑⇑⇑⇑	⇑⇑ ⇑⇑⇑	⇑⇑⇑⇑⇑	⇑⇑⇑⇑⇑

renin, aldosterone, and cortisol are drawn. Patients with idiopathic hyperplasia causing hyperaldosteronism are responsive to the angiotensin II rise elicited by the upright posture and experience an increase in aldosterone levels. The finding of similar or lower levels of aldosterone in the upright position relative to recumbence is seen in patients with an aldosterone producing adenoma, and is a predictor of response to surgical therapy. This test is helpful in approximately 85% of cases (Table 42.2).

Localization of the aldosterone producing adenoma is essential to providing adequate therapy. CT and MRI provide a very sensitive method of localizing adrenal masses but do not define the functional status of the mass. Furthermore, 3–20% of patients with hypertension have an incidental adrenal mass on CT. Therefore, a functional localizing study is necessary to determine the position of the aldosterone producing adenoma. The iodocholesterol scan is a sensitive test for lesions larger than 1 cm. If this study does not show lateralization, selective venous sampling is indicated to provide accurate localization of the tumor. Venous sampling is an invasive test; blood is drawn through a catheter guided radiologically to different levels of the vena cava and into the adrenal and renal veins. Collected blood is carefully labeled and assayed for aldosterone and cortisol levels.

In order to make an accurate diagnosis and direct appropriate therapy, evaluation of any patient with a known adrenal mass should be geared toward identifying this mass as benign nonfunctional, benign functional, or malignant.

Evaluation (Fig. 42.3) should include the following:

1. A thorough history and physical examination, looking for evidence of a functional disorder or for evidence of a cancer that may be the cause of adrenal metastases

2. Plasma samples for electrolytes (sodium, potassium), cortisol, aldosterone, and renin and 24-hour urine collection for cortisol, 17 hydroxycortisol, 17 ketosteroids, aldosterone, and VMA, metanephrine, and normetanephrine to exclude a functional tumor

3. CT scan or MRI. MRI is advocated by some authors as a means of differentiating the nature of a mass but this has not proved true in our experience. Important information gathered from these studies include size of the mass, extension into adjacent structures, status of the opposite adrenal gland, and presence of liver or other lesions

4. Nuclear scanning with iodocholesterol in certain functional masses may be helpful. MIGB scanning is only indicated if there is evidence of a catecholamine secreting tumor

5. Cytologic evaluation through CT-guided aspiration of adrenal masses is not useful to differentiate an adenoma from carcinoma. Its main role is to confirm the presence of metastasis. This should only be done after a pheochromocytoma has been excluded through biochemical analysis

Adrenocortical carcinoma should be suspected in patients with rapid progression of an endocrine syndrome or in patients who develop pain related to an adrenal mass. Size is one of the most important radiologic criteria to determine the nature of a nonfunctional adrenal mass. The risk of malignancy is proportional to the size of the mass. Approximately 90% of adrenal carcinomas are larger than 6 cm. Other criteria for malignancy are the presence of metastases or invasion of adjacent structures. Histologic criteria are not as certain as in other malignancies and careful clinical follow-up may be the only evidence of malignancy.

KEY POINTS

• Biochemical diagnosis of Cushing syndrome is based on (1) increased cortisol production, (2) loss of circadian rhythm, and (3) inability to suppress cortisol secretion by administration of dexamethasone

• Initial laboratory evaluation directed to document abnormal cortisol production

• Loss of regulation and feedback is significant component of Cushing syndrome

• Loss of feedback is more severe in patients with Cushing syndrome of adrenal origin than in patients with Cushing's disease

• Once the source of hypercortisolism has been defined, imaging studies are used to localize the pathologic process that will very likely require surgical resection

• Conn syndrome should be suspected in patients who develop hypertension and have unexplained hypokalemia

• Initial laboratory evaluation directed to documenting retention of sodium and excretion of potassium by the kidneys and to verify the increase in aldosterone production

• Patients with autonomous production of aldosterone exhibit a persistent elevation and loss of regulation of aldosterone secretion

• In patients with primary hyperaldosteronism, renin is suppressed due to the persistent autonomous elevation of aldosterone

• Patients with idiopathic hyperplasia causing hyperaldosteronism are responsive to angiotensin II rise elicited by upright posture, and experience increase in aldosterone levels; finding of similar or lower levels of aldosterone in upright position relative to recumbence is seen in patients with an aldosterone producing adenoma, and is predictor of response to surgical therapy

• Localization of aldosterone producing adenoma is essential to providing adequate therapy

DIFFERENTIAL DIAGNOSIS

The differential diagnosis of an adrenal mass includes (1) a benign nonfunctional mass such as adrenal adenomas, myelolipoma, or adenolipoma; (2) a benign functional mass such as pheochromocytomas or an adenoma causing

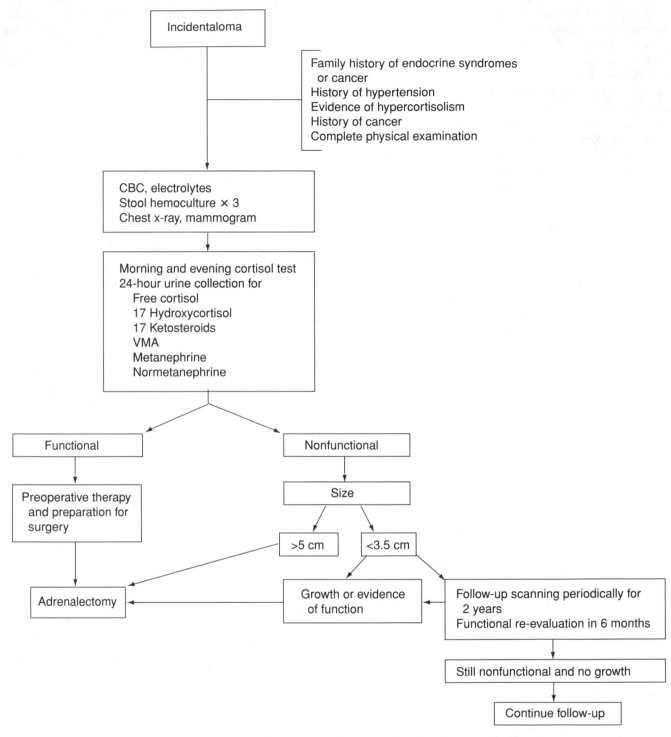

FIGURE 42.3 *Evaluation of a patient with an incidentally discovered adrenal mass.*

hypercortisolism, or hyperaldosteronism; or (3) a malignant mass, such as adrenocortical carcinoma, metastases, or malignant pheochromocytoma.

The most frequent cause of hypercortisolism is exogenous administration of steroids. The number of cases of endogenous Cushing syndrome is small by comparison. Of these, 60–70% are due to bilateral adrenal hyperplasia secondary to elevated ACTH secretion from a pituitary adenoma; this is known as Cushing's disease. Of cases, 10–20% are due to ectopic production of ACTH, characteristically by oat cell carcinoma of the lung but occasionally by pulmonary carcinoid tumors and islet cell tumors of the pancreas. A benign functional adrenal adenoma is the cause of this syndrome in approximately 20% of cases. Only 1–2% of cases are due to primary nodular adrenal hyperplasia. Rarely, it is caused by an adrenocortical carcinoma.

Pheochromocytoma should be considered in patients with poorly controlled hypertension. Patients with symptoms compatible with catecholamine release (paroxysms) should be evaluated to exclude a pheochromocytoma. Amphetamines or cocaine overdose and withdrawal from clonidine or opioids may present as an "adrenergic crisis" and should be considered in the differential diagnosis.

The most common cause of hypokalemia in patients with hypertension is the use of diuretics. Hypokalemia should be corrected and diuretics stopped in this situation before serious consideration of hyperaldosteronism. If the hypokalemia persists, hyperaldosteronism should be considered. Hyperaldosteronism may arise as a primary disorder of the adrenal gland, as discussed previously. Another condition in which aldosterone levels are elevated is secondary hyperaldosteronism, caused by processes that stimulate renin, resulting in an increase in the function of the renin-angiotensin-aldosterone axis (i.e., renovascular hypertension, congestive heart failure, cirrhosis, nephrotic syndrome).

TREATMENT

The main goals of therapy in patients who present with a functional endocrine syndrome are to (1) normalize endocrine function, (2) avoid significant hormonal deficiencies as a consequence of therapy, and (3) eradicate the tumor with the least morbid approach.

Treatment of Cushing syndrome is directed to the cause. Patients with Cushing's disease are best treated with a transsphenoidal pituitary adenoma excision. Tumors causing ectopic ACTH secretion should also be removed surgically when feasible. The treatment of choice for patients with a cortisol producing adrenal adenoma is unilateral adrenalectomy. A comparison of the different approaches is listed in Table 42.3.

Attention to detail in preoperative and postoperative management is essential. We routinely use prophylactic antibiotics in these immunosuppressed patients as well as antiembolic prophylaxis. Stress doses of steroids are necessary, and tapering over a prolonged period of time may

be required due to chronic suppression of the conralateral adrenal gland (Case 1). Patients with adrenal nodular hyperplasia require bilateral adrenalectomy and need lifelong replacement therapy with glucocorticoids and mineralocorticoids.

In patients who are not surgical candidates, or in those who refuse surgery, medical therapy with metyrapone or aminoglutethimide is an alternative. Both drugs act by inhibiting the metabolism of cholesterol into cortisol.

Definitive therapy of patients with pheochromocytoma consists of surgical resection of the tumor. This can only be accomplished safely if a meticulous preoperative preparation is observed. The objective of preoperative preparation in this setting is (1) to protect the patient from the effects of excessive catecholamine release and (2) to provide adequate fluid replacement to avoid severe hypotension following removal of the tumor. Patients with pheochromocytoma have a contracted intravascular space as a consequence of constant vasoconstriction due to α-adrenergic stimulation.

Once a diagnosis of pheochromocytoma is made, α-blockade should be started, then imaging studies and surgical planning can be done safely. Two commonly used adrenergic α-blocking agents are phentolamine and phenoxybenzamine. Phenoxybenzamine causes a noncompetitive blockage. It is given twice daily starting at low doses of 10 mg twice daily; it is the drug of choice due to its oral administration and long duration of action. The dosage should be increased gradually. As the blockade ensues, progressive peripheral vasodilatation occurs, leading to high fluid intake that restores the plasma volume. The decrease in hemoglobin (Case 2) is a consequence of hemodilution from increased fluid retention in the intravascular space that normally follows adequate α-blockade. The presence of orthostatic symptoms (dizziness upon sitting up) is also an expected consequence of α-blockade. β-Adrenergic blockade is generally not necessary, except in patients who develop tachycardia (Case 2) or present with arrhythmias. It is usually obtained with propranolol and should never be started before obtaining α-adrenergic blockade due to the risk of precipitating cardiac failure.

Blocking the synthesis of catecholamines causes a depletion of epinephrine and norepinephrine. Manipula-

TABLE 42.3 *Comparison of different surgical approaches to adrenalectomy*

SURGICAL APPROACH	POSTOPERATIVE PAIN	POSTOPERATIVE ILEUS	CONVALESCENCE	COMMENTS
Posterior	+/++	+/−	+/++	Ideal for functional cortical adenomas; small lesions
Flank	++	+/−	+++	Moderate-size lesions
Celiotomy	+++	+++	+++	Large lesions, pheochromocytoma, adrenocortical carcinoma
Laparoscopic	0	0	0	Needs high level of skills and experience
Thoracoabdominal	++++	+++	+++	Very large lesions, adrenal carcinoma invading adjacent structures

tion of the tumor can otherwise provoke an adrenergic, hypertensive crisis. Methyltyrosine (Demser) acts as a competitive inhibitor of the enzyme tyrosine hydroxylase, blocking the synthesis of epinephrine and norepinephrine. Methyltyrosine is usually used in combination with an adrenergic α-blocker. During induction of general anesthesia and through the operation, drugs and maneuvers that induce release of catecholamines should be avoided. Phentolamine or nitroprusside may be used intraoperatively to control hypertensive episodes and lidocaine and β-blockers may be used for ventricular and atrial arrhythmias. Once the tumor is removed, hypotension can occur. This can usually be treated with volume replacement but occasionally vasopressors are necessary.

Removal of the pheochromocytoma is the treatment of choice. For adrenal pheochromocytomas, an adrenalectomy is required. A transabdominal approach is recommended to allow safe removal of the gland with minimal manipulation, "dissecting the patient off the tumor," and to facilitate exploration of the abdomen to exclude multicentricity of the process. Infrequently, a pheochromocytoma is found in an extra-adrenal location; in a similar fashion, it requires surgical resection.

Patients with an aldosterone producing adenoma (Conn syndrome) are treated by unilateral adrenalectomy. Careful selection of patients for surgery is based on the orthostatic decrease of aldosterone levels, on the results of imaging studies, and, if necessary, venous sampling. Preoperative objectives are (1) control of hypertension and (2) correction of potassium depletion. These two objectives can be accomplished with the use of spironolactone, a specific aldosterone antagonist, and oral potassium replacement. If necessary, additional antihypertensive medication should be used. There is no need to use perioperative glucocorticoids. Overall, patients do well after operation and generally, no postoperative antihypertensive medication is required. Spironolactone should be stopped and potassium levels should be followed; occasionally, hyperkalemia is noted.

For patients with idiopathic nodular hyperplasia causing hyperaldosteronism in whom an orthostatic rise in aldosterone levels is noted, medical therapy is recommended. These patients are preferentially treated with spironolactone and other antihypertensive medication, and potassium placement is added as needed. Bilateral adrenalectomy in the past has provided little benefit to these patients.

Patients suspected of having an adrenal carcinoma are treated by adrenalectomy. These tumors have a mean diameter of 16 cm and require a transabdominal or a thoracoabdominal approach. An attempt should be made to resect all gross disease, including en bloc resection of tumor invading the kidney or perirenal at. When the presence of an intracaval thrombus is noted on preoperative imaging, a thrombectomy is indicated. Occasionally, cardiopulmonary bypass will be necessary if the tumor thrombus reaches the right atrium. If omental or liver metastases are found during laparotomy, especially in functional tumors,

debulking should be attempted. Treatment of patients with unresectable disease is not very rewarding. Chemotherapy has not been shown to improve survival and tumor responses are seen only in a small number of patients. The most investigated agent is ortho-para-DDD.

KEY POINTS

• Main goals of therapy in patients who present with endocrine syndrome: (1) normalize endocrine function, (2) avoid significant hormonal deficiencies as a consequence of therapy, and (3) eradicate tumor with least morbid approach

• Once diagnosis of pheochromocytoma made, α-blockade should be started, then imaging studies and surgical planning can be done safely

• Preoperative objectives are control of hypertension and correction of potassium depletion

---

FOLLOW-UP

Unilateral adrenalectomy is curative for patients with benign adrenal adenomas. Patients with Cushing syndrome will require glucocorticoid replacement therapy for variable periods, depending on the degree of suppression of the contralateral adrenal gland. This can vary from a few weeks to several months.

In the case of aldosterone producing adenomas, 85–90% of patients will experience normalization of their blood pressure following adrenalectomy. Most of the remaining patients will experience marked improvement in blood pressure control and have easily controlled hypertension.

Patients who are subjected to adrenalectomy for a pheochromocytoma require lifelong follow-up to exclude the possibility of residual tumor metastases or a metachronous lesion in the opposite adrenal gland or any sympathetic ganglia. It should include periodic visits for evaluation of symptoms, blood pressure, and catecholamine levels.

All patients who are known to have an adrenal mass that is not surgically removed need to have close biochemical and radiologic follow-up periodically, to identify a functional disorder or a growing mass, which may represent a carcinoma, as soon as possible.

Survival of patients with adrenocortical carcinoma is generally poor. Indicators that should alert to a poor prognosis are large size of the primary tumor, local invasion, or evidence of lymphatic or systemic metastasis. Histologic criteria for prognosis are not well identified, but there is some evidence that the mitotic rate might be a prognostic indicator. If untreated, mean survival is approximately 3 months. Patients who have a successful adrenalectomy face a 20%, 5-year survival. In patients who have functional adrenocortical carcinoma, urinary levels of corticosteroids can be used as a marker of recurrent disease. If recurrent disease develops, particularly in corticosteroid secreting tumors, surgical resection, if possible, is the best treatment.

SUGGESTED READINGS

Cohn K, Gottesman L, Brennan M: Adrenocortical carcinoma. Surgery 100:1170, 1986

A thorough look at an unusual tumor.

Staren ED, Prinz RA: Selection of patients with adrenal incidentalomas for operation. Surg Clin North Am 75:499, 1995

With widespread use of imaging studies, incidental adrenal masses are frequently "discovered."

Werbel SS, Ober KP: Pheochromocytoma. Update on diagnosis, localization, and management. Med Clin North Am 79:131, 1995

An excellent in-depth review.

QUESTIONS

1. Which of the following are causes of Cushing syndrome?

    A. Pituitary adenoma (Cushing's disease).

    B. Ectopic production of ACTH (by lung cancer or carcinoid tumors of the lung).

    C. Benign adrenal adenoma.

    D. Adrenocortical carcinoma.

    E. All of the above

2. Which of the following metabolic abnormalities are characteristic of Cushing syndrome?

    A. Increased cortisol secretion.

    B. Loss of circadian rhythm, regulation, and feedback.

    C. Inability to suppress cortisol secretion by the administration of exogenous corticosteroids.

    D. All of the above.

3. Which of the following is false regarding hyperaldosteronism?

    A. Is the cause of hypertension in 1% of patients.

    B. Is usually caused by a pituitary adenoma.

    C. It should be suspected in patients who develop hypertension and hypokalemia.

    D. Initial evaluation should include a 24-hour urine collection for sodium, potassium, and aldosterone levels.

    E. If an adenoma is suspected, localization is essential to provide adequate therapy.

4. Preoperative preparation of the patient with a pheochromocytoma includes?

    A. Adrenergic blockade to protect the patient from the effects of excessive catecholamine release.

    B. Provide adequate fluid replacement to avoid severe hypotension following removal of the tumor.

    C. The most commonly used agents are the α-adrenergic blockers: phenoxybenzamine and phentolamine

    D. β-Blockade should be instituted after α-blockade if necessary.

    E. Methyltyrosine acts as a competitive inhibitor of the enzyme tyrosine hydroxylase, blocking the synthesis of epinephrine and norepinephrine.

    F. All of the above.

(See p. 604 for answers.)

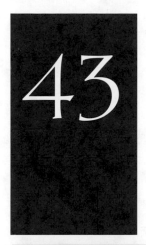

43

EXTRACRANIAL

VASCULAR

DISEASE

CHRISTIAN DE VIRGILIO

Stroke is among the leading causes of morbidity and mortality in the United States. There are approximately 500,000 new strokes each year, with 150,000 deaths. The cost of these strokes is $18 billion per year in lost productivity and direct health care expenditures. Considerable effort has been focused on identifying the underlying etiology, prevention, and treatment of stroke. Ischemic strokes currently account for the vast majority of all strokes. Despite advances in the understanding of the pathophysiology of stroke, it continues to be a formidable challenge. The aims of this chapter are to identify the more common causes of ischemic stroke, outline the diagnostic evaluation and discuss the optimal strategies for management.

CASE 1
TRANSIENT RIGHT EYE
BLINDNESS

A 64-year-old white male presented to his internist complaining of two episodes of right eye blindness, which he described as a black curtain descending over the eye that completely resolved after 5 minutes. Past medical and social history were significant for hypertension and a 50 pack/yr smoking history. Physical examination revealed bilateral carotid bruits, a regular cardiac rate and rhythm, no palpable aortic aneurysm, normal distal extremity pulses, and no neurologic deficits.

Carotid duplex scan demonstrated bilateral 80–99% ICA stenosis. The patient was placed on aspirin and im-

mediately referred to a vascular surgeon. Angiogram of the aortic arch and both carotid and vertebral arteries (four vessels), including intracranial views, confirmed 90% proximal ICA stenosis bilaterally, without lesions in the aortic arch vessels or vertebral or intracranial arteries. Preoperative ECG was normal.

The patient underwent a right carotid endarterectomy without complications. One week postoperatively, he underwent an uneventful left carotid endarterectomy. He was discharged home on aspirin.

CASE 2
RIGHT ARM AND LEG
PARALYSIS, APHASIA

A 70-year-old black female presented to the emergency room with acute onset of right arm and leg weakness that began 1 hour before admission. Past medical history was significant for diabetes and hypercholesterolemia. Physical examination revealed a regular cardiac rate and rhythm, no carotid bruits, marked right-sided weakness, and aphasia.

Diagnostic evaluation included a normal ECG, CT scan of the head that was positive for a left cerebral hemispheric infarct without hemorrhage, and a carotid duplex scan that revealed a normal right ICA and an 80–99% left ICA stenosis.

The patient was started on aspirin. The neurologic deficit gradually improved and she was discharged. Four weeks later, the aphasia had resolved and her arm and leg improved to the extent that she was able to walk again. She was referred to a vascular surgeon. Aortic arch and four vessel angiography demonstrated an 80% left ICA stenosis with an ulcerated plaque. A left carotid endarterectomy was performed. The postoperative course was uneventful and she was discharged on aspirin.

GENERAL CONSIDERATIONS

Most strokes are ischemic in origin. There are myriad causes of ischemic stroke, but the most common are carotid artery atherosclerosis and cardiac embolization.

In dealing with cerebral ischemia, it is important to understand the terminology. A transient ischemic attack (TIA) is a neurologic deficit that completely resolves within 24 hours (Case 1). A reversible ischemic neurologic deficit (RIND) lasts longer than 24 hours but less than 1 week. A completed stroke has symptoms that last beyond 1 week (Case 2).

The cerebrovascular system can be divided into the anterior and posterior circulations. The two are interconnected by the circle of Willis. The anterior circulation is represented by the carotid arteries, which divide intracranially into the anterior and middle cerebral arteries. Thus, anterior circulation symptoms are the result of ischemia to the middle cerebral and anterior cerebral artery territories (motor and sensory cortex, speech center). The carotid TIA occurs in the anterior circulation distribution and classically lasts 30 minutes or less. It results in transient motor and/or sensory symptoms limited to one side of the body, aphasia, dysphasia, or retinal ischemia (Table 43.1).

The posterior circulation consists of the two vertebral arteries that join to form the basilar artery, which supplies the cerebellum and brain stem. Posterior circulation symptoms, referred to as vertebrobasilar insufficiency, include motor and/or sensory symptoms on both sides in the same episode, ataxia of gait or clumsiness of the extremities, diplopia, dysarthria or dysphagia, and unilateral or bilateral homonymous hemianopsia. These symptoms are sometimes associated with vertigo (Table 43.2).

Most acute cerebrovascular ischemic events are the result of emboli from either a cardiac source or the carotid bifurcation. Thrombus within the cardiac chambers most often forms in the setting of atrial fibrillation or following acute myocardial infarction. The thrombus may then embolize into the cerebral circulation. The carotid bifurcation (into the internal and external carotid artery) is the most frequent site of atherosclerotic plaque deposition in the extracranial cerebral vasculature. It was previously thought that most strokes and TIAs of carotid origin were hemodynamic, due to progressive narrowing of the internal carotid artery (ICA). However, it is presently known that embolization from a carotid atherosclerotic plaque is the more common cause of neurologic events. The plaque is prone to rupture and when it does, it releases platelets and cholesterol debris into the cerebral circulation. This concept explains how even a moderate ICA stenosis, via plaque rupture and embolization, may lead to a stroke. Following rupture, an ulcer may persist in the ICA. This ulcer may be visible angiographically in the bed of the plaque (Case 2).

Once an embolus from the heart or the carotid bifurcation enters the cerebral circulation, the magnitude of the ensuing neurologic deficit is dependent on several factors. First, the duration of the ischemia is critical. The size of the embolus may determine whether it can be rapidly lysed, resulting in a TIA (Case 1), or whether it produces sufficient ischemia to cause a permanent stroke (Case 2). The patency of the contralateral carotid artery and the completeness of the circle of Willis are impor-

TABLE 43.1 *Anterior circulation symptoms*

Motor dysfunction of extremities and/or face (contralateral)

    Paralysis

    Paresis

    Clumsiness

Sensory deficit of extremities and/or face (contralateral)

Loss of vision (amaurosis fugax, ipsilateral)

Homonymous hemianopsia

Aphasia or dysphasia

TABLE 43.2 *Posterior circulation symptoms*

Motor dysfunction of extremities and/or face (ipsilateral, contralateral, or bilateral)

    Paralysis

    Paresis

    Clumsiness

Sensory deficit of extremities and/or face (ipsilateral, contralateral, or bilateral)

Unilateral or bilateral homonymous hemianopsia

Ataxia of gait

Diplopia

Dysarthria or dysphagia

Vertigo

tant, as they provide collateral circulation. The location at which the embolus lodges is likewise important. Most emboli entering the carotid system lodge in the middle cerebral artery or its branches (Case 2). However, if the embolic material lodges in the internal ophthalmic artery, temporary blindness (amaurosis fugax) may ensue until the clot dissolves or fragments, and flow to the retina is restored (Case 1).

KEY POINTS

• Ischemic strokes currently account for the vast majority of strokes

• A TIA is a neurologic deficit that completely resolves within 24 hours; RIND lasts up to 1 week; and symptoms of a completed stroke last beyond 1 week

• The carotid TIA occurs in the anterior circulation distribution, lasts 30 minutes or less, and results in transient motor and/or sensory symptoms limited to one side of the body, aphasia, dysphasia, or retinal ischemia

• Posterior circulation symptoms, or vertebrobasilar insufficiency, include motor and/or sensory symptoms on both sides in the same episode, ataxia of gait or clumsiness of extremities, diplopia, dysarthria or dysphagia, and unilateral or bilateral homonymous hemianopsia

• Most emboli entering the carotid system lodge in the middle cerebral artery or its branches; however, if embolic material lodges in the internal ophthalmic artery, temporary blindness (amaurosis fugax) may ensue until clot dissolves or fragments, and flow to retina is restored

---

DIAGNOSIS

The diagnosis of acute cerebral ischemia is made by the combination of pertinent history, physical examination, and diagnostic studies. The patient most often will complain of a focal neurologic deficit. With carotid territory ischemia (anterior circulation), this includes unilateral arm and leg paresis and/or paralysis (Case 2).

The diagnosis of a stroke can be confirmed with computed tomography (CT) of the head without contrast to look for an infarction or hemorrhage. However, the CT scan may not detect an ischemic cerebral infarct within the first 24 hours. Magnetic resonance imaging (MRI) has better resolution and is able to demonstrate smaller areas of tissue damage earlier than CT scanning, but is more expensive and not routinely available.

KEY POINTS

• Diagnosis of stroke can be confirmed with CT of the head without contrast, looking for infarction or hemorrhage

• CT scan may not detect an ischemic cerebral infarct within the first 24 hours, and MRI should be used

---

DIFFERENTIAL DIAGNOSIS

The differential diagnosis of an acute neurologic event is extensive (Table 43.3). Intracranial hemorrhage, due to trauma, arteriovenous malformation, or ruptured Berry aneurysm, should be excluded. Causes of ischemic stroke can be divided into vascular, cardiac, inflammatory, hematologic, and drug-induced disorders.

TREATMENT

Patients with a new onset neurologic deficit should be admitted to the hospital. Immediate management should focus on maintaining a patent airway and adequate breathing. If the neurologic deficit is severe, endotracheal intubation may be necessary to prevent aspiration and maintain normal oxygen and carbon dioxide levels. Hypercarbia will exacerbate cerebral edema, as carbon dioxide is a potent va-

---

TABLE 43.3 *Differential diagnosis of stroke*

Vascular
   Atherosclerosis
   Lacunar infarct
   Moyamoya (occlusion of carotid siphon)
   Fibromuscular dysplasia
Cardiac
   Arrhythmias
   Acute myocardial infarction with mural thrombus
   Prosthetic heart valves
   Rheumatic heart disease
   Atrial myxoma
   Endocarditis
Inflammatory
   Systemic lupus erythematosus
   Takayasu's arteritis
   Giant cell arteritis
   Polyarteritis nodosa
   Syphilitic arteritis
Hematologic
   Sickle cell anemia
   Polycythemia
   Leukemia
   Hypercoagulable states
Drug-induced
   Heroin
   Cocaine
   Amphetamines

sodilator. Other steps to reduce the risk of cerebral edema include elevation of the head of the bed and avoidance of excessive fluid administration. Hypotension should also be avoided as it will lower the cerebral perfusion pressure. Hypertension is commonly seen in the acute stroke setting and may be either an initiating event or secondary to the stroke. Although mild elevations in blood pressure (BP) may improve cerebral perfusion pressure, severe elevations (diastolic BP >110 mmHg) should be treated.

Following stabilization, the patient should undergo an evaluation including a complete blood cell count, prothrombin time, partial thromboplastin time, serum chemistries, erythrocyte sedimentation rate, lipid analysis, and chest x-ray. An electrocardiogram (ECG) should be obtained to detect evidence of cardiac ischemia or dysrhythmias. A CT scan of the head without contrast medium should be obtained to look for an intracranial bleed or an ischemic infarct.

Once an ischemic stroke is documented or strongly suspected, a source must be sought. If the patient has a dysrhythmia on ECG, particularly atrial fibrillation, or has other significant cardiac history, such as a dilated cardiomyopathy, a mechanical valve, or rheumatic heart disease, a cardiac source of embolus should be suspected. An echocardiogram should be obtained. If the cardiac examination and ECG are normal, and the neurologic symptoms are from the distribution of the anterior circulation, carotid disease must be suspected. A carotid duplex scan should be ordered.

The pattern of the neurologic symptoms can also give a clue as to the source of the stroke. A cardiac source is suspected if the patient has had repeated episodes of ischemia that vary in their anatomic distribution. Conversely, emboli from a carotid source tend to deposit in the same vascular bed, and as such, carotid TIAs cause similar symptoms each time. Amaurosis fugax is classically due to an embolus from a carotid plaque (Case 1).

The role of anticoagulation in the management of stroke remains controversial. For a TIA or minor ischemic stroke caused by a cardiac embolus, systemic anticoagulation with heparin followed by long-term oral coumadin should be considered. Heparin must be withheld until intracranial bleeding has been excluded by CT scanning. The value of coumadin is unknown for patients with TIA or stroke due to atherosclerotic carotid disease.

In order to develop a rational approach to carotid artery stenosis (CAS) management, one must ask several questions. What is the natural history of untreated CAS? Is it different for symptomatic versus asymptomatic CAS? What is the risk of surgical intervention? Are the risks of surgical intervention outweighed by the risks of nonoperative management? To simplify strategies, it is best to divide CAS into asymptomatic and symptomatic categories.

In patients with asymptomatic high grade CAS (>75% cross-sectional area), the annual risk of stroke is estimated to be approximately 5%. The risk of stroke or death following carotid endarterectomy performed by an experienced surgeon should be less than 3%. Thus, one can infer that surgical intervention should be considered for patients with asymptomatic high grade stenosis. However, in addition to the surgeon's expertise, patient factors need to be considered. The patient should be low risk, without significant underlying cardiac or pulmonary disease, or other medical problems that would increase the operative morbidity and mortality and thus negate the beneficial effects of the operation. The Asymptomatic Carotid Atherosclerosis Study recently examined medical (aspirin) versus surgical therapy for patients with asymptomatic CAS (≥60% cross-sectional area). They reported an aggregate risk over 5 years for ipsilateral stroke and perioperative stroke or death to be 5.1% for surgical patients and 11% for patients treated medically. There was an aggregate risk reduction of 53% in favor of surgery.

The management of symptomatic high grade (>70% cross-sectional area) stenosis also favors surgery. This was demonstrated in a controlled randomized study in which the estimated cumulative risk of ipsilateral stroke was 26% in the medical (aspirin) group versus 9% in the surgical group. Symptomatic patients included those with TIA or with nondisabling stroke in the distribution of the diseased carotid artery (Case 2). Patients with persistent dense hemiplegia were excluded, as there is no benefit from performing carotid endarterectomy in these patients.

Before carotid endarterectomy, standard angiography is recommended to confirm the findings on duplex ultrasonography (Cases 1 and 2). Angiography will detect atherosclerotic disease of the intracranial vessels, as well as proximal disease in the aortic arch, carotid, and vertebral artery origins. It will also permit more accurate calculation of the percentage of stenosis, extent of disease, and presence of ulcerations in the carotid bifurcation. Angiography also assesses the adequacy of collateral circulation from the circle of Willis, and occasionally will identify intracranial aneurysms or tumors.

The timing of carotid endarterectomy is important. Following a TIA, carotid endarterectomy can be performed expeditiously. After a stroke, however, carotid endarterectomy is rarely performed acutely, as morbidity and mortality are increased. Surgery is delayed for a period of several weeks, when an infarct is documented on CT scan. Carotid endarterectomy is not indicated if the stroke is permanently disabling (i.e., one that results in a dense hemiplegia).

During carotid endarterectomy, perfusion to the brain can be maintained with an intraluminal shunt while the carotid artery is clamped. Carotid shunting is employed routinely by some surgeons and selectively by others. Those who selectively shunt often use intraoperative electroencephalographic (EEG) monitoring to determine whether a shunt is necessary.

Postoperative management requires surveillance for new neurologic deficits. A careful examination should be performed to detect cranial nerve injuries. Nerves at particular risk of injury during carotid endarterectomy are the recurrent laryngeal, hypoglossal, marginal mandibular, and glossophayrngeal. A new neurologic deficit (not attributable to cranial nerve injury) that develops immediately postoperatively should prompt urgent exploration of the carotid artery to exclude acute thrombosis.

KEY POINTS

• Hypercarbia will exacerbate cerebral edema, as carbon dioxide is a potent vasodilator

• Hypertension commonly seen in the acute stroke setting and may be initiating event or secondary to stroke

• Cardiac source suspected if patient has had repeated ischemic episodes that vary in anatomic distribution; emboli from a carotid source tend to deposit in the same vascular bed, so that carotid TIAs cause similar symptoms each time

• In patients with asymptomatic high grade CAS (>75%), annual risk of stroke is estimated to be 5%

FOLLOW-UP

After surgery, patients should be followed on a yearly basis to detect any new neurologic symptoms, restenosis of the carotid endarterectomy site, or a new or progressive stenosis of the contralateral unoperated carotid artery.

If new neurologic symptoms develop, a carotid duplex ultrasound should be obtained to detect carotid restenosis or disease in the nonoperated carotid. However, the role of routine surveillance duplex ultrasound to detect asymptomatic restenosis following carotid endarterectomy is controversial. Early carotid restenosis (within 2 years) is typically due to myointimal hyperplasia and not recurrent atherosclerosis. Restenosis due to myointimal hyperplasia does not appear to have the same risk of stroke as does atherosclerosis. Reoperative carotid surgery carries a higher risk of cranial nerve injury and stroke.

SUGGESTED READINGS

Brown RD Jr, Evans BA, Wiebers DO et al: Transient ischemic attack and minor ischemic stroke: an algorithm for evaluation and treatment. Mayo Clin Proc 69:1027, 1994

de Virgilio C: Pathophysiology of cerebral ischemia. In White RA, Hollier LH (eds): Vascular Surgery: Basic Science and Clinical Correlations. Lippincott-Raven, Philadelphia, 1994
North American Symptomatic Carotid Endarterectomy Trial Collaborators: Beneficial effect of carotid endarterectomy in symptomatic patients with high-grade carotid stenosis. N Engl J Med 325:445, 1991
Pryse-Phillips W, Yegappan MC: Management of acute stroke: ways to minimize damage and maximize recovery. Postgrad Med 96:75, 1994
The Asymptomatic Carotid Atherosclerosis Study Group: Endarterectomy for asymptomatic carotid artery stenosis. JAMA 273:1421, 1995

QUESTIONS

1. The most common cause of cerebrovascular ischemic events is?

   A. Emboli from the carotid artery.
   B. Intracerebral hemorrhage.
   C. Proximal stenosis in the carotid artery with low flow.
   D. Vasospasm.

2. The most sensitive modality available to detect cerebral ischemia and stroke is?

   A. Duplex-Doppler.
   B. Cerebral angiography.
   C. CT.
   D. MRI.

3. In patients with asymptomatic high grade (>75%) CAS, the annual risk of stroke is approximately?

   A. 5%.
   B. 25%.
   C. 50%.
   D. 75%.

4. Surgery for TIAs, RINDs, and strokes should not be undertaken?

   A. Shortly after a resolved TIA.
   B. When TIAs are very frequent.
   C. When TIAs progress to RINDs.
   D. Within 24 hours after a complete stroke and when a fixed neurologic deficit is present.

(See p. 604 for answers.)

44

AORTIC

ANEURYSMS

CARLOS E. DONAYRE

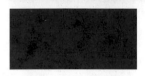

There is no disease more conducive to clinical humility than aneurysm of the aorta.

William Osler

Aneurysmal enlargement of the human aorta with aneurysm formation can occur silently without symptoms, or it can present in dramatic fashion upon rupture. The increase in age of the general population, and the widespread use of imaging modalities such as computed tomography (CT) scan and ultrasound have resulted in greater identification of this potentially lethal pathologic process. The dilemmas that are faced by physicians when dealing with aortic aneurysms are the aims of this chapter: (1) identification of patients at risk of developing aortic aneurysms, (2) definition of the etiologic factors that place patients at increased risk of aneurysm rupture, (3) comparison of the outcomes and complications encountered in an elective, an urgent, and an emergent aneurysm operation, and (4) discussion of alternative forms of therapy that may be utilized in the high risk patient who has a large aortic aneurysm.

CASE 1
ABDOMINAL PAIN AND A
PULSATILE MASS

A 68-year-old male was admitted with the chief complaint of abdominal pain. Four days before admission he developed epigastric and paraumbilical pain radiating to the back. This varied in intensity and was relieved by codeine pills. The pain in the lumbar region increased in severity 1 day before admission and began to involve the entire abdomen. He complained of nausea and vomiting, had a normal bowel movement before admission, and denied any urinary symptoms. His past medical history was significant for a prior myocardial infarction 12 years ago, and the use of nitroglycerin for the past 2 years for anginal complaints.

Physical examination revealed a well-developed, well-nourished, acutely ill man with severe abdominal pain. BP, 120/85 mmHg; pulse, 110 bpm; respiration, 22 breaths/min. The abdomen showed moderate symmetrical distention, marked tenderness, and a sensation of fullness in the left lower quadrant, with some rebound pain. The liver and spleen were not palpable. There was no shifting dullness. A pulsatile mass was palpable at the level of the umbilicus. Bowel sounds were active. Rectal examination showed no tenderness or palpable masses. Femoral and radial pulses were 2+, but the popliteal and dorsalis pedis pulses were not found. Laboratory findings were Hct, 38%; WBC count, 14,000/mm^3. Urine and stool were negative for blood. On ECG, an old inferior myocardial infarction was noted. The patient had two large IV catheters started, and he was cross-matched for 6 units of blood. An emergent abdominal CT was aborted when the patient's blood pressure fell to 90 mmHg, and he was rushed to the operating room. At exploration, a large, contained retroperitoneal hematoma was encountered. Proximal aortic control was obtained at the diaphragmatic hiatus, the aneurysm was opened, and control of the iliac vessels was achieved with Fogarty balloon catheters. A 22-mm woven graft, impregnated with collagen, was used to repair the aorta. The patient required 4 units of PRBCs, 800 ml of Cell-Saver blood, 2 units of fresh frozen plasma, and 10 units of platelets. He arrived in the surgical ICU intubated, with a BP of 110/70 mmHg, a pulse of 120 bpm, and a urine output of 100 ml/hr. He did well during the next 3 days, requiring only 2 more units of PRBCs. But on the fourth day he had a maroon stool, his blood pressure declined to 90/50 mmHg, and his urine output fell. He was also found to have rebound tenderness in the left lower quadrant. Bedside sigmoidoscopy demonstrated ischemic colonic mucosa. He was again taken to the operating room, where a gangrenous colon was found, and a left hemicolectomy with colostomy was performed. After a prolonged ICU stay, he was discharged home 7 weeks after his admission.

CASE 2
ASYMPTOMATIC AROTIC ANEURYSM

A 73-year-old, active male visited his family physician for a routine physical examination in order to qualify for a new life insurance policy. His medical history was significant only for hypertension, which was well controlled with a β-blocker. He had smoked cigarettes for 40 years, but had stopped 5 years previously. His older brother, with no known medical problems, had died unexpectedly at home 6 months previously. Physical examination was unremarkable; no abdominal masses were detected. He had strong and prominent arterial pulses, but no bruits. A screening ultrasound demonstrated a fusiform abdominal aortic aneurysm, 5 cm in greatest diameter, and a 3-cm right popliteal artery aneurysm. The patient agreed to undergo an elective aortic aneurysm repair. A preoperative abdominal CT scan confirmed the 5-cm infrarenal aortic aneurysm and also demonstrated a 3.5-cm left common iliac artery aneurysm. The patient underwent an aortic/bi-iliac bypass and synthetic graft. His postoperative course was uneventful and he was discharged from the hospital 1 week later. Three months later he underwent an exclusion and bypass of his popliteal aneurysm with a reverse saphenous vein graft.

GENERAL CONSIDERATIONS

An aneurysm is defined as a permanent, localized dilatation, 1.5 or more times the size of the normal arterial diameter. The normal aortic diameter gradually decreases in size from the thorax to the aortic bifurcation, is larger in men than women, and increases with age. The infrarenal aorta in men measures 2.2 cm in diameter compared to 1.9 cm for women; thus, 3 cm is a useful minimum size criterion. The aortic segment below the renal arteries is by far the most common location for aneurysm formation; 50% extend into and involve the iliac arteries. Dilatation of the aorta leads to vessel elongation, giving the aortic and iliac vessels a tortuous configuration. Concomitant femoral and popliteal aneurysms are present in 15% of patients diagnosed with aortic aneurysms (Case 2). The converse is also true, with 8% of patients presenting with a unilateral popliteal aneurysm having an aortic aneurysm. Over one-third are afflicted if bilateral popliteal aneurysms are present.

Atherosclerosis is the major etiologic factor associated with abdominal aortic aneurysm (AAA) formation, but an evolving view based on several observations suggests a multifactorial causation. Most patients with aneurysms are elderly, and have evidence of significant atherosclerosis in the coronary arteries and carotid bifurcation. Occlusive vascular disease of the iliofemoral segments is encountered in 25%. However, a paradoxical observation must be explained. Why does atherosclerosis lead to stenosis or occlusion in certain vessels, but to aneurysmal dilatation of the aorta in the same patient? Atherosclerosis consists of a complex series of events, ranging from smooth cell migration and proliferation to cell necrosis with calcium deposition, as a response to arterial wall injury. Atherosclerotic plaque formation is accompanied by an arterial wall remodeling response, with subsequent arterial enlargement in an effort to prevent luminal stenosis. In the superficial femoral artery this enlargement response may be restricted by anatomic factors such as a tendinous adductor canal, predisposing this artery to stenosis rather than aneurysmal dilatation. The abdominal cavity does not place any anatomic restrictions on the atherosclerotic infrarenal aorta, and aneurysmal dilatation can proceed unencumbered. The same is true in the popliteal fossa with regard to popliteal aneurysms. Thus, it can be argued that atherosclerosis is fundamentally a dilating rather than a constricting disorder of arteries.

Recent clinical observations and biochemical data suggest that aneurysm pathogenesis may be more complex than described above and possibly is related to a systemic connective tissue disorder. Patients with aneurysms are more prone to hernia formation and have a higher incidence of bilateral and recurrent hernias, as opposed to patients with aortic occlusive disease in whom inguinal herniation is unusual. This suggests that connective tissue abnormalities of both the abdominal wall and aortic wall result in hernias and aneurysms in the same patients. Elastin and collagen are structural proteins that play a critical role in the integrity of the aorta, and biochemical assays have shown decreased quantities of elastin and collagen in the wall of aneurysms. The major catabolic enzyme for the breakdown of elastin is a proteolytic enzyme, elastase. The amount of aortic elastase found in the walls of AAAs, multiple aneurysms, and ruptured AAAs is significantly higher when compared to aortas afflicted by occlusive disease. The activity of elastase is significantly modified by the proteinase inhibitor, α_1-antitrypsin, which is found in significantly lower concentrations in patients with multiple and ruptured aneurysms. The inflammatory and smooth muscle cell reaction to atherosclerotic injury appears to be altered in patients with AAA with the creation of a proteolytic environment that favors elastin and collagen degradation. Loss of structural support in the aortic media of patients with AAA renders the aorta susceptible to expansion in both diameter and length.

Other structural factors seem to favor aneurysmal formation in the infrarenal aorta. First, it has a smaller medial layer than the thoracic aorta and must tolerate a greater wall tension. Second, histologic studies have found a lack of vaso vasorum in the distal aorta. Third, laminated mural thrombus acts as a barrier to the diffusion of nutrients to the aortic wall. Under conditions in which the vasa vasorum are absent, the media is weakened by atherosclerotic plaque and impaired nutrition; atrophy of the arterial wall ensues and leads to aneurysmal degeneration.

Once an aneurysm develops, its enlargement is governed by physical principles. In order to maintain a stable diameter, the vessel wall must exert a circumferential force that opposes the distending effects of pressure. This relation is described by the law of Laplace:

$$T = P \times r$$

where T is circumferential wall tension, P is transmural pressure, and r is vessel radius. The distending force is given by the product of pressure and radius, while the retractile force offered by the arterial wall is tension. Laplace's law has to be redefined because the arterial wall is not infinitely thin:

$$S = P \times r_i/th,$$

where S is the stress force developed by the stretched vessel, P is transmural pressure, r_i is internal radius, and th is wall thickness. Using Laplace's law, tripling the aortic radius from 2 to 6 cm results in a 12-fold increase in wall tension. (It is no mystery why blowing a balloon gets easier after a certain radius is achieved.) This helps explain why large aneurysms are more prone to rupture than small ones, and why hypertension is an important risk factor for rupture.

KEY POINTS

- Inflammatory and smooth muscle cell reaction to atherosclerotic injury appears to be altered in patients with AAA with the creation of proteolytic environment that favors elastin and collagen degradation

- Loss of structural support in aortic media of patients with AAA renders aorta susceptible to expansion in both diameter and length

- Under conditions in which vasa vasorum are absent, media is weakened by atherosclerotic plaque and impaired nutrition; atrophy of arterial wall ensues and leads to aneurysmal degeneration

- Large aneurysms are more prone to rupture than small ones; thus, hypertension is important risk factor for rupture

DIAGNOSIS

Most AAAs (about 75%) cause no symptoms unless rapid expansion, leakage, or rupture occurs. They are usually detected during a routine physical examination,

when the patient undergoes an ultrasound or CT scan for an unrelated condition, during laparotomy, or by the patients themselves. It is important not to confuse an easily palpable pulsating aorta in a young, thin patient with an AAA. The lumbar-sacral curvature renders the aorta easily palpable in these individuals. In well-nourished patients, the abdominal examination can be improved if the abdominal wall is relaxed by having patients flex their knees and put their arms at their side. The presence of a prominent aortic pulsation should be searched for using light manual pressure. Most aneurysms will be palpable in the epigastrium or to the left of the umbilicus. Both lateral borders of the aneurysm should be marked and this distance measured. Physical examination overestimates the actual diameter of an aortic aneurysm by about 1 cm.

If an aortic aneurysm is found, a thorough search for femoral and popliteal aneurysms must be carried out as there is an increased association of the two. A prominent and expansile popliteal pulse with the knee flexed 30–45 degrees is highly suggestive of an aneurysm. The diagnosis can be easily confirmed with an ultrasound of the knee. Rectal examination may, on occasion, reveal the transmitted pulsations of a large internal iliac aneurysm.

Aneurysm rupture is defined as disruption of the aortic wall with extravasation of blood. The abrupt sensation of pain in the back, flank, or abdomen is characteristic of aneurysmal rupture or expansion. It is not certain why pain is produced by an expanding but intact aneurysm. The best explanation may be that sudden stretching of the layers of the aortic wall puts pressure on the adjacent somatic sensory nerves. The pain is usually severe and throbbing before rupture, but tends to become steady when rupture has occurred. It is usually located directly over the aneurysm, but radiation of the pain to the thigh, groin, or testicles is common. It must be remembered that hypotension and shock do not usually occur in the absence of rupture.

Rupture appears to occur through the posterolateral aortic wall and into the retroperitoneal space (80%) and less commonly anteriorly into the free peritoneal cavity (20%). The incidence of an anterior type of rupture is probably higher than indicated because most of these patients die abruptly and do not reach the hospital. The severity of the accompanying hypotension and shock will depend on both the extent of the blood loss and the patient's cardiovascular reserve. The classic presentation of ruptured AAAs includes abdominal and back pain, hypotension, and a pulsatile abdominal mass, but all three of these findings are present in only 20% of patients with a proven aortic rupture. However, over 90% of ruptured aneurysms produce abdominal pain of sudden onset, and over 50% of these patients also complain of back pain. In the stable patient with a ruptured abdominal aneurysm, a pulsatile mass is usually felt to the left of the midline. Since aneurysms usually rupture to the left base of the mesentery, the resulting hematoma often occurs to the left and can be palpated above the umbilicus. If the hematoma dissects downward, it can present as a tender left lower quadrant mass.

Distention in a hypotensive patient should arouse suspicion. Most patients with aneurysmal rupture will be distended from retroperitoneal or intraperitoneal blood, and a secondary intestinal ileus. Ecchymoses can result in the flank, scrotum, or thighs as blood dissects into the retroperitoneal plane. This physical finding occurs late and is usually not seen in the acute clinical scenario.

Abdominal aortic aneurysms cause symptoms not only as a result of rupture and expansion, but also due to pressure on adjacent structures. Large AAAs can cause symptoms from local compression of the duodenum (early satiety, nausea, or vomiting), ureters (hydronephrosis), or iliac veins (venous thrombosis).

Erosion of the vertebrae, which can lead to constant back pain, has also been reported, but this is more commonly seen with the now rare aneurysms of syphilitic origin. Acute ischemic symptoms can occur either from distal embolization of thrombotic debris contained within the aneurysmal sac or from aortic thrombosis. Embolism is much more common than acute thrombosis, but both combined occur in less than 5% of patients with AAA. In patients with distal emboli, a proximal aneurysmal source must always be considered, especially in those without apparent occlusive disease.

Under rare circumstances, the AAA may erode and rupture into the inferior vena cava or one of the iliac veins, producing a large aortocaval or aortoiliac fistula. These patients present with acute lower extremity swelling and cyanosis, high output cardiac failure, and an abdominal machine-like murmur. Erosion into the duodenum can also occur, resulting in massive upper gastrointestinal bleeding with catastrophic results.

Since most unruptured aortic aneurysms are asymptomatic until they expand or rupture, imaging studies are important to confirm the clinical diagnosis. Ultrasonography is the screening test of choice. Its advantages include a high degree of accuracy (95%), relatively low cost, noninvasiveness, and good patient compliance. However, the presence of intestinal gas often limits its usefulness in identifying the proximal extent of the AAA, determining iliac artery involvement, and locating the renal arteries, especially in obese patients.

CT scan is also used in the evaluation of AAAs. It yields more data than ultrasound because it can show the relationship of the aneurysm to the renal vessels, the presence of iliac artery aneurysms, and may detect other undiagnosed intra-abdominal processes. Intravenous contrast is required to obtain usable images, and thus renal complications and allergic reactions to contrast media are possible.

The use of angiography is limited in the diagnostic evaluation of AAA due to its invasiveness, documented allergic reactions, risk of dye induced renal failure, and cost.

Furthermore, because aneurysms have layers of thrombus lining the lumen, angiography cannot be relied on to determine the diameter of an aneurysm or even establish its presence. It is used in the following situations: (1) when the aneurysm is thought to extend above the renal arteries, (2) in the patient with symptomatic iliofemoral disease, (3) in those with severe hypertension or impaired renal function, and (4) in the presence of a horseshoe kidney.

A plain abdominal and lateral spine film can be obtained rapidly at the bedside, and in greater than 70% of cases the scattered plaques of calcification will outline the wall of an aortic aneurysm. Since symptomatic patients usually have an associated ileus, it is important to realize that any abdominal distention can make the ultrasound examination more difficult and often unreliable. A CT scan can be helpful but should only be obtained in the completely stable patient and only after suitable intravenous access and close monitoring have been established. Aortography is useless in this setting; it will not show the leak and may not even demonstrate an existing aneurysm. Furthermore, it is expensive, invasive, and time-consuming, and may lead to complications and volume depletion. Diagnosis is to be pursued only in the hemodynamically stable patient. In the unstable patient, rapid resuscitation and transport to the operating room take precedence.

Two aneurysmal variants merit special mention. *Inflammatory aortic aneurysms* are characterized by dense periaortic fibrosis with an abundant inflammatory reaction that contains many macrophages and often giant cells. Patients present with back pain, fever, an elevated sedimentation rate, and hydronephrosis or urinary complaints due to ureteral involvement by this intense inflammatory reaction. Although its etiology is unknown, aneurysm repair reverses the process. *Mycotic abdominal aneurysms* are AAAs that have become infected by lodgment of circulating organisms (bacteria or fungi) in the arterial wall. The most common offender is *Salmonella*. In such cases suppuration further destroys the media, potentiating rapid dilatation and rupture.

KEY POINTS

- Most AAAs (about 75%) cause no symptoms unless rapid expansion, leakage, or rupture occurs; usually detected during routine physical examination, when patient undergoes ultrasound or CT scan for unrelated condition, during laparotomy, or by patients themselves

- Physical examination overestimates actual diameter of an aortic aneurysm by about 1 cm

- Aneurysm rupture is defined as disruption of aortic wall with extravasation of blood

- Classic presentation of ruptured AAA includes abdominal and back pain, hypotension, and a pulsatile abdominal mass, but all of these three findings are found in only 20% of patients with proven aortic rupture

- Over 90% of ruptured aneurysms produce abdominal pain of sudden onset; over 50% of these patients also complain of back pain
- Abdominal aortic aneurysms cause symptoms not only as a result of rupture and expansion, but also due to pressure on adjacent structures
- Large AAAs can cause symptoms from local compression of duodenum (early satiety, nausea, or vomiting), ureters (hydronephrosis), or iliac veins (venous thrombosis)
- Erosion of vertebrae, which can lead to constant back pain, has also been reported, but this is more commonly seen with aneurysms of syphilitic origin
- Acute ischemic symptoms can occur either from distal embolization of thrombotic debris contained within aneurysmal sac or from aortic thrombosis
- Embolism much more common than acute thrombosis, but both combined occur in less than 5% of patients with AAA
- In patients with distal emboli, a proximal aneurysmal source must always be considered, expecially in those without apparent occlusive disease

DIFFERENTIAL DIAGNOSIS

The diverse and nonspecific nature of the pain caused by an expanding or leaking aneurysm all too often leads to errors in diagnosis and causes delays that may be catastrophic. The final outcome in a patient presenting with a symptomatic AAA is positively impacted if the initial diagnosis is correct. A study showed that if the initial diagnosis was correct or an aneurysm was at least suspected from the onset, a 35% mortality rate was achieved. However, if the diagnosis was incorrect or a cardiopulmonary event occurred, the mortality rose to 75%. A ruptured aneurysm should be considered in any patient past middle age who presents with sudden onset of abdominal discomfort, back pain, or hypotension. A history or signs of atherosclerosis or associated risk factors should heighten suspicion.

A normal electrocardiogram (ECG) helps to shift the focus away from the heart as the source of the patient's collapse. However, it must also be remembered that in the typical atherosclerotic patient with an aneurysm, rupture can lead to hypovolemic shock and may precipitate myocardial ischemia. A careful abdominal examination should be performed and will identify the true cause of the chest pain in most patients who arrive at the emergency room complaining of angina pectoris due to blood loss and reflex tachycardia from a ruptured aneurysm. Systolic hypertension is not uncommon in elderly patients, and the normal blood pressure of 120/85 mmHg obtained initially in the patient in Case 1 has to be redefined as hypotension.

AAA should not be confused with a dissecting aneurysm. Dissecting aneurysms usually begin in the thoracic aorta; the primary event is an erosion of the inner aortic layers, which allows hemorrhage into the media. The blood then courses along this path parallel to the main bloodstream where it may force its way back into the aortic lumen with the formation of a false channel. Although dissecting aneurysms do produce an enlarged aorta, the process is completely separate from that seen with an expanding or leaking AAA.

The main symptom of dissection is unbearable pain starting in the chest, sometimes radiating at first to the neck or back, but gradually extending down into the abdomen, and sometimes even to the hip or thigh. Diagnosis will be helped if the following points are remembered. The patient usually has a history of significant arterial hypertension of prolonged duration. A pulse examination and blood pressure determination should be carried out if possible in each limb. Discrepancies in pulses and pressures between the upper and lower or contralateral extremities are usually found and vary according to the distal extent of the dissection. If a renal artery is involved, there may be hematuria and perhaps a rise in the blood urea nitrogen (BUN) or creatinine. The limitation of blood flow to parts supplied by the affected arteries may lead to numbness, paresthesia, or even hemiplegia or paraplegia if the carotid or spinal arteries are involved.

The main differences between an aortic dissection and a symptomatic AAA are the lack of initial pain in the chest without radiation to the abdomen, the presence of strong and equal pulses in the radial and femoral locations, and the absence of numbness, paresis, or hemiplegia in an AAA.

Onset of back pain in patients with a symptomatic aneurysm is frequently initially diagnosed as renal colic. Both of these conditions can present with flank pain and radiation of the pain to the genital areas. The diagnosis of renal colic is highly questionable in the patient lacking a prior history of urinary complaints, and is found to have a normal urinalysis without microscopic hematuria, crystals, or sediments. Transient hypotension in these patients should not be attributed to a pain-mediated vagal episode or the onset of urinary sepsis. Abdominal x-rays and intravenous pyelograms should be inspected closely for the presence of calcifications outlining an aortic aneurysm.

Lumbar pain after strenuous exercise, lifting, or working is a common complaint faced by primary care and emergency room physicians. Any elderly patient who presents with the onset of back pain should be carefully examined for the presence of a pulsatile abdominal mass. Lumbar films should be carefully examined for the presence of vascular calcifications or anterior vertebral erosions. The obese elderly patient in whom a reliable examination cannot be performed should have an abdominal ultrasound to exclude the presence of an aneurysm.

The association of traumatic abdominal discomfort with hypotension can be explained by other conditions such as perforation of peptic ulcer or another viscus. However, a perforated viscus produces a board-like and exquisitely tender, rigid abdomen. Mesenteric ischemia presents with abdominal pain out of proportion to the physical examination (excruciating pain with a soft abdomen) and intestinal emptying associated with bloody diarrhea. However, shock is usually a late and often lethal manifestation of mesenteric ischemia.

Symptomatic aneurysms can also be confused with diverticulitis, since both can present with a tender left lower quadrant mass. One must remember diverticulitis is an inflammatory process, and is associated with fever, leukocytosis, and the presence of a nonpulsatile abdominal mass. Unless gross peritonitis exists, diverticulitis is not usually associated with shock.

The expanding retroperitoneal hematoma caused by a ruptured AAA can, on occasion, dissect toward the right side, mimicking right-sided renal colic or even acute cholecystitis. Albert Einstein was discovered to have a grapefruit-sized aneurysm of the distal aorta during an abdominal exploration and underwent an "omentopexy" (aneurysm wrap). For the next 10 years he complained of occasional pain in the lower abdomen and back, and suffered from intermittent episodes of pain in the right upper quadrant that were labeled as chronic cholecystitis. He was admitted to Princeton Hospital on April 15, 1955 with generalized abdominal pain, which was most intense in the right upper quadrant. A clinical diagnosis of acute cholecystitis and leaking aortic aneurysm was made, but Einstein declined the recommended aortic surgery and expired 3 days later. Autopsy revealed a normal gallbladder and a huge abdominal aneurysm that had ruptured and hemorrhaged into the tissues around the gallbladder. This historical case can be used to emphasize the dictum that any abdominal pain in a patient with a previously diagnosed AAA should be suspected of being caused by rupture of the aneurysm.

It should be remembered that

1. In elderly patients the possibility of a symptomatic AAA must be considered with any symptoms related to the abdomen or back

2. Any episode of hypotension in such patients should always be taken seriously

3. Thorough examination of the abdomen for the presence of pulsatile masses is mandatory, and should be supplemented with an abdominal ultrasound if the patient is hemodynamically stable

KEY POINTS

- Ruptured aneurysm should be considered in any patient past middle age who presents with sudden onset of abdominal discomfort, back pain, or hypotension

- In typical atherosclerotic patient with an aneurysm, rupture can lead to hypovolemic shock and may precipitate myocardial ischemia

- Main symptom of dissection is unbearable pain starting in chest, sometimes radiating at first to neck or back, but gradually extending down into abdomen, and sometimes even to hip or thigh

- Patient usually has history of significant arterial hypertension of prolonged duration; pulse examination and blood pressure determination carried out if possible in each limb

- Discrepancies in pulses and pressures between upper and lower or contralateral extremities usually found and vary according to the distal extent of dissection

- If renal artery involved, may produce hematuria and perhaps a rise in BUN or creatinine

- Limitation of blood flow to parts supplied by affected arteries may lead to numbness, paresthesia, or even hemiplegia or paraplegia if carotid or spinal arteries involved

- In elderly patients, possibility of symptomatic AAA must be considered with any symptoms related to abdomen or back

- Any episode of hypotension in such patients should always be taken seriously

- Thorough examination of abdomen for presence of pulsatile masses is mandatory, and should be supplemented with abdominal ultrasound if patient is hemodynamically stable

TREATMENT

The dilemma is which patients with asymptomatic AAA should undergo elective operative treatment or, alternatively, careful nonoperative follow-up. The only risk factors independently predictive of rupture include the initial diameter of the aneurysm (large aneurysms expand more rapidly than small ones), elevated diastolic blood pressure (Laplace's law), and the presence of chronic obstructive pulmonary disease (elastase and α_1-antitrypsin). Using these three variables alone, the 5-year predicted rupture rate increases from 2% when all three risk factors are minimal to 100% when they are all present.

Although 15–20% of small aneurysms do not expand substantially, 80% increase progressively in diameter and approximately 20% increase by more than 0.5 cm/yr. Unfortunately, it is impossible to predict the rate of expansion in any one patient; while some aneurysms are stable for years, others tend to expand rapidly. From clinical studies, it appears that for AAAs less than 4 cm in diameter the risk of rupture within 5 years is approximately 2%, with an increase to 25–40% for aneurysms larger than 5 cm. Data on risk of rupture for aneurysms in the 4–5-cm range are sparse, but such lesions have been reported to have a 5-year rupture rate of 3–12%.

The mortality risk of elective aneurysm repair has decreased in the last two decades. Mortality has fallen from 12–15% to 3–5%, with some centers reporting an operative mortality of 2% or less, with a 5-year survival of 60% and a 10-year survival of 40%. Factors increasing the risk of elective surgery include coexisting cardiac disease, peripheral atherosclerosis, hypertension, decreased renal function, chronic obstructive pulmonary disease, obesity, and multiple previous surgeries.

Elective operation is recommended for patients with AAAs that measure greater than 5 cm in diameter, are painful or tender, and have been documented to be enlarging. Distal embolization or obstruction of adjacent viscera are also indications for resection. Operations for smaller aneurysms (4–5-cm in diameter) should be performed in the low risk patient who has diastolic hypertension or who suffers from chronic obstructive pulmonary disease. Relative contraindications for small aneurysms include a recent myocardial infarction, congestive heart failure, severe angina pectoris, chronic renal failure, or life expectancy of less than 1 year.

There is no argument that the mortality rate is increased in the patient who has to undergo an emergent aneurysm repair. The mortality rates for operations performed for ruptured aortic aneurysms differ because of significant variations in the hemodynamic status of the patient at the time of presentation. Patients who are not hypotensive and have small, contained hematomas have an operative mortality rate of 20%. The mortality rate doubles to 40% in those who present with hypotension but who respond to fluid resuscitation with restoration of blood pressure and urine output.

Operative repair seeks to re-establish blood flow to the pelvis and lower extremities by utilizing a prosthetic vascular graft. Whenever possible, a tube graft is sutured below the renal arteries and above the aortic bifurcation, even in the presence of small iliac aneurysms, in order to shorten the length of the operation. If large or complex iliac aneurysms are encountered, a bifurcated graft is utilized and sutured to each iliac bifurcation.

The hemodynamically stable patient with abdominal and back pain who is found to have an aneurysm represents a challenging management problem. Since symptoms are widely believed to represent acute aneurysm expansion, and imminent rupture, immediate operation is generally accepted to be the proper course of action in an effort to avoid the complications associated with aneurysm rupture. It is recommended that once symptomatic, the hemodynamically stable AAA patient should undergo an emergent CT scan of the abdomen and pelvis under careful and close observation. The finding of blood in the retroperitoneum mandates immediate operation. In the absence of evidence of retroperitoneal bleeding, the patient at high operative risk due to pre-existing cardiopulmonary disease may benefit from a rapid and thorough preoperative assessment, and improvement of their cardiac, pulmonary, and renal function rather than from immediate operation.

Thus, the key to a better outcome in the management of a patient with ruptured and unstable aneurysm is early diagnosis, aggressive resuscitation, and an early operation

with rapid control of bleeding. It should also be remembered that nearly every complication is more likely in an emergent rather than an elective operation. The incidence of renal failure after elective aortic aneurysm resection averages approximately 3% with a mortality rate of 45%, but the incidence of acute renal failure after operation for ruptured aneurysm averages 30% with a mortality rate of 75%.

Sigmoid colon ischemia is a rare but devastating complication that is more likely to occur following repair of a ruptured AAA. It may result from embolization into, or ligation of the inferior mesenteric artery or the internal iliac arteries. Fortunately, the abundance of collateral flow to the sigmoid colon usually prevents this problem. Careful inspection of the sigmoid colon following graft replacement is essential and may be facilitated by Doppler examination of the bowel wall and mesentery. Postoperative colon ischemia should be suspected in the presence of cramping, abdominal pain, or early diarrhea (1–2 days after surgery), that usually contains blood. Prompt flexible sigmoidoscopy or colonoscopy should be performed. In most cases, patchy partial-thickness mucosal necrosis and sloughing can be detected. In the more severe cases of transmural infarction, early re-exploration is an indication of sigmoid ischemia.

Paraplegia due to AAA repair is uncommon. Recovery from this complication is unusual and the mortality rate is high.

Recently, a novel, minimally invasive approach has been introduced utilizing a stented graft to "exclude" AAA. This technique, which has been developed in animals, is now in human trials and consists of transfemoral placement of a thin walled prosthetic graft that is attached to the proximal aorta with an internal wire stent. This technique may further reduce the risk of elective AAA repair and may be especially appropriate for the high risk patient.

KEY POINTS

• Only risk factors independently predictive of rupture include initial diameter of aneurysm (large aneurysms expand more rapidly than small), elevated diastolic blood pressure (Laplace's law), and presence of chronic obstructive pulmonary disease (elastase and α_1-antitrypsin)

• Appears from clinical studies that for AAA less than 4 cm in diameter, risk of rupture within 5 years is approximately 2%, with increase to 25–40% for aneurysms larger than 5 cm

• Data on risk of rupture for aneurysms in 4–5-cm range are sparse, but such lesions reported to have 5-year rupture rate of 3–12%

• Elective operation recommended for patients with AAA measuring greater than 5 cm, are painful or tender, and documented to be enlarging

• Distal embolization or obstruction of adjacent viscera also indicate resection

• Operations for smaller aneurysms (4–5 cm in diameter) should be performed in low risk patient who has diastolic hypertension or who suffers from chronic obstructive pulmonary disease

• Relative contraindications for small aneurysms include recent myocardial infarction, congestive heart failure, severe angina pectoris, chronic renal failure, or life expectancy of less than 1 year

FOLLOW-UP

A successfully performed aneurysm repair will have little problem and generally will remain patent for the patient's lifetime. Late presenting postoperative complications include graft infection and aorto-enteric fistula formation. Both of these complications require graft resection and extracavitary arterial reconstruction; unfortunately, they have a high mortality rate, usually greater than 50% despite appropriate treatment.

Proximal or distal anastomotic disruption occurs due to arterial or graft degeneration or graft infection. A pseudoaneurysm, which is an expanding hematoma locally contained by surrounding connective tissue, is the usual end result. After 3-year follow-up, the incidence of pseudoaneurysm formation is 0.2% for the aortic anastomosis, 1% for iliac anastomoses, and 3% for femoral anastomoses. Patients should be followed with ultrasound or CT scan 5–10 years after repair to ensure that pseudoaneurysms are not forming. This can be addressed in an elective fashion before rupture occurs.

SUGGESTED READINGS

Cronenwett JL, Sargent SK, Wall MH et al: Variables that affect the expansion rate and outcome of small abdominal aortic aneurysms. J Vasc Surg 11:260, 1990

Covers the risk factors that are important to aneurysm enlargement, with an insightful audience discussion at the end.

Ernst CB: Current concepts: abdominal aortic aneurysm. N Engl J Med 328:1167, 1993

Thorough review! Will fill in and reinforce the main topics covered in the chapter, and provide you with a fairly complete list of references.

Marston WA, Ahlquist R, Johnson Jr G et al: Misdiagnosis of ruptured abdominal aortic aneurysms. J Vasc Surg 16:17, 1992

Addresses the most common errors that are made in diagnosing aortic aneurysms; surprisingly, the mortality was not negatively impacted as expected. Misdiagnosis probably preselected for patients that were able to withstand the delay and were better able to undergo surgical repair.

QUESTIONS

1. *Most abdominal aortic aneurysms?*
   A. Produce vague symptoms such as back pain.
   B. Are detected on routine physical examination.
   C. Rupture when they are 4–6 cm in size.
   D. Occur without other manifestations of atherosclerosis.

2. *The best screening test to determine whether an AAA is present is?*
   A. Angiography.
   B. CT scan.
   C. Duplex-Döppler.
   D. MRI scan.

3. *Which of the following is not predictive of the risk of AAA rupture?*
   A. Size of the aneurysm.
   B. Elevated diastolic blood pressure.
   C. Chronic obstructive pulmonary disease.
   D. Transient ischemic attacks.

4. *The most common cause of death after the successful repair of an AAA is?*
   A. Cardiac arrest/cardiac failure.
   B. Paralysis from spinal ischemia.
   C. Infection.
   D. Hemorrhage.

(See p. 604 for answers)

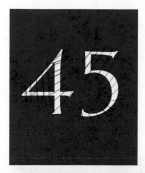

45

PERIPHERAL

VASCULAR DISEASE

RODNEY A. WHITE

This chapter reviews the pertinent pathophysiology, history, physical examination, diagnosis, and treatment of common occlusive vascular problems. The pertinent principles relevant to patient management, the pathophysiologic basis, and the important concepts of the development and consequences of vascular disease are reviewed.

CASE 1
PAINFUL BLUE TOES

A 65-year-old male presented with painful dark lesions over the toes and soles of his feet. He had had a coronary artery bypass 3 years previously.

On physical examination, he had multiple bluish gray punctate discolorations over the toes and forefeet of both legs. Peripheral pulses were palpable at all locations and there was a 6-cm pulsatile mass in the mid-epigastrium that was nontender. An abdominal ultrasound and angiogram showed a 7-cm infrarenal aortic aneurysm without involvement of the iliac vessels.

The aneurysm was repaired using an interposition graft sutured to replace the infrarenal abdominal aorta.

CASE 2
DIFFICULTY WALKING

A 72-year-old male had a 70-pack/yr history of smoking. He complained of severe aching in the left calf following one block ambulation, which progressed to involve the entire leg if he tried to walk farther. He took a drug for mild hypertension and nonprescription medications for pain in the left leg during rest at night.

Physical examination found slightly decreased bilateral femoral pulses and weak popliteal pulses. Pulses in the foot were only evident by Doppler examination. ABIs were 0.5 on the right and 0.3 on the left. There were no skin lesions on the feet.

An arteriogram of the extremities demonstrated diffuse atherosclerotic disease of the distal aorta and iliac arteries, but no areas of flow-limiting stenosis were identified. The superficial femoral arteries in both legs were occluded with flow being re-established in the popliteal arteries by collateral vessels from the profunda femoris artery (Fig. 45.1). The distal popliteal artery was occluded, with the foot being supplied by a segment of posterior tibial artery that reconstituted above the ankle via collateral vessels and connected to well-formed plantar arteries.

A left femorodistal bypass was performed using saphenous vein for the graft. Postoperatively, the ABI in the left leg was 0.8 with resolution of pain. He was able to walk approximately four blocks before experiencing claudication in the right calf.

GENERAL CONSIDERATIONS

The muscles of the lower extremities are those most commonly affected by vascular occlusive disease. As atherosclerosis in the aorta and vessels of the thigh reduces blood flow to the leg, muscle oxygen delivery is decreased. When the available oxygen supply cannot keep pace with the exercising muscle, anaerobic metabolism converts glucose into energy. The accumulation of lactic acid, one of

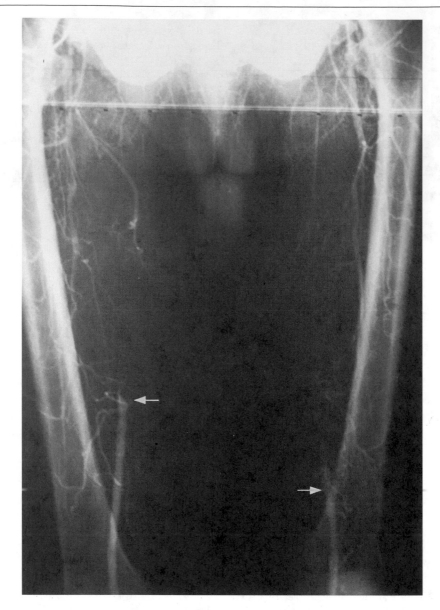

FIGURE 45.1 *Angiogram of the lower extremities demonstrating occlusion of both superficial femoral arteries (SFAs), with reconstitution of flow via collaterals of both distal SFAs and popliteal vessels (arrows).*

the major products of anaerobic metabolism, produces an aching sensation in the calf that ultimately stops the exercise. During the rest period that follows, the oxygen debt is paid back, the lactic acid is metabolized, and the pain abates. The effects of limited oxygen supply may occur in normal individuals when strenuous exercise exceeds oxygen demand. When the inflow of blood is limited by an obstructive lesion, vasodilatation in response to exercise is limited, and the muscle becomes ischemic with a smaller amount of exercise. Such flow-limited ischemia is characteristic of vascular occlusive disease. When atherosclerosis impedes the flow of blood to the muscles of the leg, simple walking may produce severe calf pain (Case 2), referred to as intermittent claudication. It is remarkably constant for each patient with respect to distance walked

before onset. After a rest period, repeat activity produces the same symptoms. Rarely, occlusive lesions may also produce effort fatigue in upper extremity muscles. As atherosclerotic disease worsens, oxygen supply to the muscles may become inadequate even with minimal or no activity. Rest pain is a manifestation of severe occlusive disease and portends limb loss. The severe ischemia of rest pain also causes changes in the skin adnexa such as the nail beds and hair follicles, which become atrophic. The skin is dry and crusted, predisposing it to infection.

Although the extremities are most commonly affected by occlusive disease, the abdominal viscera may be involved as well. Gastrointestinal angina occurs when blood flow to the bowel is reduced to a critical level and normal peristalsis results in ischemia. Patients with visceral (mesenteric) angina are afraid to eat because of the severe postprandial abdominal pain they experience. Hence, they become emaciated, frail, and wasted.

Arterial blood flow is normally orderly, with the center of the blood column moving at the greatest speed. Such laminar flow involves minimal interaction between the column of blood and the surrounding vessel wall. A stenotic lesion, such as an atherosclerotic plaque, is an obstacle to flow and creates currents that swirl through the artery and strike the vessel wall, causing it to vibrate. These vibrations produce audible bruits and palpable thrills over the affected vessel. The presence of either of these findings indicates a lesion proximal to the point of examination, since the flow alteration occurs distal to the offending lesion. Bruits may be understood by thinking about the mechanism by which Korotkoff sounds are produced when measuring blood pressure. Initially, with the blood pressure cuff fully inflated, no blood flows distal to the site of (external) stenosis. As the pressure in the cuff is reduced, blood is able to pass through the stenosis only during systole, when it has the highest kinetic energy. The flow past the cuff is not orderly, however, and strikes the arterial wall, producing a vibration that the examiner hears as a bruit. As the cuff is deflated further, the diastolic pressure is able to keep the walls of the vessel fully distended and flow is no longer disorganized; hence the bruit disappears. This important concept also explains why diabetic patients who have calcified vessels may seem to have elevated blood pressures. The calcium within the vessel wall resists collapse by the blood pressure cuff and produces a falsely elevated blood pressure.

Because ischemia occurs distal to the point of obstruction, peripheral occlusive disease usually manifests one joint lower than the location of the stenotic lesion. Hence, a lesion of the popliteal or superficial femoral artery will produce pain with exercise in the muscles of the calf (classic intermittent claudication). A lesion of the external iliac or common femoral artery will produce symptoms in the thigh and calf, while stenosis of the aorta or common iliac artery causes pain in the muscles of the buttock. Proximal lesions of this type also reduce flow to the pelvis and may produce impotence in males by reducing flow through the internal iliac arteries. The Leriche syndrome consists of the triad of impotence, buttock atrophy, and claudication.

The effects of arterial stenosis depend on the extent of the obstruction and the rapidity with which it develops. Because ischemia is an extremely potent inducer of angiogenesis, chronic ischemia promotes the growth of new blood vessels that bypass the occlusion (Fig. 45.1). The resistance to flow through a vessel is proportional to the fourth power of the radius of the vessel. Hence, even a small reduction in the cross-sectional area can cause a large decrease in flow. The tiny blood vessels that form and enlarge to allow blood flow past the obstruction can never completely alleviate the ischemia because flow resistance through them is always higher than through the native vessel. Hence, while collateral flow may be adequate to nourish muscles at rest, it cannot replace a native vessel during exercise.

The most important vessel contributing to collateral blood supply in the lower extremity is the profunda femoris artery. In patients without vascular disease, the main function of the profunda femoris artery is to supply blood to the muscles of the thigh. However, when occlusive disease exists in the external iliac or common femoral artery, the profunda femoris may *receive* blood from the internal iliac artery through collaterals around the hip. Similarly, when the superficial femoral artery is occluded, the profunda femoris may supply blood to the popliteal artery through a number of small branches that reconstitute the superficial artery distal to the occlusion (Fig. 45.1). Although these collateral pathways are important, in neither case can they completely substitute for the native vessel.

DIAGNOSIS

The vascular patient with peripheral, cerebrovascular, or myocardial ischemia usually has diffuse atherosclerosis that increases the risk of death postoperatively and subsequently from cardiovascular complications. They often have a history of cigarette smoking, diabetes mellitus, and/or a familial predisposition to vascular diseases (e.g., an inherited tendency for hyperlipidemia). Established risk factors for the development of vascular disease include cigarette smoking, hyperlipidemia, and diabetes.

Diagnosis of peripheral vascular disease begins with a history that examines risk factors, onset of disease, nature, and progression. The amount of activity required to produce symptoms is particularly important, since decreased exercise tolerance is a good indicator of progressive disease. Other pertinent items include associated cardiovascular processes such as ischemic cardiac (coronary artery) disease, cerebrovascular disease, and family history.

The physical examination should record blood pressure in both arms and the pulse status throughout. Particular attention should be paid to the symmetry of pulses and the presence of bruits and thrills. If the patient experiences pain only with activity, pulses should be examined both before and after exercise sufficient to reproduce symptoms.

The highest arterial pressure measured at the ankle with an ultrasonic flow detector (Doppler) divided by the highest arm blood pressure gives the ankle-brachial index (ABI). The severity of occlusive disease in the lower extremity is inversely related to the ABI, as is the severity of symptoms. Resting ABIs of 0.5 or less occur in patients with incapacitating intermittent claudication, 0.4 or less in those with ischemic rest pain, and 0.3 or less when gangrene or tissue loss is present. This simple measurement should be performed as part of the examination of all persons suspected of having lower extremity ischemia. In urgent or emergent cases, or in occasional patients with typical symptoms and findings, no other tests may be necessary. The ABI may be falsely elevated in patients with incompressible lower extremity arteries, which occurs with diabetes.

Treadmill walking with pre- and postexercise ankle blood pressure provides objective confirmation of the diagnosis of claudication and allows objective comparison of pretreatment and post-treatment values for the assessment of results.

Pulse volume recording is performed using a calibrated air plethysmographic waveform recording system. This test is performed at the thigh, calf, ankle, metatarsal, and toe levels. It provides semiquantitative information of arterial obstruction. Toe pulse volume recordings and toe pressures are especially helpful in diabetic patients with relatively incompressible proximal vessels that prevent accurate pressure measurements.

Physical examination and the measurement of ABIs are mandatory in all patients who present with the symptoms and signs of lower extremity occlusive vascular disease. Further diagnostic evaluation depends largely on the severity of the patient's symptoms and the degree to which they impair normal lifestyle and functioning. More invasive studies should not be obtained in patients with minimal dysfunction, those who are not candidates for operation, or those who have not had a sufficient trial of nonoperative management.

Duplex scanning is also accepted as a standard method for evaluation of lower extremity arterial disease. Color Doppler imaging is frequently used to screen patients with claudication, limiting angiography to only those who would benefit from an endovascular or surgical intervention. Duplex scanning is used to evaluate traumatic injuries, to perform completion assessment after arterial reconstruction, and postoperatively to monitor progression of recurrent lesions. It has been shown that angiography, although providing valuable morphologic data, does not yield precise information regarding residual flow abnormality or pressure gradients at the site of balloon angioplasty.

In severe disease, arteriography yields limited information regarding the morphology or extent of lesions in the arterial wall, aside from demonstrating visible calcification and topography of the luminal surface. Clinically significant atherosclerosis is usually eccentrically positioned in the arterial lumen, which may be either circular or elliptical in shape. In instances where the lumen is elliptical, biplanar angiograms more accurately define luminal cross-sectional areas and calculation of percent area stenosis.

Acute arterial occlusion stemming from trauma, embolus, or thrombosis frequently requires emergency surgery to prevent irreversible tissue loss. Symptoms are pain, analgesia or anesthesia, and discoloration of the ischemic tissue.

Embolic arterial occlusion produces symptoms that vary with the origin of the embolus. Emboli originating in the heart or ascending aorta cause central nervous system, visceral, or upper or lower extremity symptoms, whereas emboli from the abdominal aorta and from iliofemoral or popliteal lesions affect only the lower extremities. The blue toe syndrome describes multiple bilateral ischemic areas in the lower leg caused by atheromatous debris showered distally from disease in aortoiliac vessels (Case 1). Ischemic paralysis and hypalgesia may develop in acutely ischemic limbs as a result of neurovascular compression from increased fascial compartment pressure.

Thrombotic arterial occlusion usually occurs as a result of decreased blood flow in progressively narrowed, atherosclerotic vessels. Acute thrombosis of diseased arteries may be precipitated by hypovolemia or to a sudden decrease in cardiac output. Frequently, elderly patients with cardiac failure or intraperitoneal pathology have ischemic lower extremities that suggest an aortic occlusion or a dissecting aneurysm. Appropriate attention to cardiac or intra-abdominal pathology and restoration of blood volume often alleviates the ischemic symptoms. Axillary arterial thrombosis subsequent to intimal damage produced by repeated strain or trauma occurs in athletes, particularly baseball pitchers, and in individuals using crutches. Rarely, acute arterial thrombosis occurs in severely dehydrated children or in patients with hematologic disorders. Treatment of thrombotic arterial episodes requires identification and alleviation of the inciting cause (i.e., removal of the atherosclerotic obstruction, treatment of hematologic disorders), or other options, including angioplasty and/or thrombolytic therapy to lyse thrombus and restore flow by treating underlying lesions.

Chronic arterial insufficiency caused by progression of atherosclerosis is infrequently a surgical emergency. Occlusion of major arteries may not cause tissue ischemia if hypertrophic collateral vessels provide adequate vascular supply. Chronic arterial occlusive disease is typically accompanied by insidious symptoms such as wasting of the extremity, hair loss, fragile skin, and pain with activity (claudication) (Case 2). Patients may complain of a burning or warm sensation in the affected extremity, which is actually cool or of normal temperature. Decreased exercise tolerance or prolonged recovery time suggest progression of the disease.

Because chronically ischemic limbs are easily ulcerated by local irritation, patients (especially diabetics) must be instructed in meticulous foot care. Any lesions must be treated aggressively. All patients with arterial insufficiency should be encouraged to quit smoking, control their diet, and immediately visit their physician if foot problems develop. Approximately 50% of patients with claudication will experience less pain on activity if they follow these recommendations and start a supervised exercise program. The onset of rest pain heralds complications and limb loss unless surgical intervention can restore adequate tissue oxygenation.

Vascular ischemia of the upper extremity is caused by atherosclerosis, thoracic outlet compression syndromes, trauma, and systemic or local inflammatory disease. Upper extremity ischemia from acute arterial occlusions causes limb loss in 10% of lesions in the subclavian artery, 15% in the axillary artery, and less than 5% in the proximal brachial artery. Most acute arterial obstructions in the upper extremity are caused by trauma.

Thoracic outlet compression syndrome is caused by impingement of adjacent structures on all or part of the neurovascular supply to the upper extremity. Common causes include a cervical rib, fibrocartilaginous bands, scalene or subclavius muscle hypertrophy, upper thoracic or cervical trauma, and repeated strenuous hyperabduction of the arm. Accurate diagnosis of the thoracic outlet syndrome depends on reproducing symptoms with hand exercise when the arm is abducted and externally rotated (extension abduction stress test). There may be tenderness to percussion over the clavicle or brachial plexus, an audible bruit over the subclavian artery, and reduction or obliteration of pulses when the arm is in an abducted position. However, these diagnostic maneuvers are only suggestive, and many normal individuals have the same findings. Objective tests include electromyography, nerve conduction velocity, and arteriography. Relief of symptoms often follows several months of a thoracic outlet exercise program. In severe cases, resection of a cervical rib or the first thoracic rib or scalenectomy may relieve symptoms.

Upper extremity digital gangrene is infrequent. Approximately 50% of patients with digital ischemia have a correctable aneurysm, traumatic lesion, or embolic source proximal to the hand. Digital ischemia may also appear as a symptom of vasospastic or obliterative arterial disease in patients with systemic inflammatory processes. Connective tissue disorders, particularly scleroderma, are associated with progressive occlusion of medium and small diameter arteries.

Visceral ischemia is frequently not diagnosed until late in the clinical course of mesenteric arterial insufficiency. For this reason, reported mortality rates are between 55% and 100%. Laboratory and noninvasive tests are not diagnostic, and the physician must always consider mesenteric insufficiency in the initial evaluation of severely ill patients with abdominal pain, particularly elderly cardiovascular patients. Expeditious establishment and maintenance of hemodynamic stability, as well as arteriographic documentation of mesenteric vascular occlusion, are required to reduce fatal complications.

Visceral ischemia may be acute or chronic. Acute insufficiency can cause nonspecific colicky pain and guaiac-positive stools, or it may produce sepsis, acidosis, and rapid hemodynamic deterioration. The symptoms of chronic intestinal ischemia are postprandial pain and weight loss. Approximately 40% of acute ischemic events are caused by emboli; 50% are associated with low flow states and arterial thrombosis; and 10% or less are due to venous occlusion.

If the vascular supply of the gut is otherwise normal, acute occlusion of the celiac or inferior mesenteric arteries is usually compensated for by extensive collateral circulation. In general, at least two of three mesenteric vessels must be significantly obstructed for occlusion of any one vessel to impair mesenteric blood flow markedly. Occasionally, acute occlusion of the inferior mesenteric artery by thrombosis or surgical ligation causes an ischemic colitis that is characterized by severe abdominal pain in the lower left quadrant, abdominal tenderness, and bloody stools.

Although the superior mesenteric artery is subject to acute ischemia from either a thrombotic or embolic event, thrombosis usually results in more extensive ischemia because it occurs in a severely diseased artery and frequently involves the entire vessel. By contrast, emboli tend to lodge distal to the origin of the middle colic artery and may be found in otherwise normal intestinal vasculature. Mesenteric arterial emboli may only require embolectomy, whereas mesenteric thrombosis often requires resection of a large segment of devitalized intestine.

Thrombosis of the superior mesenteric veins is associated with low blood flow, hypercoagulation, portal vein thrombosis from portal hypertension, and/or splenic vein thrombosis from compression or invasion by malignancy, particularly pancreatic tumors. Splanchnic venous engorgement with edematous thickening of bowel loops produces a thumbprint pattern of gut folds, evident on upper gastrointestinal contrast radiography. Mesenteric venous thrombosis results in gut necrosis in 20–70% of patients. Mortality increases rapidly if therapy is delayed longer than 12 hours following the onset of symptoms, and approaches 100% by 48 hours. Frequently, acute mesenteric venous occlusion requires thrombectomy, resection of devitalized bowel, and anticoagulation.

KEY POINTS

- Symptoms of acute arterial occlusion are pain, pallor, pulselessness, parethesias, paralysis (the "5 P's")

- Blue toe syndrome describes multiple bilateral ischemic areas in the lower leg caused by atheromatous debris showered distally from disease in aortoiliac vessels

- Thrombotic arterial occlusion occurs due to decreased blood flow in progressively narrowed, atherosclerotic vessels

- Occlusion of major arteries may not cause tissue ischemia if hypertrophied collateral vessels provide adequate vascular supply

- Chronic arterial occlusive disease is typically accompanied by insidious symptoms such as wasting of the extremity, fragile skin, and claudication or effort fatigue

- Approximately 50% of patients with claudication will experience less pain on activity if they quit smoking, control diet, visit physician if foot problems develop, and start supervised exercise program

• Accurate diagnosis of thoracic outlet syndrome depends on reproducing symptoms with hand exercise when arm is abducted and externally rotated (extension abduction stress test)

• Physician must always consider mesenteric insufficiency in initial evaluation of severely ill patients with abdominal pain, particularly elderly cardiovascular patients

• Acute mesenteric arterial insufficiency can cause nonspecific colicky pain and guaiac-positive stools, or sepsis, acidosis, and rapid hemodynamic deterioration

• Mesenteric arterial emboli may only require embolectomy, whereas mesenteric thrombosis often requires resection of large segment of devitalized intestine

• Symptoms of chronic intestinal ischemia are postprandial pain and weight loss

• Approximately 40% of acute ischemic events are caused by emboli; 50% by low flow states and arterial thrombosis; and 10% or less due to venous occlusion

DIFFERENTIAL DIAGNOSIS

Vasculitis, vasospastic disorders, and arterial fibrodysplasias represent important causes of vascular insufficiency. Although some of these conditions are rare, they are important causes of nonatherosclerotic vascular diseases that respond poorly to operation. Vasculitis is defined as inflammation and necrosis of blood vessels producing hemorrhage, thrombosis, and vascular occlusion. Several types of vessels (veins, venules, arterioles, arteries) are affected by vasculitis. Despite attempts to characterize vasculitis, there is continued overlap in the size of blood vessels involved within the major disorders and between the syndromes as well.

TREATMENT

The treatment of peripheral vascular occlusive disease depends on the severity of the symptoms and the extent to which they interfere with the patient's lifestyle. In the least severe cases, in which symptoms are limited only to intermittent claudication, control of risk factors and graded exercise programs are usually sufficient. Patients should be advised to stop smoking and modify their diets to limit high cholesterol and fatty foods. Those who are overweight should receive nutritional consultation and help with weight loss. Blood pressure should be controlled and cardiac evaluation undertaken as necessary for the treatment of any associated heart disease. No drug or drug regimen has been shown convincingly to increase walking distance or decrease the progression of atherosclerotic disease without control of other risk factors. Pentoxyfilline is an oral agent postulated to improve flow properties of blood by decreasing viscosity. It acts primarily on red blood cell membranes to make them more deformable as they pass areas of stenosis. Since this effect occurs only in newly formed red blood cells, several weeks of treatment are required before any therapeutic benefit is observed. Because the drug is expensive and has debated efficacy, few practitioners recommend it.

Graded exercise is an important part of the treatment of lower extremity peripheral vascular disease. Patients should walk at least twice per day, increasing the distance traveled by a few steps each time. With conscientious application, most patients can double their walking distance within 3 months. This will satisfy most patients and obviate the need for further therapy. Patients should also be counseled that 5% of those with claudication only will lose the affected limb within 5 years.

When exercise and dietary/behavior modification fail to improve the situation, or in the rare case in which symptoms worsen, intervention is warranted. Therapy is also indicated for patients with rest pain. Such therapy generally takes two forms, catheter based (endovascular) or surgical, and follows analysis of the offending lesion by angiography. Transluminal angioplasty (TLA) is an endovascular technique that relies on an angiographically placed balloon catheter to disrupt the atherosclerotic plaque. Angioplasty is most applicable to short, isolated lesions that do not involve the bifurcation of vessels. Lesions in the iliac vessels and common/superficial femoral arteries may be treated successfully with balloon angioplasty. For isolated lesions, the vessel patency rate is approximately 75% at 5 years after the procedure.

When lesions are multiple, long, or involve bifurcations, surgical bypass grafting is the treatment of choice. A successful bypass has three prerequisites: (1) inflow to the bypass, (2) outflow from the bypass, and (3) a conduit for the bypass. Inflow to the bypass must provide sufficient blood flow, or the bypass will thrombose rapidly. Similarly, outflow from the bypass to the distal muscles must be present. In the vast majority of cases, inability to perform a bypass or occlusion of a bypass is due to severe outflow (distal) disease. The choice of a conduit depends on the location of the lesion. When the aorta and iliac vessels are involved, prosthetic is required because vessels of sufficient size to serve as a conduit do not exist elsewhere in the body (Case 1). For bypass of smaller vessels, such as the femoral or tibial vessels, autogenous saphenous vein is the conduit of choice (Case 2). When saphenous vein is not available (e.g., because of its prior use for cardiac bypass or severe varicosities), arm veins may be used. When placed from the common femoral vein to a distal target above the knee (femoropopliteal bypass) the patency is approximately 75% at 5 years. When the bypass extends below the knee, the patency rate falls to less than 50% at 5 years. Endovascular stenting is a new procedure that places a graft within the diseased vessel using an angiographically guided catheter. Preliminary results from these procedures have been encouraging.

Immediate thrombotic or hemorrhagic complications of vascular reconstructions can frequently be corrected during the initial postoperative period. Long-term failures are related to progression of atherosclerosis, gradual thrombotic occlusion of prostheses, infection, deterioration of prosthetic grafts with false aneurysm formation, perigraft hematoma accumulation, thrombosis from compression, or encroachment of a vascular reconstruction on adjacent organs. Many of the long-term failures are insidious, since occlusion of a reconstruction may not produce ischemia if a hypertrophied collateral circulation can provide adequate blood supply. Ankle Doppler measurements every 3 months postoperatively can detect subclinical atherosclerotic or myointimal hyperplastic stenoses in lower extremity vascular repairs. Many stenoses can be treated by surgery or transluminal balloon dilatation before occlusion of the arterial reconstruction, thus restoring flow without compromising long-term patency. Unfortunately, a significant number of long-term complications result in severe ischemia, sepsis, life-threatening hemorrhage, and/or compromised organ function.

Graft infection frequently produces fever or sepsis and can be a life-threatening complication of vascular surgery, particularly if it occurs in synthetic or nonautogenous biologic vascular prostheses. Humans do not completely heal vascular prostheses, in that a new intimal layer does not form throughout the length of the graft. Therefore, patients with prosthetic grafts in place have a lifelong increased susceptibility to graft infections. Postoperative superficial wound infections that do not involve the vascular prosthesis can be treated without removing the graft. Patients with cardiovascular implants undergoing invasive procedures or dental extractions should be prophylactically treated with antibiotics to avoid bacteremia.

Deterioration of vascular prosthetic materials may cause graft dilatation, false aneurysm formation, suture line disruption, or a perigraft hematoma formation. A pseudoaneurysm forms when the graft wall weakens, or when the suture material that secures the end of the graft to the native vessel wall pulls away. In either case, blood escapes and is contained by surrounding tissue. Over time, a fibrous capsule forms that contains the extravasated blood. Because this is a fibrous capsule that does not contain all layers of the vessel wall, it is termed a *pseudoaneurysm*. In general, any change in the configuration of a vascular reconstruction should be investigated to prevent complications.

Extra-anatomic bypasses are vascular reconstructions remote from the anatomic course of the vessel. They are usually subcutaneous or subfascial. Extra-anatomic reconstructions were originally developed to revascularize the lower extremities when repair of an aortoduodenal fistula required removal of an infected aortic bifurcation graft and ligation of the aorta below the renal vessels. Blood flow to one leg is restored by placing a prosthetic graft subcutaneously along the lateral chest wall, from the axillary artery to the ipsilateral femoral artery (i.e., axillofemoral bypass). Blood flow to the other leg is established through a second graft placed in a suprapubic subcutaneous position, from the axillofemoral reconstruction to the contralateral femoral artery (i.e., femorofemoral bypass). Long-term function of axillobifemoral reconstructions is not as good as that of an aortobifemoral interposition prostheses. An advantage of extra-anatomic bypasses is that these procedures can usually be performed using local or regional anesthesia in high risk patients. A disadvantage is that subcutaneous prostheses are easily compressed while the patient is sleeping or unconscious, causing thrombosis of the graft and distal ischemia. Early recognition of thrombosis in an extra-anatomic bypass is essential because an acute thrombus can frequently be removed, restoring flow without affecting long-term patency.

Astute clinical judgment is required to detect symptoms caused by encroachment of a vascular repair on adjacent structures. Fibrous encapsulation and stiffening of a limb of an aortobifemoral prosthesis can obstruct the ureter, producing persistent flank pain from hydronephrosis or renal infection. Compression of the iliac vein causes unilateral lower extremity venous hypertension, swelling, and discomfort. Aortoduodenal fistula is a dramatic example of a vascular repair eroding into an adjacent organ. Both infection and pulsation of the aortic anastomosis of an aortobifemoral reconstruction have been proposed as possible causes of the aortoduodenal communication. Aortoduodenal fistula should be suspected in patients with aortobifemoral bypasses who are experiencing massive upper gastrointestinal bleeding. These patients frequently have had preliminary (herald) hematemesis within the previous 24 hours. Endoscopic confirmation of bleeding from the third portion of the duodenum requires immediate laparotomy to exclude this complication; aortography is usually contraindicated because it may not demonstrate the enteric communication and because it delays laparotomy which is required to prevent exsanguination.

KEY POINTS

- In least severe cases, in which only symptom is intermittent claudication, control of risk factors and graded exercise programs are usually enough

- Graded exercise important part of treatment of lower extremity peripheral vascular disease; patients should walk at least twice per day, increasing distance by a few steps each time—most patients can double walking distance within 3 months

- Physicians should counsel patients that 5% of those with claudication only will lose affected limb within 5 years

- In vast majority of cases, inability to perform bypass or occlusion of bypass is due to severe outflow (distal) disease

- Ankle Doppler pressure measurements every 3 months postoperatively can detect subclinical atherosclerotic or myointimal hyperplastic stenoses in lower extremity vascular repairs

- Pseudoaneurysm (so-called because it is a fibrous capsule that does not contain all layers of vessel wall) forms when graft wall weakens or when suture material that secures end of graft to native vessel wall pulls away; either way, blood escapes and is contained by surrounding tissue

- Aortoduodenal fistula is a dramatic example of vascular repair eroding into adjacent organ

- Aortoduodenal fistula should be suspected in patients with aortobifemoral bypass who experience massive upper gastrointestinal bleeding; these patients often had hematemesis within previous 24 hours

- Endoscopic confirmation of bleeding from third portion of duodenum requires immediate laparotomy to exclude this complication; aortography is contraindicated because may not demonstrate enteric communication and immediate laparotomy required to prevent exsanguination

FOLLOW-UP

The general rule for following vascular patients is to maintain a high level of suspicion for development of subsequent vascular events. Since atherosclerosis and inflammatory vascular processes are generalized phenomena, complete assessment of the patient is required to diagnose emerging problems and to avert complications.

SUGGESTED READINGS

DeWeese J, Leather R, Porter J; Practice guidelines: lower extremity revascularization. J Vasc Surg 18:280, 1993

Overview of the indications for lower extremity revascularization, taking into account the natural history of untreated lower extremity ischemia, pretreatment evaluation, methods of treatment, monitoring during treatment, and post-treatment follow-up.

Hertzer N: The natural history of peripheral vascular disease. Circulation, suppl. I, 83:12, 1991

Detailed outline of the natural history of atherosclerotic vascular disease highlighting the association of multisystem involvement in patients who present with peripheral vascular symptoms.

QUESTIONS

1. *A partial stenosis in the superficial femoral artery will produce effort-related ischemia in the?*

    A. Buttock.

    B. Thigh.

    C. Calf.

    D. Foot.

2. *A patient with bilaterally diminished ankle brachial indices likely has a lesion in?*

    A. The aorta.

    B. Both iliac arteries.

    C. Both femoral arteries.

    D. Both popliteal arteries.

3. *Which of the following is inconsistent with a diagnosis of chronic mesenteric ischemia?*

    A. Anorexia.

    B. Postprandial angina.

    C. Malabsorption.

    D. Weight gain.

4. *The risk of limb loss (in 5 years) in a patient whose only symptom is claudication is?*

    A. 5%.

    B. 25%.

    C. 50%.

    D. 75%.

(See p. 604 for answers.)

46

VENOUS AND LYMPHATIC DISEASE

MARCO SCOCCIANTI

Venous disorders affect up to 20% of the adult population, and constitute an important cause of morbidity and chronic disability. This chapter reviews the most common diseases affecting the venous and lymphatic systems, including primary and secondary varicose veins, deep venous thrombosis (DVT), and lymphedema, as well as their most common complications (superficial thrombophlebitis and chronic venous insufficiency). Special attention is given to the clinical presentation and to the

differential diagnosis of each disorder as well as to the most appropriate therapeutic strategy.

CASE 1
SYMPTOMATIC VARICOSE VEINS

A 35-year-old female presented with complaints of aching discomfort and a sense of fatigue in her right leg, which developed after a vein in her right leg started to enlarge. She believed that one vein in her left leg had also become more apparent and unsightly. Her symptoms had lasted for a few months and seemed to worsen with her menstrual periods and at the end of the day. They improved by lying down with the legs elevated. She stated that her mother had a leg ulcer and her sister had had a vein stripping. On physical examination, she appeared to be healthy without abdominal or pelvic masses. No inguinal lymphadenopathy was present. The right greater saphenous vein was elongated and dilated in its entire length. Several collaterals originating from the greater saphenous vein were also dilated in both the medial aspect of the thigh and calf where some weak spots were palpated in the superficial fascia. No bruits or thrills were felt over the main

varicosities, and no areas of dermatitis or signs of previous ulceration were found over the medial malleolus. The left leg appeared normal with a minimally dilated greater saphenous vein. With the patient standing, a Valsalva maneuver was performed, and an obvious transmitted impulse was felt below the fossa ovalis bilaterally. Similarly, a Trendelenburg's test was positive and a Perthe's test was negative in both extremities. No further testing was done and she was advised to have a vein stripping on the right leg and to wear an elastic stocking on the left leg.

CASE 2
DEEP VEIN INSUFFICIENCY WITH A LEG ULCER

A 68-year-old retired maid with a history of diabetes and unstable angina attended the vascular clinic complaining of heaviness on ambulation and left ankle edema with a chronic ulcer over the medial malleolus. She stated that some years previously, her left leg became acutely swollen and some "blood thinner tablets" were prescribed. On physical examination she had a normal greater saphenous vein, a swollen ankle, a large area of induration, and marked brown skin pigmentation over the medial malleolus. At its center, a 1 × 2-cm superficial ulcer with a moist base and extensive granulation was present. A single Trendelenburg's test was negative, a double Trendelenburg's test was positive, and a Perthe's test was negative. A duplex study was done that revealed a competent saphenofemoral junction and patent femoral veins. However, the popliteal vein showed reversal of flow with the Valsalva maneuver and the Doppler probe revealed reflux in Cockett's perforators at the calf. No further tests were done and considering her surgical risks, conservative treatment was advised. An Unna boot bandage was applied.

GENERAL CONSIDERATIONS

Varicose veins are enlarged, tortuous, superficial veins. Although they are usually located in the lower extremity they can also be found in the esophagus (secondary to portal hypertension), in the spermatic cord (varicocele), or in the anorectum (hemorrhoids). It is estimated that 10–20% of the population suffers from lower extremity varicose veins. They are more common among females than males, but this difference decreases with age. Pregnancy, obesity, prolonged standing, and a sedentary lifestyle contribute to the development of varicose veins. In 50% of cases a positive family history is obtained (Case 1). Varicose veins are the result of an incompetent superficial venous system (85% greater saphenous vein, 15% lesser saphenous vein) with consequent stagnation of blood and increased resting venous pressure (Fig. 47.1). This explains the sense of heaviness in the legs and the swelling, as well as the improvement with leg elevation or compression.

Primary, or simple, varicose veins are the most common variety and are usually generalized when there is an incompetent valve at the saphenofemoral junction with subsequent progressive incompetence of several dependent valves along the greater saphenous vein. Less frequently they are localized and the incompetent valve is in one or more perforating veins. Characteristically, in primary varicose veins, the deep venous system is intact and, although the resting venous pressure is increased, it is inadequate to produce stasis dermatitis or ulcers.

Secondary varicose veins result from some abnormality of the deep and/or communicating venous systems. The most common cause is a previous episode of DVT with resultant destruction and incompetence of the valves of this system. In this situation, the pressure in the superficial system, especially in the gait area, is greatly increased and trophic changes or stasis ulceration occur (Case 2). Less frequently, varicose veins develop because of an obstruction of the deep venous system or as a result of an arteriovenous fistula with consequent increased blood flow.

DVT, phlebothrombosis, and thrombophlebitis are terms that have been used to describe blood clotting in a vein, usually of the lower extremity. In the past, the term phlebothrombosis was used when no sign of inflammation accompanied the clot, while thrombophlebitis was reserved for those instances in which a marked inflammatory reaction was present. Such a distinction is not always possible or true and therefore the term *deep venous thrombosis* is now preferred. This condition is frequent and clinically important as it can lead either to dislodgment of the thrombus and pulmonary embolism, or to organization of the thrombus and subsequent destruction of the valves of the deep and perforating venous system with consequent chronic venous insufficiency, leg swelling, and venous stasis ulceration (Case 2). Less commonly, or at least in a different milieu, thrombosis and inflammation can occur in a superficial vein, a condition referred to as superficial thrombophlebitis. It is difficult to determine the exact incidence of DVT and chronic venous insufficiency, as many of the clinical criteria or diagnostic tests used to make the diagnosis are inaccurate and many cases remain undetected. However, it has been estimated that between 250,000 and 600,000 patients are treated for DVT every year, and that over 7 million people suffer from chronic venous insufficiency, the most common sequela of DVT.

DVT may result from stasis of blood flow, alterations in the vein endothelium, or a hypercoagulable state. These three factors were first recognized by Virchow and are referred to as "Virchow's triad." Risk factors for DVT include bed rest and immobility as in postoperative states or following treatment of fractures, obesity, compression of veins by a tumor (stasis), direct trauma (vein injury), cancer, pregnancy, use of contraceptives, surgery, burns, shock or dehydration, polycythemia, or deficiency of antithrombin III or proteins S or C (hypercoagulability). It is well known that patients with cancer and those who have undergone hip replacement, prostatectomy, or pelvic surgery are at greatest risk to develop DVT and to succumb to pulmonary embolism.

DVT occurs in veins of the calf or thigh, often without producing any signs. When symptoms are present they may consist of mild swelling, pain, and tenderness of the calf, sometimes associated with a sense of stiffness in the leg. On physical examination the calf is often swollen and there may be redness and increased warmth over the affected segment. Pain on dorsiflexion of the foot (Homan's sign) implies thrombosis of the calf veins but this sign is present only 50% of the time. The natural history of DVT follows three basic patterns: (1) the thrombus may detach and cause pulmonary embolism with the inherent risk of sudden death, (2) the thrombus may progress to involve the iliofemoral vein, or (3) the thrombus becomes adherent and fibrotic (organizes), destroying the valves of the system. Several years after the acute episode, signs of chronic venous insufficiency appear.

If the thrombotic process extends to or involves the iliofemoral veins, an almost complete blockage of venous return from that limb may ensue with consequent massive swelling of the entire limb, severe pain, and marked

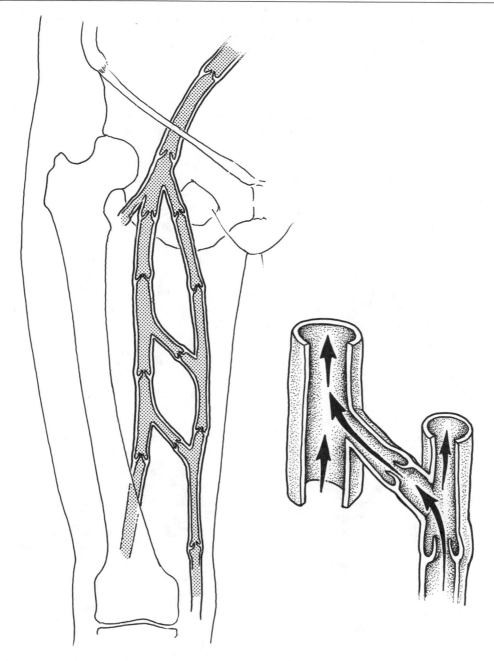

FIGURE 46.1   *Anatomy of the deep and superfical lower extremity venous system. Blood normally flows through a system of one-way valves from the superficial to the deep system.*

blanching due to subcutaneous edema of the leg, a condition called phlegmasia alba dolens or "milk leg." When the venous return becomes completely impaired, the capillary pressure may approach systemic pressure and lead to cessation of arterial inflow. In this case, the clinical picture is that of marked deep cyanosis, a condition termed phlegmasia cerulea dolens, which heralds venous gangrene and limb loss if venous return is not quickly re-established.

These extreme clinical sequelae are fortunately rare, and the most common sequela of DVT is the development

of chronic venous insufficiency (postphlebitic syndrome). This condition is characterized by persistent venous hypertension secondary to deep valvular incompetence. During ambulation, the contraction of the calf muscles (muscle pump) forces blood through incompetent deep and perforating vein valves into the superficial veins. This causes increased capillary pressure and permeability with leakage of fibrin and impaired oxygen exchange. The eventual effect is the development of edema, brownish skin pigmentation from hemosiderin-laden macrophages (stasis dermatitis), induration and fibrosis of the subcutaneous tissues (lipodermatosclerosis), and eventually skin ulceration (Case 2). Although chronic venous insufficiency is usually secondary to a previous episode of DVT, recent studies have shown that 30–40% of patients have primary valvular insufficiency rather than valve destruction due to a previous thrombotic episode.

Acute superficial thrombophlebitis is a frequent complication of varicose veins. It may follow local trauma to one of the varices with ensuing wall inflammation and thrombus formation. In this condition, the vein is inflamed but not infected. Although usually benign, if the thrombus extends into one of the deep or perforating veins, it has the potential to produce embolism and postphlebitic ulcer formation. For this reason, ultrasound evaluation (duplex study) is indicated to demonstrate the proximal extent of thrombus and the status of the deep venous system. Clinically, the affected vein appears to be tender, erythematous, and indurated with cord-like consistency. There is no peripheral edema. A mild temperature is common, but leukocytosis is rare.

Superficial thrombophlebitis may also be found in the veins of the upper extremity, where it is often a complication of the intravenous catheters used in hospitalized patients. When due to intravenous drug abuse, the vein is also usually infected and the condition is termed *acute septic thrombophlebitis*. This is usually secondary to staphylococcal colonization and is accompanied by chills, a high fever, and signs of cellulitis along the course of the affected vein.

Thrombophlebitis sometimes may recur and affect different veins at different times, a condition not associated with varicose veins, DVT, or trauma. Migratory superficial thrombophlebitis is commonly a paraneoplastic syndrome associated with mucin secreting tumors, usually of the pancreas but also of the stomach, breast, and colon. It is also found in different autoimmune diseases such as Behçet syndrome or Buerger's disease.

Lymphedema is the accumulation of high protein fluid in the extracellular space due to impaired uptake by obstructed lymphatics. It is classically divided into primary lymphedema, due to a congenital abnormality of the lymphatics, and secondary lymphedema which is acquired.

Primary lymphedema can occur sporadically or have a familial pattern (Milroy's disease). It is termed *lymphedema praecox* if it appears in patients under 30 years of age.

Secondary lymphedema is more common than primary lymphedema and is caused by conditions that remove either lymphatic tissues, such as axillary, pelvic, or inguinal lymph node dissection, or that obstruct the lymphatics, such as radiotherapy, neoplastic infiltration, recurrent lymphangitis, or *Filaria bancrofti* infection (filariasis). Prostate cancer and lymphoma are the most frequent causes of acquired lymphedema in the United States, and filariasis is most frequent internationally.

Primary lymphedema is principally encountered in young women, and starts as a slowly progressive swelling in the foot that insidiously extends to the ankle and calf and may ultimately involve the entire leg. The swelling is painless unless an infection supervenes. The edema is resistant to pressure (not pitting!) and has a rubbery consistency. Furthermore, it is not improved by leg elevation. Although usually unilateral, in advanced states both extremities may be affected. The clinical course depends mainly on the severity and level of the lymphatic obstruction. Seventy percent of patients have obstruction in the lymphatics of the leg, with edema that rarely progresses to involve the entire limb. If the iliofemoral lymphatics are occluded (20%), patients often progress to whole leg edema. With thoracic duct obstruction, the edema is usually bilateral and may involve the entire leg. The skin of these patients is particularly prone to infection and the resulting cellulitis and lymphangitis contribute to further damage of the lymphatics, which worsens the edema.

KEY POINTS

- Varicose veins are enlarged, tortuous, superficial veins; pregnancy, obesity, prolonged standing, and a sedentary lifestyle contribute to development

- Primary or simple varicose veins most common variety and usually generalized when there is an incompetent valve at the saphenofemoral junction with subsequent progressive incompetence of several dependent valves along the greater saphenous vein

- In primary varicose veins, the deep venous system is intact and, although resting venous pressure is increased, it does not produce stasis dermatitis or ulcers

- Secondary varicose veins result from abnormality of deep and/or communicating venous systems; most common cause is a previous episode of DVT with resultant destruction and incompetence of system valves

- DVT may result from stasis of blood flow, alterations in the vein endothelium, or hypercoagulable state (Virchow's triad)

- Symptoms of phlebitis may consist of mild swelling, pain, and tenderness of calf, associated with a sense of stiffness in the leg

- Natural history of DVT follows three patterns: (1) thrombus may detach and cause pulmonary emboli with inherent risk of sudden death, (2) thrombus may progress to involve iliofemoral vein, or (3) thrombus becomes adherent and fibrotic, destroying valves of system

- Most common sequela of DVT is development of chronic venous insufficiency, characterized by persistent venous hypertension secondary to deep valvular incompetence

- Ultrasound evaluation (duplex scanning) is indicated to demonstrate proximal extent of thrombus and status of deep venous system; clinically, affected vein appears tender, erythematous, and indurated with cord-like consistency

- Acute septic thrombophlebitis is secondary to staphylococcal colonization and accompanied by chills, high fever, and signs of cellulitis along course of affected vein

• Lymphedema is accumulation of high protein fluid in extracellular space due to impaired uptake by obstructed lymphatics; divided into primary (due to congenital abnormality of lymphatics), and secondary (acquired)

• Primary lymphedema is encountered in young women; starts as a slowly progressive swelling in the foot that insidiously extends to the ankle and calf and may ultimately involve the entire leg

• Lymphatic edema is resistant to pressure (not pitting) and has rubbery consistency; not improved by leg elevation

DIAGNOSIS

Although the presence of varicosities is easily recognized, the distinction between primary and secondary varicose veins sometimes may be difficult. Absence of DVT in the past medical history or lack of severe edemas, dermatitis, or ulceration strongly suggests primary varicose veins (Case 1). Some simple tests are also useful for screening patients with varicose veins before submitting them to more expensive and complex evaluation.

The single Trendelenburg's test assesses the competency of the saphenofemoral junction. With the patient supine, the superficial veins are emptied by raising the affected limb. Moderate pressure is then applied immediately below the saphenofemoral junction with a tourniquet, and the patient is allowed to stand. If on removal of the tourniquet, the saphenous vein immediately fills from above, incompetency of the saphenofemoral junction is demonstrated. The double Trendelenburg's test assesses the communicating (perforating) system (Fig. 46.2). It is similar to the previous test except that the tourniquet is not removed. If the varicosities fill from below, the perforators are incompetent. Perthe's test verifies the patency of the deep system. With the patient standing and the superficial veins dilated, a tourniquet is applied below the saphenofemoral junction and the patient is asked to walk. If pain develops and the superficial veins enlarge, the deep system is probably occluded (secondary varicose veins) and a venous stripping in this setting could be disastrous since it would remove the single path for venous return from the leg (Case 2). Noninvasive vascular laboratory testings (Doppler ultrasound, duplex, plethysmography) usually are not necessary in the evaluation of primary varicose veins but are required when secondary varicose veins are suspected or in those patients in whom surgery is contemplated.

Unilateral leg swelling, calf pain, or a positive Homan's sign are suggestive of acute DVT. Dilated superficial veins in the presence of ankle swelling, stasis dermatitis, or ulceration are indicative of chronic venous insufficiency (Case 2). These signs are inaccurate in 50% of patients with DVT and are inadequate to determine the level or the cause of chronic venous insufficiency. Several diagnostic tests are available to confirm the diagnosis and to plan appropriate therapeutic measures.

Doppler ultrasound is accurate in about 80% of cases for determining the presence of clot in the popliteal or femoral vein and for detecting the presence of incompetent valves either in the deep or in the communicating veins. This test is unreliable for detecting the presence of thrombi localized to the calf veins.

A Doppler flow probe with B-mode ultrasound allows visualization of the wall and the lumen of a superficial or deep vein in the popliteal fossa or in the thigh. It is very accurate in detecting absence or reversal of flow as well as the presence of a visible clot in the examined venous segment. In Case 2, duplex scanning did not reveal the presence of thrombus itself but did demonstrate the effects of its past presence, namely destroyed valves with reversal of flow in the popliteal vein and in some perforators of the calf (Cockett's veins).

Phlebography is the best test to confirm the diagnosis of thrombus and/or valve incompetence. Its main limitation is that it is invasive and requires injection of contrast material. Therefore, it is not suitable for screening purposes. Phlebography is now reserved for those patients in whom DVT is strongly suspected but who have equivocal noninvasive studies, or for those patients with chronic venous insufficiency in whom venous reconstructive procedures are contemplated.

Impedance plethysmography and radioactive fibrinogen scanning are other tests that are used to diagnose the presence of venous outflow obstruction. Plethysmography records volume changes in a limb during inspiration (vein filling) and expiration (vein emptying) while radioisotope scanning detects fibrinogen incorporation in a developing thrombus. These tests are accurate but are quite complex or laborious to perform and have been replaced by duplex scanning in most situations.

The diagnosis of lymphedema is primarily clinical and is based on the duration of onset (several months) of the lymphedema as well as on the distribution (forefoot, foot, ankle) and the characteristics (nonpitting, not improved by leg elevation) of the edema. Lymphangiography is reserved for those patients with whole leg edema who are considered for operative therapy, while computed tomography (CT) scanning and magnetic resonance imaging (MRI) are useful in patients with suspected secondary lymphedema (often due to cancer or lymphoma) to assess the status of the retroperitoneal lymph nodes.

KEY POINTS

• Noninvasive vascular laboratory testing (Doppler ultrasound, duplex, plethysmography) usually not necessary in the evaluation of primary varicose veins but required when sec-ondary varicose veins suspected or in those patients in whom surgery is contemplated

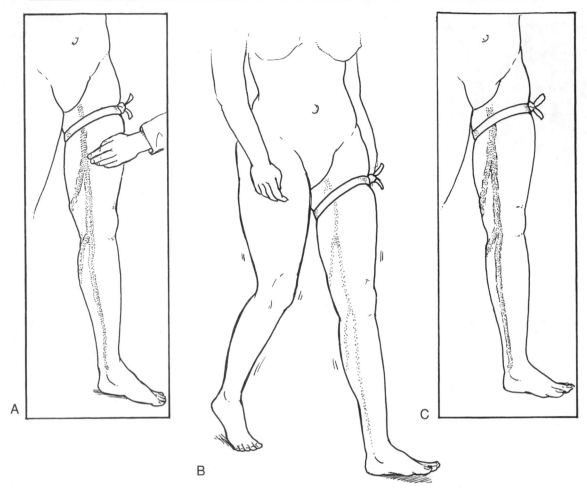

FIGURE 46.2   *The "double" Trendelenberg's test. (**A**) A tourniquet is placed at the saphenofemoral junction and (**B**) the patient is allowed to walk. (**C**) If the varicosities fill from below, incompetence of the perforating veins is demonstrated.*

• Doppler ultrasound accurate in about 80% of cases for determining the presence of clot in the popliteal or femoral vein and detecting the presence of incompetent valves either in the deep or in the communicating veins

• Phlebography best test to confirm the diagnosis of thrombus and/or valve incompetence; now reserved for those patients in whom DVT strongly suspected but who have equivocal noninvasive studies, or those with chronic venous insufficiency in whom venous reconstructive procedures are contemplated

• Lymphangiography reserved for those patients with whole leg edema who are considered for surgical therapy; CT scanning and MRI useful in patients with suspected secondary lymphedema to assess status of retroperitoneal lymph nodes

DIFFERENTIAL DIAGNOSIS

The differential diagnosis of varicose veins consists mainly in recognizing primary from secondary varicose veins and the underlying cause of the latter. If an arteri-ovenous fistula is suspected, a bruit and a thrill should be sought. In cases of iliac vein thrombosis an intraperitoneal or extraperitoneal mass should be excluded. In older patients, a femoral or popliteal artery aneurysm may cause compression and thrombosis of the adjacent vein with resultant DVT and secondary varicose veins.

The differential diagnosis of DVT is mainly related to exclusion of other conditions that cause leg swelling. If the swelling is bilateral, systemic causes of peripheral edema such as congestive heart failure, kidney failure, and hypoproteinemia should be considered. Conversely, if the swelling is unilateral and of recent onset, DVT must be confirmed. A ruptured Baker's cyst should be included in the differential diagnosis. In this case, a mass is usually palpable in the popliteal fossa and a knee effusion is present. Sometimes trauma can cause rupture of one of the calf muscles or Archilles tendon, with pain and swelling that mimic DVT. As previously noted, one or more risk factors for a thrombotic process should be identified and the presence of a pelvic tumor or an aneurysm compressing an adjacent vein should be excluded.

The differential diagnosis of chronic venous insufficiency consists of excluding other causes of leg swelling and chronic ulceration. Although many diseases can cause ulceration of the leg, decubitus ulcers and atherosclerotic ulcers are quite common and sometimes misleading in their etiology. A decubitus ulcer is usually located on the heel or lateral malleolus or above other bony prominences. They tend to be bilateral and occur in bedridden patients. They are inclined to progress and become very deep, involving muscle and bone. Arterial ulcers can be differentiated from venous ulcers by the features listed in Table 46.1.

In Case 2, the history of an old episode of popliteal vein thrombosis suggests that the leg swelling and ulcer are the result of long-standing DVT. This was confirmed by the duplex study.

Lymphedema can sometimes be confused with edema of venous origin. However, the following features help to make the correct diagnosis. Although leg elevation promptly reduces the edema of chronic venous insufficiency, several days of leg elevation are required to ameliorate lymphedema. In addition, the skin is usually normal in lymphedema while signs of chronic stasis dermatitis or a leg ulcer are common in chronic venous insufficiency. Although the foot is usually spared in venous disorders, it is always edematous in lymphedema.

KEY POINTS

• Although leg elevation promptly reduces edema of chronic venous insufficiency, several days of leg elevation are required to ameliorate lymphedema; skin is normal in lymphedema, while chronic stasis dermatitis or leg ulcer are common in chronic venous insufficiency

---

TREATMENT

The extent of involvement of the varicose process and the severity of symptoms or cosmetic disfiguration dictate the type of treatment. Patients with mild symptoms or localized varices may benefit simply by leg elevation and elastic compression. Those with more diffuse varices without main trunk involvement may benefit from compression sclerotherapy. Surgery may be indicated in those patients who have saphenofemoral junction incompetence and large varicosities, those who have suffered recurrent attacks of superficial thrombophlebitis, or those who have significant symptoms. Surgical treatment consists of removing the diseased saphenous vein with ligation of the incompetent perforators. Because varicose veins are a benign disease, only patients with severe symptoms should be considered for surgical treatment. In Case 1, the right leg became quite symptomatic. In this young patient, surgery is justified. The left leg, however, is not yet severely diseased and conservative (nonoperative) treatment should be instituted initially. When small, superficial varicosities are present and the concern is primarily over cosmetic appearance, local injection with a sclerosing agent may be all that is required.

The inherent risk of pulmonary embolism carried by DVT dictates the institution of prophylactic measures in patients at high risk of developing this complication, especially in those undergoing cancer, pelvic, or orthopaedic surgery. This can be achieved either with mechanical measures, such as intermittent external calf compression with pneumatic boots, or with anticoagulation. Several drug regimens have been proven to be effective. The antiplatelet drug aspirin (100 mg/day), or low dose heparin (5,000 units subcutaneously 2 hours before surgery and every 8 or 12 hours postoperatively) are effective. Low dose heparin is, however, inadequate after prostatectomy or hip replacement.

Once a diagnosis of DVT is established, the patient should be kept in bed with the leg elevated until the edema and the pain subside. Full anticoagulation is then instituted with intravenous heparin at a dosage that maintains the partial thromboplastin time (PTT) at 1.5–2 times normal (usually 10–25 mg/kg/hr produces a PTT of 100 seconds). After a few days, anticoagulation is continued with coumadin by mouth at a dosage that keeps the prothrombin time (PT) at 1.5–2 times normal. When an adequate PT is obtained, heparin is stopped, and coumadin is continued for at least 3 months. Thrombectomy is reserved for patients with iliofemoral thrombosis, phlegmasia cerulea dolens, or phlegmasia alba dolens. Patients in whom anticoagulation is contraindicated and who have sustained an episode of pulmonary embolism are suitable for implantation of an inferior vena cava filter.

Patients with superficial thrombophlebitis benefit from leg elevation, warm wet towels, and nonsteroidal anti-inflammatory drugs. Ambulation should be allowed to prevent clot propagation. If the thrombophlebitis extends to the saphenofemoral junction this should be ligated to prevent clot propagation into the femoral vein. If thrombophlebitis recurs, saphenous vein stripping is indicated. Patients with septic thrombophlebitis should be treated with antibiotics and excision of the infected vein.

TABLE 46.1 *Arterial versus venous ulcer*

	Venous	Arterial
Onset	Rapid	Slow
Location	Medial malleolus	Toes
Pain	No	Yes
Improved by	Elevation	Dependency
Surrounding skin	Brown pigmentation	Pale
Depth	Superficial	Deep

The management of patients with chronic venous insufficiency should control sustained venous hypertension, edema, and stasis ulceration, if present. Most patients improve with simple measures such as leg elevation and heavy-duty elastic stockings. Provided that their deep system is patent, those with recurrent ulcers or large secondary varices are best treated by saphenous vein stripping with ligation of all perforators. Young patients with recurrent ulceration in which the chronic venous insufficiency follows primary valve incompetency, may benefit from reconstructive procedures such as vein bypass, valve repair, venous cuff reconstruction, or valve transplantation. The local treatment of stasis ulceration consists, in addition to leg elevation and elastic stockings, of cleansing the ulcer with saline wet to dry dressings and application of zinc oxide paste. If cellulitis is present, oral antibiotics should be given, but topical antibiotics or medications should be avoided as they often cause contact dermatitis in this setting. Still very popular is the use of the Unna paste boot (Case 2), which is being replaced by new, more absorbent hydrocolloid dressings. An Unna boot consists of gauze that has been impregnated with zinc oxide. It serves two functions: (1) mechanical compression to the leg to reduce edema and (2) application of a topical medication.

The treatment of lymphedema is substantially nonsurgical. Hygiene of the skin of the foot is critical to prevent recurrent episodes of infection that may aggravate lymphatic obstruction. Control of the edema is achieved by periodic leg elevation during the day and at night, as well as the use of heavy-duty custom-fit elastic stockings. When the edema is difficult to control, the use of devices that produce intermittent and sequential pneumatic compression can be very helpful. Surgery is rarely indicated and is never curative. It consists of debulking operations that remove the diseased subcutaneous tissue or of reconstructive procedures that attempt to re-establish a lymphatic connection either by lymphatic-venous anastomosis or by using a pedicle of omentum or ileal mesentery.

KEY POINTS

- Surgery possibly indicated in patients who have saphenofemoral junction incompetence and large varicosities, recurrent attacks of superficial thrombophlebitis, or significant symptoms; surgical treatment consists of removing diseased saphenous vein with ligation of incompetent perforators

- Inherent risk of pulmonary embolism with DVT dictates institution of prophylactic measures in patients at high risk of developing complication; either mechanical measures such as intermittent external calf compression with pneumatic boots, or anticoagulation

- Once DVT established, patient kept in bed with leg elevated until edema and pain subside; full anticoagulation instituted with intravenous heparin at dosage that maintains PTT at 1.5–2

times normal (10–25 mg/kg/hr produces PTT of 100 seconds); after a few days, anticoagulation continued with coumadin by mouth at dosage that keeps PT 1.5–2 times normal

- Thrombectomy reserved for patients with iliofemoral thrombosis, phlegasia cerulea dolens, or phlegmasia alba dolens

- Patients with septic thrombophlebitis treated with antibiotics and excision of infected vein

- Management of patients with chronic venous insufficiency should control sustained venous hypertension, edema, and stasis ulceration

- Provided that deep system is patent, those with recurrent ulcers or large secondary varices are best treated by saphenous vein stripping with ligation of all perforators

- Local treatment of stasis ulceration consists, in addition to leg elevation and elastic stockings, of cleansing of the ulcer with saline wet to dry dressings and application of zinc oxide paste; if cellulitis is present, oral antibiotics should be given

P FOLLOW-UP

Patients who have undergone injection sclerotherapy for varicose veins should be reassessed in 1 week to check the result and the need for additional injections. After saphenous vein stripping, the legs should be supported with elastic stockings and kept elevated at night for 1 month. Patients with chronic venous insufficiency can be reassessed every 6 months. They should be instructed to return earlier if signs of dermatitis or stasis ulceration recur. Those with lymphedema should be seen whenever there is the suspicion of skin infection or recurrent lymphangitis.

SUGGESTED READINGS

Almgren B, Erikson I: Vascular incompetence in superficial, deep, and perforators veins of limbs with varicose veins. Acta Chir Scand 156:69, 1990

Reviews the pathophysiology and anatomy of varicose vein formation.

Bergan JJ, Yao JST (ed): Venous Disorders. WB Saunders, Philadelphia, 1991

A complete textbook designed primarily for practicing vascular surgeons. Contains a great deal of information on the operative management of venous disease.

Cirado E, Johnson G Jr: Venous disease. Curr Probl Surg 28:338, 1991

A recent article that details both diagnostic and therapeutic aspects. Especially useful for obtaining more information on vascular laboratory testing.

Royle JP: Recurrent varicose veins. World J Surg 10:944, 1986

A good discussion of the management of more complicated venous stasis problems.

QUESTIONS

1. Primary varicose veins?

    A. Are usually congenital.

    B. Are usually due to pathology within the saphenous vein itself.

    C. Are usually due to an incompetent saphenofemoral junction and perforating veins.

    D. Typically progress to involve the deep system.

2. DVT?

    A. Can be treated symptomatically.

    B. Should be treated initially with epinephrine.

    C. Usually results from an extension of superficial thrombophlebitis.

    D. May lead to valve incompetence.

3. Lymphedema?

    A. Usually involves the soles of the feet.

    B. Causes pitting edema.

    C. Is not relieved by leg elevation.

    D. Does not present in adulthood.

4. The most commonly used screening test for DVT is?

    A. Duplex ultrasound.

    B. Doppler.

    C. Venography.

    D. CT scan.

(See p. 604 for answers.)

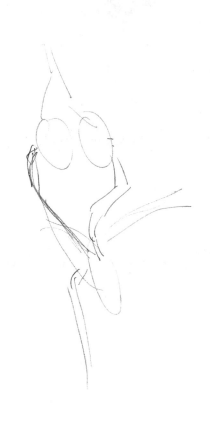

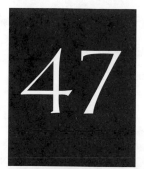

47 PULMONARY EMBOLISM

RODNEY A. WHITE

Pulmonary embolism presents with a spectrum of symptoms whose incidence increases in debilitated individuals and hospitalized patients. This chapter reviews the presentations and outlines associated risk factors. The current recommendations for therapy are also detailed along with discussions regarding more controversial issues such as long-term anticoagulation and vena cava filter placement for prevention of recurrent symptoms.

CASE 1
CHEST PAIN, SHORTNESS OF BREATH, AND HEMOPTYSIS

A 43-year-old mildly obese female was admitted for laparoscopic cholecystectomy. She had a history of recurrent episodes of acute cholecystitis.

During the laparoscopic removal of her gallbladder, the common duct was inadvertently injured and the procedure was converted to an open cholecystectomy. She had an uneventful recovery, and on the third day was ready for discharge but suffered an episode of chest pain, shortness of breath, and hemoptysis. Because of a high clinical suspicion of PE, she was given heparin, and a chest x-ray and pulmonary ventilation/perfusion scan were obtained. The chest x-ray appeared normal, but the lung scan had an area of abnormal perfusion in a well-ventilated segment of the right lower lung, consistent with PE. Duplex ultrasound study of the veins of the lower extremity showed no obvious venous obstruction as a possible source for the embolism. Based on the clinical diagnosis and positive lung scan, she was anticoagulated with heparin for 10 days and discharged on coumadin therapy for 3 months.

CASE 2
SUDDEN VASCULAR COLLAPSE

A 57-year-old male had a 24-hour history of left lower quadrant abdominal pain, fever, and malaise. He had had diverticulitis requiring hospital admission and intravenous antibiotics 1 year previously.

He was a well-developed, well-nourished male with a temperature of 38°C. There was severe tenderness and signs of localized peritoneal irritation in the left lower quadrant. His WBC count was 14,000/mm³.

He was admitted and treated with intravenous antibiotics. His symptoms persisted, and on the fourth hospital day he underwent abdominal exploration. At laparotomy, a large inflammatory mass was identified in the left lower quadrant with evidence of pericecal inflammation and abscess formation. The abscess was drained, but because of severe pelvic and pericolic inflammation, a resection was not performed. A diverting colostomy was established.

Postoperatively, he improved moderately and had low grade fever for approximately 48 hours. On the third postoperative day, while walking about, he suddenly collapsed and could not be revived.

GENERAL CONSIDERATIONS

These cases exemplify the spectrum of clinical presentation of pulmonary embolism (PE), the most feared complication of venous thrombosis. The estimated incidence varies from 285,000 to 600,000 cases each year in the United States, making it the third leading cause of mortality and one of the most common forms of respiratory death in hospitalized patients. This is perhaps not surprising, since two-thirds of the deaths from PE occur within 30 minutes of the embolism and usually are not associated with previous symptoms of deep venous thrombosis (DVT).

Although 95% of pulmonary emboli come from the major tributaries of the inferior vena cava, a small percentage originate at the cavernous sinus, the internal jugular vein, the right heart, and the deep veins of the upper extremity. Large emboli that lodge in the major pulmonary arteries may cause immediate death secondary to vasovagal shock, right ventricular failure, or pulmonary failure. Cyanosis and cardiovascular collapse are ominous consequences of massive PE. It is uncertain whether multiple smaller emboli cause death, although they can cause diffuse bronchospasm and vasoconstriction. Single, small emboli may resolve spontaneously or may be associated with pulmonary infarctions, infection, and abscesses.

KEY POINTS

• Incidence of PE varies from 285,000 to 600,000 cases each year in the United States

• PE third leading cause of mortality and a common form of respiratory death in hospitalized patients

• 95% of pulmonary emboli come from the major tributaries of the inferior vena cava

• Others originate at the cavernous sinus, internal jugular vein, right heart, and deep veins of the upper extremity

---

DIAGNOSIS

PE should be suspected in a patient with venous thrombosis who complains of dyspnea, chest pain, and hemoptysis. However, a national cooperative study reported that only 28% of 160 patients treated for PE had all three symptoms, while 65% had two of the three.

PE presents with a spectrum of findings ranging from simple agitation and anxiety to severe dyspnea (Table 47.1). Most are tachycardic and have some evidence of air hunger. Although laboratory studies are usually normal, a depressed arterial partial pressure of oxygen (PaO_2) (<60 mmHg) and a low or normal arterial partial pressure of carbon dioxide ($PaCO_2$) while breathing room air are highly suggestive. When PaO_2 is greater than 80 mmHg while breathing room air, PE is unlikely. Physical examina-

TABLE 47.1 *Symptoms and signs of pulmonary embolism*

SYMPTOMS AND SIGNS	%
Chest pain	88
Pleuritic	74
Nonpleuritic	14
Dyspnea	84
Apprehension	59
Cough	53
Hemoptysis	30
Sweats	27
Syncope	13
Respiratory rate >16/min	92
Rales	58
Increased intensity of P_2	53
Heart rate >100 bpm	44
Temperature >37.8°C	43
Phlebitis	32
Gallop	34
Diaphoresis	36
Edema	24

(From Bell WR, Simon TL, Demets DL: The clinical features of submassive and massive pulmonary emboli. Am J Med 62:355, 1977, with permission.)

tion should include evaluation of the extremities for signs of DVT. An electrocardiogram (ECG) is usually normal, although signs of right heart strain may be present. This includes right axis deviation, cor pulmonale, inverted T waves, and ST segment changes in right-sided leads. The often cited "S1 Q3 T3" and "S1 S2 S3" patterns do not occur as often as thought previously.

Approximately 50% of patients with significant PE have radiographic evidence of decreased vascularity, dilated pulmonary arteries, and/or pleural fluid. Pulmonary infarctions frequently appear as wedge-shaped infiltrates. An intravenous iodine 131 (^{131}I)-tagged microaggregated albumin ventilation/perfusion pulmonary scan frequently confirms the clinical suspicion. Pulmonary angiography is the most reliable method of diagnosis and is required before the institution of thrombolytic therapy or pulmonary embolectomy, but *not* before beginning anticoagulation with heparin.

KEY POINTS

• PE should be suspected in a patient with venous thrombosis who complains of dyspnea, chest pain, and hemoptysis

• PE presents with a spectrum of findings ranging from simple agitation and anxiety to severe dyspnea

- Most patients with PE are tachycardic and have some air hunger

- Laboratory studies usually normal, but a depressed PaO_2 (<60 mmHg) and low or normal $PaCO_2$ while breathing room air are highly suggestive

- Intravenous ^{131}I-tagged microaggregated albumin ventilation/perfusion pulmonary scan frequently confirms

- Pulmonary angiography is most reliable diagnostic method and is required before instituting thrombolytic therapy or pulmonary embolectomy, but not before anticoagulation with heparin

DIFFERENTIAL DIAGNOSIS

The differential diagnosis of PE includes pneumonia, myocardial infarction, congestive heart failure, lung abscess, tuberculosis, pneumothorax, atelectasis, and anxiety attacks. It is often difficult to differentiate from postoperative pneumonia, since both frequently occur during the same 3–5-day period after surgery. Pneumonia usually has a slower onset and is often heralded by fever, cough, and sputum production. Atelectasis is also difficult to separate since it may present with hypoxia and dyspnea as well. Those with atelectasis have chest x-ray patterns showing volume loss not seen after PE. Myocardial infarction and congestive heart failure can be diagnosed by ECG and invasive monitoring criteria. A pneumothorax should be suspected on physical examination findings.

KEY POINTS

- Treatment of PE begins with hemodynamic support, anticoagulation with continuous intravenous heparin, and bed rest

- Initial dose of intravenous heparin is 25 units/kg/hr for PE, and 10–15 units/kg/hr for thrombophlebitis

- Anticoagulation is maintained by continuous intravenous infusion of heparin in doses that keep serum PTT at 1.5–2 times normal

- Heparin does not dissolve emboli; rather, it prevents accumulation of new thrombus. Fibrinolytic agents infused into the pulmonary artery have been used to cause dissolution of emboli

- Infusion of urokinase or streptokinase directly into pulmonary artery is reserved for patients with massive PE and unstable blood pressure who require pressors (e.g., dopamine or dobutamine) to maintain adequate cardiac output

- Surgical treatment by caval clipping or ligation is indicated for recurrent PE in those receiving heparin in whom anticoagulation is contraindicated and those with septic emboli from lower extremities

- The most important step in DVT management is PE prevention; prophylaxis should be started preoperatively

- Intermittent compression devices are the preferred means of DVT prophylaxis and PE prevention

- Low dose heparin used preoperatively and postoperatively, usually in dose of 5,000 units subcutaneously every 8–12 hour

TREATMENT

Treatment of PE begins with hemodynamic support, anticoagulation with continuous intravenous heparin, and bed rest. Heparin metabolism is significantly increased by PE and, to a lesser extent, by thrombophlebitis. The initial dose of intravenous heparin is a bolus of 100 units/g, followed by an infusion of 25 units/kg/hr for PE, and 10–15 units/kg/hr for thrombophlebitis. Anticoagulation is maintained by continuous intravenous infusion of heparin in doses that keep serum partial thromboplastin time (PTT) at 1.5–2 times normal. Intravenous administration of low molecular weight dextran is effective in preventing ongoing thrombosis. Heparin does not dissolve emboli; rather, it prevents the accumulation of new thrombus. Fibrinolytic agents infused into the pulmonary artery have been used to cause the actual dissolution of emboli. At present, infusion of urokinase or streptokinase directly into the selected appropriate branch of the pulmonary artery is reserved for patients with massive PE and unstable blood pressure who require pressors (e.g., dopamine or dobutamine) to maintain adequate cardiac output. Clinical studies have shown that such patients respond rapidly to thrombolytic therapy. Patients should be kept at bed rest for 3–5 days until the thrombus at the origin of the embolus organizes and adheres to the vein wall.

Surgical treatment by caval clipping or ligation is indicated for recurrent PE in those receiving heparin, for those in whom anticoagulation is contraindicated, and for those with septic emboli from the lower extremities. Partial caval interruption by intraluminal filters entraps pulmonary emboli and prevents swelling of the lower extremities. Ligation of the vena cava is indicated to treat septic emboli. In female patients, ovarian veins should be obliterated to prevent recurrent emboli through hypertrophy of collaterals.

Pulmonary embolectomy is reserved for documented massive pulmonary emboli in patients with persistent cardiovascular collapse. The most important step in the management of DVT is the prevention of PE. This is particularly true in those at prolonged bed rest or those who require extensive operation. It is estimated that patients with hip fractures who undergo total hip replacement have a 40–70% chance of developing DVT. Virchow's triad of hypercoagulability, stasis, and endothelial damage form the cornerstone of DVT prophylaxis.

Stasis is a particularly important factor and leads to the formation of thrombi even during the intraoperative period. Hence, prophylaxis should be started preoperatively. The most effective means involves the use of a sequential compression device that consists of air bladders fashioned in the shape of a stocking. The device is connected to a pump that sequentially inflates the bladders starting at the ankle and moving proximally. This not only simulates the action of the muscle pump, but also causes the release of prostacycline from the vessel wall, which inhibits platelet aggregation, even at remote sites. These compression devices have been shown to be effective when applied to an arm of patients who have casts on both lower extremities. Presently, intermittent compression devices are the preferred means of DVT prophylaxis and hence, PE prevention.

Subcutaneous low dose heparin has been used widely for DVT prophylaxis. The mechanism of action involves saturation of the antithrombin III receptors, which prevent activation of factor X and hence, the conversion of prothrombin into thrombin. Low dose heparin, when used properly, requires preoperative as well as postoperative use. The usual dose is 5,000 units subcutaneously every 8–12 hours. Although PTT need not be monitored, the platelet count should be assessed routinely because heparin may induce an antiplatelet antibody in a small number of patients. All heparin (including line flushes) should be stopped if the platelet count falls below 100,000/mm³ in a patient with a previously normal platelet count. Low dose heparin should be used with extreme caution or not at all in patients with brain or spinal cord pathology or following trauma. Low molecular weight dextran, which prevents platelet adhesion, is a useful alternative to heparin.

Whatever form of prophylaxis is used, it should be continued until normal mobility has been restored.

M FOLLOW-UP

Most physicians anticoagulate patients with coumadin for approximately 3–6 months following resolution of uncomplicated pulmonary emboli, to prevent recurrent embolization. The frequency of recurrent embolization is not known because the primary event may have been overlooked, although the frequency of recurrent events is highest early in the course of the disease and occurs infrequently after patients recover from their illness and become active again. Most physicians agree that a documented episode of recurrent PE while a patient is being treated adequately with anticoagulation is an indication for vena cava filter placement.

SUGGESTED READINGS

Hoyt DB, Swegle JR: Deep venous thrombosis in the surgical intensive care unit. Surg Clin North Am 21:811, 1991

An excellent review of DVT and PE. Presents algorithms and treatment methods. Highly recommended.

Moser KM: Venous thromboembolism. Am Rev Resper Dis 141:235, 1990

A classic monograph on the subject, with an extensive review.

QUESTIONS

1. Most clinically significant pulmonary emboli originate in the?

    A. Calf veins.
    B. Tributaries of the inferior vena cava.
    C. Upper extremity veins.
    D. Portal vein.

2. The most accurate diagnostic technique for detecting PE is?

    A. Duplex ultrasonography.
    B. Impedance plethysmography.
    C. Pulmonary angiography.
    D. Ventilation perfusion scanning.

3. The treatment of established PE may not include which of the following?

    A. Anticoagulation with heparin.
    B. Use of a thrombolytic agent.
    C. Supplemental oxygen and mechanical ventilation.
    D. Infusion of antithrombin-III activator.

(See p. 604 for answers.)

48

CONGENITAL

CARDIAC LESIONS

FRITZ BAUMGARTNER

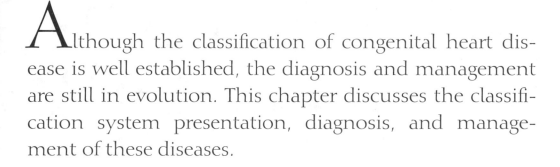

Although the classification of congenital heart disease is well established, the diagnosis and management are still in evolution. This chapter discusses the classification system presentation, diagnosis, and management of these diseases.

CASE 1
A CYANOTIC INFANT

A 1-hour-old infant was cyanotic with bluish discoloration and shortness of breath. The child was resuscitated and intubated. A chest x-ray showed a boot-shaped heart and a paucity of vascularity in the pulmonary fields. There was no evidence of diaphragmatic hernia or cystic lung disease. An arterial blood gas found a PaO_2 of 80 mmHg on 100% oxygen; $PaCO_2$, 25 mmHg; pH, 7.30; and bicarbonate, 15 mEq/dl. Bicarbonate was administered and a prostaglandin E_1 drip instituted. Echocardiography demonstrated a hypertrophied right ventricle, stenosis of the pulmonary subvalvular area, a ventricular septal defect, and "overriding" of the aorta onto the right ventricle. After resuscitation, the child underwent palliative shunt (Blalock-Taussig) the next day. Oxygenation improved substantially.

Over the next year, the child progressed physically and socially. At 2 years of age, operation was performed to correct tetralogy of Fallot. A preoperative echocardiogram demonstrated a functioning shunt. Postoperative arterial oxyhemoglobin saturation on room air was 97–99% with excellent exercise tolerance. He has been followed at 6-month intervals for routine evaluation.

CASE 2
A 3-YEAR-OLD BOY WITH POOR EXERCISE TOLERANCE

A 3-year-old male was found to have increasingly poor exercise tolerance and claudication after running a short dis-

tance. History revealed that he had frequent epistaxis progressively worsening over the past year.

He had good breath sounds bilaterally. There was no evidence of a parascapular bruit or thrill and no murmurs. A chest x-ray showed no evidence of rib notching. Although the lower extremities were warm, there were no pulses present. The blood pressure in both upper extremities was 110/80 mmHg. Arteriography revealed a coarctation of the aorta just distal to the left subclavian artery. A left 4th intercostal space thoracotomy was performed and vascular control of the subclavian artery was achieved. The aorta was opened and the coarctation excised. A primary end-to-end anastomosis was performed. One year later, his growth development and exercise tolerance were equal to those of his speers.

GENERAL CONSIDERATIONS

Congenital heart disease can be broadly classified into cyanotic and noncyanotic disorders. Generally, cyanotic disease involves a right-to-left shunt and decreased pulmonary blood flow. Noncyanotic diseases have a left-to-right shunt with increased pulmonary blood flow. There are exceptions to this broad rule (Table 48.1). Total anomalous pulmonary venous circulation and truncus arteriosus are classified as cyanotic heart diseases, although pulmonary blood flow is actually increased. Certain forms of noncyanotic congenital disease do not increase pulmonary blood flow (aortic stenosis, mitral stenosis, coarctation of the aorta, and interrupted aortic arch). Both cyanotic and

TABLE 48.1   *Classification of congenital heart disease*

CYANOTIC HEART DISEASE	NONCYANOTIC HEART DISEASE
Tetralogy of Fallot	Atrioseptal defect
Transposition of the great arteries	Ventriculoseptal defect
Double outlet right ventricle with pulmonary stenosis	Atrioventricular canal
	Patent ductus arteriosus
	Double outlet right ventricle without pulmonary stenosis
Tricuspid atresia	Aortic stenosis
Pulmonary atresia	Mitral stenosis
Total anomalous pulmonary venous circulation	Coarctation of the aorta
Truncus arteriosus	

acyanotic diseases may change with age. For example, pulmonary stenosis may become more severe, or a ventricular or atrioseptal defect may decrease in size and eventually close. Similarly, the physiologic significance of a congenital abnormality may change with time, as does the physiology of the child. One example is that with decreasing pulmonary vascular resistance, relative right-to-left shunt fractions change in a given congenital cardiac disorder. As patent ductus arteriosus closes, cyanotic congenital heart disease increases in physiologic significance because of the loss of mixed oxygenated and deoxygenated blood.

Tetralogy of Fallot is the most common cyanotic congenital heart disease. Four fundamental anatomic hallmarks define the disease: pulmonary valvular stenosis, ventricular septal defect (VSD), right ventricular hypertrophy, and overriding of the aorta onto the right ventricle (Fig. 48.1). The physiologic effect is decreased pulmonary blood flow and shunting of the blood from right to left. Early in life, a patent ductus arteriosus may mask these lesions by allowing blood to flow from the aorta to the pulmonary artery. However, when the ductus closes, the manifestations of tetralogy of Fallot worsen and children present with hypoxic or cyanotic episodes that can lead to syncope and death in severe cases. The physiology of these "spells" is constriction of an already tight right ventricular outflow tract from hypertrophied muscle bundles, resulting in an acute decrease in pulmonary vascular flow. Squatting is a frequent finding in these children and is a learned attempt to increase pulmonary vascular resistance and diminish the volume of right-to-left shunting, thus forcing more blood through the pulmonary circuit. The complications from the right-to-left shunt include strokes and brain abscesses because right heart blood flow bypasses the pulmonary circuit and embolic material is carried directly into the cerebral circulation.

Chest x-ray reveals a typical boot-shaped cardiac silhouette and paucity of pulmonary vasculature. Cardiac

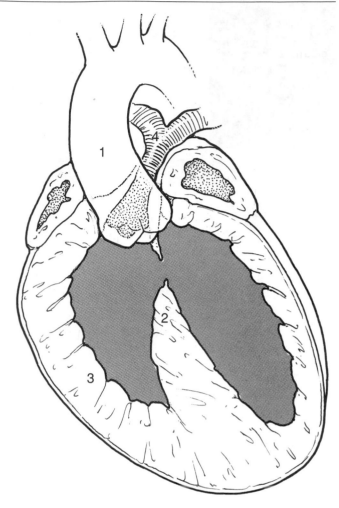

FIGURE 48.1   *Tetralogy of Fallot has four components: (1) an aorta that "overrides" both the left and right ventricles, (2) a ventriculoseptal defect, (3) right ventricular hypertrophy, and (4) stenosis of the pulmonary arterial outflow.*

catheterization defines the number and location of the ventriculoseptal defect, demonstrates the location of the pulmonary stenosis (i.e., valvular, supravalvular, or subpulmonic) and examines the pulmonary vasculature past the pulmonary bifurcation. In younger children, a palliative shunt (i.e., from the subclavian artery to the pulmonary artery [Blalock-Taussig]) should be performed (Case 1). Definitive surgery to correct the underlying anatomy should be postponed until the child reaches 2 years.

Transposition of the great arteries occurs when the aorta originates from the right ventricle and the pulmonary artery from the left. If this was the only anatomic abnormality, there could never be any survivors because only deoxygenated blood would enter the systemic circuit and only oxygenated blood would enter the pulmonary circuit. Some defect that allows mixing is necessary to permit survival, and this usually is in the form of a VSD and/or a patent ductus arteriosus (PDA). The level of cyanosis is determined by the relative amount of oxygenated blood that enters the aorta through the right ventricle. Without treatment, many of these children die within 1 month and 90% within 1 year. Multiple categories of transposition of the great arteries exist with the differing anatomy, resulting in different levels of clinical severity. Most threatening is transposition with an intact ventricular septum. These children have cyanosis within the first few hours of life. An atrial septal defect (ASD) is usually present but is inadequate to achieve satisfactory mixing. Emergency balloon atrioseptostomy (rupturing the atrial septum with a balloon catheter) is indicated to widen the ASD and permit better mixing. This can be a lifesaving maneuver.

Double outlet right ventricle is the term used for a broad category of diseases in which the aorta and the pulmonary artery arise entirely, or in a large part, from the right ventricle. Physical features vary because, morphologically, the disease is highly variable. In general, there is a large VSD and no pulmonary stenosis. Because there is adequate right ventricular mixing, cyanosis is not present. If, however, pulmonary stenosis is present, cyanosis may result.

On physical examination, electrocardiogram (ECG), and chest x-ray, there are no characteristic findings that distinguish transposition patients from the cyanotic and acyanotic condition that they simulate. Echocardiography, cardiac catheterization, and angiography are essential in reaching the diagnosis.

Ebstein's malformation occurs when portions of the leaflets of the tricuspid valve are displaced downward into the right ventricle. The remaining anterior leaflet is enlarged and "sail-like." Tricuspid regurgitation is common. The right ventricle is divided into an atrialized portion and a functional portion with displacement of the tricuspid valve into the right ventricle. This functional true right ventricle is dilated and thinner than normal. The right atrium is enormously dilated and may compress the atrioventricular (AV) node and bundle of His, producing right bundle branch block (Wolff-Parkinson-White) syndrome. The most commonly associated defect is pulmonary atresia or stenosis, occurring in one-third of patients who present later with mild dyspnea and fatigue in childhood or adult life. Cyanosis occurs in more than one-half, but usually later in infancy. These patients may present within the first week of life with shortness of breath and cyanosis, but more typically develop congestive heart failure (CHF) early on. Conduction problems are common. A child with Wolff-Parkinson-White syndrome should be suspected of harboring Ebstein's anomaly. Chest x-ray demonstrates marked cardiomegaly with a round or box-like contour of the cardiac shadow. Echocardiography is best for diagnosis. Catheterization is only needed if specific hemodynamic details need to be identified. Operation is usually delayed until adult life and involves assessing the atrialized portion of the right ventricle, excising the abnormal tricuspid valve, and performing a tricuspid valve replacement.

Tricuspid atresia occurs when the right atrium fails to open into a ventricle through an atrioventricular valve, resulting in a univentricular AV connection into the left ventricle. The left ventricle is hypertrophied, since it receives both pulmonary and systemic blood flow. Right atrial blood empties into the left atrium. The left ventricle receives blood from both the left and right atrium and may either enter the aorta or enter the right ventricle through a VSD. This results in decreased pulmonary blood flow and cyanosis. Three-quarters of patients with tricuspid atresia also have subvalvular obstruction to pulmonary flow, which worsens the cyanosis. Findings include cyanosis from birth, which may be severe. Cyanotic spells occurring within the first 6 months are a grave sign. Squatting is uncommon in this disorder, unlike tetralogy of Fallot. Chest x-ray shows decreased pulmonary vascular markings and a diminished right ventricular shadow. Treatment initially consists of a shunt to palliate the cyanotic disease followed by a procedure to connect the right atrium and the pulmonary artery.

Pulmonary atresia consists of an obstruction to pulmonary flow and some anatomic pathway for biventricular mixing (nearly always by a VSD). Newborns are typically extremely cyanotic and are best managed with infusion of prostaglandin E_1 to keep the patent ductus arteriosus open until a shunt procedure from the right ventricle to the pulmonary artery can be performed.

Truncus arteriosus occurs when one great artery arises from the base of the heart by a single truncal valve and gives rise to the aorta, pulmonary artery, and coronary arteries. Beneath this truncal valve is a ventriculoseptal defect. Presentation is typically within the first several days and consists of shortness of breath, tachycardia, irritability, and poor feeding (all manifestations of congestive heart failure). In the infants who survive, cyanosis develops from elevated pulmonary vascular resistance. Eisenmenger syndrome (reversal of shunt flow from right to left) may develop in older children due to the elevated pulmonary vascular resistance. Chest x-ray shows cardiomegaly and pulmonary plethora.

Cardiac catheterization is performed to define the anatomy of the pulmonary artery and aortic arch. Arterial oxygen saturation less than 80% is an indication that the pulmonary vascular resistance is beyond the range of standard cardiac intervention. Heart-lung transplantation may be the only surgical alternative at this stage. Operation consists of detachment of the pulmonary artery from the truncus, closure of the VSD, and placement of a graft from the right ventricle to the pulmonary artery. Without treatment, only 50% survive more than 1 month; only 10% survive to 1 year. Death in infancy is due to CHF. When pulmonary vascular resistance increases, the child has a good chance of surviving into adolescence. Truncal valve stenosis or incompetence impairs survival. Pulmonary stenosis will actually improve survival by limiting the amount of CHF and pulmonary blood flow.

Total anomalous pulmonary venous circulation is a cardiac malformation in which all pulmonary venous drainage enters the systemic venous system. An ASD or patent foramen ovale is necessary for survival after birth. In nearly all cases, the individual right and left pulmonary veins converge to form a common pulmonary venous drainage. Only 50% survive more than 3 months, and only 20% survive to 1 year. If patients survive more than 1 year, they usually have a large ASD with stable hemodynamics for 10–20 years, but then develop elevation of the pulmonary vascular resistance and eventually Eisenmenger's complex. Tachypnea is a cardinal symptom. Chest x-ray reveals a normal heart size if there is pulmonary venous obstruction, or cardiomegaly if there is minimal obstruction to pulmonary venous drainage. In partial anomalous pulmonary venous drainage, the right pulmonary veins drain into the right atrium and produce a characteristic scimitar-like configuration on a chest x-ray. The definitive diagnosis is established by cardiac catheterization and angiography. Right atrial blood will exhibit a marked step-up in hemoglobin oxygen saturation from the anomalous pulmonary venous drainage.

Operation should be immediate in any infant found to have obstructive total anomalous pulmonary circulation. In nonobstructive total anomalous pulmonary venous circulation, balloon septostomy and diuresis may be reasonable, but operation should still be performed by age 3 months.

ASD results in a left-to-right shunt with elevated pulmonary blood flow. Symptoms include shortness of breath on exertion, recurrent respiratory tract infections, and palpitations. Physical findings include left parasternal lift and a fixed and split S2. There may be a tricuspid valve murmur, as well as a pulmonic valve murmur. With large shunts, a right precordial lift may be present. Ten percent of infants with ASD are symptomatic, and of the symptomatic patients, 10% die. In older patients, there is an increased chance of death after age 40 resulting from ASD-related CHF, and an increased chance of supraventricular tachycardias after age 30. Cardiac catheterization may be done in infants to determine whether other abnormalities are present, and in adults to evaluate pulmonary hypertension. For primary closure of an ASD, a pericardial patch closure is performed (Fig. 48.2).

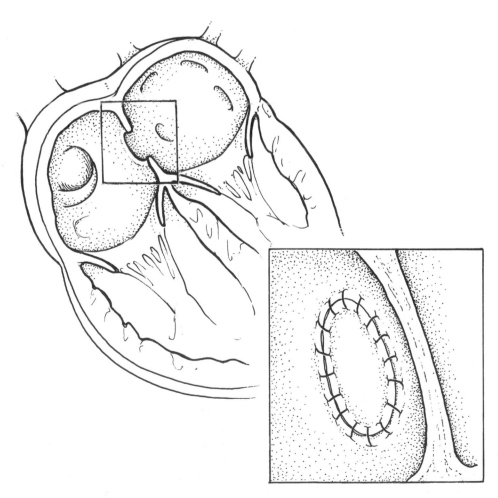

FIGURE 48.2   *An ASD and its repair with a simple patch (inset).*

VSDs include perimembranous defects, subpulmonary (conal) defects, AV canal VSDs, and muscular VSDs. Other than a pansystolic murmur, patients with small VSDs and little shunting may have no abnormal signs or symptoms and have normal chest x-rays and ECGs. Larger VSDs manifest clinically early on in infants as CHF, tachypnea, hepatomegaly, and stunted growth. Chest films in these infants show cardiomegaly and pulmonary congestion from the increased flow. The ECG demonstrates biventricular hypertrophy. The symptoms are frequently nonspecific. Echocardiography and cardiac catheterization are valuable in reaching the diagnosis. Of those VSDs diagnosed at 1 month of age, 80% will close subsequently. Of those present at age 1 year, one-quarter will close subsequently. Ten percent of infants with large VSDs die from CHF or recurrent pulmonary infections by 3 months. After 1 year, few die until 10 years, when they develop complications of pulmonary hypertension. Eisenmenger syndrome, including cerebral abscesses and stroke, polycythemia, hemoptysis, and right heart failure may occur when pulmonary pressures reach a systemic level. Chest x-ray in patients with a large VSD without elevated pulmonary vascular resistance will show cardiomegaly, increased pulmonary vasculature, and a large pulmonary artery. An ECG will demonstrate biventricular hypertrophy. When the pulmonary vascular resistance causes a bidirectional shunt, the heart reduces to normal on chest x-ray with normal appearing pulmonary vasculature. ECG will show right ventricular hypertrophy. The P2 sound is loud and there is no longer a murmur. Angiography should be performed to determine the size and location of the VSD and to determine whether other congenital anomalies are present. Repair is usually possible with a simple patch over the defect (Fig. 48.3). If the patient is very young or has other comorbid conditions or defects that will require later definitive repair, a flow restricting pulmonary artery band (which decreases pulmonary blood flow) may be placed early on to prevent the development of pulmonary hypertension.

Closure of the (patent) ductus arteriosus normally present after birth occurs in two stages. First, there is contraction of smooth muscle in the media of the vessel followed by fibrosis of the intima. Most close within 2 weeks after birth. Indomethacin and oxygen have been found to close the ductus arteriosus while prostaglandin E_1 keeps it open. When a ductus arteriosus remains patent, the infant develops CHF within 1 month. This results in tachypnea, tachycardia, poor weight gain, sweating, and irritability. By age 2 years, an untreated patent ductus arteriosus results in pulmonary hypertension and Eisenmenger syndrome. Patent ductus is particularly common in children of mothers who had rubella in the first trimester. Birth weight less than 1,000 g is a predictor of patent ductus, which occurs in 85% of these underweight children. Physical findings include a continuous machinery-type murmur. Chest x-

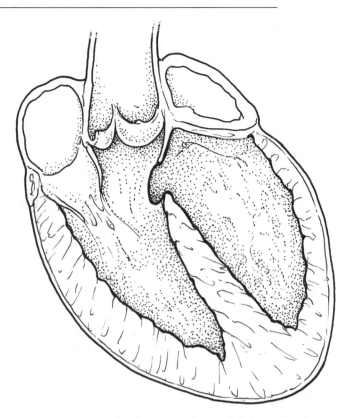

FIGURE 48.3   *A high ventriculospetal defect. This lesion lies just below the pulmonary valve, although VSDs may occur in several locations in the interventricular septum.*

rays show CHF. If pulmonary hypertension develops (with shunt reversal), a small heart without pulmonary plethora is observed. Catheterization is usually not necessary as the diagnosis can be made by echocardiography. For children less than 1 month old, patent ductus ligation is indicated only in the presence of CHF. For age greater than 1 month, patent ductus arteriosus closure may be done at any time, but generally is best accomplished before 6 months. Severe pulmonary hypertension is a contraindication to repair.

Coarctation of the aorta is a narrowing of the aorta, typically adjacent to the ductus arteriosus. A stenosis greater than 50% causes a significant pressure gradient, which can result in proximal central aortic hypertension and decreased blood pressure peripherally. The major vessels for collateral flow around the coarctation are the first two pairs of intercostal arteries just distal to the coarctation. This produces the characteristic rib notching on radiography in which increased pressure and flow in the subcostal vessel actually erodes the rib. There is a lack of rib notching in the first and second ribs because these are usually above the level of the coarctation. Bicuspid aortic valves occur in one-third to one-half of patients with coarctation. If a patient presents as a symptomatic neonate, CHF is the most common finding with tachypnea, feeding problems, and sweating during feeding. If the ductus stays widely patent, there may be a differential examination with cyanosis of the toes and a pink head and upper extremities. In older children and young adults, headaches, nosebleeds, fatigue, and claudication may be the predominant symptoms (Case 2). Collaterals may be palpable and audible on auscultation posteriorly. Chest x-ray shows marked cardiomegaly even in infancy in about one-third of patients. Rib notching is rare before the age of 3 and occurs more frequently thereafter. Angiography should be performed to determine the location and extent of the coarctation and to determine the presence of any coexistent congenital abnormalities. Approximately 75% survive to adulthood. Five percent die within the first weeks of life from CHF. Correction generally involves resection of the stenosis and primary end-to-end anastomosis of the aorta.

Congenital aortic stenosis involves a bicuspid aortic valve 70% of the time with leaflet thickening. In 30%, the valve is tricuspid. Occasionally, a unicuspid valve may be found. Left ventricular hypertrophy always results. There may be associated subvalvular or supravalvular stenosis, as well as congenital heart defects. Signs and symptoms include pallor, perspiration, inability to eat, shortness of breath, and possibly cyanosis in end-stage disease. Many children may be asymptomatic initially. In older children, the presence of symptoms (angina, syncope, or shortness of breath) signifies severe disease. In neonates and infants, a murmur across the valve may be absent if there is poor cardiac output from heart failure. In children and young adults, the signs generally are a murmur and thrill radiating to the carotid arteries, and a left systolic ejection click. ECG reveals left ventricular hypertrophy while chest x-ray demonstrates a prominent ascending aorta. Presentation in infancy nearly always represents severe disease with critically ill patients. Those that present in childhood have heart failure and may present with sudden death. In neonates with severe stenosis, emergency operation may be necessary. Prostaglandin E_1 is begun immediately to keep the patent ductus open. Aortic valvotomy is performed expeditiously.

Congenital abnormalities of the mitral valve may result in stenosis or regurgitation. Although only one component of the valve is affected, virtually the entire valve is diseased. The abnormalities occur on the atrial side of the mitral valve annulus, on the mitral annulus itself, or in the subvalvular structures, including the chordae or papillary muscles. Seventy-five percent of congenital mitral valve abnormalities coexist with other congenital heart disease, including VSD in one-third and left ventricular outflow tract obstruction in one-half of cases. Symptoms and signs include pulmonary venous hypertension such as dyspnea, orthopnea, paroxysmal nocturnal dyspnea, or recurrent pneumonias. Diagnosis is by echocardiography and cardiac catheterization. The symptoms associated with pulmonary venous hypertension are an indication for opera-

tion, at which time mitral regurgitation, valvotomy for mitral stenosis, or mitral valve replacement are performed.

KEY POINTS

- Generally, cyanotic disease involves a right-to-left shunt and decreased pulmonary blood flow

- Noncyanotic diseases have a left-to-right shunt with increased pulmonary blood flow

- Tetralogy of Fallot is the most common cyanotic congenital heart disease

- Four fundamental anatomic hallmarks define tetralogy of Fallot: pulmonary valvular stenosis, VSD, right ventricular hypertrophy, and overriding of the aorta onto the right ventricle (Fig. 48.1); physiologic effect is decreased pulmonary blood flow and shunting of the blood from right to left

- Chest x-ray reveals a typical boot-shaped cardiac silhouette and paucity of pulmonary vasculature

- Transposition of the great arteries occurs when the aorta originates from the right ventricle and the pulmonary artery from the left

- Some defect that allows mixing is necessary to permit survival; this usually is in the form of a VSD and/or a PDA

- Emergency balloon atrioseptostomy (rupturing the atrial septum with a balloon catheter) is indicated to widen the ASD and permit better mixing; this can be a lifesaving maneuver

- On physical examination, ECG, and chest x-ray, no characteristic findings distinguish transposition patients from the cyanotic and acyanotic and conditions that they simulate; echocardiography, cardiac catheterization, and angiography are essential in reaching the diagnosis

- Ebstein's malformation occurs when portions of the leaflets of the tricuspid valve are displaced downward into the right ventricle; tricuspid regurgitation is common

- A child with Wolff-Parkinson-White syndrome should be suspected of harboring Ebstein's anomaly; chest x-ray demonstrates marked cardiomegaly with a round or box-like contour of the cardiac shadow; echocardiography is best for diagnosis

- Three-quarters of patients with tricuspid atresia also have subvalvular obstruction to pulmonary flow, which worsens the cyanosis; findings include cyanosis from birth, which may be severe; cyanotic spells occurring within the first 6 months are a grave sign; squatting is uncommon; chest x-ray shows decreased pulmonary vascular markings and a diminished right ventricular shadow

- Pulmonary atresia consists of an obstruction to pulmonary flow and some anatomic pathway for biventricular mixing (nearly always by VSD); newborns are typically extremely cyanotic and best managed with infusion of prostaglandin E_1 to keep PDA open until shunt procedure from right ventricle to the pulmonary artery can be performed

- Truncus arteriosus occurs when one great artery arises from the base of the heart by a single truncal valve and gives rise to the aorta, pulmonary artery, and coronary arteries; presentation typically within first several days and consists of shortness of breath, tachycardia, irritability, and poor feeding (all manifestations of CHF)

• Without treatment, only 50% survive more than 1 month; only 10% survive to 1 year; death in infancy due to CHF; when pulmonary vascular resistance increases, child has good chance of surviving into adolescence

• Total anomalous pulmonary venous circulation is a cardiac malformation in which all pulmonary venous drainage enters systemic venous system; an ASD or patent foramen ovale is necessary for survival after birth; only 50% survive more than 3 months, and only 20% survive to 1 year

• Tachypnea is cardinal symptom; chest x-ray reveals normal heart size if there is pulmonary venous obstruction, or cardiomegaly if there is minimal obstruction to pulmonary venous drainage

• ASD results in left-to-right shunt with elevated pulmonary blood flow; symptoms include shortness of breath on exertion, recurrent respiratory tract infections, and palpitations; physical findings include left parasternal lift and a fixed and split S2

• Of infants with ASD, 10% are symptomatic and of these, 10% die; in older patients, there is an increased chance of death after age 40 resulting from ASD-related CHF, and an increased chance of supraventricular tachycardias after age 30

• VSDs include perimembranous defects, subpulmonary defects, AV canal VSDs, and muscular VSDs; other than a pansystolic murmur, patients with small VSDs and little shunting may have no abnormal signs or symptoms and have normal chest x-rays and ECGs

• Larger VSDs manifest clinically early on in infants as CHF, tachypnea, hepatomegaly, and stunted growth

• Echocardiography and cardiac catheterization are valuable in reaching the diagnosis; of those VSDs diagnosed at 1 month of age, 80% will close

• Angiography should be performed to determine size and location of VSD and whether other congenital anomalies are present; repair is usually possible with simple patch over defect (Fig. 48.3)

• When ductus arteriosus remains patent, infant develops CHF within 1 month, resulting in tachypnea, tachycardia, poor weight gain, sweating, and irritability; by age 2 years, untreated PDA results in pulmonary hypertension and Eisenmenger syndrome; physical findings include continuous machinery-type murmur; chest x-ray shows CHF

• For children less than 1 month of age, PDA ligation is indicated only in the presence of CHF; severe pulmonary hypertension is contraindication to repair

• Coarctation of the aorta is narrowing of aorta, typically adjacent to ductus arteriosus; stenosis greater than 50% causes significant pressure gradient, which can result in proximal central aortic hypertension and decreased blood pressure peripherally

• Other major congenital abnormalities include Turner syndrome, von Recklinghausen's disease, and Noonan syndrome; if patient presents as symptomatic neonate, CHF is most common finding with tachypnea, feeding problems, and sweating during feeding

• Angiography should be performed to determine location and extent of coarctation and presence of coexistent congenital abnormalities; 75% survive to adulthood

• Congenital aortic stenosis involves bicuspid aortic valve 70% of time with leaflet thickening; in children and young adults, signs generally are murmur and thrill radiating to carotid arteries, and left systolic ejection click; ECG reveals left ventricular hypertrophy, chest x-ray reveals prominent ascending aorta; those that present in childhood have heart failure and possible sudden death; prostaglandin E_1 begun right away to keep patent ductus open; symptoms include pulmonary venous hypertension, such as dyspnea, orthopnea, paroxysmal nocturnal dyspnea, or recurrent pneumonias

DIAGNOSIS

The diagnostic features of each anomaly have been presented with the pathophysiology so that anatomy can be correlated with physical findings. Classified broadly, congenital heart disease is cyanotic or noncyanotic. Cyanotic diseases generally manifest with some combination of hypoxia, cyanosis, clubbing, or cerebral abscess. Noncyanotic diseases present with increased pulmonary flow manifesting as poor feeding, heart failure, poor growth, dyspnea and respiratory distress, and frequent respiratory infections.

In some cases, the combination of history, physical findings, and chest x-ray may be so suggestive that a diagnosis can be made without further investigation. For example, a dyspneic child who squats frequently and has a boot-shaped heart on chest x-ray certainly has tetralogy of Fallot. A man complaining of lower extremity claudication with absent lower extremity pulses, a parascapular thrill and bruit, and notching of the third and fourth ribs bilaterally on his chest x-ray almost certainly has coarctation of the aorta. Features of the chest x-ray may corroborate certain findings of the history and physical examination. Patients with cyanotic congenital heart disease may have paucity of pulmonary vasculature on their chest x-rays, whereas noncyanotic congenital heart disease patients may exhibit plethora on their chest x-rays. The diagnosis is usually confirmed with echocardiography and cardiac catheterization and angiography. It is important to determine information about the specific congenital abnormality such as size and location of the VSD, pulmonary stenosis, and shunt fraction, which may be important to determine which patients undergo operation and to determine whether there are other congenital cardiac abnormalities that are coexistent.

KEY POINTS

• Cyanotic diseases generally manifest with some combination of hypoxia, cyanosis, clubbing, or cerebral abscess

• Noncyanotic diseases present with increased pulmonary flow manifesting as poor feeding, heart failure, poor growth, dyspnea and respiratory distress, and frequent respiratory infections

DIFFERENTIAL DIAGNOSIS

When patients present with cyanosis, central and peripheral components must be evaluated. Peripheral cyanosis arises from decreased cardiac output with increased oxygen extraction from the sluggish capillary flow. Central cyanosis results from a defect in oxygenation, either from pulmonary insufficiency or from an intracardiac shunt. These can be distinguished based on history, physical examination, and chest x-ray. Cyanosis from pulmonary insufficiency can be recognized by its prompt response to 100% oxygen. Peripheral cyanosis from heart failure can be demonstrated by heart failure features on chest x-ray. Chronic cyanosis from congenital shunts inevitably produce clubbing and polycythemia. The differential diagnosis of CHF, recurrent pulmonary hypertension, and chronic cough may lead one to suspect a primary pulmonary disorder and pulmonary hypertension.

The right-to-left or bidirectional shunt associated with Eisenmenger syndrome includes the complex of cerebral abscess, stroke, polycythemia, hemoptysis, and right heart failure. In patients with these symptoms, the clinical findings may be unable to distinguish whether cyanotic or noncyanotic congenital heart disease was the initial cause. Further elucidation of the specific etiology is important because cyanotic heart disease would be reparable at this point. Noncyanotic congenital heart disease and irreversible pulmonary hypertension would be irreparable at this point.

KEY POINTS

• Peripheral cyanosis arises from decreased cardiac output with increased oxygen extraction from the sluggish capillary flow

• Central cyanosis results from defect in oxygenation, either from pulmonary insufficiency or intracardiac shunt

TREATMENT

Treatment can be categorized as either palliative or definitive. Initial palliative measures usually consist of nonoperative medical management. For cyanotic congenital heart disease, this includes adequate oxygenation, institution of prostaglandin E_1 (if there is lifesaving patent ductus arteriosus present), or balloon septostomy to permit mixing of oxygenated and deoxygenated blood in conditions such as transposition of the great arteries. These maneuvers are generally only temporizing until surgical palliation or a definitive operation can be performed. Some forms of medical

management are however, definitive, as is the case with indomethacin-induced closure of a patent ductus arteriosus.

Palliative operations for congenital heart disease are classified as systemic arterial-to-pulmonary arterial shunt procedures for cyanotic heart disease or pulmonary artery banding for noncyanotic heart disease. Among the systemic-to-pulmonary artery shunting operations, the prototype is the Blalock-Taussig shunt, which involves direct anastomosis of the subclavian artery to the pulmonary artery. The modified Blalock-Taussig shunt is a graft between the subclavian and the pulmonary arteries. A pulmonary artery banding procedure is performed through a left thoracotomy in the fourth intercostal space. The main pulmonary artery is wrapped with Teflon tape to lower the pulmonary artery pressure to less than one-half of the systemic pressure.

When the child reaches adequate size for definitive operation, careful evaluation of the anatomy is undertaken to be sure changes have not occurred that may alter the surgical outcome. For example, a patient with tetralogy of Fallot may develop worsening pulmonary stenosis. Surgical maneuvers are then modified to repair the specific anatomical derangement. The pulmonary vascular resistance in the individual patient may allow for or preclude a definitive operation.

In a patient with a large VSD with CHF presenting within the first 3 months, prompt primary repair is indicated unless there are other anatomic problems that preclude definitive repair. In these cases, a pulmonary artery band is placed. Patients with elevated pulmonary vascular resistance who have a pulmonary systemic shunt ratio of less than 1.5, may have severe pulmonary hypertension. If there is no murmur or physical examination, and chest x-ray confirms a normal cardiac silhouette without cardiomegaly or pulmonary plethora, the pulmonary hypertensive changes may be irreversible. One can perform an exercise test or give oxygen to see whether this results in a decrease in the pulmonary vascular resistance. If there is no decrease, operation will be ineffective because the congenital heart disease has produced irreversible pulmonary hypertensive changes. A simple finding of a fall in arterial saturation during exercise indicates worsening of the right-to-left shunt and bespeaks of inoperability.

KEY POINT

• Palliative operations for congenital heart disease are classified as systemic arterial-to-pulmonary arterial shunt procedures for cyanotic heart disease or pulmonary artery banding for noncyanotic heart disease

FOLLOW-UP

Careful follow-up is an absolute requirement in any congenital pediatric heart surgery program. Inadequate follow-up for just a few months may convert a curable ventriculoseptal defect into irreversible pulmonary hypertensive changes, resulting in Eisenmenger syndrome. Follow-up after palliative operations is necessary to track the patient's progress and determine when definitive operation can be best performed. Times can range from several days to months, depending on the acuity of the patient's illness and the time period from the palliative and definitive operation. Follow-up with chest x-ray, echocardiography, and if necessary, angiography is a requirement.

SUGGESTED READINGS

Armstrong BE: Congenital cardiovascular disease and cardiac surgery in childhood. Part 1. Curr Opinion Cardiol 10:58, 1995

This is the first of a two-part discussion on congenital cardiovascular diseases and cardiac surgery. It is an excellent review and is highly recommended.

Armstrong BE: Congenital cardiovascular disease and cardiac surgery in childhood. Part II. Curr Opinion Cardio 10:68, 1995

This is the second of a two-part discussion on congenital cardiovascular diseases and cardiac surgery. An excellent review, and highly recommended.

Hammerman C: Patent ductus arteriosus. Clin Perinatol 22:457, 1995

This article presents a comprehensive review of the patent ductus arteriosus most commonly found in premature neonates. It includes a discussion of the anatomy and the physiology of the ductus as well as a review of the mechanisms involved in normal closure and factors leading to persistent patency. The article also discusses therapeutic options including new and innovative approaches.

Rao PS: Transcatheter management of cyanotic congenital heart defects. Clin Cardiol 15:483, 1992

This article discusses the role of transcatheter methods in the management of cyanotic congenital heart defects. Techniques such as balloon dilatation and other palliative procedures are presented with respect to the patients' cardiac anatomy and physiology.

QUESTIONS

1. Which of the following is not a manifestation of tetralogy of Fallot?
   A. Right ventricular hypertrophy.
   B. Polycythemia.
   C. Cyanosis.
   D. Increased pulmonary blood flow.

2. Which of the following is not useful in managing VSDs?
   A. Subclavian artery to pulmonary artery shunt.
   B. Pulmonary artery band.
   C. VSD patch repair.
   D. Left ventricular angiogram.

3. Patients with coarctation of the aorta do not have which of the following?
   A. Parascapular bruit.
   B. Squatting behavior.
   C. Frequent headaches and nosebleed.
   D. Lower extremity claudication.

4. The initial treatment for a neonate with a persistent PDA is?
   A. Trial of indomethacin.
   B. Pulmonary banding.
   C. Thoracotomy and ductus ligation.
   D. Pulmonary artery band.

(See p. 604 for answers.)

49

ACQUIRED CARDIAC
AND THORACIC
AORTIC DISEASE

FRITZ BAUMGARTNER

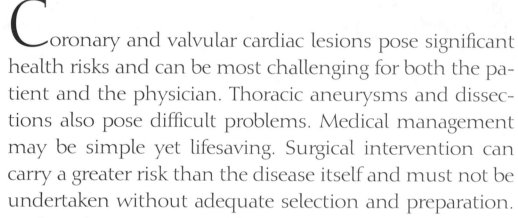

oronary and valvular cardiac lesions pose significant health risks and can be most challenging for both the patient and the physician. Thoracic aneurysms and dissections also pose difficult problems. Medical management may be simple yet lifesaving. Surgical intervention can carry a greater risk than the disease itself and must not be undertaken without adequate selection and preparation.

This chapter (1) provides information on evaluation and management of the patient with acquired cardiac disease, (2) discusses the indications for medical management, angioplasty, and surgery in coronary artery disease, (3) elucidates the etiologics, pathophysiology, and treatment of valvular heart disease, and (4) discusses the natural history of aneurysms and dissections.

CASE 1
SHORTNESS OF BREATH AND HYPOTENSION

A 62-year-old male was hospitalized for 7 days with an acute myocardial infarction. Treatment included thrombolytic therapy and intravenous heparin and nitroglycerin. He developed sudden shortness of breath that was accompanied by a BP of 80/40 mmHg and a pulse rate of 100 bpm (normal sinus rhythm). Physical examination found rales in both lung fields, mild bilateral wheezing, and a loud 4/6 systolic murmur heard best in the parasternal region in the left 4th intercostal space, which had not been present on previous examinations. He had been admitted 1 week earlier with a diagnosis of acute inferior myocardial infarction but improved with medical management and was sent home. Current medications included diltiazem 60 mg four times per day, metoprolol 100 mg twice a day, nitropatch, and enalapril 5 mg twice per day. A dopamine drip at 10 µg/kg/min was begun with increase in BP to 125/82 mmHg. The ECG demonstrated the T-wave pattern from his infarction 1 week earlier. An arterial blood gas showed a PaO_2 on room air of 50 mmHg; $PaCO_2$ of 26 mmHg; pH of 7.4; and bicarbonate of 20 mEq/L. A chest x-ray demonstrated gross pulmonary edema. Eight milligrams of intravenous furosemide was given, and the enalapril dose was doubled. The pulmonary artery catheter showed a huge V-wave in the wedge position with a mean wedge pressure of 30 mmHg and pulmonary artery pressures of 50/25 mmHg. The oxyhemoglobin saturation in the pulmonary artery was 75%, which was identical to the saturation of blood drawn from the right atrial port. He developed worsening respiratory distress and required intubation and ventilation with 100% oxygen. An echocardiogram demonstrated severe mitral regurgitation, moderate tricuspid regurgitation, and an ejection fraction of 30%. Coronary angiography showed severe triple-vessel coronary artery disease with a completely occluded right coronary artery, and a 75% stenotic left anterior descending, diagonal, and first obtuse marginal artery.

A four-vessel coronary artery bypass and mitral valve replacement with a mechanical valve was performed. Postoperatively, he continued to receive inotropic and intra-aortic balloon pump support. He was discharged home 2 weeks after surgery, and has been followed regularly in anticoagulation, surgical, and cardiology clinics.

CASE 2
SYNCOPE, SHORTNESS OF BREATH, AND CHEST PAIN

A 25-year-old Hispanic female presented with a 2-month history of progressive shortness of breath, substernal chest pain, and a fainting spell that lasted several seconds. Questioning disclosed a history of rheumatic fever as a child, but no evidence of prior cardiopulmonary problems. She had been otherwise healthy.

On physical examination, she had a 4/6 crescendo-decrescendo systolic ejection murmur, best heard in the right 2nd intercostal space parasternally and radiating to both carotids. Echocardiography demonstrated severe aortic valve stenosis with a peak gradient of 120 mmHg and a mean gradient of 80 mmHg. The valve leaflets appeared extremely thickened and fibrotic. The mitral and tricuspid valves functioned normally, although the mitral valve appeared to be mildly thickened. Various surgical options were explained, including mechanical valve replacement, a porcine bioprosthesis, and a human aortic allograft. The patient was a newlywed who desired children and requested a human allograft, which was placed electively. Postoperative transesophageal echocardiography demonstrated excellent valve function without evidence of regurgitation. Follow-up included biannual transthoracic echocardiograms that have shown excellent valve function over the course of 5 years.

CASE 3
BACK PAIN

A 65-year-old male presented to the emergency room with "tearing and ripping" mid-back pain between his shoulder blades and a cold, painful right leg. He was a heavy smoker who, 1 year ago, underwent percutaneous transluminal angioplasty of the right coronary artery. Two years before he had had bilateral carotid endarterectomies. His

hypertension was controlled with an angiotensin-converting enzyme inhibitor, but he had been out of medicine for several weeks.

Physical examination found a severely distressed male with BP of 200/90 mmHg and a pulse rate of 100 bpm. β-Blockers and afterload reducers (metoprolol and nitroprusside) were instituted, with a decrease in BP to 120/50 mmHg. Cardiopulmonary examination found a diastolic decrescendo murmur. His abdominal examination was unremarkable. The right leg was numb and cold without any femoral or distal pulses. Initial chest x-ray showed a widened mediastinum and a tortuous aorta. CT scan found a Stanford type A (DeBakey type I) aortic dissection extending to the level of the common iliac arteries. A transthoracic echocardiogram showed severe aortic regurgitation but no evidence of pericardial effusion. Aortography was performed, which showed an intimal tear in the proximal ascending aorta. The renal and visceral vessels were supplied by the true lumen and the right common iliac artery by the false lumen. The coronary arteries were patent but there was severe aortic valvular insufficiency.

The patient underwent urgent replacement of the aortic valve, the ascending aorta, and reimplantation of the coronary arteries. The dissection distal to the transverse aortic arch was not repaired but was excluded from blood flow by including the proximalmost portion of the dissection lumen in the repair. He did well and has been followed with biannual CT scans of the chest to evaluate the descending thoracic aorta, which has not enlarged beyond 6 cm.

GENERAL CONSIDERATIONS

The myocardium is supplied by the branches of the right and left coronary arteries, which arise from the sinuses of Valsalva in the root of the aorta. In 90% of cases, the right coronary artery gives rise to the posterior descending artery and branches to form an atrioventricular nodal artery and terminal posterolateral left ventricular branches. The left main coronary artery forms the left anterior descending and the left circumflex coronary arteries. The left anterior descending artery is of particular importance, since it provides many branches to the left ventricle (with its high workload) and to the interventricular septum. Blood flow through the coronary arteries to the myocardium occurs principally in diastole when the heart is at rest. Extraction of oxygen by the myocardium averages 75% and may be nearly complete under stress or during exercise.

Atherosclerosis is the principal cause of myocardial ischemia (angina pectoris) and infarction. It is a progressive disease whose beginnings can be found in infants and children. As the disease worsens, it involves multifocal lesions of more than one major coronary artery. Stenosis is short and tends to be proximal in most arteries. When a lesion reduces the cross-sectional area by more than 75%, blood flow is limited—particularly during periods of increased demand. Although vasospasm may further reduce flow, the fixed stenosis caused by plaques is the major cause of myocardial ischemia.

The natural history of coronary artery disease without treatment varies according to anatomy and left ventricular function. For single-vessel coronary artery disease, the 5-year survival is the same as a normal patient, with the exception of isolated proximal lesions of the left anterior descending coronary artery, where the survival is slightly reduced. For double-vessel disease, there is a 75% 5-year survival. In patients with coronary artery disease with normal left ventricular ejection fraction, the overall 5-year survival is 92% without treatment; for ejection fractions from 30–50%, the 5-year survival is reduced to 75%. As a general rule, the number and severity of atherosclerotic lesions progress with time. Those with unstable angina have decreased life expectancy when compared to patients with stable angina. Coronary revascularization will most benefit those with reduced ejection fractions and unstable angina, although these are the very patients that have an increased risk of morbidity and mortality from coronary revascularization.

The aortic, mitral, and tricuspid valves lie in fibrous continuity. They are separated from the pulmonary valve by the conal (infundibular) septum. Within the fibrous skeleton of the heart connecting these three valves lie the atrioventricular (AV) node and bundle of His (Fig. 49.1). Aortic valve disease may be stenosis or insufficiency. Severe calcification secondary to old age and rheumatic heart disease is an important cause of aortic stenosis. Aortic insufficiency has more varied etiologies; rheumatic disease is the most common and causes shortening of the valve cusps. Other causes include congenital bicuspid and unicuspid valves, annular ectasia from a chronic aortic aneurysm, and acute dissection. The normal area of the aortic valve is 2–3 cm². An area less than 0.8 cm² constitutes severe stenosis as does a gradient across the aortic valve of greater than 50 mmHg (Case 2). The classic symptoms of severe aortic stenosis are syncope, angina, and/or heart failure. Of these, angina is the most common and occurs in half of all patients requiring aortic valve replacement. All three symptoms are present in only about one-third of patients. The indications for surgery in aortic insufficiency are more complex. The ejection fraction taken while undergoing a stress test is the most important parameter. If a patient can increase the ejection fraction 40–50% with exercise, the valve probably does not need to be replaced. If the patient is unable to increase the ejection fraction with exercise, impending cardiac demise is imminent and valve replacement is indicated. Aortic insufficiency is a volume overload problem of the left ventricle rather than the pressure overload problem of aortic

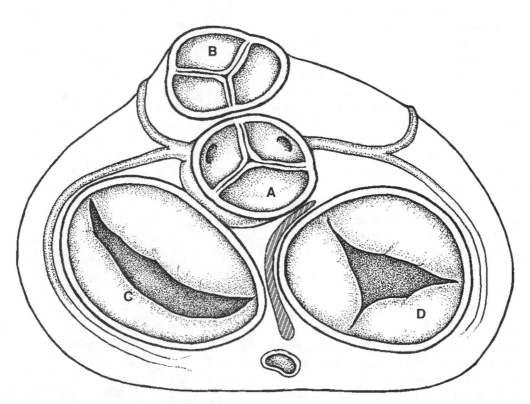

FIGURE 49.1 *A view from above the cardiac valves: aortic valve (A) pulmonic valve (B), mitral (bicuspid) valve (C), and tricuspid valve (D).*

stenosis. Aortic insufficiency progresses insidiously and, even with severe regurgitation, will not cause symptoms unless there is marked myocardial dysfunction. Once the patient develops myocardial dysfunction and worsening of the ejection fraction, aortic insufficiency has progressed to produce irreversible cardiac changes. There is a point where ejection fraction is so poor that aortic valve replacement is not feasible. On the contrary, when aortic stenosis is present, one should consider valve replacement even in patients with a severely depressed ejection fraction.

Mitral valve disease is also classified as either stenosis or regurgitation. Mitral stenosis leads to increased pulmonary vascular resistance due to spasm of the pulmonary arteries, as well as back pressure directly from the mitral valve through the left atrium and then to the pulmonary veins. Elevated pulmonary vascular resistance ultimately leads to right heart failure and tricuspid regurgitation (Case 1). Mitral regurgitation is due to a variety of causes including prolapse from myxomatous valve degeneration or localized idiopathic chordal rupture. Rheumatic heart disease is a common cause of mitral regurgitation. If a patient has combined mitral stenosis and mitral regurgitation, the cause is nearly always rheumatic. The chordae are typically shortened, thickened, fused, and sometimes so short that the papillary muscles actually appear to fuse with the valve leaflet. The normal mitral valve area is 4–6 cm². Symptoms typically begin when the area is less than 2 cm². The indication for operation for mitral stenosis is severe heart failure. Generally, in a patient who has a mitral valve area less than 1.5 cm², or a gradient across the mitral valve of greater than 15 mmHg, either commissurotomy or mitral valve replacement is desirable. Indications for surgery for mitral regurgitation are the same as that for aortic regurgitation. Like aortic insufficiency, mitral regurgitation is a condition of ventricular volume overload and surgery is required in the face of impending or established heart failure.

Part of the conceptual confusion with aortic aneurysms and aortic dissections arises from poor use of terminology. An aortic dissection is a tear in the intima resulting in a progressive separation within the walls of the media. This produces a sensation of a "tearing" or "ripping" pain in the back (Case 3). The borders of the separated media form the walls of the "false" lumen, which is distinct from the true lumen. The etiologies of aortic dissection are listed in Table 49.1. Marfan syndrome is the most common cause, although hypertension is also important. When hypertension is present, blood pressure reduction is the primary modality for both prevention and treatment.

Aortic dissection is an acute process, but if present for more than 1 month, it may be considered chronic. Aortic dissection can be classified as DeBakey types I, II, or III. Alternatively, the Stanford classification assigns dissections to groups A or B, depending on the region (Fig. 49.2). The Stanford classification is more useful, since it addresses in-

TABLE 49.1   *Etiologies of aortic diseasse*

Acute aortic dissection	Marfan syndrome
	Cystic medial necrosis
	Hypertension
Chronic aortic aneurysm	Atherosclerotic
	Chronic dissection
	Marfan syndrome
	Cystic medial necrosis
	Aortitis (syphilis or granuloma)
Aortic transection	Blunt deceleration

volvement of the ascending aorta, requires surgery because of the extremely high incidence of life-threatening complications such as occlusion of the orifices of the coronary arteries, severe aortic regurgitation, rupture with pericardial tamponade, and exsanguinating hemorrhage.

An aortic *aneurysm* is a chronic dilatation of the aorta to greater than 3 cm. Atherosclerosis is the most common etiology. A chronic dissection is appropriately called an aneurysm and is treated as such. Connective tissue degenerative disorders such as Marfan syndrome or cystic medial necrosis may cause aortic aneurysms as well as dissections. Syphilitic aortitis is an extremely rare cause of aortic aneurysm.

KEY POINTS

- Left anterior descending artery is of particular importance, since it provides many branches to left ventricle (with its high workload) and to interventricular septum

- Blood flow through coronary arteries to the myocardium occurs principally in diastole when heart is at rest

- Atherosclerosis is principal cause of myocardial ischemia (angina pectoris) and infarction

- When a lesion reduces the cross-sectional area by more than 75%, blood flow is limited—particularly during periods of increased demand

- Severe calcification secondary to old age and rheumatic heart disease is important cause of aortic stenosis

- Aortic insufficiency has more varied etiologies; rheumatic disease is the most comon and causes shortening of valve cusps

- An area less than 0.8 cm constitutes severe stenosis, as does a gradient across the aortic valve of greater than 50 mmHg

- The classic symptoms of severe aortic stenosis are syncope, angina, and/or heart failure; of these, angina is the most common and occurs in one-half of all patients requiring aortic valve replacement

- If a patient can increase the ejection fraction 40–50% with exercise, valve probably does not need to be replaced

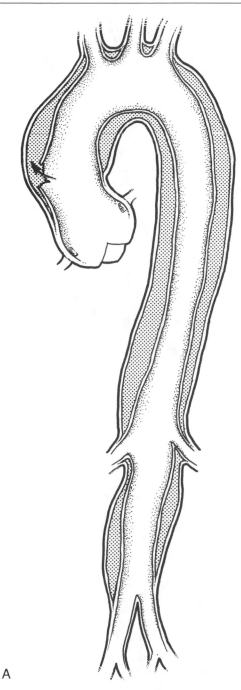

FIGURE 49.2 *The Stanford classification of aortic dissection depends on the origin of the dissection.* **(A)** *Type I dissection that begins in the ascending aortic arch and involves the entire thoracic aorta. (Figure continues.)*

• Rheumatic heart disease is common cause of mitral regurgitation

• Indication for operation for mitral stenosis is severe heart failure

• Indications for surgery for mitral regurgitation are same as that for aortic regurgitation; like aortic insufficiency, mitral re-

gurgitation is condition of ventricular volume overload and surgery is required in the face of impending or established heart failure

• An aortic dissection is a tear in the intima resulting in a progressive separation within the walls of the media; Marfan syndrome is most common cause, although hypertension is also important

• An aortic aneurysm is a chronic dilatation of the aorta to greater than 3 cm; atherosclerosis is most common etiology

DIAGNOSIS

The patient who presents with chest pain needs thorough evaluation. During the history, one should inquire specifically about the five cardiac risk factors: (1) smoking, (2) hypertension, (3) diabetes, (4) obesity, and (5) hypercholesterolemia. Physical examination should concentrate on the cardiopulmonary system with particular attention to murmurs or irregular rhythms. An electrocardiagram (ECG) and chest x-ray should be obtained. Laboratory evaluation includes the total CPK (creatine phosphokinase) and MB (myocardial band) fractions. Management may be initiated at this point with thrombolytic therapy such as urokinase or streptokinase if infarction is diagnosed. If the patient does not improve, coronary angiography should be performed. After resolution, an ECG stress test is obtained (the ECG is monitored as the patient undergoes a treadmill exercise). Any ST-segment depression of more than 1 mm is further evaluated with either coronary angiography or with a persantine-thallium test, which assesses myocardial perfusion. Thallium is taken up by perfused myocardium. When persantine (a vasodilator) is given, areas not previously perfused may now demonstrate activity. Because these areas received flow only after vasodilatation, they are at risk of subsequent episodes of ischemia. Areas that do not show uptake after persantine administration are not at risk and likely represent zones of prior infarction.

At cardiac catheterization and cine angiography, contrast is injected directly into the coronary artery orifices to image the coronary circulation in various projections. Ventriculography is also performed to evaluate left ventricular and mitral valve function (Case 2). An injection at the aortic root evaluates possible aortic insufficiency. A 50% luminal narrowing corresponds to a 75% cross-sectional area loss and puts the supplied myocardium at risk of (subsequent) infarction. Anything greater than a 50% narrowing is considered a hemodynamically significant lesion.

The diagnosis of aortic dissection starts with history, where a description of a ripping or "tearing" back pain should arouse suspicion (Case 3). Further diagnostic tests confirm the diagnosis, define the location of the intimal tear, prove whether the ascending aorta is dissected, and determine whether visceral vessels are supplied by the true

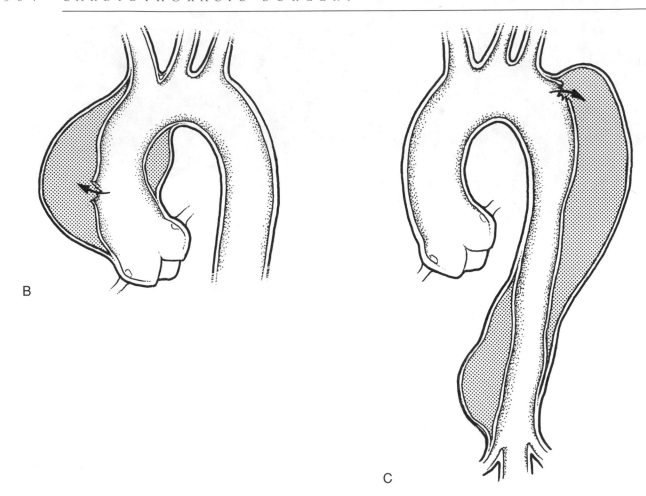

B

C

FIGURE 49.2   (Continued) **(B)** *Type II dissection that also begins in the ascending arch but stops before the origin of the great vessels.* **(C)** *Type III dissection (most common) that begins just distal to the origin of the left subclavin artery. The DeBakey classification is similar; type A dissections begin in the ascending aorta, while type B dissections begin distal to the left subclavian artery.*

or false lumens. The computed tomography (CT) scan will aid in the diagnosis and indicate whether the ascending aorta is involved. An angiogram is essential to ascertain the location of the intimal tear, which must be included in the resection. For aortic dissection involving the ascending aorta, cardiac echocardiography is important to investigate pericardial effusions or aortic insufficiency (Case 3). The CT scan, angiogram, and echocardiogram are useful for aortic aneurysms as well. Angiography is particularly important for thoracoabdominal aneurysms to determine the status of the abdominal visceral vessels and to identify the location of the spinal artery of Adamkiewicz, which usually lies between T10 and L2.

KEY   POINTS

• During the history, one should inquire specifically about five cardiac risk factors: smoking, hypertension, diabetes, obesity, and hypercholesterolemia

• A 50% luminal narrowing corresponds to a 75% cross-sectional area loss and puts the supplied myocardium at risk of infarction; anything greater than a 50% narrowing is considered hemodynamically significant

• CT scan will aid diagnosis and indicate whether ascending aorta involved

• Angiogram essential to ascertain location of intimal tear, which must be included in resection

DIFFERENTIAL DIAGNOSIS

The differential diagnosis of acute aortic dissection includes myocardial infarction, pneumothorax, and pulmonary embolus, which can be evaluated with ECG, CPK (including MB fractions), chest x-ray, and arterial blood gases. Ascending dissections may result in angina from coronary artery involvement, tamponade, or heart failure from severe aortic insufficiency. The differential diagnosis broadens with unusual presentations such as limb ischemia (Case 3) or visceral ischemia (including intestinal angina or renal failure). These occur when the orifice of a vessel, such as the superior mesenteric or common femoral artery, is sheared off by the dissection and no longer receives normal blood flow. Stroke occurs when the dissection involves the innominate or carotid arteries.

KEY POINTS

- Differential diagnosis of acute aortic dissection includes myocardial infarction, pneumothorax, and pulmonary embolus, which can be evaluated with ECG, CPK (including MB fractions), chest x-ray, and arterial blood gases

TREATMENT

The management of coronary artery disease consists of three primary modalities: pharmacologic, radiographic (angioplasty), and surgical.

Pharmacologic treatment consists of "triple therapy" including nitrates, β-blockers, and calcium channel blockers. Single- and double-vessel coronary artery disease is an indication for angioplasty. Unfortunately, up to 50% of lesions treated with percutaneous transluminal coronary angioplasty (PTCA) restenose within 6–12 months, although the procedure is initially successful in up to 90%. Emergency coronary artery bypass surgery after failed PTCA significantly increases the risk of operative death and perioperative myocardial infarction compared to elective coronary artery bypass graft (CABG) surgery. The risk of operative death and perioperative myocardial infarction after CABG without prior PTCA is between 1% and 6%. The mortality of coronary artery bypass surgery after failed PTCA increases to 5–10%, and the risk of perioperative myocardial infarction increases to 25%. The chance of failure of PTCA requiring emergency CABG is 5%. The most important factor in improving survival in patients undergoing a failed PTCA with ischemic changes is immediate coronary bypass surgery.

CABG has proven its efficacy in terms of improved patient survival and quality of life. The specific indications for CABG are (1) triple-vessel disease, particularly with a decreased ejection fraction (patients with reduced ejection fraction with coronary artery disease have a 5-year survival rate of about 75%; this increases to 90% in those undergoing CABG), (2) double-vessel coronary artery disease with a reduced ejection fraction, (3) angina refractory to triple-drug therapy, including nitrates, β-blockers, and calcium channel blockers regardless of angioplasty status, and (4) compelling anatomy, including left main coronary artery disease, in which the patients have a propensity for sudden death.

Patients who present in cardiogenic shock after acute myocardial infarction require intensive management (Case 1). If necessary, they should be intubated and mechanically ventilated. Intravenous access is established and blood obtained for enzyme and electrolyte analysis. Chest x-ray and ECG are performed. Pulmonary artery and Foley catheters should be placed, along with an arterial catheter. Pharmacologic management includes inotropes, afterload reducers, diuretics, nitrates, and calcium channel blockers. β-Blockers must be used cautiously. If shock persists, an intra-aortic balloon pump should be inserted. The balloon pump reduces the afterload against which the heart must work, thereby decreasing myocardial oxygen requirements. The decrease in afterload results in improved ejection fraction and decreased workload. Because the balloon inflates in diastole, coronary artery perfusion pressure is increased, thereby improving oxygen delivery to the myocardium. Angiography should be performed expeditiously to determine whether the patient is a candidate for surgery.

The treatment of patients with valvular heart disease differs depending on whether stenosis or regurgitation is present. The indications for surgery in aortic stenosis include syncope, angina, and heart failure. Patients with minimal heart failure may still require valve replacement if ventricular function worsens after a stress test, and if there are signs of impending cardiac failure such as an increase in the left ventricular end diastolic dimension or volume. It is important to treat these patients early before myocardial damage becomes irreversible.

For those with mitral valve stenosis, surgical treatment depends on anatomy. If the entire valve is diseased, valve excision and replacement is indicated. When mitral regurgitation is present, there is a greater role for mitral valve repair (valvuloplasty). Tricuspid valve stenosis is extremely rare, and when present, is usually rheumatic. Functional or organic tricuspid regurgitation is more common than tricuspid stenosis. Functional tricuspid disease results from annular dilatation as a result of elevated right ventricular pressure from mitral valve disease or left heart failure. Organic tricuspid regurgitation follows rheumatic fever or endocarditis. The tricuspid valve is the least common valve to be involved with rheumatic disease.

The prosthetic of choice to replace a diseased heart valve varies among patients and situations. The four basic valve replacements available are mechanical, bioprosthetic, homograft, and autograft. A mechanical valve should last for the life of the patient. A bioprosthetic valve is made from a bovine or porcine valve or from pericardial tissue, and deteriorates with time. The advantage of the bioprosthetic valve is that anticoagulation is not needed. But by 15 years, one-half of patients will require a replacement valve. The advantage of a mechanical valve is that it is permanent. The disadvantage is that patients receiving these valves require anticoagulation for the rest of their lives. Even with adequate anticoagulation, there is a 5% chance of thromboembolism within 5 years. There is also a 3% chance of developing an anticoagulation-related complication within 5 years as a result of hemorrhage from coumadin. Generally, patients less than 75 years old should undergo mechanical valve replacement. In younger people, exceptions may be made to this rule. For example, an athlete who engages in contact sports should not be anticoagulated because of the risk of hemorrhage.

Homografts come from human cadaver donors and consist of cryopreserved aorta or pulmonary artery with their corresponding valve. The advantage of a homograft is that it is more durable than bioprosthetic porcine or bovine tissue valves. The disadvantage is that these valves deteriorate with time. Alternatively, the patient's own pulmonary valve may be used to replace the diseased aortic valve. A pulmonary homograft conduit is then used to replace the donor pulmonary valve.

When there is organic tricuspid pathology, as with rheumatic disease or endocarditis, surgery of the tricuspid valve is indicated. Indications for operation on functional tricuspid regurgitation are less clear. Whether a replacement or repair of the tricuspid valve should be done depends on the status of the tricuspid valve itself. If there is organic disease involving the tricuspid valve, a replacement should be performed, usually with a bioprosthesis, although a mechanical valve may be placed. If the leaflets themselves are normal and the process is functional dilatation, an annuloplasty may be performed.

For acute thoracic aortic dissection, therapy is initially the same for both type A and B lesions. Pharmacologic management is immediately instituted for hypertension control. This includes afterload reduction and β-blockers to decrease the force of contraction and diminish the sheer stress on the aorta. Diagnostic studies are then performed. If the dissection involves the ascending aorta, urgent surgery is indicated. The type of operation must be tailored to the specific situation. For example, if the dissection is limited to the supracoronary aorta, a simple tube graft will suffice. If the dissection begins proximal to the aortic valve, a composite aortic valve replacement, ascending aortic replacement, and coronary reimplantation may be needed. If the dissection involves both ascending and descending aorta (DeBakey type III), then only that portion of the aorta involving the initial tear need be resected. The distal false lumen may be left but the proximal edge of this lumen is "tacked down" to exclude the distal dissection (Fig 49.2).

For dissections involving only the descending aorta, lifelong medical management is the mainstay of treatment. Major complications of acute type B dissection such as rupture or visceral or limb ischemia are indications for surgery, or refractory pain. For chronic aneurysms, surgery is generally indicated for dilatations greater than 6 cm. The risk of paraplegia and death must be weighed against the risk of surgery.

KEY POINTS

- Pharmacologic treatment consists of "triple therapy," including nitrates, β-blockers, and calcium channel blockers

- Most important factor in improving survival in patient undergoing failed PTCA with ischemic changes is immediate coronary bypass surgery

- Specific indications for CABG are (1) triple-vessel disease, (2) double-vessel coronary artery disease with reduced ejection fraction, (3) angina refractory to triple-drug therapy, including nitrates, and (4) compelling anatomy, including left main coronary artery disease

- Balloon pump reduces afterload against which heart must work, thereby decreasing myocardial oxygen requirements; decrease in afterload results in improved ejection fraction and decreased workload

- Indications for surgery in aortic stenosis include syncope, angina, and heart failure

- Bioprosthetic valve is made from a bovine or porcine valve or from pericardial tissue, and deteriorates with time; advantage of bioprosthetic valve is that anticoagulation not needed

FOLLOW-UP

Follow-up care after CABG requires evaluation of the patient's overall medical condition and cardiac function at periodic intervals (Case 1). The initial visits are predominantly for wound checks and to evaluate functional status. Later, it is important to assess dynamic changes using ECG, echocardiography, and chest x-ray as needed. If the pain recurs, one must consider the possibility of occlusion of a graft or development of new disease. Reinstitution of β-blockers, calcium channel blockers, and nitrates is indicated along with ECG stress testing and possibly coronary angiography. The ultrafast CT scan is a new modality that may be helpful in determining graft patency.

For patients who have had valve surgery, initial follow-up is needed to evaluate the surgical wound and determine that the level of anticoagulation with warfarin is within the therapeutic range. Anticoagulation should be evaluated once a week after discharge from the hospital and then at bimonthly intervals. Valve function is assessed by physical examination, echocardiography, and chest x-ray (Case 2).

Careful follow-up of patients with aneurysms and dissections is necessary to evaluate progression of their disease. In particular, patients with Marfan syndrome tend to develop progressive aortic involvement which may require further surgical intervention years after aortic surgery. CT scanning at 6-month intervals is reasonable as a noninvasive method for evaluating these conditions. The general vascular status of the patient as a whole should be routinely evaluated on each visit with at least a history and physical examination.

SUGGESTED READINGS

Odell JA, Orszulak TA: Surgical repair and reconstruction of valvular lesions. Curr Opinion Cardiol 10:135, 1995

This review discusses the indications and surgical management of valvular disease. It is an excellent historic and current review and is highly recommended as a general overview of valvular problems, particularly those related to the mitral valve.

Pashkow FJ: Diagnostic evaluation of the patient with coronary artery disease. Cleveland Clin J Med 61:43, 1994

This article reviews and compares the strengths and shortcomings of commonly employed noninvasive techniques for diagnosing coronary artery disease. It points out that the patient's history is still key in establishing a diagnosis and that other modalities play only a supportive role.

Patterson RE, Horowitz SF, Eisner RL: Comparison of modalities to diagnose coronary artery disease. Sem Nuclear Med 24:286, 1994

This up-to-date review compares several modalities available for the detection of coronary artery disease. Specifically, it contrasts the clinical history, rest and exercise electrocardiograms, rest and stress left ventricular function studies, myocardial perfusion imaging studies, and positron emission tomography.

Pragliola C, Kootstra GJ, Lanzillo G et al: Current results of coronary bypass surgery after failed angioplasty. J Cardiovasc Surg 35:365, 1994

PTCA is a technique in continuous development. Since its introduction, the indications for the number of lesions amenable and the outcome have changed dramatically. This study reviews the surgical results following failed PTCA. It provides a different view of the success rates of angioplasty than those you might hold.

Spittell PC, Spittell JA Jr, Joyce JW et al: Clinical features and differential diagnosis of aortic dissection: experience with 236 cases (1980 through 1990). Mayo Clin Proc 68:642, 1993

Acute aortic dissection is the most common fatal condition involving the aorta. Despite major advances in noninvasive diagnosis, the correct diagnosis is made in less than one-half the cases before the patients' demise. This study reviews a group of 235 patients in regard to their presentation, management, and outcome.

QUESTIONS

1. *Stenosis of a valve becomes hemodynamically significant when the cross-sectional area is reduced by?*
   - A. 25%.
   - B. 50%.
   - C. 75%.
   - D. 90%.

2. *The most common cause of aortic dissection is?*
   - A. Trauma.
   - B. Syphilis.
   - C. Atherosclerosis.
   - D. Marfan syndrome.

3. *Which of the following patients is the best candidate for percutaneous balloon angioplasty?*
   - A. A 60-year-old with minimal right main coronary artery stenosis.
   - B. A 70-year-old with triple-vessel disease and decreased cardiac output.
   - C. A 55-year-old with short segment stenosis in two vessels and normal ejection fraction.
   - D. A 60-year-old with angina refractory to medical management.

4. *Which of the following is a major disadvantage of tissue valves?*
   - A. Require lifelong anticoagulation.
   - B. Have limited life and require replacement.
   - C. Are not available for aortic and miral replacement.
   - D. Are common locations of vegetations and require replacement.

(See p. 604 for answers.)

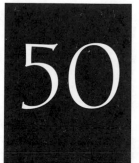

50 MEDIASTINAL MASSES

FRITZ BAUMGARTNER

Mediastinal masses present in a variety of ways and may, at times, be confused with other diseases such as lung cancer or tuberculosis. Care must be taken to avoid pitfalls in the diagnostic and therapeutic algorithms of these patients. The goals of the chapter are to (1) develop the ability to design a strategy for diagnosing mediastinal masses, (2) understand current roles of surgical management, and (3) explain the importance of radiotherapy and chemotherapy.

CASE 1
DOUBLE VISION AND MUSCLE WEAKNESS

A 30-year-old actress noted progressive double vision and muscle weakness over the past 3 months. She stated that her eyelids had begun to droop more and more lately.

Physical examination found bilateral ptosis and diplopia as well as proximal muscle girdle weakness in the upper extremities. The rest of her examination was unremarkable. Her chest x-ray showed a mediastinal mass that appeared to be anterior to the upper portion of the pericardium and ascending aorta. A CT scan demonstrated a 5-cm thymic mass that did not appear to be invading adjacent structures. A Tensilon test was performed, to which she responded dramatically and was therefore started on a course of physostigmine and steroids. A total thymectomy was performed under general anesthesia without muscle relaxants. The mediastinal mass was solid and did not invade surrounding structures. An intraoperative frozen section proved to be thymoma with clear margins. Postoperatively, she was

extubated uneventfully. Her symptoms were completely alleviated within 3 days.

CASE 2
FEVER, CHILLS, AND SWEATS

A 25-year-old nurse presented with a 1-month history of low grade fevers to 38°C, chills, and night sweats that completely soaked her bed. She lost 5 lb over the last month, but denied tuberculosis exposure, recent travel, or pregnancy.

Chest x-ray showed a middle mediastinal mass that appeared to be in the region of the carina without invasion or compression of any adjacent structures. It was irregular, measuring approximately 8 cm in diameter on CT scan. There were no other pulmonary or mediastinal lesions. She underwent mediastinoscopy and biopsy. A frozen section revealed Hodgkin's lymphoma. A CT scan of the abdomen demonstrated no intra-abdominal masses or adenopathy. A course of radiotherapy, without systemic chemotherapy, was begun with excellent symptomatic response. She has undergone routine follow-up every 3 months with a chest x-ray and biannual CT scans, and remains asymptomatic.

GENERAL CONSIDERATIONS

The mediastinum can be classified into three major anatomic regions (Fig. 50.1). The superior mediastinum lies above the plane extending from the sternal angle of Louis to the level of T4. The mediastinum, inferior to this, is divided into the anterior mediastinum, which is in front of the anterior pericardium; the middle mediastinum, which is the space between the anterior pericardium posteriorly to the anterior portion of the vertebral body; and the posterior mediastinum, which is between the anterior and posterior portions of the vertebral body and includes the region of the paravertebral gutters. In many classification systems, the superior mediastinum is considered to be a separate entity. Particular types of tumors have a propensity to be located within certain mediastinal regions.

The most common tumor of the anterior mediastinum is the thymoma. Thymomas are usually benign but may be malignant with the differentiation based on actual invasion, either radiographically or at operation. A malignant thymoma appears identical to a benign thymoma histologically. Thymomas may produce vague symptoms including shortness of breath, cough, or chest pain. They are usually not associated with systemic symptoms such as fevers, chills, or sweats. This is a very important differentiation from lymphomas, which frequently produce systemic symptoms.

Thymomas have a peculiar relationship to myasthenia gravis, a neuromuscular condition resulting from autoimmune antibodies directed against the acetylcholine receptor. Ninety percent of patients with myasthenia have adult onset disease, which affects women twice as often as men. Ten percent of patients with myasthenia gravis have thymomas; conversely, one-third to one-half of patients with thymomas have myasthenia gravis. Thymectomy in the presence or absence of thymoma may be effective in the treatment of myasthenia gravis. Approximately one-third of patients with myasthenia are cured by thymectomy. Patients with a normal thymus who undergo thymectomy for myasthenia gravis need less medication than those patients with myasthenia gravis who have a thymoma resected (Case 1).

Germ cell tumors present as anterior mediastinal masses and may be either benign or malignant. The benign germ cell tumors include benign teratomas and dermoid cysts. The malignant germ cell tumors are much more rare and may be of the seminomatous or nonseminomatous type. Those who have seminomatous mediastinal tumors must undergo careful testicular examination, including ultrasound, if physical examination is unrevealing. Seminomatous tumors have low (β-human chorionic gonadotropin (β-hCG) and α-fetoprotein levels (AFP), unlike their nonseminomatous counterparts. Nonseminomatous malignant germ cell tumors include embryonal carcinoma, malignant teratoma, choriocarcinoma, and endodermal sinus tumor (yolk sac tumor). These tumors generally produce β-hCG and α-fetoprotein.

Lymphomas may be of the Hodgkin's or non-Hodgkin's variety. A history of systemic symptoms including fever, chills, and sweats is frequently associated with lymphomas and occurs far more frequently than in patients with thymoma or germ cell tumors. Lymphomas may involve both the anterior and middle mediastinum.

Middle mediastinal tumors include lymphoma, pericardial cyst, bronchogenic cysts, and mediastinal granuloma. Pericardial cysts are generally well-tolerated, benign lesions. Bronchogenic cysts originate from the primary bronchi and require resection to prevent recurrent infection. Mediastinal granulomas may, on occasion, actually erode into the tracheobronchial tree, which leads to broncholithiasis. Lesions that may result in such intense granuloma formation include histoplasmosis, coccidioidomycosis, and tuberculosis.

Posterior mediastinal lesions are primarily tumors of neurogenic origin. The most common of these is the neurilemmoma, which is the benign counterpart of the malignant schwannoma. In children, the most common neurogenic tumor is the malignant neuroblastoma. Histologic classification is predominantly that of nerve sheath tumors and ganglionic/paraganglionic tumors. The autonomic tumors are the benign ganglioneuroma and its malignant counterparts, the ganglioneuroblastoma and the neuroblastoma. Pheochromocytomas of the posterior mediastinum are also autonomic tumors, 90% of which are benign.

KEY POINTS

- Most common tumor of anterior mediastinum is thymoma
- Thymomas have peculiar relationship to myasthenia gravis
- 90% of patients with myasthenia have adult onset disease, which affects women twice as often as men
- 10% of patients with myasthenia gravis have thymomas; conversely, one-third to one-half of patients with thymomas have myasthenia gravis
- Appoximately one-third of patients with myasthenia are cured by thymectomy
- Patients with normal thymus who undergo thymectomy for myasthenia gravis need less medication than those patients with myasthenia gravis who have thymoma resected (Case 1)
- Seminomatous tumors have low β-hCG and AFP levels, unlike nonseminomatous tumors
- Posterior mediastinal lesions are primarily tumors of neurogenic origin; most common is neurilemmoma, benign counterpart of malignant schwannoma

DIAGNOSIS

A history of fevers, chills, and night sweats makes lymphoma more likely than other types of mediastinal tumors. A history of muscle weakness, ptosis, diplopia, or known diagnosis of myasthenia gravis is important in eval-

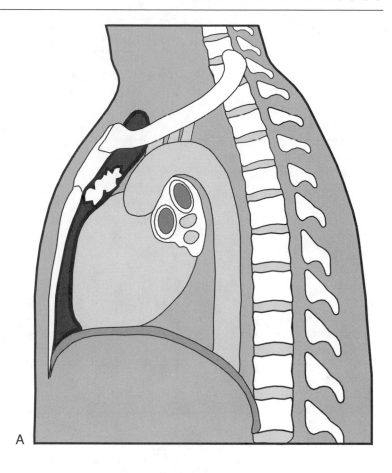

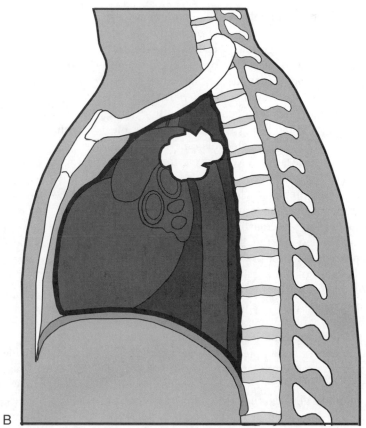

FIGURE 50.1 *Location and types of mediastinal masses. (**A**) Anterior mediastinum: thymoma, teratoma or other germ cell tumors, lymphoma, thyroid masses. (**B**) Middle mediastinum: pericardial cysts, lymphoma, bronchogenic cyst, lymphadenopathy.* (Figure continues.)

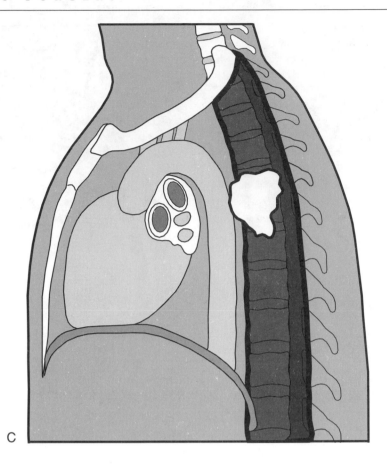

FIGURE 50.1 (Continued) *(C) Posterior mediastinum: tumors of neurogenic origin, aneurysms, hiatal hernia.*

C

uating the possibility of thymoma. Palpitations, sweats, tachycardia, and nervousness may be present in a retrosternal Graves (thyroid) goiter. A history of extensive smoking may lead one to suspect a bronchogenic carcinoma as the etiologic factor for a mediastinal mass.

A systematic physical examination is performed including careful evaluation of adenopathy. Laboratory studies should include AFP and β-hCG levels for anterior mediastinal tumors, as well as catecholamine levels and urinary vanillylmandelic acid (VMA) levels for posterior mediastinal tumors.

There are four approaches for tissue assessment of mediastinal tumors: percutaneous needle aspiration, mediastinoscopy, anterior mediastinotomy (Chamberlain's procedure), and video-assisted thoracoscopic biopsy. In general, needle aspiration of presumed thymomas is contraindicated because of the possibility of seeding the mediastinum or pleura with tumor cells. Cervical mediastinoscopy is excellent for evaluating adenopathy in the middle mediastinum; however, it does have anatomic limitations. Since the mediastinoscope is inserted anterior to the trachea, it can only sample paratracheal or carinal nodes in a plane immediately anterior to the trachea. It cannot sample the anterior mediastinum or the posterior subcarinal region. In general, the aortopulmonary window is also inaccessible. An anterior mediastinotomy will provide access to the anterior mediastinum and to the aor-

topulmonary window region. It is performed as a 2nd intercostal space minithoracotomy. All mediastinal tumors require investigation by CT scan for evaluation of the lesion itself, and to determine whether there is invasion of surrounding structures. A mediastinal tumor suspected of having a vascular component should be investigated with angiography. This is particularly useful for posterior mediastinal neurogenic tumors.

KEY POINTS

- Needle aspiration of presumed thymomas contraindicated because of possibility of seeding the mediastinum or pleura with tumor cells
- All mediastinal tumors require investigation by CT scan for evaluation of lesion itself and to determine whether surrounding structures invaded

DIFFERENTIAL DIAGNOSIS

Tuberculosis is the great imitator in the thoracic cavity, analogous to appendicitis in the abdomen. Tuberculosis, after having been in the background for decades in the United States, is exhibiting a new resurgence from the increasing number of immunosuppressed patients and alien population. Tuberculosis may, on occasion, infect isolated mediastinal structures, which would initially lead one to suspect a mediastinal tumor. Figure 50.2 shows the chest CT scan of a young student nurse with a large anterior mediastinal mass and no other pulmonary or mediastinal process. The immediate suspicion anatomically was thymoma. The mass was shown ultimately to be an isolated infection of the thymus with *Mycobacterium tuberculosis*. Tuberculosis can result in mediastinal granulomas as well.

Bronchogenic lung carcinoma, which invades the mediastinum, is a mediastinal mass, although it is not usually considered in the classification scheme. Small cell carcinoma may present with massive transmediastinal invasion from direct involvement of the mediastinal lymph nodes. Surgical intervention in these cases is limited to biopsy.

TREATMENT

The treatment for thymomas is resection. Preoperative evaluation with a CT scan can frequently identify gross invasion. For massive thymomas with surrounding invasion, preoperative radiotherapy to reduce the tumor mass is followed by resection. At operation, lack of an enveloping capsule or local invasion of adjacent tissues, including pericardium and pleura, great vessels, or phrenic nerve, indicates malignancy. If the tumor appears invasive, radical excision may be warranted. The phrenic nerves must be identified. Generally, if the patient does not have myasthenia gravis, sacrifice of one of the phrenic nerves is acceptable. If the patient does have myasthenia gravis, resection of one phrenic nerve is controversial. If the nerve appears to be invaded, it may not function, and its sacrifice may be warranted. Removal of invaded pericardium may be performed as well as removal of mediastinal pleura

and wedge excisions of invaded portions of lung. The most important aspect of thymectomy is complete removal of the thymus.

Myasthenic patients are not at significant risk of anesthesia, although no muscle relaxant should be used during the procedure (Case 1). For patients with severe myasthenia gravis, several options for treatment exist besides medication. Preoperative plasmapheresis may be a useful adjunct to reduce circulating levels of acetylcholine receptor antibodies. Thymectomy for patients with myasthenia gravis who have no evidence of thymoma should be performed if the patient is refractory to medical management. The chance of regression of myasthenia gravis is greatest in patients without thymoma.

The management of seminomatous germ cell tumors, when small and localized, is surgical resection followed by irradiation. This results in a nearly 100% cure rate; 60% of these lesions are cured with radiotherapy alone. If distant metastases are present, chemotherapy should be utilized with radiation to the primary lesion. For locally advanced disease without metastases, the treatment is controversial but should probably involve radiotherapy and chemotherapy rather than operation. For the nonseminomatous malignant germ cell tumors, the management is initially chemotherapy. If there is a response, as determined by a decrease in the β-hCG and AFP levels, resection is indicated. If, however, there is no decrease in these tumor markers with chemotherapy, a relatively aggressive tumor is present and resection is not indicated. The role of adjuvant radiotherapy is controversial.

Lymphoma is generally treated with radiotherapy and/or chemotherapy. Operation is limited to obtaining a diagnosis. If a lymphoma is suspected based on history, a much smaller diagnostic incision can be made to biopsy the

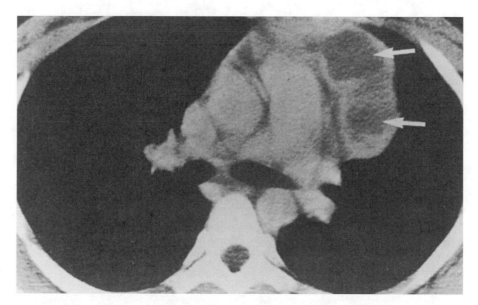

FIGURE 50.2 *CT scan of tuberculosis of the thymus gland mimicking a thymoma.*

lesion rather than a full median sternotomy. Thyroid lesions growing down into the mediastinum (Graves disease) usually require preoperative management to reduce the vascularity of the thyroid gland and reduce the production of thyroid hormone. The thyroid can usually be removed by a cervical approach, although on occasion, a median sternotomy may be necessary for massive tumors. Patients with bronchial cysts require surgical resection to prevent recurrent infection. A pericardial cyst usually needs no treatment beyond biopsy for identification. If the tumor has a classic appearance on CT scan, biopsy may not be necessary. Mediastinal granulomas do not need treatment unless they are actually eroding into the tracheobronchial tree, as is the case with broncholithiasis. Thoracotomy is required to remove the broncholith. Neurogenic tumors in the posterior mediastinum require a posterolateral thoracotomy.

KEY POINTS

- Treatment for thymomas is resection

- Preoperative plasmapheresis may be useful adjunct to reduce circulating levels of acetylcholine receptor antibodies

- Management of seminomatous germ cell tumors, when small and localized, is surgical resection followed by irradiation; this results in nearly 100% cure rate; 60% of these lesions are cured with radiotherapy alone

- Lymphoma is generally treated with radiotherapy and/or chemotherapy; operation limited to obtaining a diagnosis

---

FOLLOW-UP

Effective follow-up requires routine physical examination, radiographic evaluation, and biochemical studies if indicated (i.e., β-HCG and AFP). For presumed cures after resection of thymoma, a yearly chest x-ray and CT scan are acceptable. For benign lesions of the middle and posterior mediastinum, yearly chest x-ray alone is performed. Long-term follow-up of lymphomas or germ cell tumors treated by adjuvant therapy requires more frequent physical examination and radiographic evaluation every 1–3 months.

SUGGESTED READINGS

Blossom GB, Ernstoff RM, Howells GA et al: Thymectomy for myasthenia gravis. Arch Surg 128:855, 1993

This manuscript discusses the changes and the clinical status of patients with generalized myasthenia gravis who were treated with thymectomy. Retrospectively, it reviews 37 patients refractory to medical treatment.

Grover FL: The role of CT and MRI in staging of the mediastinum. Chest 106:391S, 1994

This article describes the roles of computed tomography and magnetic resonance imaging in the diagnostic evaluation of patients with tumors of the mediastinum. It contains a number of useful references.

Knapp RH, Hurt RD, Payne WS et al: Malignant germ cell tumors of the mediastinum. J Thoracic Cardiovasc Surg 89:82, 1985

This article reviews several of the malignant germ cell tumors of the mediastinum. Although this article is somewhat old, it is one of the best references available on the topic.

Morrissey B, Adams H, Gibbs AR et al: Percutaneous needle biopsy of the mediastinum: review of the 94 procedures. Thorax 48:632, 1993

This paper is a retrospective review of radiology-guided mediastinal biopsies over a 10-year period. It discusses the methods used in 75 patients to obtain tissue for pathologic diagnosis.

QUESTIONS

1. The most common tumor of the anterior mediastinium is a?

    A. Thymoma.
    B. Neurogenic tumor.
    C. Lymphoma.
    D. Malignant germ cell tumor.

2. Biochemical markers are useful in the diagnosis and postoperation follow-up of which of the following?

    A. Hodgkin's lymphoma.
    B. Germ cell tumors.
    C. Bronchogenic cyst.
    D. Pericardial cyst.

3. The best initial diagnostic modality for virtually all mediastinal tumors is?

    A. Mediastinoscopy.
    B. CT scanning.
    C. Lateral sternotomy.
    D. Thoracoscopy.

4. Myasthenia gravis has the best prognosis in?

    A. Patients with thymoma.
    B. Patients without thymoma.
    C. Those with absent β-hCG levels.
    D. Those who have not had prior neck irradiation.

(See p. 604 for answers.)

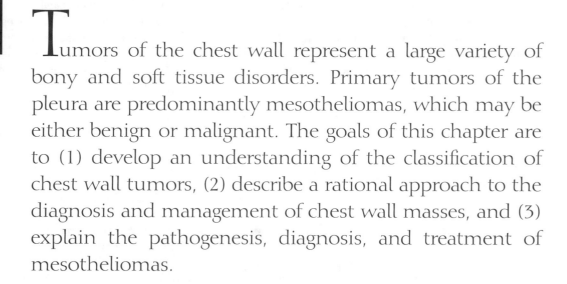

51 TUMORS OF THE CHEST WALL AND PLEURA

FRITZ BAUMGARTNER

Tumors of the chest wall represent a large variety of bony and soft tissue disorders. Primary tumors of the pleura are predominantly mesotheliomas, which may be either benign or malignant. The goals of this chapter are to (1) develop an understanding of the classification of chest wall tumors, (2) describe a rational approach to the diagnosis and management of chest wall masses, and (3) explain the pathogenesis, diagnosis, and treatment of mesotheliomas.

CASE 1
CHEST MASS

A 55-year-old male presented with a 5-year history of a slowly growing painless mass on the left chest wall. He had no other medical problems, was a nonsmoker, and had no history of radiotherapy, tuberculosis, or fungal or parasitic disease. On examination, there was an 8-cm firm chest wall mass located in the left midaxillary line at the 6th intercostal space, which was fixed, nonpulsatile, and nontender. There was no soft tissue erosion, erythema, or drainage. His laboratory evaluation was unremarkable. Chest x-ray demonstrated only a soft tissue density with no evidence of bony erosion. He had no other significant physical findings such as adenopathy or other soft tissue lesions.

Because the lesion was too large for simple excision, he underwent an incisional biopsy. The lesion was deep within the soft tissue and extended to the chest wall and the intercostal muscles. Frozen section demonstrated malignant fibrous histiocytoma. One week later he underwent chest wall resection, which included the tumor and a 5-cm margin on all sides. Frozen section found the margins clear without evidence of tumor. Chest wall reconstruction was performed using a prosthetic mesh. The patient has done well postoperatively, with serial CT scans over 6 months showing no evidence of recurrence. No adjuvant therapy was recommended.

CASE 2
MESOTHELIOMA

A 62-year-old male complained of sharp right lower chest pain and cough. He had a history of smoking in the past. Twenty years ago he had asbestos exposure while working in an insulation factory.

Physical examination found no evidence of clubbing. Breath sounds were diminished on the right. A chest x-ray demonstrated a density in the right lateral chest adjacent to the lung and pleural surface. A CT scan revealed a

10-cm pleural-based mass abutting against the lung. A pleural effusion was present.

A needle aspiration of the pleural effusion gave no cytologic diagnosis. An attempted needle biopsy of the mass was also nondiagnostic. Thoracoscopy with biopsy showed a mixed cell type malignant mesothelioma. Management options were discussed. He opted to have no therapy and expired 11 months later.

GENERAL CONSIDERATIONS

Neoplasms of the chest wall are either of bony or soft tissue origin and may be either benign or malignant. They may be either primary or metastatic and may invade the chest wall from lung, pleura, mediastinum, or breast. Benign tumors of the chest wall are rib and soft tissue tumors. The benign rib tumors include osteochondroma, chondroma, fibrous dysplasia, and histiocytosis X. Osteochondroma is the most common benign bone neoplasm. The neoplasm usually begins in childhood and continues to grow until skeletal maturity.

Chondromas constitute 15% of benign neoplasms of the rib cage. The differentiation between chondroma and chondrosarcoma is impossible on clinical and radiographic findings. Microscopically, the benign chondroma and low grade malignant chondrosarcoma may look identical. Therefore, all chondromas must be considered malignant and should be treated by wide excision. Although this approach appears excessive, the risk is negligible and may be lifesaving.

Fibrous dysplasia commonly presents as a solitary lesion. When multiple lesions are present, it is usually a part of Albright syndrome (multiple bone cysts, skin pigmentation, and precocious sexual maturity in girls) and is associated with polyostotic fibrous dysplasia.

Histiocytosis X is a disease involving the reticuloendothelial system and includes eosinophilic granuloma, Letterer-Siwe disease, and Hand-Schuller-Christian disease. Benign soft tissue chest tumors include fibromas, lipomas, neurogenic tumors, hemangiomas, and desmoid tumors.

Malignant rib tumors include multiple myeloma, osteosarcoma, chondrosarcoma, and Ewing's sarcoma. Ewing's sarcoma has a characteristic "onion skin" appearance radiographically, which is caused by elevation of the periosteum with subperiosteal new bone formation in multiple layers. Early spread to the lungs and other bones is common and occurs in about one-half of patients. Multiple myeloma is the most common primary malignant rib neoplasm, accounting for one-third of all malignant rib tumors, with chondrosarcoma being a close second. Myelomas involving the chest wall usually occur as a manifestation of systemic multiple myeloma. Solitary myeloma involving the ribs is second only to solitary vertebral involvement. Multiple myeloma is rare under the age of 30. Most patients have abnormal serum electrophoresis, and one-half have hypercalcemia and Bence-Jones protein in the urine. Chondrosarcomas usually arise in the costochondral junction or in the sternum. They are relatively uncommon under the age of 20, and most commonly appear as a slowly growing mass that has been painful for several months. All tumors arising in the costal cartilages should be considered malignant. The etiology of chondrosarcoma is unknown but may include malignant degeneration of chondromas and is known to be associated with trauma. The diagnosis of chondrosarcoma can only be made pathologically, but even this is difficult because most are well differentiated.

Osteosarcoma is more malignant than chondrosarcoma and has a less favorable prognosis. It usually occurs in adolescents and young adults who present with rapidly enlarging, painful tumors. Alkaline phosphatase levels are frequently elevated. Calcification occurs at a right angle to the cortex, producing a "sunburst" appearance on chest x-ray.

The most common malignant soft tissue tumor is the malignant fibrohistiocytoma. The tumor characteristically occurs in patients over age 50 and is rare in children. It usually presents as a painless, slowly growing mass (Case 1). It may be more common after chest wall irradiation, and spreads widely along fascial planes or into muscle, which explains the high recurrence rate after resection. Rhabdomyosarcoma is the second most common chest wall soft tissue malignancy. Wide resection followed by radiotherapy and chemotherapy results in a 5-year survival of about 70%. Liposarcoma and leiomyosarcoma are uncommon soft tissue tumors.

Mesothelioma is a primary tumor of the pleura. This is unusual since most pleural tumors are metastatic from other sites such as the breast or lung. The few primary tumors that do arise from the pleura are usually malignant. There is a strong causal relationship between asbestos exposure and mesothelioma. Nonetheless, only 7% of people exposed to asbestos actually develop mesothelioma. Conversely, 50% of patients with mesothelioma have a history of exposure to asbestos. There is characteristically a long latent period between exposure and development of the tumor. The increased risk occurs 20 years after the first exposure and continues to increase for many years thereafter.

The two histologic types of mesothelioma are localized and diffuse. Diffuse mesotheliomas are nearly always malignant, while 30% of localized mesotheliomas are malignant and 70% are benign. Benign pleural mesotheliomas usually arise from the visceral pleura on a stalk and project into the pleural space, although sessile attachment to the pleura may also occur. The tumor may also arise from the parietal pleura. Patients with localized malignant lesions usually have symptoms, while those with localized benign lesions usually do not. Symptoms include cough, pain, fever, and shortness of breath. Mesotheliomas may produce a bloody pleural effusion. A complete resection of the lesion may still be possible even if it is associated with a bloody effusion. This is an important differentiation between a mesothelioma and an intrathoracic lung neoplasm associated with a bloody pleural effusion. Solitary mesotheliomas are usually asymptomatic. Benign localized mesothelioma is also accompanied by hypertrophic pulmonary osteoarthropathy and severe hypoglycemia. Hypertrophic pulmonary osteoarthropathy occurs in about one-half of patients with mesothelioma, compared with 5% of those with bronchogenic carcinoma. Clubbing of the fingers and toes may also occur with mesothelioma and is distinct from hypertrophic pulmonary osteoarthropathy. Clubbing results from periosteal new growth and lymphocytic infiltration of the nail beds. In diffuse malignant mesothelioma, any portion of the pleura may be involved. It typically appears as sheets of tumor. Hematogenous spread to distant organs occurs in about one-half of patients. Symptoms of diffuse malignant mesothelioma include dyspnea, weight loss, cough, and severe pain. A pleural effusion is present in most cases.

KEY POINTS

- Neoplasms of the chest wall are either of bony or soft tissue origin, and may be either benign or malignant

- Benign rib tumors include osteochondroma, chondroma, fibrous dysplasia, and histiocytosis X; osteochondroma is most common

- Chondromas constitute 15% of benign neoplasms of the rib cage

- Differentiation between chondroma and chondrosarcoma is impossible on clinical and radiographic findings; therefore, all chondromas must be considered malignant and should be treated by wide excision

- Malignant rib tumors include multiple myeloma, osteosarcoma, chondrosarcoma, and Ewing's sarcoma

- Multiple myeloma most common primary malignant rib neoplasm, accounting for one-third of all malignant rib tumors, with chondrosarcoma being a close second

- All tumors arising in the costal cartilages should be considered malignant

- Osteosarcoma more malignant than chondrosarcoma, with a less favorable prognosis; usually occurs in adolescents and young adults who present with rapidly enlarging, painful tumors

- Most common malignant soft tissue tumor is malignant fibrohistiocytoma; usually presents as painless, slowly growing mass

- 50% of patients with mesothelioma have history of exposure to asbestos

- Diffuse mesotheliomas are nearly always malignant, while 30% of localized mesotheliomas are malignant and 70% are benign

- Complete resection of lesion may still be possible even if associated with bloody effusion; this is an important differentiation between mesothelioma and intrathoracic lung neoplasm associated with bloody pleural effusion

- Symptoms of diffuse malignant mesothelioma include dyspnea, weight loss, cough, and severe pain; pleural effusion present in most cases

DIAGNOSIS

The diagnosis of suspected chest wall tumors includes a careful history and physical examination followed by a plain chest x-ray and a thoracic computed tomography (CT) scan. The x-ray pattern of specific tumors such as Ewing's sarcoma and osteosarcoma aids in the diagnosis. Tumors suspected of being a primary neoplasm should ideally be diagnosed by excisional rather than by incisional biopsy. However, if the lesion is too large (Case 1), an incisional biopsy can be performed. If there is a history of a primary neoplasm elsewhere on the chest wall, the observed lesion may be a metastasis, and a needle or incisional biopsy is particularly useful.

Several factors in the history and physical examination point to mesothelioma, such as asbestos exposure. Clubbing of the fingers may be an associated finding. A CT scan of the chest may lead one to suspect a pleural-based lesion. The diagnosis is confirmed with thoracentesis of the pleural effusion. If thoracentesis fails to establish the diagnosis, aspiration of the mass and pleural biopsy may be necessary (Case 2).

KEY POINTS

- Tumors suspected of being primary neoplasm should ideally be diagnosed by excisional rather than by incisional biopsy

DIFFERENTIAL DIAGNOSIS

The differential diagnosis of a chest wall mass includes infectious etiologies, benign or malignant neoplasms, and hematomas (either spontaneous or traumatic). Infectious disorders include tuberculosis or unusual fungal organisms such as actinomycosis or nocardiosis. Intramuscular abscess cavities may present as a chest wall mass but are usually more tender than the typical chest wall tumor. Needle aspiration, culture, and appropriate skin tests support the diagnosis of an infectious etiology. Pseudoaneurysms of major vascular structures may rarely present as a chest wall mass. The presence of a pulsatile mass in the clavicular area should lead one to suspect a subclavian artery pseudoaneurysm, which typically follows penetrating injury. Angiography confirms the diagnosis.

The differential diagnosis of pleural-based lesions includes tumors of primary or metastatic etiology, or an infectious processes. Suspicion of a metastatic pleural lesion is based on history and physical examination. If these are noncontributory, it is unlikely that the lesion is a metastasis. Besides the primary pleural mesothelioma, other primary pleural tumors include a fibrosarcoma or liposarcoma. Tuberculosis or fungal infections may present with pleural aberrations and effusions. The diagnosis of these is also achieved by aspiration of the effusion, biopsy, or open thoracotomy if necessary.

KEY POINTS

- Needle aspiration, culture, and appropriate skin tests support diagnosis of infectious etiology

---

TREATMENT

After the diagnosis of a primary chest wall neoplasm is made, the objective of surgical intervention is wide excision. Combinations of adjuvant chemotherapy and radiotherapy have not been fully evaluated. Malignant fibrohistiocytoma, however, is unresponsive to radiotherapy and chemotherapy and should be widely resected. Generally, to prevent recurrence, the resection should include a 4-cm margin of normal tissue on all sides. The 5-year survival of malignant fibrous histiocytoma is approximately 40%. For rhabdomyosarcoma, the treatment is wide resection followed by radiotherapy and chemotherapy, resulting in a 5-year survival of about 70%. Chondromas should be treated as chondrosarcomas, since microscopically chondromas and low grade chondrosarcomas look identical. All chondromas should be considered malignant and treated by wide resection, which may be lifesaving. This results in cure in nearly all patients with a 10-year survival of 97%. For histiocytoma X, radiotherapy, chemotherapy, and systemic steroids are generally utilized. Ewing's sarcomas are radiosensitive, so the treatment of choice is radiotherapy. The 5-year survival is 50%.

The treatment of osteosarcoma includes wide resection of the tumor including the entire bone, rib, sternum, and adjacent soft tissue. The role of radiotherapy and chemotherapy is controversial and has been used effectively in adjuvant protocols. The prognosis is generally poor, with 5-year survival rates of 20%. Surgical intervention includes resection of the involved bone as well as resection of a 4-cm margin of normal tissue on all sides, which usually involves excising the upper and lower ribs. For tumors of the sternum and manubrium, excision of the entire involved bone and corresponding costal arches bilaterally is indicated. Metastases do not require further surgical treatment. Generally, radiation is performed for these metastatic lesions. Desmoid tumors tend to recur if inadequately excised, and

therefore should be treated with wide resection similar to primary malignant chest wall tumors.

The treatment of localized benign mesothelioma is resection. Results are generally good. The localized malignant variety is treated with wide local excision, including adjacent chest wall if arising from parietal pleura. The treatment of diffuse mesothelioma is nearly always only palliative (Case 2). Radiotherapy and chemotherapy have been inconsistent in achieving this goal. Operation for this disease is controversial. Seeding is frequent, and the tumor may actually grow out of a thoracotomy incision. Even after a radical procedure, the 2-year survival is poor and the 5-year survival is dismal.

KEY POINTS

- After diagnosis of primary chest wall neoplasm, objective of surgical intervention is wide excision

- Chondromas should be treated as chondrosarcomas, since microscopically chondromas and low grade chondrosarcomas look identical

- All chondromas should be considered malignant and treated by wide resection, which may be lifesaving

---

FOLLOW-UP

Patients with chest wall tumors who have undergone resection should be followed at 3–6-month intervals with appropriate chest x-rays and/or CT scans, yearly or biannually. The management of benign localized mesotheliomas that have been resected should be followed in a similar fashion. The management of patients with diffuse malignant mesothelioma should be compassionate, palliative measures with chemotherapy and/or radiotherapy, which may be helpful in the protocol setting.

SUGGESTED READINGS

Qua JC, Rao UN, Takita H: Malignant pleural mesothelioma: a clinicopathological study. J Surg Oncol 54:47, 1993

This paper retrospectively reviews 58 patients with malignant pleura mesotheliomas treated at one institution. Most were males who averaged 56 years at presentation. Asbestos exposure was noted in 43%. The study describes diagnosis, treatment, and outcome. This paper presents one of the large series from a single institution on plural mesothelioma.

Ryan MB, McMurtrey MJ, Roth JA: Current management of chest-wall tumors. Surg Clin North Am 69:1061, 1989

This article is an excellent review on the treatment of chest wall tumors. Although a few years old, it discusses the etiology and pathophysiology of several types of chest wall neoplasms.

Schaefer PS, Burton BS: Radiographic evaluation of chest-wall lesions. Surg Clin North Am 69:911, 1989

This article discusses the radiographic evaluation of patients with chest wall lesions and is a good companion to the article by Ryan et al.

QUESTIONS

1. The most common malignant soft tissue tumor of the chest wall is?

    A. Multiple myeloma.
    B. Ewing's sarcoma.
    C. Chondrosarcoma.
    D. Fibrohistiocytoma.

2. Mesotheliomas?

    A. Are always malignant.
    B. Are radiosensitive.
    C. When localized should be resected.
    D. Respond well to chemotherapy.

3. Chondromas and chondrosarcomas?

    A. May look similar histiologically.
    B. Arise from different sites.
    C. Become high grade malignancies.
    D. Have different presentations.

(See p. 604 for answers.)

52

BENIGN LESIONS
OF THE LUNG

FRITZ BAUMGARTNER

Common benign diseases of the lung include emphysematous disease, pulmonary sequestration, and arteriovenous (AV) malformation.

The goals of this chapter are to (1) identify those patients who would likely benefit from resection of emphysematous blebs, (2) understand the differentiation between sequestration, AV malformation, and other lung lesions, and (3) identify the current modes of therapy for sequestration and AV malformation.

CASE 1
CHEST PAIN

A 25-year-old smoker presented with severe left chest pain that occurred suddenly while mowing the lawn. He had no prior history of cardiac or pulmonary conditions. Chest x-ray revealed a 90% collapse of the left lung with a mediastinal shift to the right. A thoracostomy tube was placed in the third intercostal space in the midclavicular line, producing a gush of air with gradual resolution of the chest pain. The chest tube was placed on 20-cm water suction. There was a minimal air leak, and a chest x-ray showed full reexpansion of the lung. Over the next 48 hours, the air leak resolved. The chest tube was clamped for 4 hours, after which time a chest x-ray was obtained, revealing reaccumulation of the pneumothorax resulting in 50% lung collapse. The chest tube was placed back on suction for another 3 days and clamped once again. This time, there was no evidence of pneumothorax after 24 hours. The chest tube was removed without evidence of subsequent pneumothorax.

One year later, he returned with identical symptoms, at which time chest x-ray revealed a 90% pneumothorax, again on the left side. Another chest tube was placed. The

next day he underwent resection of a left apical bleb. There has been no recurrence of the pneumothorax.

CASE 2
SHORTNESS OF BREATH

A 55-year-old male visited his primary care physician complaining of shortness of breath. He had an extensive history of smoking but denied hemoptysis, fever, chills, sweats, and had only intermittent coughing and sputum production. He became dyspneic after climbing one flight or stairs. He had no known cardiac or peripheral vascular history and was on no medications. He was barrel-chested and had hyperinflated lung fields.

Chest x-ray revealed a huge left apical bulla with compression of the left hilum inferiorly. The right lung, although hyperinflated, had no gross abnormalities. There were no pulmonary lesions. His arterial blood gas showed a PaO_2 of 55 mmHg, $PaCO_2$ of 42 mmHg, and pH of 7.40. A CT scan showed a giant left apical bulla compressing the vasculature of the left lower and left upper lobes. Pulmonary angiography confirmed compression of the pulmonary vasculature. A ventilation/perfusion scan demonstrated that 55% of ventilation was going to the right lung and 45% to the left lung. However, 80% of perfusion was to the right lung and 20% to the left lung. At thoracotomy, a giant bulla was removed with prompt expansion of the left upper and lower lobes. A mild air leak resolved postoperatively after 48 hours. One year later his chest x-ray remained normal.

GENERAL CONSIDERATIONS

Spontaneous pneumothorax is quite frequent among tall, asthenic, smoking young males, but may occur in females (Case 1). The incidence is approximately 1 per 10,000. Chest pain is the most common symptom, occurring in over 90%. The disorder is usually caused by small bullae located in the apical portion of the lung, although it may also arise from the superior segmental portions of the lower lobes. In older patients, a spontaneous pneumothorax is usually from more diffuse cystic disease, which often cannot be completely resected and may require repeated chest tube insertion. The rate of spontaneous pneumothorax recurrence ranges between 20% and 50% after the initial event. After a second pneumothorax, the chance of additional pneumothoraces is much higher, and is between 50% and 80%.

The differentiation between a bleb and a bulla is made on size alone. A bleb is generally less than 1–2 cm, while bullae are much larger. Bullae ventilate poorly because they are not subjected to the normal recoil mechanism of the lung. Larger bullae compress surrounding normal lung, resulting in collapse and poor ventilation and perfusion. Emphysematous giant bullae are nearly always found in patients with extensive smoking histories.

Sequestrations may be either intralobar or extralobar. The intralobar variety is much more common than the extralobar type. The sequestered lung lies invested within the patient's own pulmonary pleura and is surrounded by normal pulmonary tissue. The location is usually within the left lower lobe. Intralobar sequestrations include a patent bronchus that enters the affected area lung, as well as a systemic artery rather than a pulmonary artery and drains through the pulmonary venous system. An extralobar sequestration is also found most commonly in the left lower lobe. In this case, however, a patent bronchus is not present and the incidence of recurrent pulmonary infection is decreased. Small systemic arteries supply the sequestration. The venous drainage is to systemic rather than to pulmonary veins and usually enters the hemiazygos vein. That there is no communication with the tracheal bronchial tree is significant and dramatically reduces the incidence of recurrent pulmonary infections. Coexisting abnormalities are frequent and include cardiac anomalies, pectus excavatum, and AV malformations. Figure 52.1 shows a large anomalous artery supplying an intralobar sequestration that passes through the left hemidiaphragm. The surgical specimen demonstrates the lesion's intraparenchymal extent and containment within the visceral pleural envelope.

AV malformations are extremely rare; however, they are an important part of the differential diagnosis of lung masses and especially the solitary pulmonary nodule. They are usually asymptomatic and are identified on routine radiographic studies, being located subpleurally. Symptoms, when present, consist of dyspnea, cyanosis, and clubbing. Hemoptysis, hemothorax, or stroke may occur. About onehalf of patients have the Osler-Weber-Rendu syndrome (pulmonary AV malformations associated with hereditary

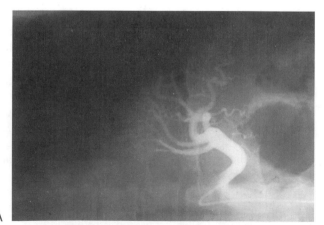
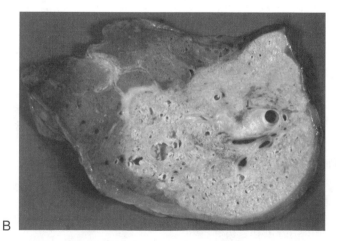

FIGURE 52.1   *(A) Angiogram showing vessels originating from the abdominal aorta passing from the abdominal aorta through the diaphragm to supply the sequestration. (B) Cross-section of pathology specimen showing sequestration of Fig. A.*

hemorrhagic telangiectasia). Strokes and/or brain abscess occur because particulate matter passes through the pulmonary arterial system directly into the pulmonary venous system and into the left heart and systemic circulation.

DIAGNOSIS

When a spontaneous pneumothorax is suspected, one should obtain a chest x-ray to confirm the diagnosis. A previous history of the disorder is of critical importance. Physical examination will demonstrate decreased breath sounds on the affected side along with dullness to percussion. If the patient has a tension pneumothorax (intrapleural air under pressure causing a mediastinal shift), signs of respiratory distress will be present. In this instance, a needle catheter should be inserted immediately to decompress the chest. Under these emergency circumstances, a chest x-ray is not required before definitive therapy is instituted.

The diagnosis of emphysematous bulla is usually made in patients who have long-standing emphysematous disease. The history and physical examination should detect chronic obstructive pulmonary disease, while the chest x-ray usually shows hyperlucent areas consistent with emphysematous bullae. If respiratory compromise is present (based on the emphysematous bullae), then suitability for operation must be evaluated. This is accomplished by evaluating lung structure and function. Initially the chest x-ray will provide information regarding suitability for resection. Patients in whom more than one-third of the hemithorax is filled with a bullous cavity generally can be helped substantially by operation. Further radiographic evidence is provided by computed tomography (CT) scan, which shows compression of the pulmonary vessels and

parenchyma by the bullous lesion. An angiogram will diagnose compression of the pulmonary vasculature. Finally, a ventilation/perfusion scan will reveal both decreased ventilation and perfusion on the affected side. Ventilation will be impaired because neither the compressed lung nor the bulla ventilates normally.

The diagnosis of pulmonary AV malformations is easiest in those patients who present with clubbing, cyanosis, and polycythemia. A chest x-ray usually shows the lesion, and its diagnosis is confirmed on pulmonary angiography. Diagnosis in the asymptomatic patient without cyanosis is more difficult. The chest x-ray abnormality, which frequently appears as a solitary pulmonary nodule, often undergoes extensive workup for other disorders before the diagnosis of AV malformation is considered. The Osler-Weber-Rendu syndrome accounts for about one-half of all cases, in which there are multiple small lesions with capillary abnormalities associated with hemorrhagic telangiectasia elsewhere.

Intralobar sequestration may be suspected by pulmonary abnormalities on chest x-ray. The diagnosis is confirmed by angiography, which visualizes an aberrant artery leading to the affected area. Additionally, aberrant systemic venous drainage can be seen. The vessels may arise from the descending thoracic aorta at any point and may even originate from the intra-abdominal aorta with the artery traversing the diaphragm. CT scan demonstrates these abnormal vessels well and may be used in lieu of arteriography. Extralobar sequestration may be detected on routine chest x-ray as a triangular mass pointing toward the hilum. The diagnosis is confirmed by arteriography, which shows small systemic arteries arising from the aorta leading to the abnormal extrapulmonary lobe. The venous drainage is systemic, similar to that for intralobar sequestrations.

DIFFERENTIAL DIAGNOSIS

The differential diagnosis for spontaneous pneumothorax includes causes of chest pain such as angina or acute myocardial infarction, pulmonary embolus, dysphagia, and aortic dissection. These may be excluded by history alone, since this condition usually occurs in young and healthy individuals. A simple chest x-ray confirms the diagnosis of spontaneous pneumothorax.

The differential diagnosis of emphysematous bullae is generally limited after review of the chest x-ray. The problem with emphysematous bullae comes not with establishing the diagnosis, but rather in determining which patients are operative candidates and can be expected to benefit from resection. The differential diagnosis of sequestration differs between the intralobar and extralobar varieties. Infection of the intralobar sequestration may be indistinguishable clinically from bronchiectasis and lung abscess, both of which result in fever and productive cough. Generally, however, sequestration occurs in the lower lobe on the left side, while most lung abscesses (particularly those arising from aspiration) occur on the right. A CT scan identifying the large anomalous vessel from the descending thoracic aorta confirms the diagnosis. For extralobar sequestration, suspicion is aroused by its frequent association with other congenital abnormalities, including heart defects, foregut malformations, and congenital diaphragmatic hernia. Radiologic evaluation, including selective angiography and/or CT scan, will help in the diagnosis. Aortography is generally not useful because the arterial supply tends to be rather small. The differential diagnosis of an AV malformation is that of any coin lesion and includes neoplastic etiologies, infection, and old granulomatous disease. Evaluation of a solitary pulmonary mass is discussed in detail in the section on lung cancer. Among the one-third of patients who present with cyanosis, clubbing, and polycythemia, a high index of suspicion for AV malformations should be maintained.

TREATMENT

The initial management of a spontaneous pneumothorax consists of re-expanding the lung with chest tube insertion. A small chest tube can generally be used and is inserted anteriorly (rather than chest tube positioning for effusion or trauma, which is usually posterior). The management of a small (<10%) spontaneous pneumothorax is somewhat controversial, since these patients may be managed effectively and safely with observation and oxygen administration alone. Oxygen will cause the nitrogen in the air contained within the pneumothorax to diffuse out through the pleura, thus decreasing its size. This management should be done cautiously with periodic chest x-rays to be sure that the pneumothorax does not enlarge, in which case immediate chest tube insertion is required. Subsequent management depends on the patient's course. Persistence of an air leak longer than 5 days generally requires surgical intervention. Most cases of spontaneous pneumothorax, however, can be managed expectantly. The chance of a spontaneous pneumothorax recurring after the initial episode is 20–50%. The patient must stop smoking. There are certain conditions for which operation is indicated after the initial episode. These include occupations as a pilot or scuba diver, where rapid changes in atmospheric pressure may result in a pneumothorax. It is generally accepted that a second pneumothorax is an indication for bleb resection and apical pleurodesis. Resection of the apical bleb can be performed by open thoracotomy or by video-assisted thoracoscopic stapling of the bleb. The video thoracoscopic methods are less invasive. A pleurodesis can be performed by abrading the surface of the parietal pleura with a cautery scratch pad. Most blebs causing spontaneous pneumothoraces are in the apices of the upper lobes, although they may arise from the superior segments of the lower lobes. Some advocate the use of sclerosing agents for spontaneous pneumothorax to facilitate pleurodesis and prevent future pneumothorax formation. Unfortunately, this causes intense and diffuse scarring of the pleural space whose long-term effects are not known. In young individuals who have a long lifespan and who may need future thoracotomy for other diseases, pleurodesis may not be a wise choice. Pleurodesis is usually reserved for patients with malignant pleural effusions.

The most important part of the management of emphysematous bullae is selection of those patients most likely to benefit from resection. Once that decision has been made, a thoracotomy is performed and a stapler is used to resect the bullous portion of the lung. Care is taken to ensure that normal lung is not injured or removed. The re-expansion of the lung is generally quite dramatic. The operation can be expected to improve pulmonary function markedly because of the decrease in extrinsic compression on normal lung tissue.

The treatment of both intralobar and extralobar sequestration is resection. There is a more compelling reason to resect an intralobar sequestration—because of the increased incidence of infection and lung destruction. The guiding principle of resection lies in achieving control of the anomalous pulmonary vessel, which usually courses through the inferior pulmonary ligament. Lobectomy is the usual form of treatment. Surgery for extralobar sequestration is indicated to allow re-expansion of remaining normal lung tissue. Since the extralobar sequestration has its own visceral pleural envelope, resection of the abnormal lung alone is indicated.

The treatment of a pulmonary AV malformation is primarily by resection, which should completely remove the lesion while limiting the amount of normal resected lung. Multiple lesions require careful attention to conservation of lung tissue. In these cases, the use of angiographic embolization may be considered. Recanalization of the AV malformation after angiographic embolization has been described and may be a disadvantage when compared with resection.

KEY POINTS

• Initial management of spontaneous pneumothorax consists of re-expanding lung with chest tube insertion; small chest tube used and inserted anteriorly

• Persistence of air leak longer than 5 days requires surgical intervention

• Chance of spontaneous pneumothorax recurring after initial episode is 20–50%

• Most important part of management of emphysematous bullae is selection of patients most likely to benefit from resection

---

FOLLOW-UP

After an initial episode of spontaneous pneumothorax, follow-up can be as needed or at yearly intervals. The same is true after resection of an apical bleb. Follow-up of a bulla is usually every 3 months, but depends on the extent of the patient's emphysematous disease. Follow-up for the congenital pulmonary disorders is every several months or more frequently as needed. Follow-up is needed for AV malformation patients who undergo angiographic embolization. They require careful evaluation for the presence of cyanosis as evidenced by desaturation on arterial blood gas testing.

SUGGESTED READINGS

Kravitz RM: Congenital malformations of the lung. Pediatr Clin North Am 41:453, 1994

This recent manuscript describes multiple types of congenital malformations in the pediatric population. The article is well written and contains a number of references that are useful for further reading.

Rappaport DC, Herman SJ, Weisbrod GL: Congenital bronchopulmonary diseases in adults: CT findings. AJR 162:1295,1994

This article describes congenital lung diseases that present in adults. These lesions can be divided into those that arise from the primitive foregut (bronchopulmonary malformations) and those that originate in the pulmonary vasculature. While the latter group is usually found early in life, those arising from the primitive foregut may present later. This article describes a number of radiologic findings that are useful in making the differential diagnosis.

Vigneswaran WT, Townsend ER, Fountain SW. Surgery for bullous disease of the lung. Eur J Cardiothorac Surg 6:427, 1992

This article describes 22 patients who underwent operative procedures for bullous disease at one institution. The presentation, diagnosis, and management are discussed in detail. This is one of the larger series on this topic.

QUESTIONS

1. *A 28-year-old male presents with shortness of breath. The symptoms occurred shortly after completing a 10-mile jog. His past medical history is not contributory. The chance of this process recurring is?*

    A. Less than 10%.
    B. Between 20–50%.
    C. 75%.
    D. Greater than 90%.

2. *Intralobar emphysematous blebs?*

    A. Are less common than the extralobar variety.
    B. Have pulmonary arterial blood supply.
    C. Rarely present with pulmonary infections.
    D. Are best diagnosed by pulmonary angiography.

3. *AV malformations are usually discovered?*

    A. On physical examination.
    B. On routine chest x-ray.
    C. On presentation for hemoptysis.
    D. After a stroke.

4. *A young patient with recurrent pneumothorax from apical blebs should?*

    A. Have the blebs resected.
    B. Be evaluated for Marfan syndrome.
    C. Undergo pleurodesis.
    D. Have a CT scan to evaluate the contralateral lung.

(See p. 604 for answers.)

53

LUNG

CANCER

FRITZ BAUMGARTNER

Lung cancer is increasing in incidence and severity, placing treatment in constant evolution. This chapter (1) discusses the etiology and demographic of lung cancer, (2) develops a strategy for the evaluation and diagnosis of patients who present with a solitary pulmonary nodule, (3) reviews the staging and prognosis of different types of lung cancer, and (4) discusses available therapies and their indications and outcomes.

CASE 1
HACKING COUGH

A 57-year-old male had had a hacking cough productive of nonbloody sputum for the past 2 months. He smoked two packs per day for the past 30 years. He had known COPD and stable angina, for which he took nitrates and β-blockers.

On examination he had hyperexpansile lung fields, but there were no other gross abnormalities. A chest x-ray revealed a solitary pulmonary nodule, 1 cm in diameter, located in the left lateral midlung field. A chest x-ray performed 3 years prior was normal. The lung fields were hyperexpanded. Sputum cytology was normal. A CT scan of the chest and upper abdomen showed a pretracheal lymph node 0.5 cm in diameter. The pulmonary nodule was a 2-cm peripheral lesion located in the superior segment of the left lower lobe, without evidence of chest wall invasion. Pulmonary function testing found an FEV_1 of 1.0 L/sec. Arterial blood gas on room air was PaO_2 of 70 mmHg; $PaCO_2$, 44 mmHg; pH, 7.38; and bicarbonate, 26 mEq/L. Although he was able to climb half a flight of stairs easily, a full flight of stairs made him short of breath. A ventilation/perfusion scan found that 45% of both ventilation and perfusion went to the left lung and 55% to the right lung.

Only erythema consistent with COPD was seen on bronchoscopy. Brushings and washings of the left superior segmental bronchus returned as squamous cell carcinoma. Mediastinoscopy showed anthracotic lymph node tissue without cancer. Several days later, a left posterolateral thoracotomy was performed with a left superior segmentectomy. The patient did well postoperatively and had been followed with chest x-rays every 4 months, CBC and liver function tests every 4 months, and a yearly CT scan of the chest and upper abdomen. He had completely stopped smoking and was able to walk at a reasonable pace without becoming short of breath, although inclines were still troublesome.

CASE 2
SHOULDER PAIN AND A DROOPY EYELID

A 60-year-old male presented with the chief complaint of progressive left shoulder pain and a droopy left eyelid for the past month. He smoked heavily until 2 years before, when he quit because of claudication. Medical management included aspirin and graduated exercise. He denied recent weight loss.

He was found to have ptosis and miosis of the left eye, with decreased sweating of the left face and arm. He also exhibited mild decreased sensation in the ulnar aspect of his left upper extremity, although there was no weakness in the ulnar distribution. He had pain with left shoulder or neck motion. There was no adenopathy. There was dullness to percussion of the left upper chest. A chest x-ray showed a mass in the left upper lobe in the superior sulcus (Fig. 53.1A). A CT scan confirmed these findings and showed the mass to be abutting the lowermost portion of the brachial plexus. There did not appear to be vertebral body or vascular involvement, although a portion of the first rib posteriorly was eroded (Fig. 53.1B). A CT scan of the upper abdomen, liver function tests, and CBC were normal. Sputum cytology was nondiagnostic. Bronchoscopy revealed no evidence of lesions; brushings and washings of the left upper lobe orifice and segmental bronchi were unremarkable. A CT-guided needle aspiration of the mass demonstrated squamous cell carcinoma. He received 3,500 cGy of radiotherapy to the left upper lobe and chest wall over the course of 3 weeks. One week after completion, a repeat chest x-ray and CT scan demonstrated some resolution of the tumor without evidence of mediastinal adenopathy, or liver or adrenal metastases.

An en bloc resection of the superior sulcus, chest wall, and left upper lobe tumor was performed. The subclavian artery and vein were preserved. The T1 nerve root was found to be surrounded by tumor and was sacrificed with the specimen. Frozen section showed squamous cell carcinoma with clear margins. The patient did well postoperatively with worsening of his symptoms of ptosis, miosis, and anhydrosis on the left side. Although his shoulder pain had improved markedly, he noticed some shoulder droop but moved his arm quite well with nearly normal motor strength.

GENERAL CONSIDERATIONS

Lung carcinoma is the most common cancer and the most common cause of death from cancer in men. It is the most common cancer in women and is equal to breast cancer as the most common cause of death in women.

Malignant lung lesions can be classified under various systems, although the most useful is small cell and nonsmall cell carcinoma. Differentiation is important in terms of prognosis and treatment. The nonsmall cell varieties include squamous cell carcinoma, adenocarcinoma, and large cell carcinoma. Low grade malignant lesions such as carcinoid tumor and adenoid cystic carcinoma are less common forms of nonsmall cell carcinoma. Rare primary malignant tumors include sarcomas, which may be parenchymal or endobronchial; lymphomas, which may be either Hodgkin's or non-Hodgkin's variety; and bronchoalveolar carcinoma. Small cell (formerly called "oat cell") carcinoma is classified separately from nonsmall cell carcinoma, denoting differences in prognosis and treatment.

Adenocarcinoma of the lung is the most frequent histologic type and is responsible for 50% of lung carcinomas. Squamous cell cancer is the next most common and accounts for 30%. Small cell cancer represents approximately 15% of lung carcinomas, while large cell carcinomas make up less than 5%.

Carcinoid tumor is a low grade malignant lesion occasionally found in the lung. There is a histologic continuum

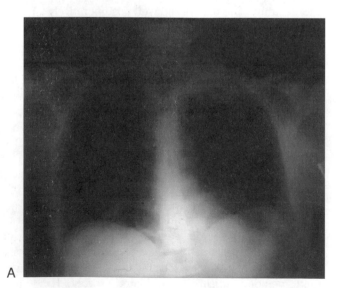

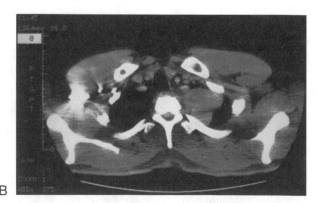

FIGURE 53.1 *(A) Chest x-ray showing a left lung apical mass. (B) CT scan confirming a left superior sulcus mass.*

of carcinoid up to small cell carcinoma, constituting a family of "Kulchitsky" tumors. The other low grade malignant lesion is the adenoid cyctic carcinoma, which is characterized by submucosal spread and perineural invasion. The staging of nonsmall cell lung carcinoma is illustrated in Table 53.1 and Figure 53.2.

Small cell lung carcinoma is likely a systemic disease. At initial presentation, nearly two-thirds of the patients have metastases outside the thorax that involve at least one other organ. Small cell lesions are generally unresectable independent of size or presence of mediastinal lymph nodes. Chemotherapy is generally considered the first line of treatment for small cell carcinoma. The TNM classification is frequently not used for small cell carcinoma, because it is presumed that most cases have systemic micrometastases. Resection, in combination with adjuvant chemotherapy, may result in cure. Some groups have reported a 5-year survival of almost 33% following surgical management of carefully selected patients with small cell lung carcinoma. Without any form of treatment, small cell lung carcinomas are rapidly fatal with a mean survival time of less than 12 weeks.

Extrathoracic paraneoplastic syndromes are neuroendocrine phenomena associated with lung carcinoma. These include (1) Cushing syndrome, (2) excessive ADH production, and (3) hypercalcemia caused by parathyrin (parathyroid hormone [PTH]).

TABLE 53.1 *Nonsmall cell abbreviated staging of lung carcinoma*

Stage	Survival
I (T1, T2)	85%
II (N1)	60–70%
III	
IIIa (T3 or N2)	25–35%
IIIb (T4 or N3)	10–20%
IV (M1)	<10%

Tumor size

T1 <3 cm

T2 >3 cm or visceral pleura involvement or atelectasis/pneumonitis

T3 Invasion of nonessential chest structures

T4 Invasion of essential chest structures or malignant effusion

Nodal status

N1 Intrapulmonary nodes

N2 Mediastinal nodes

N3 Contralateral or supraclavicular nodes

Metastases

M0 Alometastases

M1 Metastatic disease

KEY POINTS

• Malignant lung lesions are classified under various systems, although most useful is small cell and nonsmall cell carcinoma; differentiation is important to prognosis and treatment

• Nonsmall cell varieties include squamous cell carcinoma, adenocarcinoma, and large cell carcinoma

• Small cell (formerly oat cell) carcinoma classified separately from nonsmall cell carcinoma, denoting differences in prognosis and treatment

• Adenocarcinoma of lung most frequent histologic type, responsible for 50% of lung carcinomas; squamous cell cancer accounts for 30%; small cell cancer, 15%; and large cell, less than 5%

• Small cell lung carcinoma is systemic disease; at initial presentation, two-thirds of patients have metastases outside thorax that involve at least one other organ

• Small cell lesions generally unresectable independent of size or presence of mediastinal nodes; chemotherapy first line of treatment

DIAGNOSIS

A history of cough, hemoptysis, chest pain, fever, chills, weight loss, and smoking habits are important. Travel to the San Joaquin Valley or Mississippi River Valley are important in establishing exposure to coccidioidomycosis or histoplasmosis. Appropriate skin testing should be performed. Similarly, exposure to tuberculosis should determined.

Physical examination, concentrating on the cardiopulmonary system, is essential. Attention should be paid to the lymph nodes and evidence of systemic tumor spread. Abdominal and rectal examinations are important because the observed lung lesion may be a pulmonary metasasis. If the patient has no evidence of another primary, the lung lesion has only a small chance of being a metastasis. A high quality pulmonary artery and lateral chest x-ray should be compared with previous studies to look for any recent change. If a coin lesion is observed on chest x-ray, cancer and tuberculosis should be considered and appropriate evaluation undertaken to exclude these diagnoses. A sputum cytology must be obtained since it may establish the diagnosis. PPD (purified protein derivative) skin testing with controls is important to exclude tuberculosis. Bronchoscopy should be performed early to search for the primary lesion and obtain biopsies. If the lesion is peripheral, brushings and washings of the suspected segmental bronchus are appropriate. Percutaneous-guided needle aspiration of a peripheral lesion may save the patient an invasive diagnostic procedure and allow more rapid institution of radiotherapy.

The evaluation of the tumor does not end with establishing the diagnosis, since staging is vital in therapeutic

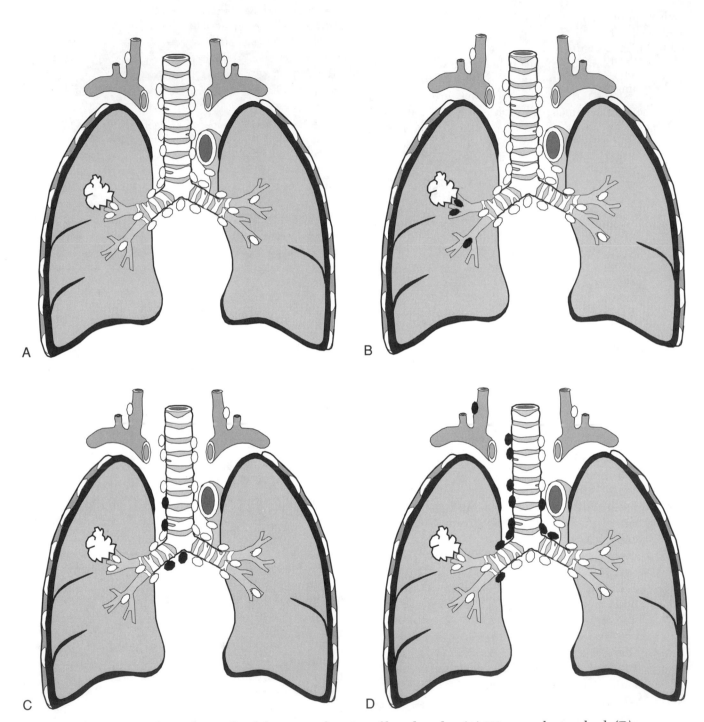

FIGURE 53.2   *Dependence of nodal status on location of lymph nodes. (**A**) N0, no nodes involved; (**B**) N1, involvement of intrapulmonary nodes; (**C**) N2, involvement of ipsilateral mediastinal and/or sub-carinal lymph nodes; (**D**) N3, involvement of contralateral or ipsilateral supraclavicular/scalene nodes.*

planning. Lung carcinomas are best staged by CT scan. Nodes less than 1 cm usually do not harbor malignant cells. Mediastinal nodes greater than 1 cm require further evaluation. Node enlargement may represent either reactive inflammation or involvement with carcinoma. Assessment is by cervical mediastinoscopy, anterior mediastinotomy (Chamberlain procedure) or by video-assisted thoracoscopic methods. The sensitivity and specificity of CT scanning in the staging of lung cancer is only 90%. Therefore, many perform mediastinal lymph node sampling whether or not the CT scan reveals enlarged lymph nodes. This impacts subsequent treatment since mediastinal lymph node involvement generally indicates an unresectable process.

Staging is performed to determine whether a tumor is resectable. Typically, tumors up to stage IIIa are considered resectable and possibly curable. Therefore, it is vitally important to stage the tumor accurately before embarking on major surgery. Once a tumor has been deemed resectable, the patient's ability to withstand the procedure and its sequelae must be addressed. This is determined in part by the cardiopulmonary and vascular status. Routine electrocardiogram (ECG) is necessary, and a stress ECG may be indicated for those with suspected cardiac disease. An evaluation of pulmonary status mandates pulmonary function tests and an arterial blood gas analysis. Assessment of exercise tolerance can be made simply by having the patient walk up a flight of stairs. Generally, if this is tolerated without overt shortness of breath, exercise tolerance is such that a thoracotomy and partial pulmonary resection can be tolerated. Among pulmonary function tests, predicted postoperative forced expiratory volume in 1 second (FEV_1) is particularly important. If 0.8 L or less, resection may be contraindicated. Preoperative activity is an important consideration, however, because a sedentary elderly patient with an FEV_1 of less than 0.8 L may tolerate the procedure, while a younger, otherwise healthy, and active patient may do poorly. Although clinical judgment is important, the value of 0.8 L is generally considered a boundary that should not be crossed. The postoperative FEV_1 should be estimated. If a patient has a preoperative FEV_1 of 2.0 L, a pneumonectomy will presumably reduce the FEV_1 by one-half with a resultant postoperative value of 1.0 L. Using these determinants and the segmental anatomy of the lungs, one will be able to determine what the resultant FEV_1 will be after resection of a lobe or segment. On arterial blood gas measurement, a $PaCO_2$ above 45 mmHg indicates severe hypoventilation and may preclude surgery.

The segmental anatomy of the lungs is important in planning pulmonary resections. On the right, there are three segments in the upper lobe, two segments in the middle lobe, and five segments in the lower lobe. On the left there are four segments in the upper lobe (two segments in the upper lobe proper and two segments in the lingula) and four segments in the lower lobe. Overall, approximately 55% of total lung function is from the right lung and 45% from the left lung. One can thus assess whether to perform a resection based on postoperative function predicted by the number of segments removed. For example, if one performs a right upper lobectomy in a patient with a preoperative FEV_1 of 1.1 L, three segments will be removed. Of the 18 segments in the lung, 15 will remain after surgery. The remainder (15 of 18) multiplied by 1.1 L equals 0.91 L as a predicted postoperative FEV_1; therefore, a lobectomy would be acceptable in this patient if other factors, including the arterial blood gases, are within normal limits.

If the postoperative FEV_1 will be marginal, a quantitative ventilation/perfusion scan ($\dot{V}/\dot{Q}$) may be useful (Case 1). This will help determine which portions of the lung are not functional and do not contribute to overall pulmonary function. For example, if a patient has a right upper lobe lesion and a marginal predicted postoperative FEV_1, a ventilation/perfusion scan that shows little ventilation or perfusion of the right upper lobe indicates that these nonfunctioning segments can be resected without further compromising overall FEV_1. If the perfusion and ventilation data differ, the perfusion information should be used.

KEY POINTS

- Bronchoscopy should be performed early to search for primary lesion and obtain biopsies

- Percutaneous-guided needle aspiration of peripheral lesion may save patient invasive diagnostic procedure and allows more rapid institution of radiotherapy

- Lung carcinomas best staged by CT scan; nodes less than 1 cm usually do not harbor malignant cells; mediastinal nodes greater than 1 cm require further evaluation

- Mediastinal lymph node involvement generally indicates unresectable process

- Evaluation of pulmonary status mandates pulmonary function tests and arterial blood gas analysis

- Assessment of exercise tolerance can be made by having patient walk up flight of stairs

- Among pulmonary function tests, predicted postoperative FEV_1 is particularly important; if 0.8 L or less, resection may be contraindicated

- Overall, approximately 55% of total lung function is from right lung and 45% from left lung; one can thus assess whether to perform resection based on postoperative function predicted by number of segments removed

---

DIFFERENTIAL DIAGNOSS

The solitary pulmonary nodule is on an important list of differential diagnoses. The history and physical examination are critical in determining which processes are more likely. For example, an extensive smoker is more likely to have lung cancer than a nonsmoker who just returned from a region heavily infested with tuberculosis or coccidioidomycosis. A tumor may be benign or malignant. The malignant variety may be primary or metastatic, with likelihood determined by history and physical examination, as well as by histology. If a patient has no systemic evidence of an extrathoracic primary cancer, the chance of a lung lesion being a metastasis from an extrapulmonary source is less than 2%. The presence of tuberculosis should never be underestimated, since it wears many disguises, and should never be less than second on a list of differential diagnoses for lung pathology. A tuberculosis skin test with controls should be conducted.

The chest x-ray is very helpful. Generally, tuberculosis is found in the apices of the lung, although it may be in any location. Cavitary lesions associated with carcinoma are generally squamous cell carcinomas. Squamous cell carcinomas and small cell carcinoma are usually, but not universally, centrally located, whereas large cell tumors and adenocarcinomas are typically more peripherally located. The presence of "popcorn," lamellar, or target calcifications implies benign disease such as granuloma, although carcinoma should not be excluded. Other benign lesions include plasma cell granulomas (inflammatory pseudotumors), which are postinflammatory reactions and not true neoplasms; granular cell myoblastoma (granular cell tumors), which originate from Schwann cells usually found in larger bronchial origins (although they may occur as peripheral lesions); and leiomyomas, lipomas, and fibromas, which are benign mesenchymal tumors. Congenital causes of pulmonary masses include arteriovenous (AV) malformations, sequestrations, and other benign lesions. An arterial blood gas analysis in a patient with an AV malformation will show a decrease in saturation due to right-left shunting. Arteriography is diagnostic. Sequestration can also be diagnosed by arteriography. Pulmonary infarction may appear as a pulmonary mass and often has a classic wedge-shaped appearance on CT scan.

KEY POINTS

• If a patient has no systemic evidence of extrathoracic primary cancer, chance of lung lesion being metastasis from an extrapulmonary source is less than 2%

• Cavitary lesions associated with carcinoma are generally squamous cell carcinoma; squamous cell and small cell carcinomas are usually centrally located, whereas large cell tumors and adenocarcinomas are more usually more peripheral

---

TREATMENT

The treatment of small cell versus nonsmall cell carcinomas is fundamentally different. Nonsmall cell lung carcinoma is generally considered a surgically curable disease

up to stage III. Small cell lung carcinoma, with the exception of certain early stage I lesions, is considered systemic and incurable, and is managed with chemotherapy. Stage I and stage II nonsmall cell lung carcinomas are curable by surgical resection. This requires exploratory thoracotomy to exclude disease not apparent on preoperative evaluation such as small miliary, pulmonary, or parietal disease; pleural metastases; synchronous lesions; or evidence of mediastinal node involvement or biopsy.

Overall, the prognosis for stage 1 nonsmall cell carcinoma managed by surgical resection is a 5-year disease-free survival of 85%. Survival for stage II is 60%. Generally, adjuvant chemotherapy or radiotherapy are not given for stage I or stage II nonsmall cell lung carcinoma. Stage IIIa divides surgically curable from nonsurgical incurable disease. Stage IIIa lung carcinomas invading the chest wall (T3 lesions) are curable as long as there is no mediastinal lymph node involvement. Tumors that invade the chest wall other than in the region of the superior sulcus are managed by en bloc lobectomy with chest wall resection, including a 5-cm margin around the tumor of the chest wall. The superior sulcus tumor is a special type of lung carcinoma that invades the chest wall. This is usually a squamous cell carcinoma arising at the apex of the upper lobes, although other histologic types are possible. The tumor invades the endothoracic fascia and may involve the lower roots of the brachial plexus, the sympathetic chain and adjacent ribs, and often the vertebral bodies (Case 2). Radiotherapy alone for superior sulcus tumors has been reported to relieve pain and prolong survival (Case 2). Therefore, preoperative radiation of 3,000–4,000 cGy over 3–4 weeks is followed by a 1–3 week period of rest and recuperation followed by resection of the tumor. Five-year disease-free survival is approximately 30%.

For small cell carcinoma, attempted curative surgery is limited to about 10% of patients. Currently, resection of stages I and II small cell lung cancer with preoperative or postoperative chemotherapy is recommended, followed by additional mediastinal radiotherapy for N1 disease. No resection is indicated for N2 disease. Prophylactic cranial radiation is performed in cases of small cell lung cancer because of the high risk of brain metastases. Chemotherapy regimens generally used for small cell lung cancer include cyclophosphamide, doxyrubicin, and vincristine.

The standard lung cancer operation for tumor confined to a lobe of the lung is a lobectomy rather than a segmental resection or wedge resection. There is evidence, however, that segmentectomy may result in similar long-term survival. This is important in those with limited pulmonary function when a lobectomy will result in poor predicted postoperative FEV$_1$ (Case 1). In these situations, a segmentectomy may permit anatomic resection, yet limit the amount of pulmonary compromise. In patients with squamous cell carcinoma, segmentectomy and lobectomy appear equal. However, there is a 20% survival benefit for lobectomy compared to segmental resection overall. In particular, adenocarcinomas do poorly with limited resections. Videothoracoscopic techniques are becoming more and more common. Some attempts have been made to perform wedge resections of primary lung carcinomas, but studies have found the incidence of recurrence unacceptably high. Wedge resection is an even more inferior operation than segmentectomy and should only be used as a last resort.

The role of radiotherapy in stages I and II lung cancer is debated. Even though radiotherapy decreases the recurrence rate, this has not translated into improved survival. Currently, therefore, resection alone is indicated for stages I and II nonsmall cell lung carcinoma. Radiation is extremely useful preoperatively for superior sulcus tumors and has been shown to improve disease-free survival.

The incidence of brain metastases is higher in patients who have adenocarcinoma or small cell carcinoma of the lung than in any other histologic types. Patients with untreated brain metastases have a mean survival of only 1 month. This is doubled if steroids alone are used and is improved to 4 months with the addition of cranial radiation. For small cell carcinoma, brain metastases signify incurable disease, and the patient should be treated with chemotherapy and cranial radiation. In some instances, a solitary brain metastasis may be resectable in nonsmall cell carcinoma in the absence of other contraindications. Excluding solitary brain metastases, the presence of extrathoracic metastatic lesions in nonsmall cell lung carcinoma precludes resection of the primary tumor. The role of postoperative cranial radiotherapy is debated.

The management of pulmonary metastases varies depending on the number of lesions, duration, attempted curative resection of the primary, and whether control of the primary has been established. Wedge resection of metastatic lesions from primary extremity sarcomas is effective. Similarly, solitary pulmonary metastases from primary colon carcinomas have been successfully treated. Hepatomas metastatic to the lung, breast tumors with pulmonary metastases, or lung primaries that have metastasized to other portions of the lung have extremely poor prognoses and are not candidates for surgical resection. The number of simultaneous metastases is important. Generally, it is believed that six or fewer lesions can be resected, depending on the patient's preoperative and predicted postoperative pulmonary function. The time from resection of the primary is important because the longer the time period between the identification of a pulmonary metastasis and the time of resection of the primary, the greater the chance that surgical resection of the lung lesion will be effective. If a pulmonary metastasis appears at the same time as a primary lesion is diagnosed, the chance of surgical cure is markedly diminished.

KEY POINTS

- Nonsmall cell lung carcinoma generally considered surgically curable disease up to stage III; small cell lung carcinoma, with the exception of certain early stage I lesions, is considered systemic and incurable, and is managed with chemotherapy; stage I and stage II nonsmall cell lung carcinomas are curable by resection

- Overall, prognosis for stage I nonsmall cell carcinoma managed by surgical resection is 5-year disease-free survival of 85%; survival for stage II is 60%

- Superior sulcus tumor is special type of lung carcinoma that invades chest wall; this is usually squamous carcinoma arising at apex of upper lobes, although other histologic types possible

- For small cell carcinoma, attempted curative surgery is limited to about 10% of patients

- Standard lung cancer operation for tumor confined to lung lobe is lobectomy rather than segmental resection or wedge resection

- Although radiotherapy decreases recurrence rate, this is not translated into improved survival; currently, therefore, resection alone is indicated for stages I and II nonsmall cell lung carcinoma

- Wedge resection of metastatic lesions from primary extremity sarcomas is effective; similarly, solitary pulmonary metastases from primary colon carcinomas have been treated successfully

FOLLOW-UP

The patient should undergo at least biannual physical examinations with chest x-rays and yearly CT scans of the chest. Yearly liver function tests should be performed to evaluate possible hepatic metastases. Bronchoscopy is not performed postoperatively except for specific indications such as suspected recurrence or evaluation of a new primary.

SUGGESTED READINGS

Midthun DE, Swensen SJ, Jett JR: Clinical strategies for solitary pulmonary nodule. Ann Rev Med 43:195, 1992

The solitary pulmonary nodule is a classic dilemma both for the practicing clinician and for the student undergoing college examination. Questions that arise include whether the lesion is malignant or benign, and whether it should be observed, biopsied, or removed. This article reviews the current body of knowledge about the solitary nodule and discusses the clinical approach to its evaluation. Highly recommended.

Petersen GM: Epidemiology, screening, and prevention of lung cancer. Cur Opinion Onco 6:156, 1994

This overview article discusses the causes, diagnosis, and prevention of lung cancer. It takes a slightly different approach to the problem than the student might be familiar with.

Pugatch, RD: Radiologic evaluation in chest malignancies. A review of imaging modalities. Chest 107:294S, 1995

Radiographic evaluation of the chest is a critical part of lung cancer diagnosis and follow-up. This article discusses radiologic techniques, including computed tomography and magnetic resonance imaging. It reviews the importance of solitary nodules as well as diagnostic patterns in patients with lung cancer.

QUESTIONS

1. *The treatment of choice for a diagnosed stage II squamous cell lung carcinoma is?*

    A. Lobectomy.
    B. Wedge resection alone.
    C. Preoperative mediastinal irradiation followed by wedge resection.
    D. Pneumonectomy.

2. *The survival (5-years disease free) for all surgically treated cases of stage I nonsmall cell carcinoma of the lung is?*

    A. 30%.
    B. 55%.
    C. 5%.
    D. 85%.

3. *In a patient with lung cancer, a mediastinal lymph node on CT of what size would warrant preoperative mediastinoscopy for staging?*

    A. Less than 1.0 cm.
    B. Greater than 1.0–1.5 cm.
    C. Greater than 1.5–2.0 cm.
    D. Greater than 2 cm.

4. *The following is the least reasonable treatment plan for a patient with a 1-cm, peripheral small cell carcinoma?*

    A. Lobectomy alone.
    B. Lobectomy and chemotherapy.
    C. Chemotherapy alone.
    D. Routine preoperative mediastinoscopy regardless of mediastinal node size.

(See p. 604 for answers.)

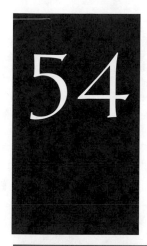

54

INFECTIONS OF
THE LUNG AND
PLEURAL SPACE

FRITZ BAUMGARTNER

The etiology, treatment, and prognosis of thoracic infections have changed dramatically during this century. The triumph of medical science over tuberculosis (TB) has been tempered recently by the dramatic rise in the incidence of this disease in the United States, as more and more immunocompromised patients live longer lives. Other pulmonary and plueral infections are also increasing in importance. The purpose of this chapter is to (1) appreciate the types of bacterial and fungal lung infec-

tions and their medical and surgical treatment, (2) review the treatment of TB and the indications for operation, and (3) become familiar with the complexity of empycma and appropriate management schemes.

The pulmonary infections manifested by AIDS and the opportunistic pathogens associated with it are discussed in Chapter 10.

CASE 1
MASSIVE HEMOPTYSIS

A 54-year-old Hispanic male presented to the emergency room with hemoptysis. His blood pressure was 80 mmHg systolic with a pulse rate of 100 bpm. Large bore intravenous catheters were placed while blood was drawn for a blood count and type and cross-match. Although he was not actively coughing blood when first seen, he had fresh blood staining in his mouth and on his lips. A chest x-ray demonstrated a right upper lobe infil-

trate. He was placed in the right lateral decubitus position. Further questioning and physical examination revealed exposure to TB through a family member. He denied history of cancer or lung infections, but smoked several cigarettes a day. He reported coughing up at least two cups of blood before coming to the emergency room.

During his evaluation, he had an episode of hemoptysis that produced another 100 ml of bright red blood. At that point, with blood being infused, he underwent rigid bronchoscopy with blood aspirated from the right mainstem bronchus. Blood could be seen trickling from the right upper lobe orifice. A balloon-tipped embolectomy catheter was placed into the bleeding lobar bronchus. Doses of INH, rifampin, and ethambutol were given. An arterial blood gas was obtained that revealed (on 100% inspired oxygen) pH, 7.45; PaO_2, 325 mmHg; and $PaCO_2$, 35 mmHg. The surgeon thought that the patient could withstand a pulmonary resection at that time, and the right upper lobe was removed.

Postoperatively, he did well and was treated successfully with a course of INH, rifampin, and ethambutol with negative sputum on three separate occasions. His postoperative TB skin test was strongly positive with a 15-cm wheal and induration and erythema. He is followed on a biannual basis with sputum cytology and chest x-rays.

GENERAL CONSIDERATIONS

Approximately 7% of the population is infected with the tubercle bacillus. With more and more immunodeficient patients surviving longer, and a growing immigrant population, it is likely that TB will again emerge as a disease in the forefront of thoracic surgery. The clinical manifestations of TB arise more often in the elderly and among new immigrant groups. The bacilli are airborne and result in an initial pulmonary infection that most often produces a primary complex (Ghon's tubercle) with a secondary focus of TB in the hilar lymph nodes. This results in a hypersensitivity reaction to the organism manifested by a positive purified protein derivative (PPD) skin test defined as an area of induration and erythema greater than 1 cm in diameter within 48 hours. In the primary infection, the PPD skin test is negative for 8 weeks after the infection and subsequently becomes positive when the hypersensitivity reaction occurs. Only 10% of these patients develop clinically significant disease, while 90% are limited to a Ghon complex. The 10% who advance exhibit some or all of the five clinical manifestations:

1. Pleural effusion: if the patient has a positive PPD skin test and a pleural effusion, the chance of TB being the source is 90%

2. Miliary TB: multiple pulmonary nodules are present. The patients are usually anergic with a negative TB skin test. One-half will die of their disease

3. Tuberculous pneumonia: tuberculous pneumonia results from aerosolizing the bacteria into the lung parenchyma. The TB skin test is typically positive

4. Extrapulmonary latent disease: this may involve multiple organ systems, including the kidney, brain, epididymis, liver, or joint surfaces. The knee, bladder, appendix, cecum, or terminal ileum are commonly involved

5. Local erosion: this may involve lung destruction, hemoptysis, rupture of an abscess into the pleura bronchus, or a bronchopleural fistula. These constitute indications for operation

Other myobacteria are becoming more and more prevalent in the immunocompromised population. These include *Mycobacterium kansasii*, *intracellulare*, and *avium*. Cavitation with multiple thin-walled cavities are more common than when *Mycobacterium tuberculosis* is the causative organism. However, pleural effusions are uncommon with atypical forms. Patients with atypical mycobacteria are often clinically less ill than their sometimes impressive chest x-rays would imply. With postprimary pulmonary TB (i.e., reactivation TB), the disease is localized primarily to the apical and posterior segments of the upper lobes and the superior segments of the lower lobes, but other areas may be involved as well. The process consists of caseous necrosis which may coalesce, liquify, and empty into a bronchus.

KEY POINTS

- Bacilli are airborne and result in initial pulmonary infection that most often produces primary complex (Ghon's tubercle) with secondary focus of TB in hilar lymph nodes

- Five clinical manifestations of TB are pleural effusion, miliary TB, tuberculous pneumonia, extrapulmonary latent disease, and local erosion

- Cavitation with multiple thin-walled cavities are more common than when *Mycobacterium tuberculosis* is causative organism

BACTERIAL AND FUNGAL INFECTION

In the past, pulmonary infections frequently required surgical intervention. Although still common, medical treatment today is often able to prevent infections from progressing. At least one-half of all cases of pneumonia are bacterial, with most due to pneumococcus. Chronic hospitalized patients on ventilators tend to develop gram-negative or anaerobic lung infections, which may result in lung abscess formation. The most common cause of a lung abscess is aspiration. Other causes include necrotizing pneumonia, bronchial obstruction (from carcinoma or foreign body entrapment), or infection of cysts. The segments of the lung in which aspiration pneumonia and abscess are most common are on the right side, since the right mainstem bronchus leaves the trachea at a more acute posterior angle than does the left mainstem bronchus. Material tends to enter the posterior segment of the right upper lobe or the superior segment of the right lower lobe, as these are the most dependent portions of the lung when lying supine. Bronchiectasis is an infectious dilatation of the bronchial tree. The problem often begins with a pneumonia and is frequently associated with chronic bronchitis. One-half of patients have bilateral disease, which is usually in the lower lobes.

The middle lobe syndrome is a manifestation of partial kinking or obstruction of the middle lobe bronchus. It may also be caused by enlarged sclerotic hilar nodes impinging on the middle lobe orifice, and leads to repeated middle lobe infections.

Mycotic infections of the lung include coccidioidomycosis, histoplasmosis, actinomycosis, aspergillosis, and *Candida pneumonia*. *Coccidioides immitis* is a fungal organism endemic to the Southwest. The spores are inhaled from the soil. One-half of the population living in endemic areas have positive skin tests. Although most are asymptomatic, flu-like symptoms occur in one-third of individuals, and of these, 1% develop a protracted illness. Additionally, there may be pleuritic chest pain, and mucus or bloody sputum. The diagnosis is made by sputum culture. Coccidioidomycosis may result in cavitation of the lung, which can rupture and produce hemoptysis.

Histoplasma capsulatum is found in soil contaminated by bird or bat droppings and occurs most frequently in the Mississippi River valleys. The symptoms of histoplasmosis are similar to TB, although the disease tends to progress less rapidly. Cough, malaise, hemoptysis, weight loss, and fevers may all coexist. It is frequently associated with TB as well. Granulomatous involvement of the mediastinum is quite common and may result in compression of the superior vena cava, middle lobe bronchus, middle lobe syndrome, or dysphagia. It is frequent etiology for broncholithiasis or actual erosion of mediastinal lymph nodes into the bronchus. The severe scarification of the mediastinum may result in traction diverticulum of the esophagus. Histoplasmosis should be considered in the evaluation of a solitary pulmonary nodule.

Actinomyces israelii normally inhabits the human mouth. Immunosuppression may lead to opportunistic infection by this organism involving three forms: cervicofacial, thoracic, or abdominal. All result in a marked fibrotic response, formation of sulfur granules through draining sinuses, or nonspecific pulmonary infiltrates.

Nocardia asteroides is also a slow growing organism and may mimic TB with its acid-fast bacillus. The symptoms of human infection are often flu-like, with empyema developing in 25% of cases. It often forms multiple fistulas and sinuses as does actinomyces. Nocardia may also be a cause of broncholithiasis.

Candida albicans is a normal inhibitant of the human body but may lead to an opportunistic infection, particularly in chronically ventilated, bedridden intensive care unit patients who are malnourished. Candidiasis localized to the bronchopulmonary regions is extremely rare and is usually a terminal event in systemic disease.

Pneumocystis carinii is an opportunistic infection leading to progressive pneumonia and respiratory insufficiency in patients with acquired AIDS or other immunodeficiency syndromes.

Empyema is most often a result of a lung abscess or pneumonia. It also occurs after lobectomy or pneumonectomy. Other causes include spontaneous pneumothorax, retained foreign body, or a subdiaphragmatic process resulting in a supradiaphragmatic empyema. Thoracentesis provides the diagnosis, and depends on the gross characteristics of the effusion and chemical evaluation to distinguish between exudate and transudate. The complexity of an empyema increases dramatically when there has been a previous lung resection, because the nonfilled pleural space makes it much more difficult to eradicate an empyema. Empyemas after lung resection are rare but catastrophic.

KEY POINTS

- At least one-half of all cases of pneumonia are bacterial, with most due to pneumococcus

- Chronic hospitalized patients on ventilators tend to develop gram-negative or anaerobic lung infections, which may result in lung abscess formation; most common cause of lung abscess is aspiration

- Segments of lung in which aspiration pneumonia and abscess most common are on right side, since right mainstem bronchus leaves trachea at more acute posterior angle than does left mainstem bronchus

- Although most patients with mycotic infections are asymptomatic, flu-like symptoms occur in one-third of individuals, and of these, 1% develop protracted illness; diagnosis made by sputum culture

- Symptoms of histoplasmosis are similar to TB, although disease tends to progress less rapidly; should be considered in evaluation of solitary pulmonary node

- Empyema most often results from lung abscess or pneumonia, and also after lobectomy or pneumonectomy; thoracentesis provides diagnosis, and depends on gross characteristics of effusion and chemical evaluation to distinguish between exudate and transudate

DIAGNOSIS

The diagnosis of TB is established by various methods, although a characteristic radiographic pattern and positive PPD skin test strongly suggest and warrant the institution of antitubercular medications. The actual diagnosis requires microscopic visualization of acid-fast bacilli in the sputum, or culture of the organism from the sputum or from nasogastric secretions. Other etiologies of pneumonias and lung abscesses also require actual culture of the organism from the sputum or bronchoscopic brushings or washings. The radiographic manifestations of primary *Mycobacterium tuberculosis* may appear in the pulmonary parenchyma or in the hilar or mediastinal lymph nodes in the pleural space. Parenchymal involvement occurs most often in the midzone of the lung and resembles pneumonia. Cavitation is not common in primary TB. Hilar or paratracheal nodal enlargement may occur in adults but is much more frequent in the young and occurs in nearly all affected children. Effusion on chest x-ray is more common in adults than in children.

The diagnosis of bronchiectasis can be made on radiographic grounds. The computed tomography (CT) scan is characteristic and reveals ectatic dilatations of the obstructed, destroyed bronchial segments. In the past, a bronchogram was performed to diagnose bronchiectasis;

however, the CT scan has nearly obviated the need for this uncomfortable and sometimes dangerous procedure. The diagnosis of middle lobe syndrome can be established by a sequence of radiologic and endoscopic findings, including atelectasis of the middle lobe on chest x-ray, CT scan evidence of compression of the middle lobe bronchus from enlarged sclerotic lymph nodes, and bronchoscopic evidence of compression of the middle lobe orifice with potential erosion into the bronchus from broncholiths.

The diagnosis of mycotic infections relies on a high index of suspicion based on the patient's history and physical examination, including prior travel history. Confirmation of the diagnosis is based on radiographic findings, skin test results, and culture of the organism.

Empyema is diagnosed by sampling the pleural fluid, either by thoracentesis or by chest tube insertion. Either watery fluid or pus is generally obtained. For clear watery fluid, culture and chemistries are obtained. A positive culture implies an empyema. Chemistry evaluation suggests an empyema if the specific gravity is greater than 1.020, white blood count greater than 500/cm³, protein greater than 2.5/dl, pH less than 7.0, glucose less than 40 mg/dl, or lactate dehydrogenase (LDH) greater than 1,000.

Clues to the presence of a lung abscess include development of pulmonary symptoms 1–2 weeks after an aspiration or pneumonia. Symptoms include fever, sweats, chills, and production of foul-smelling, purulent sputum. Hemoptysis is common. Radiographic findings demonstrate an abscess cavity with an air fluid level.

KEY POINTS

- Diagnosis of TB requires microscopic visualization of acid-fast bacilli in sputum, or culture of organism from sputum or from nasogastric secretions

- Diagnosis of bronchiectasis can be made on radiographic grounds; CT scan is characteristic and reveals ectatic dilatations of obstructed, destroyed bronchial segments

- Diagnosis of middle lobe syndrome can be established by sequence of radiologic and endoscopic findings, including atelectasis of middle lobe on chest x-ray, CT scan evidence of compression of middle lobe bronchus from enlarged sclerotic lymph nodes, and bronchoscopic evidence of compression of middle lobe orifice with potential erosion into bronchus from broncholiths

- Chemistry evaluation suggests empyema if specific gravity is greater than 1.020, white blood count greater than 500/cm³, protein greater than 2.5 g/dl, pH less than 7.0, glucose less than 40 mg/dl, or LDH greater than 1,000

DIFFERENTIAL DIAGNOSIS

TB is the great imitator in the chest and should, in general, never be less than second on the list of differential diagnoses for a pulmonary process. Carcinoma may also be an imitator, and one should never assume TB is the cause of a pulmonary lesion unless the possibility of carcinoma has been carefully excluded. Radiographic characteristics of the lesion may be helpful in establishing the etiology. For example, a cavitary lesion is usually an infectious process, either mycobacterial, pyogenic, or fungal. Squamous carcinoma, however, can also present as a cavitary lesion.

The differential diagnosis of empyema is similar to that for any exudate, which must be separated from a transudate that can result from congestive heart failure, nephrotic syndrome, hypoproteinemia, cirrhosis, or myxedema. These disorders usually result in bilateral pleural effusions, although unilateral effusions are possible. They can generally be excluded based on appropriate history, physical examination, and laboratory tests. The differential diagnosis of exudative pleural effusions includes carcinoma, subdiaphragmatic infection, pancreatitis, trauma, and pulmonary infarction. Appropriate laboratory testing is particularly helpful for malignant pleural effusions since cytology of the pleural fluid is usually diagnostic.

KEY POINTS

- Differential diagnosis of exudative pleural effusions includes carcinoma, subdiaphragmatic infection, pancreatitis, trauma, and pulmonary infarction

- Appropriate laboratory testing is particularly helpful for malignant pleural effusions since cytology of pleural fluid is usually diagnostic

TREATMENT

The primary management of TB is medical. Before the availability of antitubercular medications, patients with TB were pulmonary cripples who frequently required deforming chest operations to treat their disease. The management of TB in the modern era has been simplified by the use of antitubercular regimens such as INH (300 mg/day PO) rifampin (600 mg/day IV or PO), and ethambutol (900 mg/day to 15 mg/kg/day). Streptomycin, pyrazinamide, and ethionamide are other antituberculous drugs used infrequently. Atypical mycobacterial infections are generally more refractory to medical management than is *Mycobacterium tuberculosis*.

The indications for operation in TB include the presence of massive pulmonary destruction, hemoptysis, rupture of an abscess into the pleural space or into a bronchus, bronchopleural fistula, the inability to exclude carcinoma, and failure of standard medical management. TB may produce such massive pulmonary destruction that resection is required. This is usually in the form of a lobectomy. Hemoptysis is an important indication for surgical intervention (Case 1).

The sequence of priorities in a patient with hemoptysis is resuscitation followed by chest x-ray. The patient should be placed with the affected side down, to prevent blood from being aspirated into the normal bronchus. Early bronchoscopy should be performed. A balloon catheter is sometimes useful to seal the affected bronchus and prevent aspiration of blood into normal segments. Treatment strategy should include either angiographic embolization of the bleeding pulmonary arterial branch or immediate thoracotomy and lobectomy. Embolization has an initial success rate of 85%; however, bleeding recurs in 25%. There is a danger of spinal cord infarction from intercostal artery embolization. For these reasons, if the patient is sufficiently stable, a lobectomy of the involved lung should be performed. Antitubercular medication should be instituted immediately, as peak levels of the antibiotic can be achieved while the operation is underway. Rupture of a tubercular abscess into the pleural space generally requires chest tube placement at a minimum, followed by resection of the abscess cavity.

The inability to differentiate carcinoma from TB is critical. Carcinoma can form in tubercular cavities. Patients whose radiographic findings do not significantly improve after administration of antituberculous drugs should undergo evaluation for lung carcinoma.

Medical management involves an extended duration of combined antituberculous chemotherapy. Failure of standard medical management is defined as persistent acid-fast bacilli in the sputum after 6 weeks of antibiotic treatment. Even a transient cessation of one drug may result in resurgence of the disease. The management of extrapulmonary TB may require surgical intervention (resection) of the affected organ.

Bacterial infections of the lung and lung abscesses are primarily managed medically. Percussion and postural drainage are particularly important in abscess drainage. Institution of appropriate antibiotics based on the culture of the offending organism is essential. Patients will nearly always respond to such regimens with the abscess cavity diminishing in size within 2 or 3 weeks. Failure of the radiographic picture to improve within this time period frequently leads to the diagnosis of cavitating lung carcinoma. Operation is rarely required for lung abscess unless there is concomitant carcinoma or massive hemoptysis. Medical therapy is successful in over 95% of cases.

Bronchiectasis is a curable disease, although it was previously thought to be irreversible. It will heal with appropriate medical management, which includes percussion, postural drainage, and treatment with appropriate antibiotics. Improvement can usually be documented on repeat CT scan. Surgical intervention (lobectomy) may be necessary for localized severe disease that is refractory to strict medical management.

The treatment of middle lobe syndrome consists of treating the underlying etiology. If the obstruction is extrinsic (such as a mediastinal granuloma), then medical management similar to bronchiectasis is initiated and operation is rarely required. If operation is needed for chronic collapse of the middle lobe with recurring infection, lobectomy is indicated. Another indication for operation is the inability to exclude carcinoma or the finding of carcinoma as the cause of middle lobe syndrome. Most cases of broncholithiasis are adequately managed nonoperatively with or without bronchoscopic removal of the broncholith. Some patients require operation when there is severe hemoptysis or when malignancy cannot be excluded, at which time a lobectomy is usually performed.

Symptomatic coccidioidomycosis may be treated with amphotericin-B or ketoconazole. Resection for cavitary coccidioidomycosis is performed for the same indications as tuberculosis. Histoplasmosis, in symptomatic cases, is treated with a course of amphotericin-B. Cavitary histoplasmosis generally is not effectively treated with antifungal drugs and requires resection. However, preoperative and postoperative amphotericin-B therapy should be instituted. Ketoconazole is an alternative antibiotic with less toxicity. The treatment of aspergillomas (fungus balls) is controversial. Although medical therapy (i.e., amphotericin-B) is often thought to be unsatisfactory, it is used frequently. Aspergillomas generally should be resected. An aspergilloma may erode into a pulmonary artery branch, resulting in severe hemoptysis. Empyemas resulting from aspergillus may require chest tube drainage and possibly resection of the infected lung. Actinomycosis is treated with penicillin. Surgical treatment may be necessary for complications of severely draining sinuses due to *Nocardia asteroides* infections. Sulfadiazine is the treatment of choice. Surgical management is generally restricted to draining empyemas and abscesses. The treatment of candida pulmonary infection is administration of amphotericin-B.

The management of empyema can be difficult and often confusing (Table 54.1). The fundamental questions that must be answered are

1. Is it acute or chronic?
2. Is there dead space that requires obliteration?
3. Is there a bronchopleural fistula?
4. Is this a postoperative problem?

For empyema that does not resolve after pulmonary resection (i.e. following lung abscess or pneumonia), thoracentesis should be performed initially. This accomplishes both therapeutic and diagnostic purposes and distinguishes a transudate from an exudate. Appropriate broad spectrum antibiotics are initiated if exudative or frankly purulent, until identification of the organism allows specific antibiotic regimens to be instituted. Figures 54.1 to 54.3 depict the subsequent management scheme. If the effusion is found to be an empyema, a chest tube is

TABLE 54.1 *Assessment of empyema in the postoperative patient*

Empyema
- Is there adequate drainage?
- Is there a space problem?
- Is there a bronchopleural fistula?
- Is this a postoperative infection?
- Is this acute or chronic?

Drainage procedures
- Chest tube
- Rib resection
- Clagett window/Eloesser flap

Airspace filling procedures
- Thoracoscopy
- Fill space with muscle and omentum

Bronchopleural fistula after surgery
- Early reoperation
- Transpericardial approach to close fistula
- Muscle flap over fistula

placed and connected to suction drainage. After 10 days, this is converted to open drainage as an empyema tube. A sinogram is then obtained by placing radiopaque dye through the chest tube. If no cavity is present, the chest tube can be slowly withdrawn over a period of several days to weeks. If a small cavity is found, and if the chest tube is draining it well, the tube may be slowly withdrawn. If the cavity is not draining well through the chest tube, a new thoracostomy tube should be placed. Alternatively, rib resection is performed to facilitate drainage. If there is a

large cavity that appears to be well drained, the tube may be advanced slowly. If the lung does not re-expand fully, then decortication is indicated 6–8 weeks later. Decortication is a process by which restrictive debris around the lung is removed to allow the lung to expand fully. If there is a large cavity that is not well drained, rib resection is indicated to facilitate drainage, or a Clagett window is performed. A Clagett window involves resection of several ribs and tacking the skin down to the intercostal muscle to permit good drainage through a large space. The physician or nurse, and ultimately the patient, can irrigate and pack this wound. The Eloesser flap is a specific form of drainage in which a tube of skin is literally laid down into the cavity to facilitate drainage.

The management of empyema occurring after lung resection differs somewhat from that of a nonresection empyema. The issues are more complex in terms of filling residual air space with surrounding tissue and the danger of breakdown of suture lines resulting in a bronchopleural fistula. The problem of empyema is more common after a pneumonectomy than after a lobectomy. Generally, following pneumonectomy, an additional procedure is necessary if an empyema occurs, because of the difficulty in eradicating a pleural space infection with so much dead space. Such empyemas are usually managed with a Clagett window, although the space may be packed with omentum or muscle. A bronchopleural fistula changes the management scheme drastically. With early empyema and bronchopleural fistula (i.e., within 6 days postoperatively), chest tube drainage is indicated followed by immediate re-exploration to repair the technical problem. Included in the repair is an intercostal muscle flap. For late post-pneumonectomy empyema with bronchopleural fistula, chest tube drainage is the initial procedure followed by a

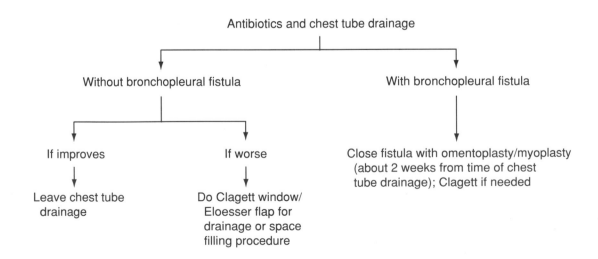

(Empyema with lobectomies can usually be managed simply with chest tube and possibly rib resection)

FIGURE 54.1 *Management of postresection empyema.*

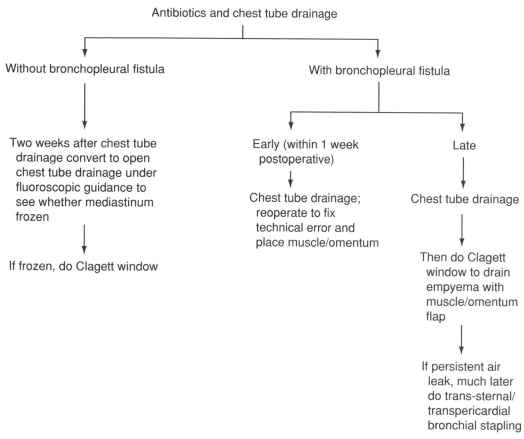

Antibiotics and chest tube drainage

Without bronchopleural fistula

Two weeks after chest tube drainage convert to open chest tube drainage under fluoroscopic guidance to see whether mediastinum frozen

If frozen, do Clagett window

With bronchopleural fistula

Early (within 1 week postoperative)

Chest tube drainage; reoperate to fix technical error and place muscle/omentum

Late

Chest tube drainage

Then do Clagett window to drain empyema with muscle/omentum flap

If persistent air leak, much later do trans-sternal/transpericardial bronchial stapling

FIGURE 54.2   *Management of postpneumonectomy empyema.*

Clagett window to drain the empyema along with a simultaneous muscle flap.

KEY POINTS

• Management of TB in modern era simplified by use of antitubercular regimens such as INH (300 mg/day PO), rifampin (600 mg/day IV or PO), and ethambutol (900 mg/day–15 mg/kg/day)

• Sequence of priorities in a patient with hemoptysis is resuscitation followed by chest x-ray; patient should be placed with affected side down, to prevent blood from aspirating into normal bronchus; early bronchoscopy performed; balloon catheter sometimes useful to seal affected bronchus and prevent aspiration of blood into normal segments

• Embolization has initial success rate of 85%; however, bleeding recurs in 25%

• Inability to differentiate carcinoma from TB is critical; carcinoma can form in tubercular cavities; patients whose radiographic findings do not improve after administration of antituberculous drugs should undergo evaluation for lung carcinoma

• Failure of standard medical management is defined as persistent, acid-fast bacilli in sputum after 6 weeks of antibiotic treatment

• Percussion and postural drainage are particularly important in abscess drainage; institution of appropriate antibiotics based on culture of offending organism is essential; patients will nearly always respond to such regimens with abscess cavity diminishing in size within 2 or 3 weeks

• Medical therapy successful in over 95% of cases

• Symptomatic coccidioidomycosis may be treated with amphotericin-B or ketoconazole

• Treatment of candida pulmonary infection is administration of ampohotericin-B

• For empyema that does not resolve after pulmonary resection (i.e., following lung abscess or pneumonia), thoracentesis should be performed initially

• Generally, following pneumonectomy, additional procedure is necessary if empyema occurs, because of difficulty in eradicating pleural space infection with so much dead space

• With early empyema and bronchopleural fistula (i.e., within 6 days postoperatively), chest tube drainage is indicated followed by immediate re-exploration to repair the technical problem

FOLLOW-UP

Follow-up of TB involves careful radiologic evaluation (bimonthly) of the patient while medication is being given, usually over 9 months to 1 year (Case 1). It is important to

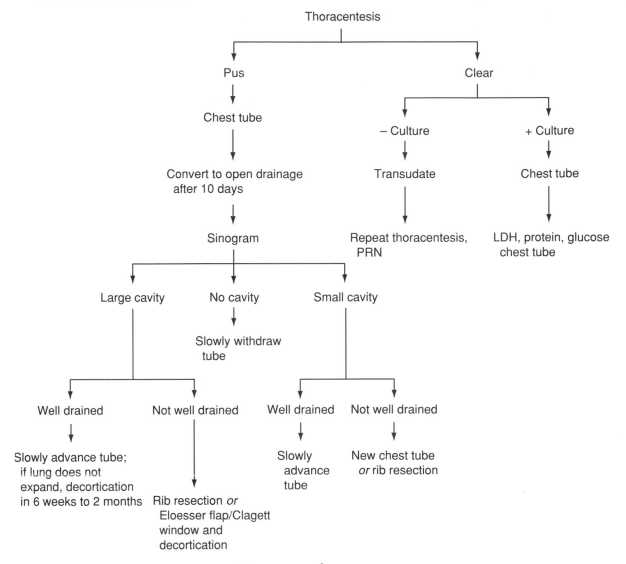

FIGURE 54.3   *Management of nonpostresection empyema.*

obtain sputum cultures to follow the progress of treatment on a routine basis. If there is persistent positive sputum after 6 weeks of presumably adequate medical management, surgical intervention may be necessary. Careful radiologic follow-up is needed also to exclude the presence of a tumor. If there is no response in the radiologic pattern soon after initiation of antitubercular medications, evaluation for carcinoma should be instituted immediately.

Follow-up of patients with pulmonary infections depends on the extent of their disease. If the lung infection results in an abscess without empyema formation, follow-up with chest x-ray on a monthly basis and then biannually after 6 months is acceptable depending on the severity of disease and progress of treatment.

Follow-up of empyema demands scrutiny of not only the radiologic picture, but also withdrawal of the chest tube if open chest drainage has been initiated. Chest tubes converted to open drainage can be withdrawn about 1–2 cm on a weekly basis as an outpatient once it is known that the empyema cavity is indeed closing as documented by sinogram. Repeat CT scans should be performed before removing the chest tube completely to be sure that another cavity not being drained by the chest tube is not present. A plastic bag placed over the chest tube serves as an adequate collection chamber. Generally, chest tubes can be removed over a course of about 2 months. Follow-up should be on a biannual basis or more frequently if necessary.

KEY POINTS

• If no response to radiologic pattern soon after initiation of antitubercular medications, evaluation for carcinoma should be instituted immediately

SUGGESTED READINGS

Barker AF: Bronchiectasis. Sem Thoracic Cardiovasc Surg 7:112, 1995

This article is an excellent tutorial on infectious bronchiectasis. This complex subject is reviewed in depth by the author.

Cordice JW Jr, Chitkara RK: The role of surgery in treating pleuropulmonary suppurative disease—review of 77 cases managed at Queens Hospital Center between 1986 and 1989. J Natl Med Assoc 84:145, 1992

Despite the generally favorable experience in recent years regarding the management of suppurative pleuropulmonary disease, empyemas and lung abscesses are still important surgical problems. This is particularly true in hospitals that serve large numbers of disadvantaged patients. This study from New York describes the etiology, clinical presentation, treatment, and results of therapy of pleuropulmonary disease.

LeMense GP, Strange C, Sahn SA: Empyema thoracis. Chest 107:1532, 1995

This excellent review describes the diagnoses and management of empyema. It is up-to-date and complete and highly recommended.

Nicotra MB: Bronchiectasis. Sem Respir Infect 9:31, 1994

This article is complementary to the one by Barker. It is complete and includes a literature review.

Polkey MI, Rees PJ: Tuberculosis: current issues in diagnosis and treatment. Br J Clin Pract 48:251, 1994

Although the incidence of tuberculosis began to decline in the early 1800s, it has recently emerged as a significant problem. This article reviews the diagnosis and management of tuberculosis. It is an excellent review that contains multiple references for further reading.

QUESTIONS

1. *Empyema occuring after an episode of aspiration pneumonia?*
   A. Is best treated by pulmonary resection.
   B. Should be treated with antibiotics selected on the basis of thoracentesis.
   C. Requires bronchoscopy for diagnosis.
   D. Usually can be treated without a chest tube.

2. *Pulmonary tuberculosis?*
   A. Is usually treated after mediastinoscopy.
   B. Is best treated with thoracoplasty.
   C. Is most commonly due to atypical species.
   D. May cause severe hemorrhage and bronchopleural fistulas.

3. *The most common pulmonary mycotic infection in immunocompromised patients is?*
   A. Histoplasmosis.
   B. Coccidioidmycosis.
   C. *Candida albicans.*
   D. Asperigillosis.

4. *Which of the following is not characteristic of a pulmonary (pleural) exudate?*
   A. High specific gravity.
   B. Low pH.
   C. Low protein.
   D. High glucose.

(See p. 604 for answers.)

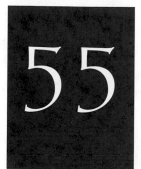

55

THORACIC

TRAUMA

FRED S. BONGARD

FRITZ BAUMGARTNER

The major vascular, respiratory, digestive, and neural structures traversing the chest make it a vulnerable area. The management of thoracic trauma is complex not only because of these major anatomic structures, but also because it must be integrated with the concomitant care of abdominal, neurologic, and orthopaedic injuries.

The purpose of this chapter is to (1) provide an understanding of the types of penetrating and blunt trauma and their presentation, (2) develop an index of suspicion for the presence of life-threatening injuries, and (3) integrate the management of thoracic trauma with injury to other organ systems.

CASE 1
A GUNSHOT WOUND

A 25-year-old male presented to the emergency room after sustaining a single gunshot wound to the left 3rd intercostal space in the midclavicular line. His BP was 50 mmHg with a pulse of 150 bpm. As the patient was intubated, large bore resuscitation catheters were placed in both femoral veins and 2 L of lactated Ringer's solution was infused rapidly. He remained lethargic, although his BP rose to 100 mmHg with a pulse of 120 bpm. He was extremely diaphoretic and ashen. A left chest tube was placed in the 6th intercostal space in the mid-axillary line, which produced 150 ml of blood. A chest x-ray showed a minimal left hemothorax, and a large right hemothorax. A

right tube thoracostomy was placed, which produced 500 ml of blood. A posterior wound was found immediately under the tip of the right scapula. No other injuries were noted. The cardiac shadow on the chest x-ray was normal in size.

Despite continued resuscitation, he had poor capillary refill, distended neck veins, and plethoric facies. Pulsus paradoxus was not evident. In the operating room, a pericardial window showed gross blood with tense pericardial tamponade. A midline median sternotomy was performed, the blood evacuated, and an injury to the left ventricle identified and repaired. The patient's hemodynamics immediately improved with decompression of the tamponade. There were mild bilateral peripheral pulmonary parenchymal injuries that were not bleeding actively and were not repaired further. Flexible bronchoscopy found no evidence of tracheobronchial injury, and esophagoscopy demonstrated no evidence of esophageal injury. A subsequent barium swallow confirmed the absence of esophageal injury.

CASE 2
DISTENDED ABDOMEN AFTER A
CAR WRECK

A 42-year-old male unbelted driver was involved in a car accident from which he had to be extricated. His BP was 80 mmHg in the field and 90 mmHg on arrival to the emergency room. He was unconscious and intubated. Large bore intravenous catheters were placed and saline infusions rapidly given. His abdomen was grossly distended and tense. A chest x-ray showed a hazy mediastinum. After a "one-shot" IVP, a midline laparotomy was performed, revealing a splenic rupture. A splenectomy was performed. A postoperative head CT scan found no evidence of intracranial injury. An aortic arch angiogram was done because of the mechanism of injury and the hazy mediastinum. It demonstrated complete transection of his aorta at the level of the ligamentum arteriosum. He was brought back to the operating room, where an interposition graft was placed in the distal thoracic artery. He recovered uneventfully.

GENERAL CONSIDERATIONS

The *immediately* life-threatening chest injuries include airway obstruction, tension pneumothorax, open pneumothorax, massive hemothorax, flail chest, and cardiac tamponade. Other *potentially* life-threatening injuries include aortic disruption, pulmonary contusion, tracheobronchial rupture, myocardial contusion, esophageal rupture, and diaphragmatic disruption. Hypoxia is the most important life-threatening consequence of chest injury, and the first step in the care of these patients should be to ensure adequate airway control, ventilation, and oxygenation. The management of traumatic airway obstruction varies with the type of trauma. Massive oral and facial injury require cricothyroidotomy or tracheostomy for airway control. Endotracheal intubation in the presence of these injuries is ill-advised and may worsen an already delicate situation by completely disrupting partial injuries. All others should be intubated initially.

The pleural space between the lungs and the chest wall normally is at a slightly negative pressure. This helps overcome the elastic recoil of the lung parenchyma and prevents alveolar collapse at end expiration. An injury to the chest wall or lung that permits air to enter this space removes the pressure gradient (intrapleural pressure becomes equal to atmospheric pressure) and allows the lung to collapse on itself. This "simple" pneumothorax affects respiration because blood is shunted through the collapsed lung without participating in gas exchange. If the contralateral lung is functioning normally, the resultant hypoxia may be minimal with only minor complaints. On physical examination, the affected side will not exhibit breath sounds, and there will be a dullness to percussion because the usually resonant air-filled lung has completely or partially collapsed into a more solid mass. If severe chest wall or pulmonary parenchymal injury occurred, hemorrhage may partially fill the pleural space, resulting in a hemopneumothorax.

An injury to a lung may produce a one-way valve such that air enters the pleural space on inspiration but does not exit on exhalation. Similarly, patients who are receiving positive pressure mechanical ventilation may have air forced through such an injury into the pleural space under relatively high pressure. Unlike a simple pneumothorax, this mechanism causes compression of the lung under supra-atmospheric pressure. The condition is referred to as a tension pneumothorax (Fig. 55.1). It may occur following either blunt or penetrating trauma. The danger of a tension pneumothorax is not only the hypoxia associated with compression of the ipsilateral lung, but also a mediastinal shift that collapses the contralateral lung, and "kinks" the superior and inferior vena cavae. This vascular compression decreases venous return to the heart and results in hypovolemic shock.

An open "sucking" pneumothorax may occur with a large open chest wound. Rapid decompensation results in death in minutes. Equilibration occurs between intrathoracic and atmospheric pressure, resulting in ineffective ventilation because air enters the pleural space from the environment. A flail chest occurs when a portion of the chest wall (ribs) does not have bony continuity with the remainder of the thoracic cage (i.e., when ribs are fractured in two different places and multiple ribs are involved). This leaves the chest wall unstable. The free or "flail" segment now moves in response to underlying pleural pressure, rather than with the chest wall as a whole. As the chest expands during inspiration to decrease intrathoracic pressure, the free segment moves inward while the rest of the ribs move outward. The flail segment, therefore, exhibits "paradoxical" motion. The hypoxia associated with flail chest is less a result of the actual mechanical paradoxical movement and is more related to underlying pulmonary injury and contusion.

Cardiac tamponade is a great imitator and is sometimes difficult to diagnose. Classic findings result from restricted venous return to the heart. Tamponade usually follows penetrating injuries, although it is occasionally caused by blunt injury. Pulsus parodoxus is an inconstant but important finding. This is defined as a decrease in systolic blood pressure by 10 mmHg or more, with inspiration. Physiologically, inspiration increases venous return to the right side of the heart, which shifts the intraventricular septum toward the left side, resulting in decreased volume and filling of the left ventricle. The net result is decreased cardiac output. Normally, the heart is able to distend within the pericardium, but when tamponade occurs, the heart is externally compromised, which allows respiration to affect blood pressure. This is true only for spontaneously breathing patients, as mechanical ventilation provides positive pressure rather than the normal negative pressure of spontaneous breathing (Fig. 55.2).

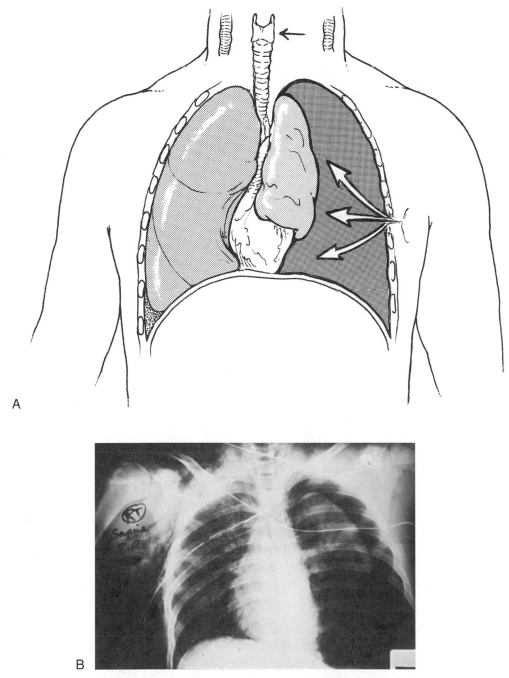

FIGURE 55.1 (*A*) *A tension pneumothorax not only causes ipsilateral lung collapse but also shifts the mediastinum and associated structures to the contralateral side. This causes both respiratory and circulatory embarrassment.* (*B*) *Chest x-ray showing the findings depicted Fig. A. Note how the left lung is displaced to the upper portion of the chest in association with rightward displacement of the mediastinum.*

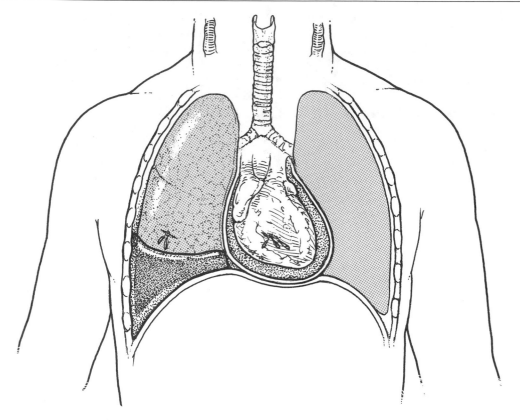

FIGURE 55.2   *Pericardial tamponade is most commonly caused by penetrating injuries of the right or left ventricle. As the indistensible sac fills with blood, venous return is impeded, the heart cannot fill, and the cardiac output decreases. This is an immediately life-threatening condition. The patient shown also has a right hemothorax from a stab wound to the right lower lobe.*

Traumatic rupture of the aorta most commonly occurs just distal to the ligamentum arteriosum in the proximal descending thoracic aorta. It may range from an intimal tear of the aorta to a complete transection, with exsanguinating hemorrhage or containment of the injury by the periadventitial connective tissue, which maintains the aortic lumen. Ninety percent of traumatic ruptures of the aorta are fatal at the time of the accident. Initial survivors can usually be saved if the aortic rupture is identified expeditiously. Of the 10% who survive the initial aortic injury, one-half will die in the hospital if left untreated. Some of these patients may live for years with a traumatic transection of the aorta and not present until much later with a progressive false aneurysm. The most common cause of traumatic aortic injury is the rapid deceleration that occurs when the chest is crushed against the steering wheel during a high speed motor vehicle accident. The downward shear induced during falls from heights may also disrupt the aorta.

Tracheobronchial tree injuries usually occur between the larynx and the subsegmental bronchi. They can result from either blunt or penetrating injury. Generally, segmental and subsegmental bronchial injuries do not require treatment, but laryngeal, tracheal, and mainstem bronchial or lobar injuries must be repaired. Injuries to the trachea may follow blunt deceleration injuries that occur by impacting the chest or neck against the steering wheel. The most common location of tracheobronchial injuries from blunt trauma is within 2.5 cm of the carina (i.e., at the level of a mainstem bronchus). Esophageal trauma may accompany a tracheobronchial injury. Following blunt trauma, this typically manifests several days after the tracheobronchial injury, when necrosis of the anterior portion of the esophageal wall results in a traumatic tracheoesophageal fistula. Esophageal trauma, however, is most commonly caused by penetrating mechanisms such as transmediastinal gunshot wounds and may be difficult to diagnose.

Myocardial contusion has traditionally been overrated in importance. Although blunt cardiac injury can lead to rupture of the heart and death (which is immediately evident), simple contusion does not result in major life threatening hemodynamic sequelae. On occasion, it may cause severe myocardial dysfunction and/or arrhythmias. In general, a patient with blunt chest trauma who has no evidence of electrocardiographic (ECG) changes on his initial ECG has an extremely low risk of developing future arrhythmias related to a myocardial contusion. Right ventricular dysfunction may occur since the right ventricle is the most anterior portion of the heart and is most susceptible to compression from a direct sternal blow. Diagnostic studies (such as echocardiography) are usually not indicated.

- Immediately life-threatening chest injuries include airway obstruction, tension pneumothorax, open pneumothorax, massive hemothorax, flail chest, and cardiac tamponade

- Potentially life-threatening injuries include aortic disruption, pulmonary contusion, tracheobronchial rupture, myocardial contusion, esophageal rupture, and diaphragmatic disruption

- Hypoxia is most important life-threatening consequence of chest injury; first step in care should be to ensure adequate airway control, ventilation, and oxygenation

- On physical examination, affected side will not exhibit breath sounds, and there will be a dullness to percussion because the usually resonant air-filled lung has completely or partially collapsed into a more solid mass

- Tension pneumothorax causes compression of lung under supra-atmospheric pressure; danger is not only hypoxia associated with compression of ipsilateral lung, but also mediastinal shift that collapses the contralateral lung, and "kinks" the superior and inferior vena cavae; this vascular compression decreases venous return to the heart and results in hypovolemic shock

- Flail chest occurs when a portion of chest wall does not have bony continuity with remainder of thoracic cage; this leaves chest wall unstable; the flail segment now moves in response to underlying pleural pressure, rather than with the chest wall as a whole; as chest expands during inspiration to decrease intrathoracic pressure, free segment moves inward while rest of ribs move outward, exhibiting "paradoxical" motion

- Pulsus paradoxus is inconstant but important finding, defined as decrease in systolic blood pressure by 10 mmHg or more with inspiration

- Traumatic rupture of aorta most commonly occurs just distal to ligamentum arteriosum in proximal descending thoracic aorta; initial survivors can usually be saved if aortic rupture is identified expeditiously; of 10% who survive initial aortic injury, one-half will die in hospital if untreated

- Tracheobronchial tree injuries usually occur between larynx and subsegmental bronchi; most common location is within 2.5 cm of carina

- Patient with blunt chest trauma and no evidence of ECG changes has extremely low risk of developing future arrhythmias related to myocardial contusion

DIAGNOSIS

Airway obstruction and respiratory compromise are always the most important and immediate concerns. Patients with facial or cervical trauma must be approached with extreme caution because attempts to insert an endotracheal tube may result in complete transection of a partially torn trachea. Stridor is the key to diagnosis. Those with airway obstruction will be stridorous and lying or sitting in a position of maximum comfort. They must not be forced into the supine position, but rather should be allowed to remain sitting or leaning to minimize discomfort. Palpation of the neck and chest may reveal crepitus, which should also arouse suspicion of an associated tracheobronchial injury. A chest x-ray typically reveals marked subcutaneous emphysema and a pneumothorax (Fig. 55.3). Flexible bronchoscopy by an experienced operator will confirm the diagnosis. An endotracheal tube threaded over the bronchoscope may be placed at the time of examination. The procedure must be done under carefully controlled conditions and must never be attempted haphazardly by a novice. If the patient deteriorates, cannot be transported to the operating room for bronchoscopy, or is in distress, immediate tracheostomy or cricothyroidotomy is indicated. Bronchscopy can be performed later to establish the diagnosis.

A pneumothorax should be suspected based on the mechanism of injury and clinical presentation. Penetrating injuries most commonly produce a pneumothorax, although blunt trauma-created rib fractures are often responsible. The presentation depends on the type of pneumothorax as well as associated injuries that may distract the examiner's attention. A simple pneumothorax in a young person may produce few signs or symptoms, while an older person may complain of severe respiratory distress and be markedly dyspneic. Dullness to percussion and decreased breath sounds are the usual findings. When a hemothorax is present, blood loss into the chest may reach several units of blood and produce signs of systemic hypotension. Tension pneumothorax is life threatening and presents with distended neck veins, displaced trachea (away from the injured side) dyspnea, hypotension, decreased breath sounds, and hyperresonance to percussion. Patients who are hypovolemic from blood loss elsewhere may not have distended neck veins. If a tension pneumothorax is suspected, a decompressing catheter (large bore intravenous cannulae) should be placed, based on clinical findings, before a chest x-ray is obtained. In the case of a simple hemopneumothorax, a chest x-ray is indicated and will help to confirm the diagnosis. There are times, however, when the chest x-ray may be misleading. Complete transections of the trachea or mainstem bronchus, or cardiac rupture with tamponade can occur with a "normal" chest x-ray. Cardiac tamponade presents like tension pneumothorax, with distended neck veins, hypotension, tachycardia, muffled heart tones, pulsus paradoxus, and obvious distress. Unlike tension pneumothorax, breath sounds are normal, the trachea is not deviated, and respiratory distress is not present.

Cardiac tamponade may be overdiagnosed in trauma patients who have had massive and excessive volume resuscitation resulting in overhydration with distention of the neck veins. It is frequently erroneously assumed that blunt or penetrating injury of the heart with cardiac tamponade will result in dilatation of the cardiac shadow. This does not occur since the pericardium is nondistensible. A patient in distress with elevated neck veins and high cen-

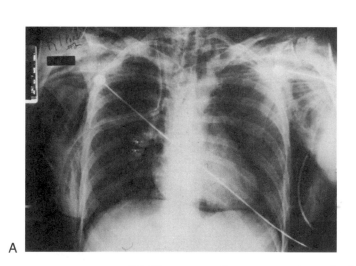

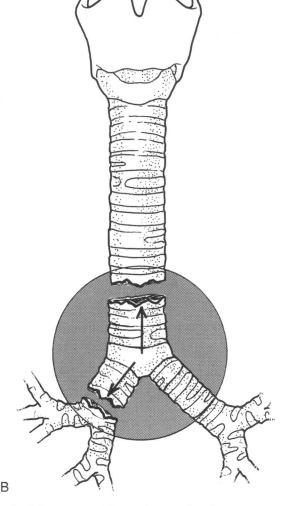

FIGURE 55.3   *(A) Chest x-ray of a patient with tracheobronchial disruption. Notice the streaks of air in the soft tissue, which even reach to the axilla. (B) A diagrammatic represention of a tracheobronchial disruption. Most take place within 2 cm of the carina, as shown here.*

tral venous pressure should be suspected of having cardiac tamponade despite a normal cardiac shadow.

The physical findings of aortic rupture at the ligamentum arteriosum from blunt trauma include diminished blood pressure in the left upper extremity compared to the right upper, due to a hematoma compressing the left subclavian artery. Rarely, lower extremity pulses may be diminished. The radiologic manifestations can be subtle or characteristic. Widening of the mediastinum and blunting of the aortic knob are the two most common and most reliable characteristics of blunt traumatic aortic injury on chest x-ray (Fig. 55.4). These two findings may be present normally in obese individuals. Therefore, it is useful to obtain a second chest x-ray with the patient sitting upright (assuming the spine is stable and the patient is not hypotensive), to determine whether the mediastinum normalizes and a sharp aortic knob is visualized. Depression of the left mainstem bronchus, a pleural apical cap, and deviation of the nasogas-

tric tube to the right are other common radiographic findings. Aortography is the most accurate method available for the diagnosis of aortic disruption (Fig. 55.5). Although CT scans have gained popularity for this purpose, they still are not as reliable as angiography. Because sudden rupture carries a high risk of death from exsanguination, arch aortography should always be performed in patients with widened mediastinal silhouettes on plain x-ray.

The diagnosis of esophageal injury is made by endoscopy or by esophagography. Esophagoscopy may use either a flexible or a rigid endoscope. If esophagoscopy is uninformative, but there is a high clinical index of suspicion, esophagography with water soluble contrast should be performed. Gastrografin is preferred to barium because, if there is a leak, Gastrografin will be less toxic to the mediastinum. If the Gastrografin study is negative, it should be followed by a barium swallow that provides finer detail and resolution.

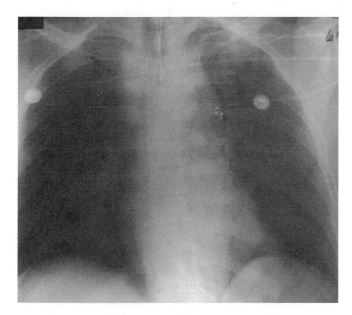

FIGURE 55.4 *Chest x-ray of a patient with blunt aortic injury demonstrating the characteristic widened mediastinum (greater than 8 cm across at the tracheal bifurcation) and the indistinct aortic knob.*

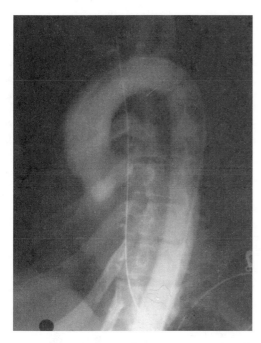

FIGURE 55.5 *Aortogram showing a transverse line across the aorta just below the origin of the left subclavian artery. The contrast distal to this point becomes less concentrated. These are classic findings of a (descending) aortic disruption.*

KEY POINTS

• Patients with facial or cervical trauma must be approached with extreme caution, because attempts to insert endotracheal tube may result in complete transection of partially torn trachea; stridor key to diagnosis—those with airway obstruction will be stridorous and lying or sitting in a position of maximum comfort; they must not be forced into supine position

• Simple pneumothorax in young person may produce few signs or symptoms; older person may complain of severe respiratory distress and be markedly dyspneic; dullness to percussion and decreased breath sounds are usual findings; when hemothorax presents, blood loss into chest may reach several units of blood and produce systemic hypotension

• Tension pneumothorax is life threatening and presents with distended neck veins, displaced trachea, dyspnea, hypotension, decreased breath sounds, and hyperresonance to percussion; patients who are hypovolemic from blood loss elsewhere may not have distended neck veins

• If tension pneumothorax suspected, a decompressing chest catheter should be placed based on clinical findings

• Cardiac tamponande presents like tension pneumothorax, with distended neck veins, hypotension, tachycardia, muffled heart tones, pulsus paradoxus, and obvious distress; unlike tension pneumothorax, breath sounds are normal, trachea not deviated, and respiratory distress not present

• Blunt or penetrating injury of the heart with cardiac tamponade will not result in dilatation of cardiac shadow

• Widening of mediastinum and blunting of aortic knob are two most common and most reliable characteristics of blunt traumatic aortic injury on chest x-ray (Fig. 55.4)

• Aortography is most accurate method available for diagnosis of aortic disruption (Fig. 55.5); because sudden rupture carries high risk of death from exsanguination, arch aortography should always be performed in patients with widened mediastinal silhouettes on plain x-ray

• Diagnosis of esophageal injury made by endoscopy and esophagography

DIFFERENTIAL DIAGNOSIS

The different types of chest injury are distinct and require early recognition so that appropriate therapy can be instituted. For example, a patient who sustains blunt chest trauma and is in shock, distended neck veins may be due to either a blunt cardiac injury with tamponade, or to a tension pneumothorax with mediastinal shift and impeded venous return to the heart. Rapid physical examination will demonstrate the absence of breath sounds on one side, tympany to percussion, and respiratory distress if tension pneumothorax is the cause. Treatment must be instituted before obtaining a chest x-ray if there are diminished breath sounds, since delay may be fatal. If a tube thoracostomy or decompressing catheter is placed when the patient does not have a tension pneumothorax, it can be removed shortly thereafter. It is far better to place an unnecessary tube thoracostomy than to delay one needed critically. Apparent "cardiac tamponade" may be caused by overzealous fluid resuscitation. This typically occurs in a young trauma patient with minimal injuries, and results in distention of neck veins. A central venous catheter helps establish a diagnosis of elevated central venous pressure, although the etiology may not be immediately apparent.

TREATMENT

The treatment of chest trauma begins with initial resuscitation, during which the airway is secured. This may require cricothyroidotomy for massive orofacial injuries, or fiberoptic bronchoscopy with endotracheal intubation over the bronchoscope in cases of tracheal injury. If the patient is asphyxiating and a flexible fiberoptic bronchoscope is not immediately available, emergency cricothyroidotomy should be performed immediately.

The patient who clinically has a tension pneumothorax and is hemodynamically compromised should be managed by immediate insertion of a large bore intravenous catheter (16 gauge or larger) into the chest through the 2nd intercostal space at the midclavicular line. If this results in a release of air, the diagnosis of tension pneumothorax is confirmed and a formal tube thoracostomy can be placed. The needle should not be placed too far medially (i.e., parasternally), lest the internal mammary artery be injured. A chest tube should be inserted for all patients with a pneumothorax after blunt or penetrating trauma, because these pneumothoraces frequently enlarge subsequently, when a physician may not be immediately available. Also, the patient may require operation and undergo intubation with positive pressure ventilation, which will increase the size of the pneumothorax. A chest tube for a traumatic pneumothorax should be placed posteriorly in the mid- or posterior axillary line, with the tube directly posterior to permit drainage of any blood that may have accumulated. An open pneumothorax is best managed immediately with a large vaseline gauze placed to overlap the wound edges. This is anchored firmly on three sides, leaving one side open to create a one-way "flap" valve, so that trapped air inside the pleural space can be expelled, without permitting air to enter from the outside. A chest tube should be placed and expeditious operative management performed to close the chest wound. When a hemothorax is present, a "cell saver" collection apparatus should be used so that blood can be transfused back to the patient. Operation should be performed for immediate loss of 1,500 ml or more of blood on placement of a chest tube. Blood loss exceeding 1,000 ml over the first hour, or more than 500 ml each hour over the next 2 hours, or more than 250 ml each hour over the next 3 hours are all indications for thoracotomy, since a surgically correctable problem can usually be identified.

Pericardiocentesis should rarely, if ever, be performed following trauma. For suspected tamponade with hemodynamic compromise, the patient should undergo an operative subxiphoid window to permit visual inspection of the pericardial sac and heart. In extreme cases, a left anterolateral thoracotomy with decompression of the tamponade should be performed in the emergency room. The most important aspect of the initial management of cardiac tamponade is adequate intravenous volume resuscitation. This increases the preload of the heart and offsets the compressive effect of the tamponade.

Management of traumatic disruption of the aorta is surgical. The affected portion is replaced with a Dacron prosthetic graft (Fig. 55.6). Paralysis of the lower extremities is the major complication (<5%) because the procedure interferes with blood flow to the spinal cord. Generally, spinal cord protection methods are not necessary.

Tracheobronchial injuries require early intervention. Fifty percent of deaths from this injury occur within 1 hour after trauma. If the patient survives the initial injury, the chance of subsequent serious complications is extremely high, which include persistent atelectasis with pneumonia, bronchiectasis, empyema, stenosis, and stricture of the injured segment. A patient with major tracheobronchial injuries will eventually develop a pneumothorax or subcutaneous emphysema. The initial management should be directed at securing the airway, either by cricothyroidotomy or endotracheal intubation over a flexible bronchoscope. A chest tube is inserted if there is evidence of pneumothorax. If there is a large air leak with subcutaneous emphysema, a tracheobronchial injury should be suspected. Flexible bronchoscopy should be performed, preferably in the operating room, to identify the tracheobronchial injury. If one is found, operative repair should be done at that time.

The management of traumatic esophageal injury is early thoracotomy and primary repair with placement of a pleural flap over the injury. The management of pulmonary contusion consists predominantly of mechanical ventilation.

Trauma involving the chest, abdomen, and neurologic systems requires aggressive and skillful diagnosis and management. General priorities must be established. Abdominal trauma should take precedence over all other injuries except those involving the airway and breathing. A surgically correctable problem in the abdomen is a much more common source of shock than a surgically correctable problem in the chest or brain.

KEY POINTS

- Patient who clinically has tension pneumothorax and is hemodynamically compromised should be managed by immediate insertion of large bore intravenous catheter (16 gauge or larger) into chest through 2nd intercostal space of midclavicular line

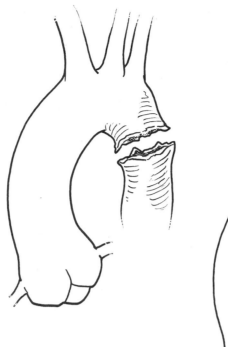
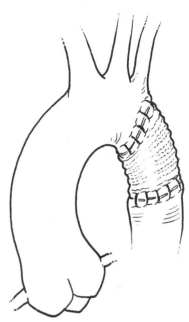

FIGURE 55.6 *Descending thoracic aortic injuries are repaired by inserting a prosthetic graft into the defect created by the injury. This procedure carries a 2–5% incidence of paraplegia because clamping of the aorta during the operation interrupts flow to the spinal artery, which brings blood to the spinal cord.*

- Pericardiocentesis should rarely, if ever, be performed following trauma; for suspected tamponade with hemodynamic compromise, patient should undergo operative subxiphoid window to permit visual inspection of pericardial sac and heart; most important aspect for initial management of cardiac tamponade is adequate intravenous volume resuscitation

- Initial management should be directed at securing airway, either by cricothyroidotomy or endotracheal intubation over flexible bronchoscope

- Abdominal trauma should take precedence over all other injuries, except those involving airway and breathing

FOLLOW-UP

The inpatient management of a tube thoracostomy following trauma depends on the volume of drainage and whether air continues to leak from the pleural space. A chest evacuation device has three chambers, one for collection of fluid, a water seal, and a suction regulator. Output from the chest should be quantitated daily. When there is no evidence of air leak in the water seal chamber, the device is removed from suction. Simple water seal should be maintained for 12–24 hours more to ensure that the lung remains fully expanded and that an air leak does not recur. A chest x-ray should be obtained before removing the chest tube, and repeated several hours later to ensure that the pneumothorax has not reaccumulated.

SUGGESTED READINGS

Minard G, Kudsk KA, Croce MA et al. Laryngotracheal trauma. Am Surg 58:181, 1992

This article reviews the mechanisms, diagnosis, and treatment of laryngotracheal trauma. It contains valuable information about an infrequently seen but very dangerous injury.

Symbas PN, Justicz AG, Ricketts RR: Rupture of the airways from blunt trauma: treatment of complex injuries. Ann Thoracic Surg 54:177, 1992

Tracheobronchial injuries usually result from blunt trauma and are often a complex constellation of individual injuries. This paper summarizes 183 cases of airway rupture previously reported in the literature. Additionally, it discusses the diagnosis and repair of these injuries.

Weiman DS, Walker WA, Brosnan KM et al: Noniatrogenic esophageal trauma. Ann Thorac Surg 59:845, 1995

Early diagnosis and proper management are essential if good outcome is to be expected in management of patients with esophageal trauma. These injuries are particularly treacherous and require careful diagnosis and management to avoid empyema and death.

QUESTIONS

1. *Which of the following is not characteristic of pericardial tamponade?*
   A. Hypotension.
   B. Tachycardia.
   C. Distended neck veins.
   D. Tympany on thoracic percussion.

2. *The test of choice to diagnose an aortic arch rupture is?*
   A. A CT scan.
   B. An aortogram.
   C. An ultrasound.
   D. A thallium scan.

3. *For a suspected tension pneumothorax, the initial management consists of?*
   A. Inserting a 16-gauge angiocatheter in the pleural space.
   B. Inserting a 32 F chest tube.
   C. Intubation and mechanical ventilation
   D. A confirmatory chest x-ray.

4. *Which one of the following injuries should be managed first?*
   A. Splenic disruption.
   B. Diaphragmatic injury.
   C. Esophageal tear.
   D. Thoracic aortic dissection.

(See p. 604 for answers.)

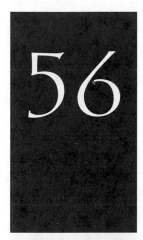

56

MAJOR RESPIRATORY

DIFFICULTIES IN

THE NEWBORN

THOMAS C. MOORE

Respiratory distress in the newborn may result from airway obstruction, reduction in lung volume, or parenchymal disease. The newborn is an obligate nose breather, and the airway is small and soft. The major causes of respiratory difficulty are intrathoracic.

This chapter reviews several of the major causes of infantile respiratory distress, including (1) esophageal atresia and tracheoesophageal fistula, (2) congenital diaphrag-

matic hernia, (3) pulmonary sequestration, (4) congenital lobar emphysema, and (5) congenital cystic adenomatoid malformation. All of these can present with cyanosis shortly after birth, making knowledge of their pathophysiology particularly important in arriving at the correct diagnosis and management.

CASE 1
A CHOKING NEWBORN

A female newborn (39-week gestation, complicated by polyhydramnios) began coughing and choking shortly after birth. Although she was suctioned repeatedly with a bulb aspirator, she continued to salivate excessively and gag on her secretions. For a few moments, she became deeply cyanotic, but regained her pink color with vigorous suctioning. There were rhonchi and gurgling in both lung fields on auscultation and a loud cardiac murmur.

Her abdomen became distended within a few hours after delivery. Attempts to place a small nasogastric tube failed when the catheter would not pass. A plain radi-

ograph showed air in the stomach, with the nasogastric tube coiled in the midthoracic portion of the esophagus. Because only a short segment of esophagus was absent, she underwent early surgery with primary anastomosis of the proximal and distal esophageal segments.

CASE 2
WORSENING CYANOSIS AND A
DISTENDING ABDOMEN

A male infant seemed fine at birth, but over the next 24 hours he became progressively dyspneic and cyanotic. His abdominal girth increased, almost in direct proportion to how much he cried. There were no breath sounds on the left and normal sounds on the right. A chest/abdominal x-ray demonstrated a hazy left hemithorax with a large air bubble. A nasogastric tube was inserted, and a subsequent radiograph showed the tip of the tube was lying in the left chest.

Despite an oxygen face tent, his cyanosis worsened, requiring endotracheal intubation and mechanical ventilation. High airway pressures necessitated readjustment of the ventilator to deliver small tidal volumes at high respiratory rates. An arterial blood gas was pH, 7.22; $PaCO_2$, 55 mmHg; and PaO_2, 70 mmHg on 100% oxygen. Sodium bicarbonate was given intravenously, and the respiratory rate increased even more. A vasodilatator improved the situation somewhat, but ECMO was ultimately required when his PaO_2 level deteriorated even further. Despite aggressive support, the extreme pulmonary hypoplasia prevented weaning from ECMO and he died 2 weeks later.

GENERAL CONSIDERATIONS

One of the great triumphs in pediatric surgery has been the repair of esophageal atresia and tracheoesophageal fistulas, which were once uniformly fatal malformations. The mortality rates have progressively decreased due to advances in diagnosis, surgical technique, anesthesia, and neonatal care.

The incidence of esophageal atresia is about 1 in 3,000 births. There is a strong familial incidence with cases occurring in twins, siblings, and children of parents born with esophageal atresia. However, no specific genetic mechanism has yet been determined.

Esophageal atresia occurs in several forms. In the most common cases a fistula connects the trachea to a portion of the esophageal remnant. In this type, air can pass through the fistula from the trachea into the stomach. A number of classification systems exist, but all may be divided into "air-in-the-stomach" and "no-air-in-the-stomach" categories, where the presence of air is indicative of a fistula. The "air-in-the-stomach" variety is the most common, occurring in approximately 85% of cases (Case 1). Almost all have a blind upper esophageal pouch, with a fistula connecting the trachea and the distal esophagus. Among the "no-air-in-the-stomach" variety, 92% are due to proximal esophageal atresia without a tracheoesophageal fistula. About 4% of all cases have a fistula without atresia forming an H-type variation (Fig. 56.1).

Approximately one-half of infants born with esophageal atresia have additional congenital malformations. This association has been termed the VACTERL syndrome, which consists of malformations in any of the following areas: *v*ertebral, *a*nal, *c*ardiac, *t*racheo*e*sophageal, *r*adial (and/or *r*enal) and *l*imbs. Although associated, these anomalies do not necessarily all occur in any given case. Cardiac problems (Case 1) and imperforate anus are the most commonly found additional malformations.

A maternal history of hydramnios or polyhydramnios may be the first clue in the diagnosis of a child with esophageal atresia. Excessive levels of amniotic fluid are indicative of a blockage of the upper gastrointestinal system, which interferes with the baby's ability to swallow amniotic fluid. Prenatal ultrasonography assists in antenatal diagnosis. A child that froths at the mouth and is unable to swallow shortly after birth should be suspected of having esophageal atresia. Other findings include repeat episodes of coughing, choking, and cyanosis. Feeding may provoke these symptoms. Attempts to pass a nasogastric tube are met with resistance as the tube curls in the proximal esophageal pouch (Case 1). Abdominal distention results from air passing through the tracheoesophageal fistula into the stomach, while a scaphoid abdomen suggests esophageal atresia without a fistula. An upright roentgenogram of the entire abdomen should be taken. The position of the nasogastric tube will demonstrate the esophageal atresia and may also suggest associated anomalies such as gastrointestinal atresias or malrotations and skeletal disorders. The use of contrast materials should be avoided because they may be aspirated into the lungs. Although additional malformations such as imperforate anus and radial dysplasia can be seen, an echocardiogram is required to evaluate cardiac anomalies. Diagnosis of the H-type fistula without atresia is more difficult. A child that coughs or chokes during feeding with frequent pneumonitis should undergo cinefluoroscopy to determine the presence of a fistula. Bronchoscopy is also useful.

Congenital diaphragmatic hernias occur when the transverse septum fails to fuse completely during the 8th week of embryonic development. Some congenital diaphragmatic hernias may be diagnosed antenatally by ultrasound. Although it may be difficult to detect abdominal viscera in the chest, polyhydramnios, mediastinal displacement, and absence of an intra-abdominal stomach silhouette are clues to the diagnosis.

The most common form of congenital diaphragmatic hernia is the posterolateral (Bochdalek) type, which occurs through a defect in the pleuroperitoneal membrane. These hernias are found on the left side in over 80% of patients. Right-sided hernias are less common and less severe because the liver prevents bowel from passing into the thorax. Bilateral defects are extremely uncommon. Hernias may rarely occur through an anterior defect in the foramen of Morgagni.

The stomach, small bowel, colon, spleen, and left hepatic lobe may all enter the pleural cavity through a left-sided diaphragmatic defect, while the liver, small bowel, and colon are found in right-sided hernias. A hernia sac is found in about 20% of cases, since the viscera enter the pleural cavity before the pleuroperitoneal membrane is fused. While a sac is uncommon in Bochdalek hernias, it is typically present in hernias through the foramen of Morgagni.

The most serious defect associated with a congenital diaphragmatic hernia is hypoplasia of the ipsilateral lung. This results from compression of the pulmonary parenchyma by the visceral contents of the hernia and the contralateral displacement of the mediastinum. The degree of lung hypoplasia determines the infant's chance for survival (Case 2). After birth, attempts at lung re-expansion

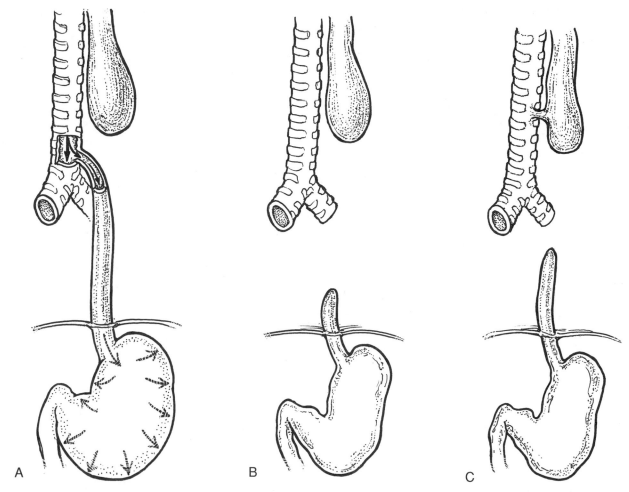

FIGURE 56.1. *(A) The most common type of esophageal atresia includes a tracheoesophageal fistula that allows air to pass into the stomach (arrows). As the child cries, air fills the stomach and distends the abdomen. (B) The second most common type has "no air in the stomach" and consists of a blind proximal esophageal pouch. A proximal (diverting) esophagostomy should be performed quickly so that the child does not aspirate saliva. (C) A proximal fistula with either a complete or an incomplete esophagus forms the H-type fistulas. These are relatively uncommon.*

with mechanical ventilation must be gentle, since excessive force will overdistend the hypoplastic lung resulting in rupture and tension pneumothorax.

Postnatally, infants with congenital diaphragmatic hernia develop dyspnea and cyanosis, which worsens as swallowed air further distends the herniated stomach (Case 2). Respiratory distress manifests as gasping respirations and cyanosis. Infants with respiratory distress within 6 hours of birth are most likely to have severe lung hypoplasia and a lower chance of survival. These infants have minimal normal lung tissue and decreased pulmonary reserve, hence their respiratory insufficiency manifests rapidly. Dextrocardia and lack of breath sounds on the left side are strong indications of a diaphragmatic hernia. Auscultation of bowel sounds in the chest with a scaphoid abdomen should arouse suspicion. An upright plain film of the chest and abdomen will demonstrate intestinal gas patterns in

the chest and rightward displacement of the mediastinum (Case 2). Radiography will not be helpful if insufficient air has entered the bowel. Congenital diaphragmatic hernia may be differentiated from cystic adenomatoid malformations of the lung and mediastinal cysts by the finding of an intestinal gas pattern in the chest.

A portion of the lung receiving an arterial blood supply but unconnected to the bronchial tree is said to be sequestered. An extralobar sequestration occurs when the anomalous lung tissue is separate from the normal lung, while an intralobar sequestration lies within the lung. Extralobar sequestrations are typically asymptomatic and can be found in the chest or in the abdomen. They are often discovered accidentally during diaphragmatic hernia repairs or other thoracic procedures. Unless the sequestration is large enough to cause respiratory difficulties, it will likely go unnoticed.

Intralobar sequestrations usually occur in the lower lobes and may include only a portion or the whole lobe. The sequestered lung often receives its blood supply from the thoracic or abdominal aorta or from the intercostal arteries. An entire lung may be sequestered. Although cystic malformations and inflammation are uncommon in extralobar sequestrations, they are common occurrences with intralobar sequestrations.

Diagnosis of extralobar sequestrations is often accidental, occurring during other operations. A plain radiograph will show what appears to be a mediastinal tumor. Intralobar sequestrations should be suspected in patients with recurrent respiratory infections or pneumonia. Pulmonary aniography will show the anomalous blood supply to the sequestered lung tissue. A computed tomography (CT) scan also demonstrates the sequestrum as well as its blood supply.

Congenital lobar emphysema manifests as gross overinflation of the lung. This typically involves a single pulmonary lobe. The lobe is unable to deflate due to bronchial obstruction, which is often caused by bronchomalacia (deficient bronchial cartilage). This leads to collapse of the bronchus, aspirated mucus, and bronchial atresia. Congenital heart malformations are commonly associated. The condition is relatively rare and occurs more frequently in boys than in girls.

Respiratory difficulties resulting from congenital lobar emphysema become apparent within 4 weeks of birth in 50% of patients. Symptoms include dyspnea, coughing, and wheezing. In more advanced cases, cyanosis is present. Physical examination reveals absent or diminished breath sounds, hyperresonance to percussion on the affected side, and mediastinal shift to the contralateral side. The affected lobe is more translucent on chest radiographs. In the case of an emphysematous upper lobe, the shadow of the collapsed lower lobe may be seen. Similarly, with an affected right middle lobe, opaque areas representing the compressed upper and lower lobes are evident. In all cases, a mediastinal shift is apparent. In some instances, radiographs taken shortly after birth will show an enlarged but opaque lung due to retention of fetal pulmonary fluid. Studies over several days demonstrate resolution of the opacity as the translucent lung becomes evident. Chylothorax, diaphragmatic hernia, and congenital adenomatoid degenerative disease must be differentiated. Bronchography and bronchoscopy should be avoided as they may damage the bronchial tree and cause worsened air trapping.

Often confused with congenital lobar emphysema, congenital adenomatoid malformation (CAM) is characterized by multiple variably sized pulmonary cysts without bronchial cartilage or glands. The air and fluid-filled cysts often occupy an entire lobe and may occur throughout the entire lung. Bilateral cases are rare. Patients with CAM typically present within 3 months of birth. Those with malformations encompassing larger portions of the lung present earlier. Three types of CAM have been identified. Type I contains single or multiple cysts greater than 1 cm in diameter. Type II (intermediate CAM) consists of multiple small cysts with diameters less than 1 cm each. Type III consists of solid bronchial and alveolar structures. Associated malformations include the prune belly syndrome and pectus excavatum, but are rare.

Postnatally, cysts may enlarge as they entrap greater volumes of air. Expansion of the affected lobe often leads to respiratory distress, which occurs with intralobar pulmonary sequestration and congenital lobar emphysema (dyspnea, coughing, and eventual cyanosis). Because of the multiple air and fluid levels observed on chest x-rays, CAM mimics diaphragmatic hernia radiographically. Radiographs showing the full abdomen are required to demonstrate the normal abdominal gas pattern in CAM. Physical and radiographic findings may prove indistinguishable from those of lobar emphysema, and the distinction is often not made until operation.

KEY POINTS

- Newborns are obligate nose breathers, and the airway is small and soft

- Incidence of esophageal atresia is 1 in 3,000 births

- In most cases, fistula connects trachea to portion of esophageal remnant; in this case, air passes through fistula from trachea into stomach

- "Air-in-the-stomach" variety atresia is most common (85%); almost all have blind upper esophageal pouch with fistula connecting trachea and distal esophagus

- Among "no-air-in-the-stomach" variety, 92% are due to proximal esophageal atresia without tracheoesophageal fistula

- Cardiac problems and imperforate anus most commonly found additional malformations

- A child that froths at the mouth and is unable to swallow shortly after birth should be suspected of having esophageal atresia; other findings include repeat episodes of coughing, choking, and cyanosis

- Abdominal distention results from air passing through tracheoesophageal fistula into the stomach, while a scaphoid abdomen suggests esophageal atresia without a fistula

- Although it may be difficult to detect abdominal viscera in the chest, polyhydramnios, mediastinal displacement, and absence of intra-abdominal stomach silhouette are clues to diagnosis of diaphragmatic hernia

- Most common form of congenital diaphragmatic hernia is posterolateral (Bochdalek) type, which occurs through defect in pleuroperitoneal membrane; these hernias are found on left side in over 80% of patients

- Most serious defect associated with congenital diaphragmatic hernia is hypoplasia of ipsilateral lung; degree of lung hypoplasia determines infant's chance for survival

- Postnatally, infants with congenital diaphragmatic hernia develop dyspnea and cyanosis, which worsen as swallowed air further distends herniated stomach; infants with respiratory distress within 6 hours of birth most likely to have severe lung hypoplasia and lower chance of survival
- Portion of lung receiving arterial blood supply but unconnected to bronchial tree said to be sequestered; sequestered lung often receives its blood supply from the thoracic or abdominal aorta or from the intercostal arteries
- Congenital lobar emphysema manifests as gross overinflation of lung, leading to collapse of bronchus, aspirated mucus, and bronchial atresia
- Respiratory difficulties resulting from congenital lobar emphysema become apparent within 4 weeks of birth in 50% of patients; symptoms include dyspnea, coughing, and wheezing; physical examination reveals absent or diminished breath sounds, hyperresonance to percussion on the affected side, and mediastinal shift to the contralateral side
- Patients with CAM typically present within 3 months of birth

DIFFERENTIAL DIAGNOSIS

The appropriate management of newborns with respiratory distress depends largely on timely recognition of their signs. These consist of copious production of secretions, tachypnea, cyanosis, and agitation. Differential diagnosis is best accomplished based on time of presentation.

TREATMENT

Infants with esophageal atresia should have a suction catheter placed in the proximal esophageal stump to prevent aspiration pneumonia (Case 1). A humidified incubator will promote hydration of secretions while frequent repositioning will aid in drainage. Antibiotic therapy consists of ampicillin (75 mg/kg) and gentamicin (1.5 mg/kg), which should be given every 8 hours.

Although mortality rates have significantly declined over the past few decades, postoperative morbidity continues to remain high. Problems with anastomotic leakage, esophageal stricture, recurrent fistula, and gastroesophageal reflux occur.

Congenital diaphragmatic hernias require operative repair when the infant is stable. The hypoplastic lungs demand delicate resuscitation to prevent barotrauma. The infant should be paralyzed and endotracheally intubated. Frequent blood gas measurements are required to keep the blood pH above 7.4 to alleviate respiratory acidosis, which leads to increased pulmonary vascular resistance and further hypoxia. Respiratory alkalosis should be achieved by ventilation, with 100% oxygen administered at high rates and low volumes (Case 2). Intravenous

sodium bicarbonate may be necessary. Use of pharmacologic vasodilatators may be helpful in decreasing pulmonary vascular resistance and right-to-left shunting. In the most serious cases, extracorporeal membrane oxygenation (ECMO) is an invaluable tool for artificial oxygenation. Alveolar growth and a decrease in pulmonary vascular resistance have been observed in patients on ECMO over a 3-week period. If the child is mature and does not have other severe anomalies, the defect can be repaired early with a primary esophageal anastomosis. If the child is premature, or has associated anomalies, repair must be staged. In the first step, the tracheoesophageal fistula is divided to prevent further aspiration, and a feeding gastrostomy is placed to aid in nutrition. The second step consists of primary anastomosis of the two ends of the esophagus. If the child has only a tracheoesophageal fistula, this can be divided simply. When atresia is present without a fistula, a cervical esophagostomy is needed to prevent aspiration. Repair usually requires complex reconstruction. An abdominal approach is used to replace the bowel in the abdominal cavity and repair the diaphragmatic defect. Occasionally, the abdominal wall cannot be closed and a silo is required to return the abdominal contents gradually without adversely affecting respiration by displacing the diaphragm upward. The silo consists of a cone of prosthetic material sewn to the edges of the abdominal incision. The volume of the silo is reduced gradually, forcing the viscera back into the abdomen.

Postoperative care is directed at maintaining respiratory alkalosis and low pulmonary vascular resistance. When the space-occupying viscera are removed and the diaphragm is closed, the hypoplastic lung may expand with alveolar growth. In cases diagnosed antenatally, the infant may be delivered by cesarean section and immediately placed on ECMO.

Extralobar pulmonary sequestrations are typically found when thoracic procedures are performed for other indications. At that time, the blood supply to the sequestered lung tissue may be ligated and the anomalous lung removed. Intralobar sequestrations may become cystic and inflamed leading to recurrent infections, lung abscesses, and pneumonia. Because it is difficult to isolate the portion of the lung not communicating with the bronchial tree, a lobectomy may be required to remove the sequestered lung tissue.

Although lobar emphysema may resolve in some cases without lobectomy, rapid progression of respiratory symptoms demands emergency treatment. Lobar emphysema is readily treated surgically with a thoracotomy and lobectomy of the affected lobe. The postoperative course is normally uneventful, and follow-up studies show a compensation in lung growth resulting in normal or close-to-normal lung volume.

As with pulmonary sequestration and lobar emphysema, congenital cystic adenomatoid malformation is often treated operatively under emergency conditions because of respiratory distress. A lobectomy or pneumonectomy is the operation of choice. Type III, solid CAM, may be segmentally excised from normal parenchymal tissue.

KEY POINTS

- Infants with esophageal atresia should have suction catheter placed in proximal esophageal stump to prevent aspiration pneumonia; humidified incubator will promote hydration of secretions, while frequent repositioning will aid drainage

- Congenital diaphragmatic hernias require operative repair when infant is stable

- Hypoplastic lungs demand delicate resuscitation to prevent barotrauma

- Respiratory alkalosis should be achieved by ventilation with 100% oxygen administered at high rates and low volumes

- If child mature and without other severe anomalies, defect can be repaired early with primary esophageal anastomosis

- If child premature or has associated anomalies, repair must be staged

---

SUGGESTED READINGS

deLorimer AA, Harrison MR, Adzick S: Pediatric surgery. In Way L (ed): Current Surgical Diagnosis and Treatment. 10th Ed. Appleton & Lange, E. Norwalk, CT, 1994

A thorough and authoritative chapter that covers the major portions of pediatric surgery. The chapter is well written and contains a number of useful references. Highly recommended.

German JC, Mahour GH, Woolley MM: Esophageal atresia and associated anomalies. J Pediatr Surg 11:299, 1976

A very good review of the more common types of esophageal atresia. One of the classic references.

Puri P (ed): Congenital diaphragmatic hernia. Mod Probl Paediatr 24:142, 1989

This review covers the pathophysiology as well as the diagnosis and the management of the disease. A very good reference source.

QUESTIONS

1. *The most common type of tracheoesophageal fistula?*
   A. Has a proximal esophageal pouch and a fistula between the trachea and the distal esophagus.
   B. Is an H-type fistula with a normal esophagus.
   C. Is an H-type fistula with a proximal esophageal pouch.
   D. Connects the proximal esophageal pouch to the trachea.

2. *Survival in congenital diaphragmatic hernias is related to?*
   A. Associated cardiac anomalies.
   B. The gestational age at delivery.
   C. The extent of lung hypoplasia.
   D. Associated spinal cord defects.

3. *Which of the following is* not *appropriate in the management of an infant with a congenital diaphragmatic hernia?*
   A. Use of extracorporeal membrane oxygenation.
   B. High pressure, low volume mechanical ventilation.
   C. Pulmonary artery vasodilatators.
   D. Intravenous sodium bicarbonate.

(See p. 604 for answers.)

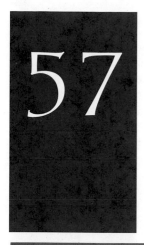

57

NEONATAL

GASTROINTESTINAL

OBSTRUCTION

THOMAS C. MOORE

Developmental abnormalities of the intestinal tract can occur anywhere along its length, with the presentation/discovery closely related to the location and completeness of the obstruction. Esophageal abnormalities are discussed in Chapter 15.

CASE 1
IMPERFORATE ANUS
WITH FISTULA

A newborn, full-term female was noted to have no apparent anus at birth. Review of the prenatal care was unremarkable, and an ultrasound at 34 weeks' gestation was normal without hydramnios. Family history revealed an aunt who had had a similar defect. Examination revealed an anal fistula opening into the low posterior vaginal wall, with subsequent spontaneous meconium passage. Radiograph and ultrasound scan showed normal vertebral development, a normal heart, and a low rectal pouch. An esophageal contrast study was normal. On day 5, the child had a posterior sagittal anoplasty reconstruction.

CASE 2
DUODENAL ATRESIA

A full-term male vomited bile stained material at 6 hours of life. Efforts at feeding brought continued vomiting, and radiographs showed a paucity of gas in the gastrointestinal tract. No prenatal care had been received, although the mother reported a normal pregnancy. Family history was noncontributory. Examination was remarkable for facial features consistent with Down syndrome and an abdomen

that was scaphoid, nontender, and without masses. A nasogastric tube was inserted after the radiographs and 20 ml of air instilled. A repeat radiograph showed air in the stomach and proximal duodenum only ("double-bubble" sign), confirming suspicion of duodenal atresia. Intravenous fluids and electrolytes were needed to correct the deficits caused by vomiting and lack of intake. Cardiac evaluation was normal. Operative findings were of an atretic segment just distal to the ampulla of Vater. Duodenoduodenostomy was done, and no other sites of atresia were found.

GENERAL CONSIDERATIONS

Congenital developmental defects of the intestinal tract are relatively uncommon, occurring in approximately 1 of 1,000 live births in the United States. Their importance stems not only from their obvious implications regarding the patient's ability to aliment themselves, but also because not infrequently there are associated birth defects (Case 2). Failure to recognize these associated birth defects may have serious impact on the outcome. Indeed, these associated birth defects are often the main determinant of the patient's morbidity and mortality.

Hypertrophic pyloric stenosis is one of the most common and readily diagnosed forms of gastrointestinal obstruction, and is due to a relative narrowing at the pylorus.

Intestinal atresias result from events in utero in the second month that interfere with the blood supply of the developing segment of the gut. Imperforate anus and its many variations (Case 1) represent a failure of the normal progression from a cloacal origin to separate genitourinary and gastrointestinal systems. Malrotation, or mid-gut volvulus, occurs because of an incomplete or inadequate fixation of the intestines into the retroperitoneal position, an event that occurs later in time at 10–12 weeks of gestation.

KEY POINTS

• Developmental abnormalities of intestinal tract can occur anywhere along its length, with presentation/discovery closely related to location and completeness of obstruction

• Failure to recognize associated birth defects may have serious impact on outcome; often are main determinant of patient's morbidity and mortality

DIAGNOSIS

With the exception of pyloric stenosis and malrotation/mid-gut volvulus, most congenital gastrointestinal defects present within the first few days of life and often within the first 12–24 hours of life (Case 2). The more distal the intestinal segment of involvement, the later the presentation. The most common presenting symptom is vomiting, although with distal atresia, abdominal distention and failure of passage of normal meconium are additional symptoms to be expected.

Pyloric stenosis typically becomes symptomatic 3–6 weeks after birth. At this time, the baby begins to vomit increasingly forcefully (often projectile) after each feeding. Because of the location of the obstruction, the vomitus is always nonbilious, although it may have a brownish "coffee-grounds" appearance from the presence of blood due to gastritis. After vomiting, the child remains hungry.

The diagnosis of congenital hypertrophic pyloric stenosis is made by careful examination of the abdomen for the typical "olive" or pyloric "tumor." This is best done in a quiet examining room with no parent present. The infant is placed on a comfortable examination table with the examiner comfortably seated on the infant's right side. An assistant gives the infant 10% sugar water by bottle and nipple to serve as a type of relaxer as the starving baby eagerly swallows the sugary "treat." The examiner gently uses the right hand to propel the viscera of the epigastrium and left flank toward the left hand, which palpates lateral to and over the right rectus muscle. At times, the olive is readily palpable; other times it takes longer. A careful examination should reveal the olive nearly 100% of the time. Ultrasound is unnecessary if examination reveals an olive. It is highly operator dependent, but in skilled hands may be beneficial in equivocal cases. Another alternative is an upper gastrointestinal radiograph with barium, which will show a narrow, elongated pyloric channel (string sign).

Imperforate anus and its variations (Case 1) are usually obvious on physical examination at birth while most other forms of intestinal malformations are not (Figs. 57.1 and 57.2). Physical examination in patients with intestinal atresia varies with the level of obstruction. If the obstruction is proximal in the duodenum or proximal jejunum, abdominal distention is relatively minor and is limited to the upper abdomen or epigastrium. Distal obstructions, not surprisingly, produce significantly more intestinal and thus abdominal distention, frequently noted before the onset of vomiting.

Often the first clue that an intestinal atresia exists will be the finding of hydramnios on a prenatal ultrasound. Up to 75% of cases of intestinal atresia will produce evident hydramnios on ultrasound. Although the detection of hydramnios on prenatal ultrasound may predict the likelihood of intestinal atresia, it does not change the obstetric course of the patient. The specific prenatal diagnosis of intestinal atresia is not often made because the lack of gas in utero does not allow easy visualization of the intestinal tract due to similar acoustic characteristics between the fluid-filled loops of bowel. Following delivery, vomiting is the most common early symptom, although vomiting in the newborn due to nonanatomic causes is a relatively frequent and nonspecific symptom. Persistence of the vomiting (Case 2) should lead to suspicion of either a functional gastrointestinal problem or sepsis. Radiographic evaluation is usually suggestive of an intestinal obstruction, although if the neonate has recently vomited, air may need to be insufflated into the intestinal tract (Case 2) to delineate the obstructed bowel and the level of obstruction.

The typical double-bubble sign seen with duodenal atresia is related to the presence of a gas bubble within the stomach and within the duodenum. More distal obstructions show a typical radiographic pattern of dilated loops of bowel, often with air-fluid levels on lateral films. The main concern would be to differentiate a jejunal or ileal atresia from a malrotation or mid-gut volvulus. The finding of a normal appearing cecum in the right lower quadrant on a contrast enema makes a malrotation or volvulus very unlikely, although infrequently this can occur.

Contrast studies of the small bowel performed by instilling small amounts of contrast through a nasogastric tube can also be used. The decision for a lower versus upper gastrointestinal contrast study is frequently made on the basis of the quantity of dilated intestines seen on the plain abdominal films.

Duodenal atresia typically occurs distal to the ampulla of Vater (Case 2), although occasional cases can involve the first portion of the duodenum. The hallmark of this latter presentation is nonbilious vomiting occurring within the first 12–24 hours of life. When duodenal atresia is diagnosed,

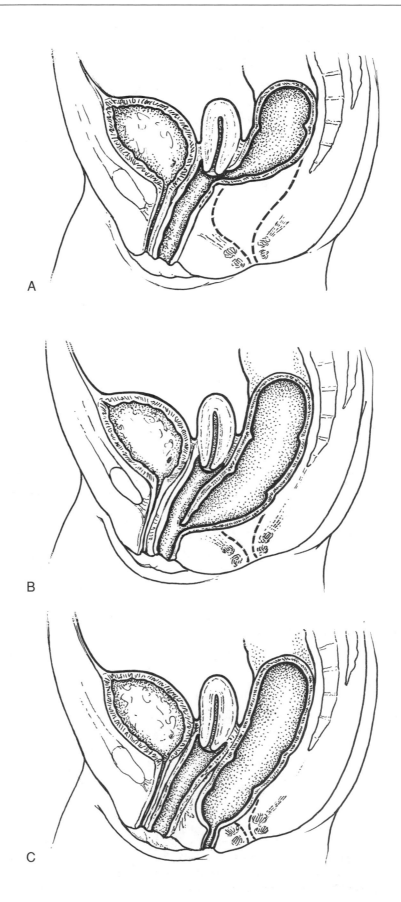

FIGURE 57.1 *Imperforate anus (female). (A) High malformation; (B) mid-malformation; (C) low malformation.*

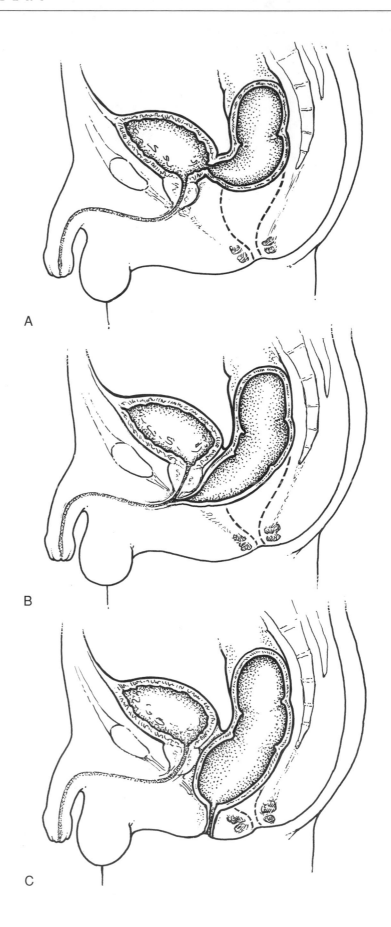

FIGURE 57.2 *Imperforate anus (male). (**A**) High malformation; (**B**) mid-malformation; (**C**) low malformation.*

associated birth defects should be considered. Down syndrome is the most common of these (Case 2), occurring 30–40% of the time. Other commonly associated abnormalities include malrotation/mid-gut volvulus, congenital heart anomalies, and esophageal atresia (hence the esophageal swallow in Case 2).

More distal atresias have been classified into five types: type 1 is an intraluminal diaphragm with continuity of the bowel wall (Fig 57.3); type 2 has a cord-like segment attaching two blind ends of intestine (Fig. 57.4); type 3 is a complete separation of the blind ends in addition to a mesentery defect (Fig. 57.4); type 4 is multiple atresias; and type 5, extremely rare, is amputation or absence of the entire mid-gut. Overall bowel length is typically shortened in cases of type 2 atresia and is definitely so with types 3 through 5 atresias. Jejunal or ileal atresias can be found in cases of gastroschisis, omphalocele (see Ch. 60), volvulus, and intussusception, but are rarely (<10%) associated with additional congenital defects. Malrotation, nonrotation, and mid-gut volvulus are problems of fixation with the potential for a twisting or volvulus along the superior mesenteric artery. The urgency of a mid-gut volvulus is that the bowel becomes gangrenous very rapidly if not corrected, due to occlusion of the blood supply.

Infants with malrotation typically vomit bile-stained contents, suggesting a duodenal obstruction. Despite this apparent obstruction, there may be passage of meconium and milk stools. Blood staining of the bilious vomitus or of the stool, associated with apparent abdominal tenderness, should heighten consideration of a volvulus and compromised or strangulated gut. Plain abdominal x-rays may show an apparent double-bubble, but an upper gastrointestinal contrast study will typically show a corkscrew-like appearance of the distal duodenum. Other radiographic findings include the appearance of the small intestine isolated to the right side of the abdomen with the large intes-

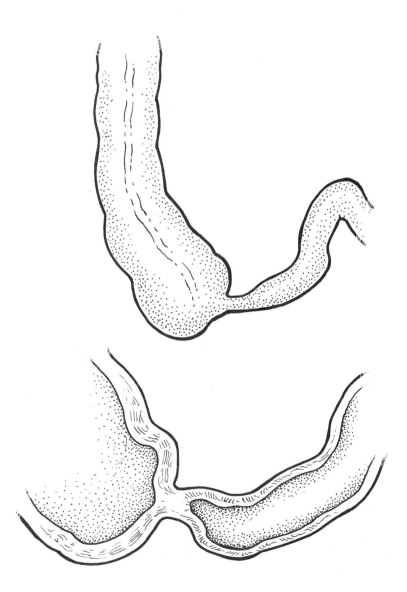

FIGURE 57.3 *Type 1 atresia. Lower image shows lumenal appearance.*

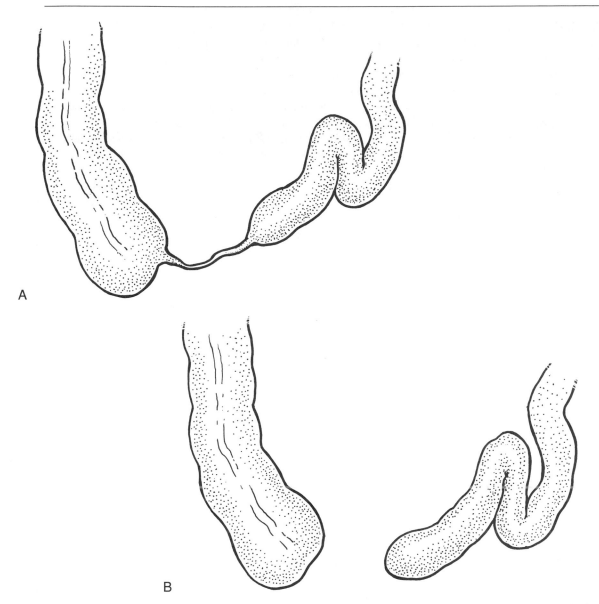

FIGURE 57.4   *Intestinal atresia. (**A**) Type 2 atresia with cord-like continuity. (**B**) Type 3 atresia lacks this connection.*

tine on the left, and/or the cecum located in the right upper quadrant. Alternatively, ultrasound findings may indicate a malrotation by examining the relative positions of the superior mesenteric vein and artery.

Imperforate anus is actually a broad spectrum of congenital anorectal malformations. For the matter of simplicity, these are divided into high, intermediate, and low defects (Figs. 57.1 and 57.2). More comprehensive nomenclature systems exist to cover the variety of rectal, urinary tract, genital fistulas, stenosis, and atresias for the interested reader. Low malformations almost always involve cutaneous fistulas. The rectum is contained within the sphincter mechanism but is anteriorly displaced from the actual anal opening. The fistula may run subcutaneously through the perineum to open into the base of the scro-

tum or penis in males or near the vagina in females. Lower deformities are readily diagnosed by physical examination. Meconium typically comes through the fistula, although it may appear at the site of the anal opening.

Intermediate malformations involve fistulization between the rectum and urethra in males and between the rectum and vagina in females (Case 1). The intermediate classification implies that the rectum is contained within the striated muscle complex of the levator ani, while higher defects typically imply poor development of the sphincter mechanism and levator ani complex, which portends a discouraging prognosis of future continence. The presence of an anal dimple with an apparent anal "wink" or contraction on cutaneous stimulation is a strong predictor of ultimate continence following appropriate and successful surgery.

Occasionally, high and intermediate deformities occur without fistula, a term known as *anal agenesis.*

High malformations may occur with fistulas between the rectum and bladder neck in males (rectoprostatic), while in females the high malformation problem results in a persistent cloaca. This cloacal defect involves fusion of the rectal, urinary, and genital tracts. These high fistulas in both males and females are frequently found in conjunction with sacral and other vertebral defects. In general, the higher the malformation the more likely associated defects will be found. These include genitourinary defects, congenital heart defects, esophageal atresia, tracheoesophageal fistula, renal dysplasia, and upper extremity (radial) limb dysplasia.

Coexistence of several of these defects are sometimes seen in families and are referred to as the VATER complex (vertebral anal tracheoesophageal radial/renal). The familial tendency of these coexisting defects suggests an anosomal recessive genetic mechanism. The awareness of the frequent cardiac abnormalities has led some to change the terminology to VACTERL (vertebral anal cardiac tracheoesophageal renal limb). Ultrasound (Case 1) is a particularly useful modality to investigate these defects as it can adequately visualize not only the upper urinary tract (kidneys), but also is frequently able to identify the distance between the anal opening and the rectal pouch, aiding in classification and ultimately therapy.

KEY POINTS

- Most congenital gastrointestinal defects present within first few days of life and often within first 12–24 hours of life

- Diagnosis of congenital hypertrophic pyloric stenosis is made by careful examination of abdomen for typical "olive" or pyloric "tumor"

- Often, first clue that an intestinal atresia exists will be finding of hydramnios on prenatal ultrasound

- Following delivery, vomiting is most common early symptom

- When duodenal atresia is diagnosed, associated birth defects should be considered

- Imperforate anus is actually broad spectrum of congenital anorectal malformations

---

DIFFERENTIAL DIAGNOSIS

The differential diagnosis primarily includes necrotizing enterocolitis (NEC), meconium ileus, and Hirschsprung's disease. NEC almost exclusively affects preterm infants, and its clinical course typically becomes evident after attempts at early feeding of these low birth weight, immature neonates. Clinical symptoms may include vomiting or intolerance of foods as well as abdominal distention. Additionally, evidence of sepsis, including thrombo-

cytopenia, is usually evident and radiographic appearance will show an ileus pattern. The observation of pneumatosis intestinalis (gas within the bowel wall) on radiograph, coupled with the aforementioned clinical scenario, make the diagnosis straightforward.

Hirschsprung's disease is due to an aganglionic segment of rectum and/or colon. The disease may involve the entire colon and rectum or a variable amount of the distal colon and rectum. A pseudo-obstruction is caused by a lack of peristaltic activity due to the hyperexcited neuronal activity that results in continuous contraction of the bowel musculature in the aganglionic segment. Additionally, the spastic internal sphincter muscle contracts under rectal distention rather than exhibiting normal relaxation. The typical clinical finding is that of constipation after birth with delayed passage of meconium for more than 24 hours. Other clinical findings may include bile-stained vomiting that, as the disease progresses, can become feculent. It is usually associated with abdominal distention as well.

Physical examination will often reveal fecal material on rectal examination, especially in cases of more distal involvement only. Radiographs will vary depending on the level of pseudo-obstruction, with total colonic aganglionosis mimicking a distal small bowel obstruction. Contrast enema will be diagnostic, showing the characteristic distended colon tapering into the aganglionic segment or, in the case of a total colonic aganglionosis, a proximally dilated small bowel tapering down at or around the ileocecal valve into a microcolon. Rectal suction biopsy will be definitive in the diagnosis of Hirschsprung's disease by showing the lack of ganglions in the rectal segment. Operative correction of Hirschsprung's disease involves resection of the entire aganglionic segment of colon and rectum, with a pull-through technique the most frequent procedure performed in the United States.

Meconium ileus is frequently confused with distal small bowel atresias, with abdominal distention and vomiting and failure of passage of meconium the most common early findings. The disease has a very strong association with cystic fibrosis and it is due to a viscus meconium, high in protein content, which obstructs the lumen of the ileum and colon. This strong correlation necessitates the performance of a sweat test in cases of suspected meconium ileus to diagnose cystic fibrosis. As with other midgut obstructions, the proximal ileum is dilated. The distal ileum is clogged with viscus meconium and the narrow distal end contains taffy-like meconium pellets. Findings of microcolon require the diagnosis to be differentiated from Hirschsprung's disease. Occasionally, the increased weight of the distal ileum containing the thickened meconium can result in perforation or volvulus of the bowel. Additionally, atresia or meconium peritonitis can complicate the clinical scenario.

A family history of cystic fibrosis, which is autosomal recessive, is the first clue to accurate diagnosis of meconium ileus. Onset of symptoms can occur within hours of birth and in complicated cases of meconium ileus, abdominal distention may be present at birth. These complicated cases may have additional findings of pneumoperitoneum and peritonitis. Physical examination may reveal loops of bowel that may indent on palpation of the abdomen, but most commonly is nonspecific. Radiographic findings may be similar to those in cases of distal ileal atresia, but the trapped air in the distal ileum can impart a ground glass appearance. More proximal loops of dilated intestine are also frequently seen. A gastrograffin enema is diagnostic as well as therapeutic, as the hypertonic solution will pull fluid into the intestinal lumen, loosening the adhesive meconium. Often a second administration is necessary to sufficiently evacuate the meconium. Intravenous fluid support is necessary during this process, as the high osmolarity of the gastrograffin solution will cause significant third spacing within the intestinal lumen.

KEY POINTS

- Family history of cystic fibrosis, which is autosomal recessive, is first clue to accurate diagnosis of meconium ileus

TREATMENT

Due to vomiting of intestinal contents and inability to ingest fluids and food, most infants with intestinal obstruction have fluid or electrolyte deficiencies, or both. Restoration of these pre-existing losses should precede operative intervention. The operative approach to the infant with hypertrophic pyloric stenosis is pyloromyotomy. A longitudinal incision is made from the distal stomach (antrum) extending onto the proximal duodenum, and the muscle is then bluntly separated to allow outpouching of the mucosa.

The treatment of duodenal atresia will vary with the type of atresia present. A simple diaphragmatic obstruction, remote from the ampulla of Vater, can be excised or divided to allow continuity of the intestinal tract. More commonly, a duodenoduodenostomy (Case 2) is necessary, which allows anastomosis and establishment of continuity between the proximal obstructed duodenum and the distal duodenum, without interfering with the ampulla or pancreas. More distal atresias (jejuno or ileal) are usually managed by anastomosis between the proximal dilated segment and the distal "decompressed" segment. Functional return of intestinal activity may be delayed due to the sometimes massive dilatation of the proximal segment. Prolonged nasogastric suction or gastrostomy drainage, combined with tube or parenteral feeding will be required in a small number of cases.

Malrotation, or mid-gut volvulus, if diagnosed before the onset of gangrene, is treated by derotation of the involved intestinal segment with re-establishment of blood flow. All adhesions or Ladds bands (congenital adhesions) should be taken down and the entire intestinal tract assessed for potential occult atresias. Passage of a tube through the duodenum is recommended to fully evaluate this region. Following this, the cecum is placed in the left upper quadrant to prevent further incidences of volvulus, and an appendectomy is frequently performed to prevent further confusion in this high risk, young population. The more common finding of gangrenous bowel on exploration is usually approached by resection of the gangrenous segment. Unfortunately, this often leaves the infant with a short gut syndrome and a potential lifelong dependence on total parenteral nutrition. The recent strides in intestinal transplantation may prove to be of benefit in this subgroup. An alternative approach, which has found recent success, is the "patch, drain, and wait" technique, in which the intestines are left in situ and multiple drains are placed, creating functional enterostomies from any perforated segments. A later re-exploration will often surprise the operating surgeon with preservation of intestinal segments previously thought to be nonsalvagable.

Imperforate anus is most commonly treated through a perineal or posterior sagittal approach. Popularized by Pena, posterior sagittal anoplasty has a good record of success, and the recent trend toward early operation seems to allow improved ultimate neural function, a previously problematic area when the operation was staged and performed at a later age.

FOLLOW-UP

Operation for duodenal atresia is usually successful in restoring normal gastrointestinal continuity and function. Therefore, no special follow-up is necessary beyond the postoperative period. Associated birth defects may, however, warrant further intervention. Restoration of intestinal continuity is also highly successful with more distal atresias. Normal intestinal function may not be achieved, however, as insufficient intestinal length to support nutritional needs may not remain, especially in types 3–5. Parenteral nutrition may be necessary as a supplement for caloric requirements. Hypertrophy of intestinal villi and/or bowel lengthening procedures will allow some patients to be weaned off parenteral nutrition, while others will remain "short-gut cripples." A similar problem occurs when malrotation results in extensive bowel ischemia and gangrene.

Imperforate anus patients, especially the high level abnormality group, have frequent, ongoing problems with defecation (especially incontinence). Although secondary ("salvage") operative procedures are occasionally indicated and beneficial, most of these problems are effectively dealt with by bowel training regimens, psychosocial counseling, and true peer interactions available at specialized centers.

KEY POINTS

• Operation for duodenal atresia usually successful in restoring normal gastrointestinal continuity and function

• Restoration of intestinal continuity also highly successful with more distal atresias

• Normal intestinal function may not be achieved, however, as insufficient intestinal length to support nutritional needs may not remain (especially in atresia types 3–5)

• Imperforate anus patients, especially high level abnormality group, have frequent, ongoing problems with defecation (especially incontinence)

SUGGESTED READINGS

Cook RCM: Gastric outlet obstructions. p. 406. In Lister J, Irving IM (eds): Neonatal Surgery. 3rd Ed. Butterworths, London, 1990

An overview of proximal congenital gastrointestinal obstruction.

Groff D III: Malrotation. p. 320. In Ashcraft DW, Holder TM (eds): Pediatric Surgery. 2nd Ed. Harcourt Brace Jovanovich, Philadelphia, 1993

Discusses etiology as well as presentation and treatment.

Pena A: Imperforate anus and cloacal malformations. p. 373. In Ashcraft KW, Holder TM (eds): Pediatric Surgery. 2nd Ed. Harcourt Brace Jovanovich, Philadelphia, 1993

An extensive treatise from the foremost authority on the subject.

QUESTIONS

1. Duodenal atresia is commonly associated with?

    A. Hirschsprung's disease.

    B. Down syndrome.

    C. Cystic fibrosis.

    D. Esophageal duplication.

    E. All of the above.

2. The best test for the initial assessment of imperforate anus is?

    A. Ultrasound.

    B. Detailed physical examination.

    C. Plain radiographs.

    D. Contrast studies.

    E. CT scan.

(See p. 604 for answers.)

58

A B D O M I N A L

T E N D E R N E S S

THOMAS C. MOORE

EDWARD PASSARO, JR.

Abdominal pain and/or tenderness is one of the most frequent complaints in both children and adults. Key elements in determining whether the symptoms represent a benign self-limiting process or one indicative of a serious disease are the history and the observed progression of the disease. In the pediatric age group this differential by these key elements is often hampered by a lack of history, and a more rapid progression of the disease.

This chapter outlines the evaluation of abdominal tenderness/pain in three distinct age categories: the neonate, ages 1–4, and ages 5–10. Three distinct disease processes are presented to illustrate the salient features of each age.

CASE 1
NECROTIZING ENTEROCOLITIS

A 2,000-g premature male infant was intubated in the ICU because of mild respiratory distress. On the 8th day following extubation, enteral feedings had just begun when the infant developed abdominal distention and respiratory distress. The feedings were stopped and the infant reintubated. His temperature was 38.1°C. There was intramural bowel gas and a small amount of free air on abdominal plain films. Antibiotics were given and the infant was operated on. Throughout the distal portion of the small bowel there were patchy areas of dilated hemorrhagic segments, intermingled with patches of gray, shrunken, flaccid bowel. The bowel was crepitant in these regions, and two segments had small punctate perforations. The perforations were closed in one instance by simple suture,

and in the other by bringing the scant omentum to the perforation and tacking it in place. Drains were placed and the abdomen closed. There was a small amount of drainage for the first 4 days and then it stopped. His abdomen became soft and he was afebrile. The drains were slowly advanced. On day 21, enteral feedengs were started again. On day 23, the infant passed a normal stool.

CASE 2
INTUSSUSCEPTION

A 1-year-old male infant developed colicky abdominal pain and anorexia. He had tenderness in both lower abdominal quadrants, and some examiners felt a mass in the right lower quadrant. A stool guaiac test was negative. He was sedated, IV catheters were started, and a barium enema examination was done under fluoroscopy. With gradual instillation of the contrast, an ileocolic intussusception was seen. Hydrostatic pressure and manual massage in the right lower quadrant reduced the intussusception. The following day the child ate and subsequently had a bowel movement and was discharged.

CASE 3
APPENDICITIS

A 6-year-old male was noted by his parents to have a loss of appetite. He otherwise appeared healthy and active. The following day, despite a limited intake of food, he had frequent loose bowel movements. He was taken to the family physician, who found him to be afebrile, with an abdomen that was flat and not tender. He was given some methylcellulose granules to be taken with water to reduce the frequency of the bowel movements. The following day the boy's abdomen appeared distended, and he appeared tired and apathetic to his mother. Taken back to the family doctor, he now had a temperature of 38.1°C. His abdomen was slightly distended but not tender to palpation. On rectal examination he was more tender on the right than the left. His WBC count was 12,600/mm³.

He was thought to have appendicitis, probably lying in the pelvis, and he was brought to the hospital for operation. He was given antibiotics preoperatively. The surgeons found a long appendix with an acutely inflamed tip lying in the pelvis. The appendix was removed and the pelvis irrigated locally with warm saline. He was discharged afebrile the following day.

GENERAL CONSIDERATIONS

Abdominal pain and tenderness, although common and usually benign in children, can portend significant illness. As exemplified in the three case presentations in this chapter, each age group has a unique set of abdominal diseases most often encountered within it. Abdominal tenderness or distention in the neonatal patient is a grave finding. It signifies a significant developmental or anatomic abnormality ranging from hypertrophic pyloric stenosis proximally to imperforate anus distally (see Ch. 55). These anatomic abnormalities are not amenable to medical therapy. Operation is invariably required both to diagnose (intestinal bands or malrotation) and to treat the condition.

Necrotizing enterocolitis (NEC) is a notable exception to this generalization (Case 1). Developing in premature infants and neonates, it is not associated with any particular anatomic abnormality, and its cause remains unknown. Current hypotheses center on mucosal injury of an ischemic nature that allows bacterial invasion of the submucosa and muscularis of the bowel, leading to the profound bowel necrosis characteristic of this disease. Ischemic injury may be caused by hypoxia. Enteral feedings, especially those of high osmolarity, have also been a proposed source, providing substrate for bacterial growth while damaging the integrity of the mucosa.

Beyond the neonatal period and extending up to approximately age 5, the causes of abdominal tenderness/distention can be thought of as due to abnormal physiol-

ogy, sometimes related to a developmental anomaly. In Case 2, for example, the cause of the intussusception can be either hyperperistalsis or a lead point from a Meckel's diverticulum. Similarly, hyperfunctioning of gastric mucosa found on occasion in a Meckel's diverticulum can produce abdominal tenderness from mucosal ulceration, occasionally leading to bleeding. Depending on the nature of the abnormality, it may be corrected nonoperatively (Case 2).

In the later years of childhood, again as a generalization, abdominal pain and distention are most often associated with infectious causes. Every child can be expected to have this type of abdominal pain and tenderness during life. While the vast majority of these episodes are benign, a few are early stages of significant disease (Case 3).

KEY POINTS

- Each age group has a unique set of abdominal disease most often encountered within it

- Abdominal tenderness/distention in the neonatal patient is a grave finding

- Operation invariably required both to diagnose (intestinal bands or malrotation) and to treat the condition

- NEC a notable exception to this generalization

- Beyond the neonatal period and extending up to age 5, the causes of abdominal tenderness/distention can be thought of as due to abnormal physiology related to developmental anomaly

- Depending on the nature of the abnormality, it may be corrected nonoperatively

- In the later years of childhood, again as a generalization, abdominal pain and distention often associated with infectious causes

- Although the vast majority of these episodes are benign, a few are early stages of significant disease

DIAGNOSIS

The congenital defects leading to abdominal tenderness/distention in the neonatal period can usually be diagnosed by physical examination (hypertrophic pyloric obstruction, imperforate anus) and abdominal x-rays. A precise diagnosis can usually be made on clinical findings in this group, as each anatomic defect will produce a characteristic set of clinical findings.

NEC is suggested by the rapid development of abdominal tenderness/distention in the premature infant or neonate. These findings, along with the presence of intramural gas in the bowel (Case 1), establishes the diagnosis.

Diagnosis of abdominal pain/tenderness in the second age category (1–4) is more difficult. Melena, or "currant-jelly" stool, or the suggestion of an intra-abdominal mass in the right lower quadrant are important diagnostic clues (Case 2). Diagnostic studies may be useful (pertechnetate scans for Meckel's diverticulum, barium enema under fluoroscopic control for intussusception). The latter is particularly important, because it can be therapeutic (Case 2).

In the third age category (5–12 years), diagnosis of a specific condition is particularly difficult. Fortunately, in this age group, a history is generally available. Observation when the etiology is not known helps to define a progressive disorder requiring operation for diagnosis and treatment (Case 3) or a self-limiting process not requiring treatment.

KEY POINTS

- Congenital defects leading to abdominal tenderness/distention in the neonatal period can usually be diagnosed by physical examination (hypertrophic pyloric obstruction, imperforate anus) and abdominal x-rays

- Diagnosis of abdominal pain/tenderness in ages 1–4 is more difficult

- In ages 5–12 years, diagnosis of a specific condition is particularly difficult

DIFFERENTIAL DIAGNOSIS

In the neonatal age group, the primary consideration in diagnosis is developmental abnormalities of the gastrointestinal tract. These include obstructions for anomalies at the pylorus (hypertrophic pyloric stenosis), intestinal atresias (most commonly at the duodenum), and imperforate anus. Additionally, there may be malrotations of the bowel or internal or external hernias, which produce abdominal tenderness and distention. However, as indicated above, among the most common of these is NEC, which is unique in not having an anatomic basis. The anatomic abnormalities can be identified by physical examination (feeling the gastric "olive" of hypertrophic pyloric stenosis) or radiographic studies, that demonstrate intestinal obstruction related to the level of the affected bowel.

Beyond the neonatal period and up to approximately 5 years of age, the causes of abdominal pain are often related to abnormal physiology. Intussusception develops because of increased peristalsis of the terminal ileum (Case 2) (Fig. 58.1). Beyond the first year of life there is often an anomaly such as Meckel's diverticulum or polyps as the lead point for the formation of the intussusception. A barium study is often both diagnostic and therapeutic (Case 2).

Meckel's diverticulum, producing bleeding and occasionally diverticulitis, is the other major differential diagnosis. It is suggested by passage of dark, bloody stool. The bleeding is not associated with pain or distention, which is an important point in its differentiation from other causes of hematochezia or melena such as obstruction and bowel

necrosis from adhesive bands or duplications of bowel segments. Bleeding from a Meckel's diverticulum can be detected by a technetium-99 pertechnetate scan with concomitant cimetidine administration. The radioactive tracer is concentrated in the ectopic gastric mucosa found in the Meckel's diverticulum, which produces the bleeding by eroding the adjacent bowel mucosa.

In the older child (5–10), the major differential concerns infectious causes of disease. At times the diagnosis is very difficult to establish (Case 3). Here, a good history (generally available) and a period of observation are critical in both ascertaining the cause of the abdominal tenderness and in suggesting the appropriate diagnostic and therapeutic maneuvers.

Although appendicitis is the major consideration in this age group, other causes include urinary tract infections and nonspecific inflammation of mesenteric lymphatic systems (Brennan syndrome).

Urinary tract infections can be detected by careful kidney palpation and percussion, and urinalysis. Nonspecific mesenteric lymphadenitis presently cannot be detected preoperatively.

There are many other less frequently encountered causes of abdominal tenderness and distention. Careful observation of the patient is often the most important step in ascertaining which patients require treatment and which patients have a self-limiting disease process ("gastrointestinal flu") that requires no further investigation or treatment.

KEY POINTS

- In neonatal age group, primary consideration in diagnosis is developmental abnormalities of gastrointestinal tract

- At times diagnosis difficult to establish; a good history and period of observation are critical in ascertaining cause of abdominal tenderness and appropriate diagnostic and therapeutic maneuvers

- Careful observation of patient often most important step in ascertaining which patients require treatment and which have self-limiting disease process (gastrointestinal flu) that requires no further investigation or treatment

TREATMENT

In the neonatal period, abdominal tenderness and/or distention usually requires operation for both diagnosis and treatment. Anatomic anomalies are treated by procedures to excise or relieve the obstruction.

NEC is currently best treated by simple closure of perforations where possible, drainage of the peritoneal cavity, nutritional support, and waiting. These conservative measures have been highly successful in tiding the infant through the disease process, which is not understood (Case 1).

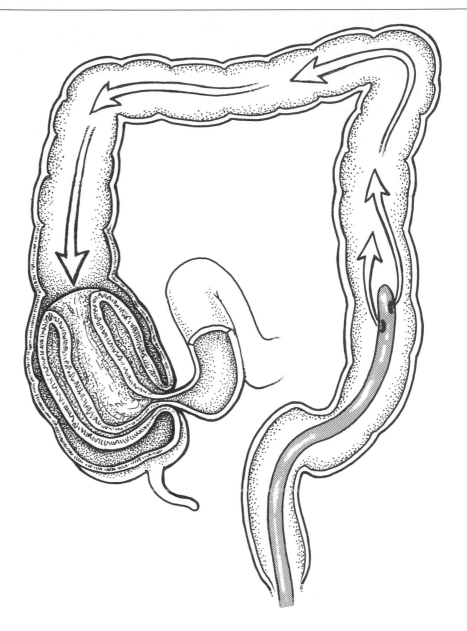

FIGURE 58.1 *Intussusception due to increased peristalsis of the terminal ileum.*

Intussusception can be treated nonoperatively in some patients by using a hydrostatic column of barium or air to reduce the intussusception (Case 2). When this cannot be done, or a lead point is found, then operative reduction and resection of the lesion producing the intussusception is required.

Appendicitis is best treated by appendectomy. Intra-abdominal purulent collections from either a perforated appendix or other causes is best treated by initial antibiotics and percutaneous drainage of the abscess. Subsequently, definitive treatment (appendectomy, bowel resection) can be done.

K E Y   P O I N T S

• In the neonatal period, abdominal tenderness/distention usually requires operation for diagnosis and treatment

FOLLOW-UP

To ensure that relief of the disease process has been achieved (Case 2) or that no complication of the operation (Case 3) has occurred, patients require frequent visits during the first year. Of concern is recurring abdominal tenderness and distention following operation because of intra-abdominal adhesions (see Ch. 21). Rarely, intussusception can recur following reduction during a barium enema study.

K E Y   P O I N T S

• To ensure that relief of disease process has been achieved or that no complication of operation has occurred, patients require frequent visits during first year

SUGGESTED READINGS

Oberlander TF, Rappaport LA: Recurrent abdominal pain during childhood. Pediatr Rev 14:313, 1993

Reviews this complex problem and emphasizes importance of careful, repeated evaluations and waiting.

QUESTIONS

1. *In the neonate, abdominal tenderness/distention?*
   A. Is a grave sign.
   B. Is related to a congenital anomaly.
   C. Is found in NEC without a concomitant congenital anomaly.
   D. All of the above.

2. *In the age group of 1–5 years, abdominal tenderness and distention?*
   A. Will always require operation for diagnosis and treatment.
   B. Are associated with diseases having high mortality and morbidity rates.
   C. Are invariably related to infectious causes.
   D. May be related to abnormal physiology, and some lesions can be treated without operations.

3. *Among children age 5–12 years?*
   A. Infectious disease processes are the major causes of abdominal tenderness.
   B. Abdominal tenderness/distention will require operation for diagnosis and treatment.
   C. Abdominal tenderness and distention occur, but rarely.
   D. Observation of the child rather than urgent operation is dangerous.

(See p. 604 for answers.)

59

NEONATAL
JAUNDICE

THOMAS C. MOORE

Mild jaundice is a common abnormality in the first weeks of life. This "physiologic jaundice" clears rapidly. Jaundice that fails to clear or that develops after the first week or two of life is of more concern, often indicating an anatomic biliary tract abnormality.

CASE 1
LIVER TRANSPLANT

An 18-month-old white male infant presented with deepening jaundice and fevers. His past medical history was significant for a Kasai procedure at 10 weeks of age and multiple admissions following that for jaundice and sepsis, including a second Kasai at 6 months of age. Due to the increasing frequency of episodes of cholangitis and later, progressive liver failure, the patient was considered for liver transplant, which was successfully performed 1 month before the patient's second birthday.

CASE 2
BILIARY ATRESIA

A 6-week-old black female infant was found to have worsening jaundice. The mother reported otherwise normal development and only had noticed the jaundice for the previous 3 days. Dark urine and pale bowel movements were also reported. Initial examination revealed hepatomegaly, and blood tests were significant for elevated bilirubin of 9 and an elevated alkaline phosphatase of 650 (NL, <110). Ultrasound showed dilated intrahepatic ducts consistent with biliary atresia. Operation was done with hepatic portoenterostomy (Kasai procedure). The patient subsequently did well, with only one mild episode of cholangitis 1 month postoperatively.

GENERAL CONSIDERATIONS

Biliary atresia is an acquired condition of obstruction of the extrahepatic bile ducts and progressive fibrosis of the intrahepatic ducts, often culminating in cirrhosis, liver failure, and death if not treated. Early attempts at surgical repair of biliary atresia resulted in the classification of "correctable" and "noncorrectable" obstructions. These distinctions were based on the appearance of the extrahepatic ducts at operation. Patency of the proximal extrahepatic ducts with fibrinous obliterative obstruction of the gallbladder, cystic duct, and distal common bile duct was deemed "correctable." Since the introduction of the Kasai operation (hepatic portoenterostomy) in 1959, this terminology was rendered obsolete as all forms of biliary atresia are treatable with some degree of success.

Biliary atresia affects approximately 1 in 10,000 children, most commonly females. Previously considered as a congenital defect, current evidence points to a viral etiology. The progressive fibrosis of the liver after birth without operative intervention, the occurrence in only one of monozygotic twins, and clusters of cases—all point to an infectious etiology, with reovirus and cytomegalovirus (CMV) being two leading candidates.

Choledochal cysts (saccular dilatations of the extrahepatic bile ducts) and Caroli's disease (intrahepatic biliary duct dilatation) also commonly present with jaundice. These diseases are also currently thought to be of viral origin and, along with biliary atresia, may represent a spectrum of diseases of the bile ducts.

DIAGNOSIS

Jaundice in the infant with biliary atresia typically becomes evident within the first few weeks of life. Choledochal cysts or Caroli's disease may present later in life, even in adulthood, depending on the extent and location of the ductal abnormalities. Infants with these biliary diseases manage to eat regularly, gain weight, and grow normally for the early part of their life (Case 2). In addition to jaundice, other common symptoms include abdominal pain, vomiting, and anorexia. Hepatomegaly is common early in the course (Case 2).

The prognosis of the infant with untreated biliary atresia decreases markedly by the 10th week of life. Prompt diagnosis is therefore crucial. Although a battery of blood tests can be useful to look for other causes of infantile jaundice, ultrasound and radionuclide isotope scans are the most useful tools in differentiating biliary tract abnormalities from hepatocellular causes. The dilated intra- and occasionally extrahepatic ducts can be detected by ultrasound. Absorption and clearance of technetium-99 IDA derivates into the biliary ducts is normal in patients with biliary atresia as hepatocellular function is not compromised initially, while poor hepatocellular uptake and excretion are observed with primary hepatocellular disease.

DIFFERENTIAL DIAGNOSIS

α_1-Antitrypsin deficiency and neonatal hepatitis are important considerations in the differential diagnosis of biliary atresia. Imaging studies, primarily ultrasonography and radionuclide scanning, can usually differentiate between these diverse classes of neonatal jaundice, and α_1-antitrypsin deficiency can be diagnosed by laboratory evaluation. Neonatal hepatitis is often a diagnosis of exclusion. It more commonly occurs in premature, low birthweight infants. Liver biopsy, if performed, will reveal inflammation, fibrosis, and multinuclear giant cells. It is important to recognize that neonatal hepatitis and biliary atresia may coexist.

TREATMENT

Preoperative administration of fluids and vitamin K are used to correct any deficiencies. Kasai's hepatic portoenterostomy or a modification thereof is usually done. A liver biopsy is first taken and evaluated to ensure the patency of the intrahepatic ducts, and a cholangiogram is performed by injecting a radiopaque solution into the gallbladder. If the cholangiogram cannot be obtained because of a fibrous gallbladder, the operation proceeds. A hepatojejunostomy is then performed connecting a defunctionalized (Roux-en-Y) segment of the jejunum to the portal area of the liver and thus connecting the liver/biliary tract to the intestines.

Despite the use of a defunctionalized intestinal segment, the most common postoperative cause of morbidity and mortality is ascending cholangitis (Cases 1 and 2), which affects most patients within the first month after operation. Patients with cholangitis experience fever, recurrence of jaundice, reduced bile duct flow, and leukocytosis. Persistent ascending cholangitis has often been treated by a repeat operation in an attempt to improve the drainage of bile (Case 1).

Liver transplantation is seldom the initial approach to the management of biliary atresia in infants under 10 months of age. Not only is the patient's own liver the best functioning one available, the proposed viral etiology of biliary atresia, combined with the resultant immunosuppression of transplantation, invokes even an greater risk of ultimate malignant transformation (cancer) of remaining portions of the intrahepatic and extrahepatic biliary tract. Liver transplantation is considered when repeat portoenterostomy operations prove unsuccessful or the liver has become too hardened and cirrhotic in infants past 10 months of age (Case 1).

Choledochal cysts are preferentially treated by excision of the cyst and hepaticojejunostomy. Simple drainage of the cyst into the duodenum or jejunum is a largely abandoned operation because of the high incidence of late carcinoma development.

SUGGESTED READINGS

Moore TC: Pathogenesis of biliary atresia. Pediatrics 78:182, 1986

A look at the evidence for a viral etiology of the disease.

Ohi R, Nio M, Chiba T et al: Long-term follow-up after surgery for patients with biliary atresia. J Pediatr Surg 25:442, 1990

Highlights outcome, including need for reoperation and transplant.

Yamaguchi M: Congenital choledochal cyst. Analysis of 1,433 patients in the Japanese literature. Am J Surg 40:653, 1980

An extremely large and comprehensive series of a disease that is uncommon in North America.

QUESTIONS

The best test for differentiating biliary atresia from other causes of jaundice is?

    A. Serum bilirubin measurement.

    B. CT scan.

    C. Liver biopsy.

    D. Ultrasound.

    E. Cholangiogram.

2. The treatment of biliary atresia by hepatic portoenterostomy may result in?

    A. Progressive liver failure.

    B. A normal life.

    C. Repeated episodes of cholangitis.

    D. Temporary improvement only.

    E. All of the above.

(See p. 604 for answers.)

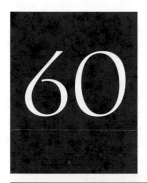

60

ABDOMINAL WALL
MALFORMATIONS

THOMAS C. MOORE

EDWARD PASSARO, JR.

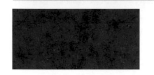

Abdominal wall defects occur at two sites where organs pass through: the umbilicus, where viscera formed in the amniotic sac outside the abdomen pass into the abdominal cavity; and the inguinal region, where testes migrate from their retroperitoneal abdominal location to the scrotum outside or external to the body. Of the two, the latter is far more common.

This chapter describes the defects to be found at these two sites and emphasizes the points in their differentiation and treatment.

CASE 1
OMPHALOCELE

A 30-year-old female was seen in the 6th month of her second pregnancy. An abdominal ultrasound showed a male fetus with what was interpreted as extra-abdominal viscera. No other congenital defect was noted. An α-feto-protein level later returned markedly elevated. She was informed of the findings and accepted that a cesarean section delivery would be done before term. At operation, a 2,800-g male was delivered. At the base of the umbilical cord was an intact 8-cm sac containing most of the small bowel and a portion of the colon. The bowel appeared normal. There was no cardiac murmur. The following day the neonate underwent operation. The sac was excised and the defect repaired primarily. On follow-up examination 2 months later, there was normal growth and development of the infant.

CASE 2
GASTROSCHISIS

A 4-hour-old female neonate was referred because of extra-abdominal viscera. She was delivered vaginally to a 32-year-old mother of three. The external bowels were edematous, reddened, and covered in patches with a yellow-gray peel. They had been placed in a plastic sac for transport.

On arrival, the neonate appeared cold but otherwise healthy. She was placed on a warming blanket in the neonate ICU. The abdomen was flat and underdeveloped. To the right of the umbilicus was a 4-cm defect through which passed most of her intestines. She was brought to operating room where a plastic tube (chimney) was sewn to the skin edges around the defect with the bowels inside the tube. The other end of the plastic chimney was closed and maintained vertically by a line attached to the end, and brought through a pulley with a weight at the end. During the following week, the edema in the extra-abdominal loops of bowel receded and the intestines gradually slid into the abdomen. On the 9th day, a primary repair of the abdominal wall defect was done. There was normal growth and development of the neonate on follow-up visit at 2 months.

CASE 3
INGUINAL HERNIA

The mother of a 2-month-old male infant noted a bulge in the right inguinal region when the infant cried. When the infant was relaxed and not crying, the mass disappeared. The mass was not noticeably tender or firm when the mother touched it. The pediatrician confirmed the presence of a right inguinal hernia, probably indirect. No hernia or dilatated inguinal rings could be felt on the left side. A right inguinal hemography was done. On follow-up examination 4 months later, no inguinal masses or bulges were found.

GENERAL CONSIDERATIONS

During embryonic development the viscera develops in the amniotic sac outside of the abdominal cavity. With maturity the sac is gradually reabsorbed and the viscera (liver and bowels) are relocated into their proper intra-abdominal sites. This generally takes place by the 8th week of prenatal life.

When this process is interrupted, usually because of genetic defects, the abdominal contents remain in the amniotic sac. The abdominal cavity is then severely underdeveloped. The sac may remain intact but is usually ruptured during birth. The viscera tends to be dilated, edematous, and covered with a gelatinous "peel" (Fig. 60.1). The genetic factors responsible may involve other organs, in particular the heart. Omphalocele is thus indicative of a very serious problem. It has a high mortality rate because of the associated congenital defects, in particular those of the heart.

Another defect to be found about the umbilicus, invariably to the right of it (Fig. 60.2), is gastroschisis. Here again, there is bowel outside of the abdominal cavity. The

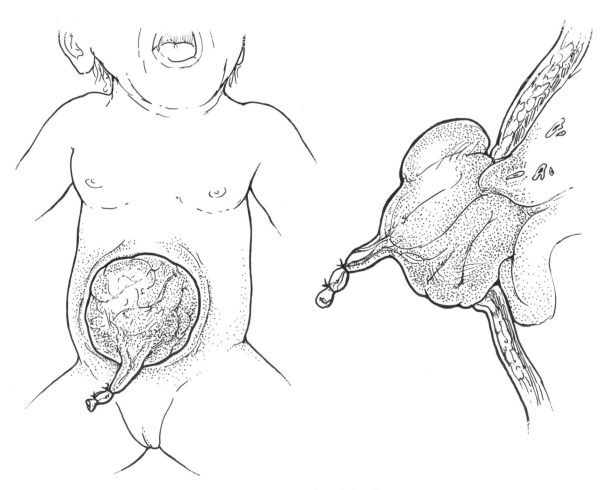

FIGURE 60.1 *Omphalocele.*

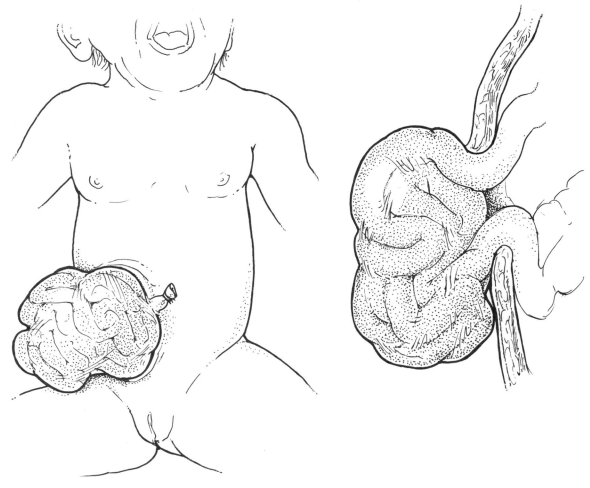

FIGURE 60.2   *Gastroschisis.*

bowel is similarly edematous, dilated, and covered with a thick, gelatinous peel. Although there may be associated defects, they are exclusively of the bowel and include such things as atresias, volvulus, or areas of stenosis. These defects are thought to result from vascular injuries and the effect of pressure on the bowel. However, other organs are normal. This, together with a recently recorded significant increase in the incidence of gastroschisis, implies that environmental rather than genetic factors are responsible for its development. Gastroschisis has a much lower mortality rate than omphalocele.

Remnants of the connection between the bowel and the yolk sac may persist at the umbilicus, namely, the omphalomesenteric duct remnants. Because a duct may persist or remain as an atrophic fibrous band, it can produce intestinal obstruction as a segment of bowel gets caught or wrapped about the band.

The other remnant to be found in the umbilicus is a remnant of the urachal duct connecting the umbilicus to the urinary bladder. The urachal duct and bladder are retroperitoneal and therefore not associated with intestinal obstruction.

The last and most common benign defect of the umbilicus is an umbilical hernia. Common in blacks, they usually close as the infant grows.

Overall, inguinal hernias are the most common abdominal wall malformation. The testis, as it descends from its retroperitoneal site of origin, is usually accompanied by a finger of the peritoneum (see Ch. 13), the processus vaginalis. Although this remnant coursing along the cord structures is relatively common, only a few develop into indirect hernias. In neonates and newborns, these usually occur on the right and, not infrequently, bilaterally.

KEY POINTS

• When developmental process interrupted, usually because of genetic defects, abdominal contents remain in amniotic sac

• Viscera tends to be dilated, edematous, and covered with gelatinous "peel" (Fig. 60.1)

• Omphalocele is indicative of very serious problem; high mortality rate because of associated congenital defects, in particular those of the heart

• Another defect to be found about umbilicus, invariably to the right of it (Fig. 60.2) is gastroschisis

• Although there may be associated defects, they are exclusively of the bowel and include such things as atresias, volvulus, or areas of stenosis; these defects are thought to result from vascular injuries and effect of pressure on the bowel

• Gastroschisis has much lower mortality rate than omphalocele

• Overall, inguinal hernias are most common abdominal wall malformation

DIAGNOSIS

The diagnosis of congenital abdominal wall malformations can be made on careful inspection.

Large defects with the presence of extracorporeal bowel are obvious. Grossly similar omphalocele and gastroschisis can be further differentiated by careful examination as discussed below.

The general use of ultrasonography during pregnancy has made possible prenatal detection of these defects. Screening for elevated levels of serum α-fetoprotein (AFP) also detects these defects.

The discharge of bile-stained or feculent-like material suggests persistent omphalomesenteric duct. Contrast studies showing the dye in the ileum confirm the diagnosis. A granulating, non-healing umbilicus may contain a gastric mucosa found in these ducts.

Clear fluid expressed from the umbilicus suggests a urachal duct or cyst. Contrast die injected into the sinus shows the course of the tract, often to the bladder.

Umbilical hernias are usually evident on gross inspection; less commonly, the defect is only found on palpation. Hernias may become obvious when the child cries or strains.

Inguinal hernias are evident as bulges or masses in the groin that become visible or more pronounced when the child cries and increases the intra-abdominal pressure. When not visible, a hernia should be considered in the infant who cries when moving bowel or who appears restless or uncomfortable for no discernible reason. Careful palpation of the cord structure bilaterally will give the feeling of a thickened, smooth structure ("silk-glove" sign) beneath the examining finger.

KEY POINTS

• Clear fluid expressed from umbilicus suggests urachal duct or cyst

• Inguinal hernias evident as bulges or masses in groin that become visible or more pronounced when child cries and increases intra-abdominal pressure

DIFFERENTIAL DIAGNOSIS

The finding of extracorporeal bowel covered with a thick, gelatinous peel at birth is due to either omphalocele or gastroschisis.

Omphaloceles are readily diagnosed by the presence of the omphalosac remnant in which the viscera are contained. The sac is found at the base of the umbilical cord (Fig. 60.2). The sac is rarely intact. More frequently, a portion of it remains after the trauma of birth. The intestines are covered by thick, gelatinous peel. The finding of an associated cardiac defect suggests the diagnosis.

Gastroschisis, by contrast, lacks a sac, and is found always to the right of the umbilicus. It is not associated with cardiac or other defects, other than those of the bowel.

Omphalitis, infection of the umbilicus, can produce a discharge that resembles that of omphalomesenteric duct remnant or of a urachus. Omphalitis, however, responds promptly to local hygiene and topical antibiotics, whereas the drainage from the congenital duct elements persists.

Bulges in the groin include hydroceles and undescended testes. The scrotum must be carefully examined, therefore, when the infant is thought to have an inguinal hernia. Hydroceles contain clear peritoneal fluid. In a darkened room they transilluminate light readily, whereas hernias and undescended or retractile testes do not. The retractile testes can be replaced down into the scrotum, whereas the undescended testis cannot.

KEY POINTS

• Omphaloceles readily diagnosed by presence of omphalosac remnant in which viscera are contained

• Gastroschisis lacks a sac and is found to right of umbilicus; not associated with cardiac or other defects, other than bowel

• Omphalitis, infection of umbilicus, can produce discharge that resembles that of omphalomesenteric duct remnant or of urachus

• Bulges in groin include hydroceles and undescended testes; in darkened room, transilluminate light readily, whereas hernias and undescended or retractile testes do not

TREATMENT

Omphalocele can be treated by gradual inversion of the sac, allowing the viscera to slowly be returned to the abdominal cavity. Alternatively, when most of sac has been lost, the viscera can be contained in a plastic bag anchored to the abdominal wall, which serves the same function as the intact sac.

The treatment of this and other congenital disorders is undergoing change because of accurate antenatal diagnosis by ultrasonography. Omphalocele and associated cardiac defects discovered early in the pregnancy pose the question of terminating the pregnancy. When the pregnancy is continued, delivery by cesarean section is preferable, as the intestines are normal in these instances. The thick, gelatinous peel is related to normal labor and vaginal delivery.

Gastroschisis, similarly, is best treated by cesarean section delivery to avoid the morbidity from otherwise edematous bowel covered by a peel. At delivery, the normal-appearing bowel is returned to the abdominal cavity, and the abdominal wall defect is closed primarily. Gastroschisis found during labor and vaginal delivery is treated by placing the swollen peel-covered bowel in a plastic sac sewn to the edges of the defect. Gradually the swelling subsides, the peel is slowly reabsorbed, and the bowel is returned to the abdominal cavity. The abdominal wall defect is then repaired. Omphalomesenteric duct remnant is excised along with a short segment of the ileum into which it leads.

Urachal duct remnant is excised and the bladder and umbilical defects closed.

Umbilical hernias are observed until the child is about 5 years of age, as most will have closed by then. Those that persist or become enlarged or systematic are treated by repair of the defect.

Inguinal hernia repair is perhaps the most common operation done in neonates and infants. In contrast to adults (see Ch. 13), these are invariably indirect hernias. Simple excision of the hernia sac, processus vaginalis, suffices in neonates. In other infants, a repair of the inguinal region may be necessary.

KEY POINTS

- When most of sac lost, viscera can be contained in plastic bag anchored to abdominal wall, which serves same function as intact sac
- When pregnancy is continued, delivery by cesarean section is preferable, as intestines are normal in these instances

R FOLLOW-UP

Repairs of abdominal wall defects need to be observed over the following year to ensure that the repair does not fail and a defect recur. In addition, neonates born with extracorporeal viscera are followed to ensure that intestinal complication of obstruction or malabsorption do not occur.

SUGGESTED READINGS

Bethel C, Seashore J, Touloukian R: Cesarean section does not improve outcome in gastroschisis. J Pediatr Surg 24:1, 1989

A consideration of the pros and cons of cesarean section in the prevention of bowel complications in this condition.

Hatat V, Baxter R: Surgical options in the management of large omphaloceles. Am J Surg 153:449, 1989

Elucidates the last treatment plans for these large, difficult lesions.

QUESTIONS

1. The thick, gelatinous peel found covering the extracorporeal intestines in either instance of omphalocele or gastroschisis is?

    A. Due to genetic or viral infections responsible for the development of both conditions.

    B. Related to the extracorporeal location of the bowel antenatally in both conditions.

    C. Related to the biochemical changes and trauma associated with normal labor and delivery.

    D. Cannot be prevented by any present means.

2. Of the two, omphalocele and gastroschisis?

    A. Omphalocele is the more lethal condition because of associated cardiac defects.

    B. Gastroschisis is the more lethal condition because of the lack of the amino sac to protect the exposed bowel from injury and infection.

    C. The prognoses are similar inasmuch as extracorporeal bowel is found in each and the difference is primarily in the size and location of the abdominal wall defect.

    D. None of the above.

3. Umbilical hernias are?

    A. Particularly common in premature infants and black infants.

    B. Benign, as most will close spontaneously with growth and development.

    C. Treated when they fail to close in the first 5 years, enlarge, or become symptomatic.

    D. All of the above.

(See p. 604 for answers.)

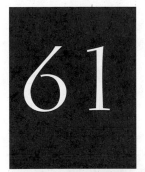

61

TRAUMA IN CHILDREN

FRED S. BONGARD

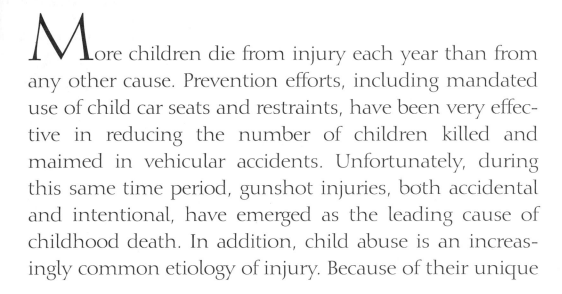

More children die from injury each year than from any other cause. Prevention efforts, including mandated use of child car seats and restraints, have been very effective in reducing the number of children killed and maimed in vehicular accidents. Unfortunately, during this same time period, gunshot injuries, both accidental and intentional, have emerged as the leading cause of childhood death. In addition, child abuse is an increasingly common etiology of injury. Because of their unique

anatomic and physiologic makeup, children frequently sustain multisystem injuries that can rapidly become fatal if not recognized and treated expediently.

This chapter reviews the basic steps in pediatric resuscitation, including airway and fluid management. Furthermore, it discusses the management of shock as well as the treatment of thoracic, abdominal, central nervous system, and extremity injuries. Thorough familiarity with these principles is required to provide efficient and quality care for the injured child.

CASE 1
A GUNSHOT WOUND TO THE LEG

A 10-year-old gang member was involved in a gunfight with a rival gang. During the encounter, he sustained a single gunshot wound to the right thigh. On arrival in the emergency room, his BP was 90/80 mmHg with a heart rate of 140 bpm. His pants were saturated with blood and had to be removed with scissors. Both feet were cool to palpation. No other injuries were present.

A large bore intravenous catheter was inserted in an antecubital vein, and an 800-ml bolus of warmed lactated Ringer's solution was infused over 15 minutes to this 40 kg patient. His heart rate slowed and pulse pressure increased. The extremities became warmer.

Radiographs of the right thigh showed a badly comminuted fracture with extensive soft tissue damage and swelling. Operative fixation was required.

CASE 2
SOME STRANGE ECCHYMOSES

A 2½-year-old female was brought to the emergency room by her mother after falling down stairs. Her mother reported that the child was sitting on a step while playing with the family dog. In a moment of excitement, the dog bumped her, resulting in a fall of five steps onto a marble floor. On examination, she was persistently irritable ("V" score = 3) and crying vigorously with no signs of respiratory distress. After several minutes of agitation, she vomited greenish yellow liquid.

Examination found multiple ecchymoses of differing size and age throughout her body. Two ribs on the right side had palpable fractures. A radiograph demonstrated an old and partially healed left radial fracture. A head CT scan was performed because of the child's increasing lethargy. No mass lesions were detected.

When questioned about the number and extent of injuries, the mother responded that the child was constantly active and was always falling. After consultation with a social worker, the treating physician decided to contact the local child protection authorities.

GENERAL CONSIDERATIONS

Childhood victims of trauma undergo the same basic physiologic responses as older patients. Several factors are unique to this age group, however, and require special attention. Because children are smaller, they are exposed to a greater amount of force per unit of body surface area than are adults. Also, because the ratio of body surface area to weight is highest at birth, heat is lost rapidly by infants, making them hypothermic within a short period. These patients must be kept warm during diagnosis and management with particular attention paid to the use of warmed solutions whenever possible. Furthermore, because they have less fat and connective tissue than older patients, kinetic energy is more easily transmitted to the viscera, resulting in multiple organ injuries. Because their skeletons are soft and incompletely calcified, internal organ injury may occur in the absence of fractures. This is of particular importance in the thorax, where the soft ribs provide little protection for the lungs and mediastinum. Rib fractures are evidence of high energy transfer and should arouse suspicion of underlying injury (Case 2).

Childhood injury may have long-term consequences that affect both physical and psychological development. As many as 60% of children who sustain severe multisystem trauma have residual personality changes 1 year later, while up to 50% exhibit cognitive and physical handicaps. The injury often goes beyond the child victim by affecting parents and siblings. Financial and social hardships may follow an injury, resulting in long-term disability. The importance of these consequences must be remembered when dealing with young patients and their families.

KEY POINTS

- Pediatric trauma patients must be kept warm during diagnosis and management, with particular attention paid to use of warmed solutions whenever possible

- Internal organ injury may occur in absence of fractures

- Rib fractures are evidence of high energy transfer and should arouse suspicion of underlying injury

---

DIAGNOSIS

The diagnostic approach to the injured child is not fundamentally different than that for the adult. Injured infants are unable to provide a history regarding their injury, while young children are so agitated or frightened that pertinent information cannot be obtained. Parents, relatives, or bystanders become vital sources of information regarding the circumstances of injury. Emotional, crying children are often impossible to evaluate until they are calmed and reassured.

The initial evaluation should center around the Airway, Breathing, and Circulation (ABCs). Once done, the level of consciousness should be assessed using either the Glasgow Coma Scale or the "V" score (Table 61.1). Once identified, brain injuries should be treated immediately, since they are a major source of subsequent morbidity and mortality.

Multiple injuries are very common in children, making a methodical survey mandatory. The chest can be evaluated with a plain radiograph, while the abdomen requires a computed tomography (CT) scan. If a head injury is suspected, a CT evaluation of the head is required. Both oral and intravenous contrast should be used for the abdominal scan, while the head scan is best performed without contrast enhancement. Radiographs of the neck, spine, pelvis, and extremities should be obtained as the clinical situation warrants. Interpretation of these studies is often difficult because ossification centers may be confused with fractures.

Hemorrhage is common following injury in children. Fortunately, their physiologic reserve allows compensation even in the face of severe hypovolemia. The presence of relatively normal vital signs (Case 1) may mislead the physician into thinking that the injury is relatively minor. Tachycardia and decreased skin perfusion (presenting as mottling and/or coolness) are important early findings that should warn of the true extent of injury. Although tachycardia is the initial response to hypovolemia, it may also be caused by pain and fear. For this reason, evaluation of organ perfu-

TABLE 61.1 *Pediatric Verbal Score*

Verbal Response	V Score
Appropriate words or social smile, fixes, and follows	5
Cries, but consolable	4
Persistently irritable	3
Restless, agitated	2
None	1

(From American College of Surgeons, Committee on Trauma: Advanced Trauma Life Support Manual. American College of Surgeons, Chicago, IL, 1993, with permission.)

sion (e.g., skin color and urinary output) and blood pressure is mandatory. In general, a child's blood pressure should be 80 mmHg plus twice his or her age in years. The diastolic blood pressure should be two-thirds of the systolic blood pressure. A decrease in pulse pressure (systolic minus diastolic pressure) is indicative of vasoconstriction (increased peripheral vascular resistance) in response to hypovolemia (Case 1). A blood volume loss of about 25% is required before clinical signs appear (Table 61.2). Initial treatment consists of a 20 ml/kg bolus of warmed fluid (usually lactated Ringer's solution) given over 10–15 minutes (Case 1). Evidence of appropriate resuscitation includes (1) a decrease in the heart rate to less than 130 bpm, (2) an increase in the pulse pressure to more than 20 mmHg, (3) a return of skin color and warmth, (4) improved mental status, (5) an increased urine output (>1 ml/kg/hr), and (6) an increased systolic blood pressure (>80 mmHg). If the child does not improve after the first bolus of fluid, a second bolus may be given *after* consultation with a surgeon. Because the child may require emergent surgical intervention, consultation is mandatory when the initial fluid bolus fails to return vital signs to normal. If improvement does not occur after two boluses, blood transfusion will likely be necessary. Until type-specific blood is available, type O Rh-negative packed red blood cells (10 ml/kg) is used.

Venous access for children with multiple injuries, especially infants, is problematic. When possible, percutaneous access is preferred. The common femoral veins should be avoided in infants and young children because of the high incidence of ischemic limb loss and venous thrombosis. When venous cutdowns are required, the preferred sites are the greater saphenous vein at the ankle, the median cephalic vein at the elbow, and the median cephalic vein in the upper arm. The external jugular vein can often be cannulated percutaneously. Intraosseous infusion into the marrow cavity of an uninjured long bone is an acceptable alternative in children less than 6 years of age. Complications are uncommon but include cellulitis and osteomyelitis.

Hypothermia can occur quickly during the resuscitation of an undressed child. This may increase coagulation times, depress central nervous system functioning, and render the patient refractory to pharmacologic therapy. Warmed fluids should be used whenever possible, and the child should be kept covered when not undergoing examination. Heat lamps should be used around small children and infants.

Blunt injuries of the chest are common in childhood. A compliant chest wall permits the ready transfer of energy to the intrathoracic organs, frequently without external evidence of trauma. When rib fractures are present, this implies massive kinetic energy transfer and is usually associated with multisystem injury (Case 2). The mobility of the mediastinum makes children more susceptible to the hemodynamic effect of tension pneumothorax.

The treatment of thoracic injuries is similar to that for adults, with special attention paid to the possibility of concealed injuries. Decompression and drainage with a tube thoracostomy is required when a pneumo- or hemothorax is present.

Abdominal injuries may be caused by either blunt or penetrating mechanisms. The key to management is thorough examination and accurate diagnosis. The examiner should calmly ask the child about the accident and whether pain is present. If the patient is too young or cannot answer, a relative or witness should be questioned. Examination should proceed only when the child is calm and at ease. Because young children tend to swallow air, rapid increases in abdominal girth must not be mistaken for intra-abdominal hemorrhage. Placement of an orogastric tube will decompress the stomach and facilitate examination.

Peritoneal lavage or CT scan may be used to evaluate the abdomen. CT scans are particularly useful because the identification of some intra-abdominal injuries (e.g., liver or splenic lacerations in a stable patient) may allow nonoperative management in selected cases. Surgical consultation is mandatory during the decision-making process. Peritoneal lavage is accomplished by instilling 10 ml/kg of

TABLE 61.2 *Systemic responses to blood loss in the pediatric patient*

	<25% Blood Volume Loss	25–45% Blood Volume Loss	>45% Blood Volume Loss
Cardiac	Weak, thready pulse; increased heart rate	Increased heart rate	Hypotension, tachycardia to bradycardia
Central nervous system	Lethargic, irritable, confused	Change in level of consciousness, dulled response to pain	Comatose
Skin	Cool, clammy	Cyanotic, decreased capillary refill, cold extremities	Pale, cold
Kidneys	Decreased urinary output; increased specific gravity	Minimal urine output	No urinary output

(From American College of Surgeons, Committee on Trauma: Advanced Trauma Life Support Manual, American College of Surgeons, Chicago, IL, 1993, with permission.)

warmed lactated Ringer's solution into the peritoneal cavity. Up to 1 L (the usual adult dose) may be used. Because children generally have thin abdominal walls, catheter placement must be carried out with extreme caution to prevent penetration of the bowel with the lavage catheter. The CT scan is the preferred modality because it provides anatomic information. Peritoneal lavage may be the test of choice in situations such as (1) severe brain injury requiring immediate surgery, when time does not permit an abdominal CT, and (2) a physical examination that suggests peritonitis (the lavage fluid will exhibit white blood cells or fecal material, while the CT scan is not sensitive for bowel injuries).

Head and spinal cord injury are common among children and often result from pedestrian accidents. Unlike the situation in adults, survival among children following head trauma is more related to associated injuries than to the head injury itself. This is not the case among those younger than 3 years, in whom outcome from severe head trauma is worse than in older children. Children are very susceptible to the effects of secondary brain injury that occur in the face of hypotension, hypoxia, seizures, and hypothermia. The prompt and thorough resuscitation of head injured children is critical to optimum management.

Vomiting is common among head injured patients and does not necessarily imply increased intracranial pressure (Case 2). Children with fontanels that have not yet fused are relatively tolerant of increased intracranial pressure and expanding mass lesions because they can accommodate more volume. When a bulging fontanel is present in a noncomatose patient, one should be suspicious that a severe head injury is present with increased intracranial volume. Seizures are common and are usually self-limited. If seizures occur, CT scanning is indicated.

Classification and treatment of head injuries is similar to that for adults with a few exceptions. The Glasgow Coma Scale is useful for monitoring the progress of older children who are able to verbalize. The Pediatric Verbal Score ("V" score, Case 2) should be used for those less than 4 years of age (Table 61.1). Intracranial pressure monitoring must be instituted early in those with a Glasgow Coma Score of 8 or less, or in those with multiple injuries who need other operations. Antiseizure drugs commonly used in children with head injuries include (1) phenobarbital, (2) diazepam, (3) phenytoin, and (4) mannitol (used to reduce intracerebral swelling). Repeated careful assessment of the child's progress is mandatory. Neurosurgical consultation should be obtained at the beginning of treatment. Intervention must be undertaken if the child fails to improve or begins to deteriorate.

Extremities are among the most common locations for injuries in children. They are often difficult to diagnose accurately because of lack of mineralization around the growth plate. Children tend to lose more blood from long bone fractures than adults do. Even small children can

lose several hundred milliliters of blood from pelvic and long bone fractures. Proportionately, this amount is greater than that seen in adults. The volume is sequestered around the bone within the fascia and may present as a compartment syndrome (Case 1). Fractures should be immobilized and treated definitively either with casting or operative reduction and fixation.

KEY POINTS

• Initial evaluation should center around airway, breathing, and circulation (ABCs)

• Tachycardia and decreased skin perfusion (presenting as mottling and/or coolness) are important early findings that should warn of true extent of injury

• Child's blood pressure should be 80 mmHg plus twice their age in years

• Blood volume loss of about 25% required before clinical signs appear (Table 61.2)

• Initial treatment consists of 20 ml/kg bolus of warmed fluid, usually lactated Ringer's solution, given over 10–15 minutes

• Evidence of appropriate resuscitation includes (1) a decrease in heart rate to less than 130 bpm, (2) an increase in pulse pressure to more than 20 mmHg, (3) a return of skin color and warmth, (4) improved mental status, (5) an increased urine output (>1 ml/kg/hr), and (6) an increased systolic blood pressure (>80 mmHg)

• Common femoral veins should not be used for venous access in infants and young children because of the high incidence of ischemic limb loss and venous thrombosis; when venous cutdowns required, preferred sites are greater saphenous vein at ankle, median cephalic vein at elbow, and median cephalic vein in upper arm

• CT scans useful in identification of some intra-abdominal injuries (e.g., liver or splenic lacerations in a stable patient), to allow nonoperative management in select cases

• Unlike adults, survival among children following head trauma is more related to associated injuries than to head injury, except among children younger than 3, in whom outcome from severe head trauma is worse than in older children

• Children are very susceptible to effects of secondary brain injury that occur in face of hypotension, hypoxia, seizures, and hypothermia

• When a bulging fontanel presents in a noncomatose patient, one should suspect severe head injury with increased intracranial volume; if seizures occur, CT scan is indicated

• Intracranial pressure monitoring must be instituted early in those with Glasgow Coma Score of 8 or less, or in those with multiple injuries who need other operations

• Children tend to lose more blood from long bone fractures than adults; even small children can lose several hundred milliliters of blood from pelvic and long bone fractures

TREATMENT

Management of the airway and ensuring breathing and circulation are the three cardinal first steps in the care of any trauma victim, young or old. This is often difficult in children who have a disproportionately larger cranium than midface. The airway is best protected in the "sniffing position" in which the midface is brought into a slightly anterior and superior relationship. Attention to in-line traction of the cervical spine is important during this maneuver. Intubation is difficult in infants because of the anterior position of their larnyx. Furthermore, because an 18-month-old infant's larnyx is only 7 cm long, overzealous insertion of an endotracheal tube may result in a right mainstem intubation with possible injury to the tracheobronchial tree and/or inadequate ventilation. Tracheostomy and cricothyroidotomy are needed infrequently, but when required, cricothyroidotomy or insertion of a needle through the cricothyroid membrane for jet ventilation is preferred.

Children should be mechanically ventilated at about 20 breaths/min (infants require 40), with a tidal volume of 7–10 ml/kg. Care must be taken to avoid respiratory alkalosis developing from hyperventilation. When adequately volume resuscitated, children have little problem maintaining normal pH. Sodium bicarbonate should be used with extreme caution, since it may aggravate respiratory acidosis. This occurs when the HCO_3^- moiety combines with a proton to provide carbonic acid H_2CO_3. Carbonic acid dissociates into H_2O+CO_2, thus increasing the load of carbon dioxide that must be eliminated by the lungs.

FOLLOW-UP

Childhood victims of trauma typically develop normally both physically and psychologically unless they have sustained a debilitating injury. Special attention must be paid to the emotional needs of both the patient and family, as this often forms the limiting step in the patient's recuperation.

Of particular importance are battered children. The abused child syndrome refers to any child who sustains a nonaccidental injury as the result of acts by parents, guardians, or acquaintances. Child abuse is one of the major causes of mortality among infants less than 1 year of age. A history and physical examination inconsistent with each other should alert the physician to the possibility of child abuse. Historic items include (1) a prolonged interval between the time of injury and presentation for medical care, (2) a history of repeated presentations for injury in different clinics or emergency departments, (3) failure to comply with medical advice, and (4) a history that changes or varies between parents or guardians. Physical findings of significance include (1) multiple subdural hematomas, especially without a new skull fracture, (2) retinal hemorrhage or perioral injuries, (3) ruptured viscera without a clear history of major trauma, (4) injury to the genital or perianal areas, (5) evidence of old scars or healed fractured on radiograph, (6) fractures of long bones in children under 3 years of age, (7) unusual skin injury patterns consistent with bites, burns, or rope marks, and (8) sharply demarcated (e.g., from a cigarette) second- and third-degree burns.

All states currently require that physicians report cases of child abuse (even when only suspected) to authorities. Provisions are usually made to protect physicians who report suspected abuse from legal liability.

KEY POINTS

- History and physical examination inconsistent with each other should alert physician to possibility of child abuse

SUGGESTED READINGS

American College of Surgeons (Committee on Trauma): Advanced Trauma Life Support Manual. p. 26. American College of Surgeons, Chicago, IL, 1993

This chapter from the American College of Surgeons Trauma Life Support Manual is an excellent step-by-step reference on the management of pediatric injuries. A number of the protocols presented in this chapter come from the Committee on Trauma guidelines. For those interested in emergency medicine and trauma, the Advanced Trauma Life Support Manual is an invaluable reference.

Choong RK, Grattan-Smith TM, Cohen RC et al: Splenic injury in children: a 10 year experience. J Pediatr Child Health 29:192, 1993.

This article retrospectively reviews the management of splenic trauma at a large Australian referral center over a 10-year period. Forty-nine patients with splenic injury are discussed. The manuscript includes presentation, diagnosis, management, and outcome.

Doueck HJ: Screening for child abuse: problems and possibilities. Appl Nurs Res 8:191, 1995.

This article discusses some excellent points on screening for child abuse. This is an unfortunate problem that all practicing physicians need to be aware of.

Mitchell KA, Fallat ME, Raque GH et al: Evaluation of minor head injury in children. J Pediat Surg 29:851, 1994.

This excellent review describes the evaluation and early diagnosis of children with minor head injury. It is a short and easily readable article.

Roche BG, Bugmann P, Le Coultre C: Blunt injuries to liver, spleen, kidney, and pancreas in pediatric patients. Eur J Pediat Surg 2:154, 1992

This article discusses 96 children with blunt injuries to the liver, spleen, pancreas, and kidney. The review determines the accuracy of radiologic imaging and defines clinical factors present on admission that are predictive of major injuries requiring operative intervention. The current trend toward nonoperative management of injuries in children makes this article of particular importance.

QUESTIONS

1. Which of the following is the first priority in the management of an injured child?

    A. Establish a large bore intravenous catheter.
    B. Secure an adequate airway.
    C. Stabilize the cervical spine.
    D. Perform a peritoneal lavage.

2. Which of the following would not be expected with an acute loss of circulating blood volume of less than 25%?

    A. Cool and clammy skin.
    B. Decreased urine output.
    C. Lethargy and confusion.
    D. Hypotension.

3. Which statement is not true?

    A. Children are more susceptible to a tension pneumothorax than adults.
    B. Children have higher surface area/weight ratios than adults.
    C. Children bleed less from fractures than adults.
    D. Intraosseous catheters for venous access are restricted to patients less than 6 years of age.

4. Which of the following findings would most likely be indicative of the abused child syndrome?

    A. An 8-year-old boy with a broken femur. His mother states that he was hurt while playing football with the neighbors.
    B. While examining a 3-year-old with a scald burn, the nurse informs you that she saw the child 2 months ago at another hospital with a similar injury.
    C. A 9-year-old girl with a subdural hematoma. The father states that she has trouble on her bicycle and has fallen several times but has never needed medical attention.
    D. An 18-month-old boy, easily comforted by his mother, who brings him in after he fell down a flight of stairs.

(See p. 604 for answers.)

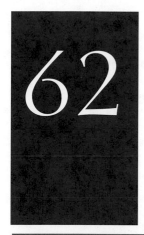

62

KIDNEY AND

PANCREAS

TRANSPLANTATION

MILAN KINKHABWALA

DAVID K. IMAGAWA

Kidney transplantation is the treatment of choice for most patients with end-stage renal disease (ESRD). In the United States, diabetes mellitus, hypertension, and chronic glomerulonephritis are the most common causes of renal parenchymal damage leading to dialysis depen-

dence. Patients who are eligible for kidney transplantation may wait up to 4 years for a cadaveric donor organ, reflecting the overall shortage of organ donors compared to potential recipients. Overall graft survival exceeds 85% at 1 year for both cadaveric and living allografts.

Patients with severe complications of type 1 diabetes mellitus may be eligible for whole organ pancreatic transplantation. Most commonly, pancreatic transplantation is performed together with renal transplantation in diabetic patients with ESRD. One-year graft survival after whole organ pancreas transplantation is approximately 80%.

The aims of this chapter are to (1) elucidate the indications for kidney and pancreatic transplantation, (2) briefly describe the organ donation process, (3) describe the transplant operation, and (4) describe the diagnosis and treatment of common postoperative complications. More comprehensive discussions of the mechanisms of immunosuppressive agents are provided in Chapter 63.

CASE 1
RENAL TRANSPLANTATION
FOLLOWED BY CMV INFECTION

A 36-year-old male with ESRD due to hypertension required hemodialysis for 1 year before undergoing transplant evaluation. The patient had two brothers, aged 33

and 39, who were potential living donors. However, one brother was the sole supporter of a large family and the other brother was found to be ABO incompatible. Eighteen months later, a suitable cadaveric organ was obtained. The organ was delivered to the transplant center 24 hours after procurement. The transplant operation was uneventful. Postoperatively, the kidney made minimal urine. A renal ultrasound demonstrated patent renal artery and vein. Renal scan showed good uptake but poor excretion. Because of the desire to avoid cyclosporine nephrotoxicity in the setting of poor initial graft function, OKT3 was started for immunosuppression. The patient was dialyzed on postoperative day 2. On postoperative day 3, the kidney began to excrete urine. Urine flow steadily increased from less than 200 ml/day to over 1,500 ml/day over the next several days. The creatinine level fell slowly to 2.0, where it stabilized. Because of the concern for undiagnosed rejection, a renal biopsy was obtained on postoperative day 6, which demonstrated only resolving ATN. OKT3 was discontinued and cyclosporine was started. The Foley catheter was removed on postoperative day 7. Once the cyclosporine dose was adjusted to maintain a serum trough level of approximately 250–300, the patient was discharged. One month postoperatively, he was readmitted for fevers, pancytopenia, diarrhea, and an increase in creatinine. He was hydrated with intravenous crystalloid solution. Flexible sigmoidoscopy revealed colitis, with a biopsy demonstrating intracellular viral inclusion particles. CMV disease was diagnosed and intravenous ganciclovir initiated. Symptoms slowly resolved over several days. His creatinine returned to baseline. He was discharged and completed a 2-week course of ganciclovir at home.

CASE 2
KIDNEY AND PANCREAS TRANSPLANTATION

A 42-year-old male with ESRD due to insulin-dependent diabetes mellitus developed profound nephrotic syndrome secondary to diabetic nephropathy at the age of 39. He had been dialysis-dependent for 2 years. Since starting dialysis, he was hospitalized for a life threatening episode of diabetic ketoacidosis. In addition, his diabetes was complicated by peripheral neuropathy, gastroparesis, and retinopathy. He was believed to be a potential candidate for combined renal and whole organ pancreas transplantation and underwent evaluation. A suitable donor became available 1 month later. At operation, the kidney was first implanted, followed by the pancreas. Both grafts functioned immediately. Postoperatively, the patient did not require supplemental insulin. Immunosuppression was based on OKT3 and steroids for 7 days, after which cyclosporine and Imuran were started. Steroids were tapered over several days. Urinary amylase averaged 2,000 units/L/hr. Serial electrolytes revealed a serum bicarbonate level of 16; therefore, sodium bicarbonate was added to his intravenous solution with resolution of his acidosis. On postoperative day 5, the urinary amylase level was noted to have decreased by 50%, and the creatinine had increased from 1.6 to 1.9. A renal biopsy was obtained and 1,000 mg of corticosteroids were administered. The results of the biopsy were available the next day, confirming rejection. Another 1,000 mg of corticosteroids were given. The urine amylase level increased to 1,700 units/L/hr, and the creatinine decreased to 1.8. Steroids were tapered over 5 days during which the urinary amylase and creatinine continued to improve. The Foley catheter was removed and the patient voided without difficulty. There was minimal drainage from the surgical drains and the drainage fluid amylase level was only 300. Therefore, the drain was removed. The patient was discharged on postoperative day 11, tolerating a regular diet without insulin coverage.

GENERAL CONSIDERATIONS

All patients with ESRD on dialysis should be considered for renal transplantation. In the United States, diabetes, hypertension, and chronic glomerulonephritis are the most common disorders leading to chronic renal failure. Chronic dialysis becomes necessary when the glomerular filtration rate (GFR) falls below 5 ml/min. GFR is approximated by measuring creatinine clearance from a 24-hour urine collection. Two options for dialysis exist: hemodialysis and peritoneal dialysis. Hemodialysis is performed at a dialysis center two to three times weekly and requires placement of a vascular access catheter or a surgically created arteriovenous shunt. Peritoneal dialysis may be performed at home, but requires daily dialysis and placement of a peritoneal catheter. The specific dialysis regimen is individualized according to medical and social requirements. Although dialysis can allow indefinite survival in ESRD patients, it is a poor substitute for normally functioning kidneys: solute removal is only 10% that of normal kidneys, even with the most efficient hemodialysis. Most patients with ESRD therefore suffer chronic malaise. In addition, time spent on dialysis, complications of uremia, and complications of vascular or peritoneal access all contribute to chronic disability. Kidney transplantation is therefore the treatment of choice for most ESRD patients.

Proper recipient selection is crucial to optimal outcome with respect to patient survival, quality of life, and allocation of scarce organs. Evaluation of the potential recipient begins with a complete history and physical examination as well as complete laboratory profile. Incurable malignancy or chronic infection are contraindications to transplantation because of the likelihood that immunosuppression will exacerbate these conditions. Psychiatric illness or poor social supports likely to cause noncompliance may also exclude a recipient because of the stringent requirement for lifelong immunosuppression and follow-up care. Although age alone is not a determinant, many elderly patients will be excluded because of advanced cardiopulmonary disease that may be a prohibitive risk for operation. After evaluation is completed, the patient's case is presented before a multidisciplinary selection committee. The task of the committee is to assess suitability based on the patient's medical condition as well as the need to allocate scarce organs efficiently. If selected, the patient is placed on a waiting list at the transplant center until a donor organ is available.

Availability of a potential living donor, either related or unrelated (e.g., spouse), may preclude the lengthy wait for a cadaveric organ. Currently, short term (1-year) results are equivalent with cadaveric or living donor transplantation; however, because morbidity and mortality of living donation is low (mortality <0.05%), most transplant centers encourage living donation. Donation must be completely voluntary. Recipients should be protected from pressure to solicit from family members, and donors should be protected from pressure to donate. Evaluation of the living donor is extensive; potential donors are excluded when there is overt or potential underlying renal disease. History, physical, and laboratory examination, and renal angiography are required for assessment of renal vascular anatomy. If the living donor candidate is acceptable, the donor nephrectomy and recipient operation are planned together. The donor nephrectomy is performed extraperitoneally through a flank incision. The kidney graft is immediately placed in cold preservation solution and transported to the recipient operating room for immediate implantation. Postoperatively, the donor is able to eat within 24-48 hours and is discharged after approximately 5 days.

Eighty percent of renal transplantation in the United States is from cadaveric (brain-dead) donors. Organ procurement from these donors is a complex process involving multiple institutions, physicians, and families. Organ procurement organizations (OPOs) coordinate donation and placement of organs through regional offices and field coordinators. The most important individual in the donation process is the referring nurse or physician who contacts the OPO with a potential donor. All subsequent evaluation and assessment is performed by the OPO so that the referring physician has little burden other than the initial phone call. The field coordinator actively manages the donor candidate and arranges the operation if the candidate is a suitable donor. The organ procurement operation is performed by transplant surgeons from regional transplant centers. The organs that are removed are stored at 4°C in University of Wisconsin solution, designed to minimize ischemic damage. Thus stored, kidneys will generally function with up to 48 hours of cold ischemia, but most transplant centers prefer implantation within 24-36 hours. Upon procurement, it is the responsibility of the OPO to place the kidneys with suitable ABO matched recipients, based on a point scale that stresses length of waiting time on the list and histocompatibility (HLA).

The recipient who has been selected is contacted by the transplant center and immediately admitted to the hospital. In addition to standard laboratory assessments, blood is sent for assay of cytotoxic antibodies in the recipient against antigens (cross-match) derived from a sample of donor blood. Reactivity of recipient serum against donor lymphocytes indicates the presence of preformed cytotoxic antibodies in the recipient. Transplantation of the donor kidney in the presence of a positive cross-match may result in hyperacute rejection and therefore should not be performed. If the cross-match is negative, transplantation may proceed. Most patients undergo preoperative dialysis for clearance of solutes, but patients are intentionally not depleted of intravascular volume to avoid hypovolemic insult to the allograft.

In the operating room, a central venous line is placed for assessment of intravascular volume. Hypovolemia is corrected with albumin and crystalloid infusion. A Foley catheter is placed and the bladder irrigated with antibiotic solution. Exposure is obtained most commonly through an oblique incision in the lower abdomen, allowing placement of the graft in the extraperitoneal pelvis. The kidney

graft renal artery and vein are anastomosed to the iliac vessels in the recipient, usually in end-to-side fashion (Fig. 62.1). After revascularization, the graft changes appearance from bloodless pale to perfused pink, and urine may begin to flow from the ureter. The donor ureter is next implanted into the bladder by ureteroneocystostomy, in which the ureter is spatulated and anastomosed to the inside of the bladder (Fig. 62.1).

Postoperatively, the patient is monitored in an intensive care unit (ICU) for 24-48 hours. Significant extracellular fluid shifts and electrolyte changes may occur due to the large volume diuresis that characterizes the first 24 hours after transplantation. This diuresis may reach 1,000 ml/hour and must be replaced with crystalloid solution on an hourly basis to prevent hypovolemia. Once the kidney regains normal concentrating ability, the patient is discharged to the transplant ward. Diet is advanced as tolerated and ambulation encouraged. Immunosuppression is begun immediately after transplantation, requiring daily therapeutic drug levels for dose adjustment. Foley catheter

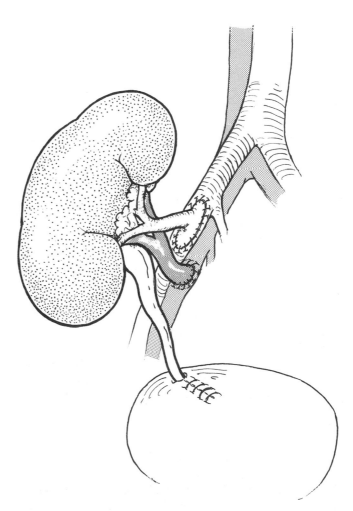

FIGURE 62.1 *Renal transplantation, showing anastomoses to the iliac vessels and inside of the bladder.*

drainage of the bladder is continued for 3–5 days, allowing the ureteral anastomosis to heal. If there are no complications, patients may be discharged after removal of the Foley catheter with close outpatient follow-up.

Whole organ pancreatic transplantation has been used in the treatment of type 1 diabetes and is the only therapy available that normalizes levels of glycated hemoglobin (Hgb A_{1c}). Although functioning pancreatic transplantation allows freedom from insulin dependence, it is unclear whether it reverses established secondary complications of diabetes. These secondary complications include peripheral and autonomic neuropathy, retinopathy, nephropathy, and cardiovascular disease. In most cases, whole organ pancreas transplantation is performed together with kidney transplantation in diabetic patients with ESRD in whom the need for immunosuppression is a requirement, regardless of the pancreatic allograft. In rare patients with profound brittle diabetes, the risk of life threatening hypoglycemic unawareness may justify intervention with isolated pancreas transplantation. Evaluation and exclusion criteria are similar to kidney transplantation and include screening for coronary artery disease in patients older than 45 years because of the increased prevalence of ischemic cardiac disease in patients with type 1 diabetes.

The pancreatic allograft is procured from cadaveric donors and includes the entire gland together with a portion of duodenum, superior mesenteric and splenic arteries, and splenic vein (Fig. 62.2). The graft is placed in the right iliac fossa, utilizing the recipient iliac artery and vein for anastomosis. When a kidney is also being transplanted (most of the time), the kidney is placed in the opposite iliac fossa (Fig. 62.2). The pancreatic exocrine secretions are most commonly drained into the bladder, using the attached duodenum to fashion an anastomosis to the bladder wall. Intestinal drainage of pancreatic secretions is also possible but less commonly performed because the urinary amylase in bladder-drained grafts is a useful parameter with which to follow allograft function (Case 2). Before closure, a Jackson-Pratt drain is placed near the anastomosis.

Postoperatively, patients are monitored in the ICU for 24–48 hours. Generally, insulin independence occurs immediately with graft revascularization, reflecting endocrine function of the allograft (Case 2). Exocrine pancreatic secretion can be monitored in the urine and provides a useful method of monitoring graft function: urine collections are sent daily for amylase concentrations and recorded on bedside charts. Decreases in urine amylase (Case 2) may reflect graft dysfunction, most commonly rejection, in the absence of other factors. Diet is advanced cautiously because of the concern for diabetic gastroparesis. Foley catheter drainage is maintained for 7 days. The Jackson-Pratt drain is then removed if there is no evidence of leakage of urine or pancreatic secretions (Case 2). Total initial hospital stay is generally 8–10 days.

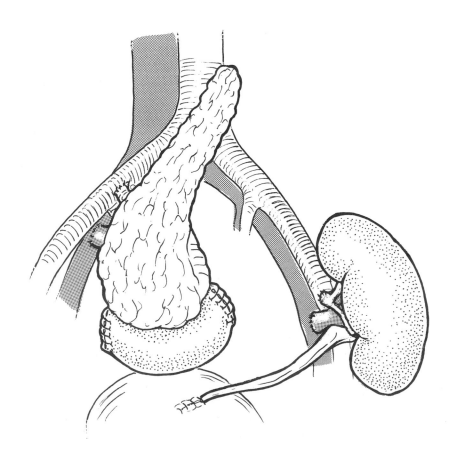

FIGURE 62.2 *Multiple organ transplantation, including kidney and pancreas.*

KEY POINTS

- Kidney transplantation treatment of choice for most ESRD patients

- Overall graft survival exceeds 85% at 1 year for both cadaveric and living allografts

- Patients with severe type 1 diabetes mellitus complications may qualify for whole organ pancreatic transplant; 1-year graft survival is 80%

- In United States, diabetes, hypertension, and chronic glomerulonephritis are most common disorders leading to chronic renal failure

- Solute removal in hemodialysis only 10% that of normal kidneys; kidney transplantation only treatment of choice for most ESRD patients

- Incurable malignancy or chronic infection contraindicate transplantation because immunosuppression exacerbates these conditions

- Short-term (1-year) results are equivalent between cadaveric or living donor transplant, but morbidity and mortality of living donation is low (mortality <0.05%)

- 80% of U.S. renal transplants are from cadaveric (braindead) donors

- Most important individual is referring nurse or physician who contacts OPO with a potential donor

- OPO must place kidneys with suitable ABO matched recipients, based on a scale that stresses length of wait on list and histocompatibility (HLA)

- Kidney transplantation with positive cross-match may result in hyperacute rejection and should not be performed

- Although pancreatic transplantation allows freedom from insulin dependence, it is unclear whether it reverses established secondary complications of diabetes

- Pancreatic exocrine secretions are most commonly drained into bladder

- Exocrine pancreatic secretion can be monitored in urine and provides useful method of monitoring graft function: urine collections sent daily for amylase concentrations and recorded on bedside charts

DIAGNOSIS OF COMPLICATIONS

The post-transplant course can be characterized by early and late periods during which different complications confront the clinician. Complications can be further categorized as technical complications and those arising as a result of immunosuppression. Immunosuppression-related complications are primarily infection and malignancy and occur in direct proportion to the degree of immunosuppression.

Accurate and timely diagnosis requires vigilance and a familiarity with the diagnostic modalities available. Useful noninvasive imaging studies include ultrasonography and radionuclide scanning. Ultrasound provides rapid assessment of obstruction to urine flow or leakage of urine or lymph fluid around the allograft. In addition, duplex sonography combines real time imaging with Doppler analysis to provide information on flow within the blood vessels (Case 1). From this information, a resistive index can be obtained. Changes in the resistive index may herald graft dysfunction. Radionuclide renal scanning provides information on renal parenchymal function by measurement of uptake and excretion of tracer. When imaging studies and clinical course suggest graft dysfunction, renal allograft biopsy may be required to establish a diagnosis (Case 1). Biopsy is performed percutaneously at the bedside under sterile technique. Histologic study of the tissue is then performed by a transplant pathologist.

Occasionally, the transplanted kidney does not function immediately (Case 1). This delayed graft function is manifested by initial oliguria or anuria and is most commonly caused by acute tubular necrosis (ATN). ATN may reflect preservation injury or other undiagnosed insult to the donor organ. ATN usually resolves over several days, but dialysis may be necessary until the graft begins to function. When ATN is present, early cases of rejection may be missed. Initial ATN is an important predictor of poorer long-term graft survival compared to patients with normal initial function.

Acute allograft rejection is mediated by a host cellular immune response against alloantigens. Clinically, graft dysfunction manifested by oliguria and rising creatinine may be seen. Fever and malaise may be present as well as pain over the graft. Diagnosis may be suggested by an increase in resistive index on ultrasound or decrease in excretion of tracer on renal scan, but confirmation requires biopsy and histologic examination of tissue. Even with biopsy, rejection may be difficult to differentiate from cyclosporine toxicity. Initial treatment is with high dose steroids followed by OKT3 for steroid-resistant rejection. Episodes of acute rejection predict diminished long-term graft survival compared to patients who do not have episodes of rejection.

Vascular complications include thrombosis and bleeding, both of which are rare (<1%) Sudden loss of urine output in the absence of other factors (e.g., hypovolemia), fever, and pain over the graft suggests acute arterial thrombosis. Management requires urgent ultrasound or renal scan and immediate surgical exploration. In most cases, irreversible ischemia is present at exploration, requiring graft removal.

Infections that characterize the early post-transplant period include viral, fungal, and bacterial infections. Bacterial infections may be relatively innocuous (wound or urinary) or severe (gastrointestinal perforation or intra-abdominal abscess); early empiric antibiotics are therefore initiated in all patients with suspected bacterial sepsis. Fungal organisms cause opportunistic infection in direct proportion to the degree of immunosuppression and the illness of the host. Severely ill patients hospitalized in the ICU are at highest risk of systemic fungal infections, which are associated with high mortality. The most common post-transplant viral infection is caused by cytomegalovirus (CMV) (Case 1). Invasive CMV infection presents with a wide spectrum of potential signs and symptoms, most commonly fever, hepatitis, pneumonitis, and enterocolitis. Because of the high incidence of CMV disease, many transplant centers administer prophylaxis against CMV in the early post-transplant period in those patients at risk. The highest risk group are patients who were serologically negative for CMV who received an organ from a CMV-exposed donor.

Urologic complications in the early post-transplant period include obstruction to urine flow and urine leak. Obstruction and urine leak often present with graft dysfunction (oliguria and rising creatinine) and may be diagnosed by ultrasound findings of hydronephrosis, hydroureter, or a fluid collection. Urine leak may reflect ischemic necrosis of the renal pelvis or ureter, or disruption of the ureteroneocystostomy; surgical exploration is therefore mandatory.

After 1 year, allograft function generally stabilizes and the risk of technical complications decreases. Cumulative effects of long term immunosuppression, however, become more prevalent. Slow decline in renal allograft function may suggest cyclosporine nephropathy, chronic rejection, or recurrence of the underlying disease that led to ESRD. Malignancies that are normally controlled by intact immune mechanisms may require cessation of immunosuppression and graft loss. The most common immunosuppression-induced malignancy is a spectrum of Epstein-Barr virus-induced lymphoproliferative disease, which in its most severe form presents as frank monoclonal lymphoma.

In addition to immunosuppression-related complications that afflict all recipients of organ transplants, recipients of whole organ pancreatic grafts are at risk of additional complications. Metabolic acidosis is almost always present (Case 2) and reflects urinary loss of bicarbonate from pancreatic exocrine secretions. Generally, acidosis is corrected with oral bicarbonate, but occasionally life-threatening acidosis requires hospitalization for correction with intravenous therapy. Vascular complications (thrombosis and bleeding) occur with increased frequency compared to renal transplants. Leakage of pancreatic exocrine fluid may reflect disruption of the duodenal-bladder anastomosis from ischemia or technical error and can result in life threatening sepsis. Activation of pancreatic enzymes may result in severe cystitis and urethritis. Poor bladder emptying from neurogenic bladder dysfunction may result in reflux pancreatitis.

Rejection of the pancreatic allograft is often manifested by decreasing urinary amylase (Case 2). In many cases, pancreatic allograft rejection occurs together with renal allograft rejection, so that a rising creatinine may also be present. Biopsy of the pancreatic allograft is not easily performed; confirmation of rejection is obtained by renal biopsy. Islet cell dysfunction resulting in hyperglycemia is a late finding and may reflect irreversible damage to the pancreatic allograft.

KEY POINTS

- Immunosuppression-related complications are primarily infection and malignancy and occur in direct proportion to degree of immunosuppression
- Delayed graft function manifested by initial oliguria or anuria and most commonly caused by ATN
- Initial ATN important predictor of poorer long-term graft survival compared to patients with normal initial function
- Episodes of acute rejection predict diminished long-term graft survival compared to patients who do not have them
- Fungal organisms cause opportunistic infection in direct proportion to degree of immunosuppression and illness of host
- Most common post-transplant viral infection caused by CMV
- Metabolic acidosis almost always present and reflects urinary loss of bicarbonate from pancreatic exocrine secretions
- Rejection of pancreatic allograft often manifested by decreasing urinary amylase
- Islet cell dysfunction resulting in hyperglycemia is late finding and may reflect irreversible damage to pancreatic allograft

DIFFERENTIAL DIAGNOSIS

Early postoperative renal allograft dysfunction is manifested by oliguria and rising creatinine. Differential diagnosis includes hypovolemia, mechanical problems (obstruction/leakage), ischemia, acute rejection, drug toxicity (most commonly cyclosporine), and infection. Hypovolemia is corrected by fluid challenge; if oliguria persists, additional diagnostic intervention is necessary. Additional findings may suggest the etiology of graft dysfunction, including fever, wound swelling or tenderness, or elevated drug levels. Early noninvasive diagnostic intervention includes ultrasound and renal scanning, both of which will rapidly exclude acute arterial thrombosis and are helpful in diagnosing mechanical complications. When a perigraft fluid collection is identified, urine can be differentiated from lymphatic fluid by simple aspiration of the fluid and measurement of fluid creatinine. Differentiation between rejection and cyclosporine toxicity generally requires biopsy, but empiric treatment for rejection may be initiated before biopsy results are available (Case 2).

Persistent fever and leukocytosis suggesting infection requires pan-culture and empiric broad spectrum antibiotics, as well as a diligent search for the source. Viral, fungal, or bacterial organisms may be responsible. Imaging studies are directed by findings on history and physical examination. Early ultrasound of the renal allograft is obtained when findings are nonspecific. Patients presenting with abdominal pain require urgent surgical exploration when peritonitis is present. Because steroids may blunt signs and symptoms of the acute abdomen, early abdominopelvic computed tomography scan is often obtained in patients with abdominal complaints and equivocal examination.

DRUG TREATMENT

Immunosuppressive management is based on a balance between adequate suppression of the immune response preventing allograft rejection and avoidance of excessive immunosuppression leading to drug toxicity, infection, and malignancy. In order to achieve this balance, combinations of agents with synergistic effects are used. The most common regimen in renal and pancreatic transplantation utilizes cyclosporine, azathioprine (Imuran), and steroids. Some centers utilize the murine monoclonal anti-T cell antibody OKT3 as an initial immunosuppressive agent ("induction immunosuppression"), delaying cyclosporine in the immediate perioperative period in order to minimize nephrotoxicity.

Rejection is routinely treated with high dose steroids ("pulse") followed by a taper over several days (Case 2). Steroid resistant rejection may require treatment with OKT3. OKT3 therapy causes rapid T-cell clearance and abolition of the immune response, but also causes massive cytokine release that may result in fever, malaise, pulmonary edema, or hypotension.

Most patients are discharged from the hospital on prophylaxis for viral and fungal infections, which includes acyclovir (an antiviral agent), Nystatin (an antifungal agent), and trimethoprim-sulfamethoxazole (Bactrim) for *Pneumocystis carinii*. Additional prophylactic measures may be required in some patients, such as long term ganciclovir or CMV immunoglobulin in patients at risk of CMV disease.

FOLLOW-UP

One-year graft survival after cadaveric renal transplantation is approximately 85%. Long-term graft survival is greater for living donors compared to cadaveric transplants and for completely HLA identical ("six-antigen match") transplants compared to those with greater histologic disparity. Other variables such as number of rejection episodes, initial nonfunction (ATN), and previous failed transplant are also predictors of poorer long term graft function. The most common reason for late kidney graft loss is chronic rejection. One-year pancreatic graft survival after combined kidney-pancreas transplantation is approximately 80%, but less than 60% for isolated pancreatic transplants.

All patients are followed closely after transplantation. Upon discharge, most centers follow patients weekly for the first month. During outpatient visits, blood is drawn for assessment of graft function and measurement of cyclosporine levels. Acute rejection manifested by graft dysfunction (rising creatinine, oliguria) occurs most commonly in the first few months after transplantation and always requires admission for treatment. Most infections and febrile episodes in the early postoperative period require inpatient treatment. Stress steroid coverage is required for any major operation because of chronic adrenal suppression by exogenous oral steroids. Oral antibiotic prophylaxis is required for dental and other outpatient procedures.

Within the first year after transplantation, maintenance steroid doses are generally reduced if graft function remains normal. Steroids are generally not completely withdrawn, although investigation of steroid withdrawal is ongoing at some centers. Cyclosporine must be continued lifelong unless prohibitive toxicity is seen, in which case alternative regimens are designed.

SUGGESTED READINGS

Barker C, Naji A, Dafoe D, Perloff L: Renal transplantation. In Sabiston D (ed): Textbook of Surgery: The Biological Basis of Modern Surgical Practice. WB Saunders, Philadelphia, 1991

Brayman K, Najarian J, Sutherland DER: Transplantation of the pancreas. In Cameron J (ed): Current Surgical Therapy. Mosby–Year Book, St. Louis, 1992

Sollinger H, Knechtle S, Reed A et al: Experience with 100 consecutive simultaneous kidney-pancreas transplants with bladder drainage. Ann Surg 214:704, 1991

QUESTIONS

1. The major limiting factor for increased numbers of renal transplants is?

    A. Lack of suitable recipients.

    B. Lack of suitable donors.

    C. Backup renal dialysis capabilities.

    D. Costs.

2. The major long range complication of combined renal/pancreas transplantation is?

    A. Kidney failure.

    B. Pancreatic graft failure.

    C. Progressive diabetic vascular disease.

    D. None of the above.

(See p. 604 for answers.)

63

LIVER

TRANSPLANTATION

DAVID K. IMAGAWA

The first clinical attempt at orthotopic liver transplantation (OLT) was made by Thomas Starzl and colleagues at the University of Colorado in 1963. Although the first seven patients died, the procedure met with success in 1967. It was, however, the introduction of the immunosuppressive agent cyclosporine (CsA) that led to 1-year survival rates of 80%. At a National Institutes of Health (NIH) consensus conference in 1983, it was agreed that liver transplantation was "a therapeutic modality for end

stage liver disease that deserved broader application." Since that time the number of liver transplant centers and transplants has risen dramatically. In 1994, in the United States, 92 centers performed 3,574 OLTs. Worldwide, 196 centers performed 6,058 OLTs. The aims of this chapter are to (1) elucidate the indications for OLT in the adult and pediatric population, (2) briefly describe the surgical procedure, (3) characterize the immunosuppressive agents that are used to prevent and treat allograft rejection, and (4) describe the diagnosis and treatment of frequent postoperative complications.

CASE 1
REJECTION FOLLOWING TRANSPLANTATION

A 43-year-old white male presented to the emergency department with complaints of shortness of breath, increasing abdominal girth, and lower extremity edema. His past medical history was remarkable for a 2-unit blood transfusion for a leg fracture following a motorcycle accident. He consumed alcohol on a regular basis until 1 year ago and had one arrest for driving under the influence of al-

cohol. He denied intravenous drug use or tattoos. His temperature was 38.7°C and his sclerae were icteric. He had muscle wasting and a large amount of ascites. The liver span was 7 cm and the edge was not palpable. The spleen tip was palpable. There was 2+ pitting edema of the lower extremities. Laboratory values were significant for a WBC of $12.6 \times 10^3/mm^3$, bilirubin of 2.6 mg/dl, SGOT of 114 units (NL 10–40 units), SGPT 87 units (NL 10–35 units), alkaline phosphatase 267 units/L (NL 45–115 units/L), albumin 2.2 g/dl (NL 3.5–5.5 g/dl) and a PT of 18.2 seconds (NL 12–14 seconds). Hepatitis C antibody was positive.

A chest x-ray showed a moderate right pleural effusion and abdominal ultrasound showed a small cirrhotic liver, splenomegaly, and ascites. A paracentesis gave cloudy ascitic fluid that subsequently grew *E. coli*. On endoscopy there were moderate esophageal and gastric varices. He was treated with intravenous antibiotics and diuresis. The patient was evaluated for OLT and was believed to be a candidate if he attended Alcoholics Anonymous as an outpatient.

Three months later, an appropriate liver donor became available and he underwent an uneventful OLT. He was started on CsA, Imuran, and prednisone. On the seventh postoperative day he developed a fever, right upper quadrant pain, and elevated serum liver enzymes. A duplex examination showed a patent portal vein and hepatic artery. A liver biopsy showed acute rejection. A "steroid pulse" was administered but liver chemistries remained elevated. A repeat liver biopsy showed persistent rejection. A 14-day course of the monoclonal antibody OKT3 was administered with resolution of the symptoms and serum chemistries and the patient was discharged on the 26th postoperative day.

Two weeks after discharge the patient was again found to have elevated liver enzymes. Repeat liver biopsy showed both acute and chronic rejection. He was admitted to the hospital and the immunosuppressive regimen was changed from CsA, Imuran, and prednisone to FK506 and prednisone.

CASE 2
SUCCESSFUL TRANSPLANTATION

A 3-year-old white female was admitted to the hospital with fever, increasing jaundice, ascites, and failure to thrive. She had been the product of a normal pregnancy and had done well until 3 weeks of age. At that time she was noted to be jaundiced with a total bilirubin of 9 mg/dl and a conjugated bilirubin of 6 mg/dl. Physical examination revealed hepatomegaly. HIDA scan showed good uptake of tracer by the liver but no excretion into the gallbladder or intestinal tract. A diagnosis of biliary atresia was made and she underwent a portoenterostomy for biliary enteric drainage.

Upon admission, the patient was started on intravenous antibiotics for presumptive cholangitis, which was treated and resolved. She was considered to be a candidate for OLT due to obvious failure of her portoenterostomy. Because of her declining health she remained hospitalized. One month after admission, an OLT was done. On postoperative day 2, the patient developed a fever of 39°C, was lethargic, and had an SGOT of 2,400 units and an SGPT of 1,820 units. Duplex examination failed to demonstrate a hepatic artery. A celiac angiogram showed a thrombosed hepatic artery. Emergency operation was performed and hepatic artery thrombosis and liver necrosis were found. The patient was returned to the ICU and plans for emergency retransplantation were made. Twelve hours later, a liver from an 8-year-old donor became available. At operation the donor liver was divided and the left lobe of the liver transplanted into the patient.

The patient slowly improved, but 14 days after the second transplant she developed fevers and neutropenia. Blood cultures were positive for CMV. Ganciclovir was administered for 2 weeks and lower doses of immunosuppression (CsA, Imuran, prednisone) administered.

She was ultimately discharged 30 days following the second transplant.

GENERAL CONSIDERATIONS

The indications for OLT are (1) progressive hyperbilirubinemia, (2) portal hypertension as manifested by intractable ascites, hypersplenism, and/or bleeding varices, (3) uncontrollable encephalopathy, (4) poor synthetic function as expressed by decreased albumin and fibrinogen or an elevated prothrombin time (PT), (5) inability to function or maintain normal activity, (6) pediatric metabolic disease associated with chronic liver disease, and (7) unresectable hepatic malignancy. The latter is usually reserved for primary hepatic tumors (hepatoma, hepatoblastoma) without extrahepatic metastases. In rare instances, patients with primary neuroendocrine tumors and metastatic liver disease may be candidates for resection with OLT.

Depending on the specific type of end stage liver disease, each of these criteria may influence a candidate for OLT. However, in general, a severe manifestation of one of these conditions, or a combination of various complications that cannot be controlled with alternate modalities, are considered indications for OLT. Table 63.1 lists common diseases that can be treated by OLT.

The operation itself can be divided into three phases: (1) the donor hepatectomy, which is usually performed at an outside hospital and takes 2 hours, (2) the recipient hepatectomy, which takes 2–4 hours, and (3) transplantation of the donor liver into the recipient, which takes 2–4 hours.

Although local and regional donors are preferred due to logistical considerations, the introduction of University of Wisconsin preservation solution allows for cold ischemic times of up to 24 hours, although less than 12 hours is ideal. During the donor operation, the anatomy of the donor liver must be examined and any anomalies recognized.

The recipient hepatectomy can be the bloodiest and most dangerous part of the operation. The major vascular structures and common bile duct are isolated, and the recipient liver is removed. In adult patients, many centers utilize venovenous bypass to decrease portal hypertension and to prevent severe decreases in cardiac output (CO) during the anhepatic phase.

The vascular anastomoses are performed in a specific order: (1) suprahepatic cava, (2) infrahepatic cava, (3) portal vein, and (4) hepatic artery. The biliary anastomosis is performed last. In adults, a choledochocholedochostomy is used, except in cases where the bile duct is found to be diseased (sclerosing cholangitis). In children or adults with sclerosing cholangitis, a Roux-en-Y choledochojejunostomy is created because these recipients have either no common bile duct or a very small common bile duct.

TABLE 63.1 *Diseases commonly treated by OLT*

Adult Diseases	Pediatric Diseases
Posthepatic cirrhosis (chronic active hepatitis B or C)	Intrahepatic and extrahepatic biliary atresia
Primary biliary cirrhosis	Inborn errors of metabolism
Primary sclerosing cholangitis	α_1-Antitrypsin deficiency
Autoimmune chronic active hepatitis	Tyrosinemia
α_1-Antitrypsin deficiency	Protoporphyria
Budd-Chiari syndrome	Galactosemia
Hemochromatosis	Glycogen storage disease
Fulminant subacute hepatitis (A, B, or C)	Wilson's disease
Wilson's disease	Crigler-Najjar syndrome
Toxic hepatitis	Fulminant subacute hepatitis (A, B, or C)
Alcoholic liver disease (in selected patients)	Toxic hepatitis
	Primary hepatic tumor (in selected patients)

KEY POINTS

• OLT indications are (1) progressive hyperbilirubinemia, (2) portal hypertension as manifested by intractable ascites, hypersplenism, and/or bleeding varices, (3) uncontrollable encephalopathy, (4) poor synthetic function as expressed by decreased albumin and fibrinogen or an elevated PT, (5) inability to function or maintain normal activity, (6) pediatric metabolic disease associated with chronic liver disease, and (7) unresectable hepatic malignancy

• OLT divided into three phases: (1) donor hepatectomy, performed at an outside hospital, taking 2 hours, (2) recipient hepatectomy, taking 2–4 hours, and (3) transplantation of donor liver into recipient, taking 2–4 hours

• University of Wisconsin preservation solution allows for cold ischemic times of up to 24 hours—less than 12 hours is ideal

DIAGNOSIS

Management of the patient following OLT is challenging. All patients will experience at least one or more of the complications listed in Table 63.2. Prompt diagnosis and treatment are necessary in order to avoid graft failure or death.

Approximately 5–10% of donor livers will not function when transplanted into the recipient. The causes of primary nonfunction (PNF) are not well understood, but may relate to poor donor selection, hemodynamic instability in the donor, harvest injury, ischemic injury, or complications in the recipient operation. Recent studies have also implicated the role of an accelerated antibody-mediated rejection process. A patient with PNF will not regain consciousness in the intensive care unit (ICU), will continue to exhibit coagulopathy, and will have no or very poor bile output. Laboratory values will show a PT of more than 20 seconds, and serum glutamic oxaloacetic transaminase (SGOT), serum glutamic pyrovic transaminase (SGPT), and lactate dehydrogenase (LDH) values of over 5,000 and rising. A few of these livers may spontaneously recover function. Administration of prostaglandin E_1 may be useful. However, most patients exhibiting PNF will require emergent retransplantation. Three common technical failures are bleeding, hepatic artery thrombosis (Case 2), and bile duct leak; all require reoperation.

Intra-abdominal bleeding immediately following OLT is a common occurrence. The patient is usually profoundly coagulopathic before and during the operative procedure. During the operative and perioperative period packed red blood cells (RBCs), fresh frozen plasma (FFP), platelets, and cryoprecipitate are administered. If coagulopathy persists aminocaproic acid (Amicar), or aprotinin (Trasylol) may be administered. In the postoperative period the patient's hematocrit (Hct) level central pressures, abdominal girth, and drain outputs are monitored. If bleeding persists the patient is returned to the operating room (10% of cases).

TABLE 63.2 *Postoperative complications following liver transplantation*

Primary nonfunction
Bleeding
Hepatic artery thrombosis
Acute rejection
Infection
Biliary obstruction or leak
Perforated viscus
Metabolic abnormalities
Chronic rejection

Early thrombosis of the hepatic artery following OLT is relatively common in the pediatric population (10–18%) but less common in the adult population (<3%). Although the hepatic artery may be ligated in the native liver, often without sequelae (i.e., during control of bleeding in liver trauma), the transplanted liver is exquisitely sensitive to hepatic arterial flow. If hepatic artery thrombosis (HAT) occurs during the immediate postoperative period the usual clinical presentation is that of fulminant hepatic necrosis and sepsis. Urgent retransplantation is always required. HAT may also present with a syndrome of hepatic abscesses and relapsing bacteremia. These patients may rapidly progress to hepatic necrosis.

The presence of a T-tube stenting the choledo-chocholedochostomy in the majority of OLT patients allows for direct access to the biliary tree. A T-tube cholangiogram will show dislodgement of the tube from the duct or mechanical obstruction of the duct by stones, sludge, or blood. HAT can also lead to necrosis of the bile duct and a subsequent leak. In patients without a T-tube a bile leak can be confirmed with a DISIDA (technetium-99 diisopropyl imunodiacetic acid) scan. Diagnosis of a bile leak requires emergent operative exploration. In most cases the choledochocholedochostomy will require conversion to a Roux-en-Y choledochojejunostomy. If the degree of bile duct necrosis is severe, retransplantation may be required.

Most OLT recipients will exhibit some evidence of cellular-mediated rejection episodes. Unlike kidney transplants, OLT patients are matched only for liver size and blood type. In emergent situations the blood type matching may even be forgone. The pathophysiology of rejection involves the reaction of helper and cytotoxic T cells against class I, II, and other allogenic determinants on the surface of hepatocytes, bile duct epithelium, and vascular endothelium.

Mild acute rejection usually occurs between the 4th and 10th postoperative days (Case 1). The clinical presentation is usually that of fever, increased liver function tests, and right upper quadrant or back pain. A percutaneous liver biopsy is diagnostic.

As OLT patients are immunosuppressed, they are quite susceptible to bacterial, fungal, and viral infections. Preoperative and perioperative antibiotics (for at least 24 hours) are used to prevent bacterial infections. Specific organisms may require adjustment of the antibiotic regimen. Nystatin swish and swallow (500,000 units three times daily) is given for fungal prophylaxis; systemic fungal infections require amphotericin. The most common and potentially devastating viral infection is CMV (Case 2). This virus may infect the graft, blood, bowel, or lung. The incidence of CMV infection has been decreased by the administration of the intravenous antiviral agent ganciclovir during the hospital stay, followed by oral acylovir until postoperative day 100.

OLT patients may develop an acute abdomen from lesions such as a perforated gastric or duodenal ulcer. Diagnosis and treatment are similar to the nontransplant patient.

Hyperkalemia, hyperglycemia, and hypomagnesemia are common in OLT patients. These derangements are side effects of the immunosuppressive agents used to prevent allograft rejection. Diagnosis and treatment are identical to the nontransplant patient.

Histologic changes in chronic rejection are more variable than in mild acute rejection. Features include intimal proliferation, fibrosis, and disappearance of the bile ducts ("vanishing bile duct syndrome"). This form of rejection is usually seen after the third month posttransplant. Conversion from CsA-based immunosuppression to FK506 (see Treatment) is occasionally successful (Case 1). Other patients may proceed to liver failure and require retransplantation.

KEY POINTS

- Approximately 5–10% of donor livers will not function in recipient

- Most patients exhibiting PNF require emergent retransplantation

- Early thrombosis of the hepatic artery following OLT occurs in 10–18% of pediatric patients but less than 3% of adults; hepatic artery may be ligated in the native liver, often without sequelae (i.e., during control of bleeding in liver trauma)

- Transplanted liver exquisitely sensitive to hepatic arterial flow

- Diagnosis of a bile leak requires emergent operative exploration

- Pathophysiology of rejection involves reaction of helper and cytotoxic T cells against class I, II, and other allogenic determinants on the surface of hepatocytes, bile duct epithelium, and vascular endothelium

- CMV the most common and potentially devastating viral infection

---

DIFFERENTIAL DIAGNOSIS

The majority of OLT patients with complications will present with the triad of fever, elevated liver enzymes, and abdominal pain. The presence of refractory hypotension suggests the occurrence of a catastrophic intra-abdominal process. Workup and therapy must be performed in a systematic and timely manner. Once adequate intravenous access has been established, routine laboratory studies (complete blood count [CBC], electrolytes, liver enzymes) should be sent. Blood cultures for bacteria, fungus, and virus should be drawn. Empiric antibiotic coverage for gram-negative organisms and anaerobes should be started. An upright chest x-ray to rule out the presence of free air is useful.

If the patient has an acute abdomen, then immediate surgical exploration is required. Failure to demonstrate any intra-abdominal pathology should not be considered a "negative exploration."

The usual clinical situation requires differentiation between rejection and HAT. Although a percutaneous liver biopsy is diagnostic, it takes 24–48 hours to obtain the results. If a T-tube is present, a cholangiogram performed under antibiotic coverage should be obtained. The study is diagnostic for T-tube dislodgement, biliary leak, or an anastomotic stricture. It may also demonstrate intrahepatic biliary strictures or the presence of common duct stones or sludge.

A duplex ultrasound study should be obtained next. Although this test is highly user-dependent, it can demonstrate intra-abdominal fluid collections, intrahepatic biliary dilatation, and most importantly, the patency of the portal vein and hepatic artery anastomoses. Confirmation of HAT, however, requires either angiography of the celiac axis (Case 2) or exploratory laparotomy.

TREATMENT

Although refinements in surgical technique have led to some of the improvements in survival following OLT, the seminal development was the introduction of CsA into clinical usage. Current immunotherapy is based on triple therapy utilizing CsA, Imuran, and corticosteroids.

Azathioprine (Imuran) is a 6-mercaptopurine analog that exerts its immunosuppressive effect by interdiction of mitosis in stimulated lymphoid cells by interfering with nucleotide synthesis. The major side effect is severe leukopenia from myelosuppression.

The synergistic immunosuppressive effect of steroids with azathioprine acts by inhibiting antigen-driven T-cell proliferation by blocking release of interleukin (IL-1) from monocytes.

CsA is a metabolite of the fungal species *Tolypocladium inflatum Gams*. Although CsA interferes with both B- and T-cell activation its major effect is interference with the function of helper T cells. This is accomplished by inhibiting transcription of the IL-2 gene and therefore the release of IL-2 from activated T cells.

Despite the increased graft survival seen with CsA, side effects are common. Even with careful monitoring of serum levels, nephrotoxicity may occur. Concomitant rejection may also occur, often making the diagnosis difficult. Other side effects include cholestasis, hirsutism, hypertension, and neuropathy. Infection with cytomegalovirus (CMV) or other opportunistic organisms can be life threatening in the immunosuppressed patient. Finally, there is a predilection for the development of B-cell lymphoproliferative diseases in patients receiving CsA. Treatment is a reduction in the immunosuppressive regimen,

with spontaneous regression and long-term survival in many cases.

Tacrolimus (FK506) is a neutral macrolide isolated from a soil fungus, *Streptomyces tsukubaenis*. FK506 appears to effect the same common early pathway as CsA on cytokine transcription but does so at doses 10–100 times lower than CsA. Early results following liver kidney transplantation demonstrated high graft survival and apparently less toxicity than CsA. A recent multicenter study has shown FK506 to be more effective than CsA in preventing allograft rejection when used as induction therapy.

At the present time there is only one monoclonal antibody (OKT3) licensed for use in clinical organ transplantation. OKT3 Muromonab-CD3 is a murine monoclonal antibody directed against the human CD3 antigen. The CD3 complex is a 20,000-dalton protein located on the surface of all peripheral T cells; binding of OKT3 apparently interferes with the transduction of the signal from the adjacent antigen recognition site. This prevents T-cell proliferation and activation of cytotoxic activity.

KEY POINTS

- Azathioprine (Imuran), a 6-mercatopurine analog, exerts immunosuppressive effect by interdiction of mitosis in stimulated lymphoid cells by interfering with nucleotide synthesis; major side effect is severe leukopenia from myelosuppression

- Corticosterioids inhibit antigen-driven T-cell proliferation by blocking release of IL-1 from monocytes

- CsA interferes with both B- and T-cell activation, but major effect is interference by inhibiting transcription of IL-2 gene and therefore release of IL-2 from activated T cells

- FK506 appears to effect same common early pathway as CsA on cytokine transcription but at doses 10 to 100 times lower than CsA

- CD3 complex is a 20,000-dalton protein located on the surface of all peripheral T cells; binding of OKT3 interferes with signal transduction from adjacent antigen recognition site

FOLLOW-UP

The majority of deaths following OLT occur within the first month. An overall 1-year survival rate of 80% for all patients (1,200 transplants) is seen at our institution. Similar results are reported from most large centers.

Once a patient is discharged from the hospital they are followed closely for the first several months. Readmission for rejection is not uncommon. If a T-tube has been placed, it is electively removed 3 months after transplant. The patient is then returned to the referring physician and liver enzymes followed on a 1–3-month basis. Long-term complications include chronic rejection, increased risk of lymphoma and skin cancers, renal failure from the nephrotoxic drugs, and cardiovascular morbidity from elevated cholesterol levels.

KEY POINTS

• Overall 1-year survival rate of 80%

• Long-term complications include chronic rejection, increased risk of lymphoma and skin cancers, renal failure from nephrotoxic drugs, and cardiovascular morbidity from elevated cholesterol

---

SUGGESTED READINGS

Busuttil RW, Klintmalm GB (eds): Transplantation of the Liver. WB Saunders, Philadelphia, 1995

A textbook devoted solely to liver transplantation. Detailed chapters on specific issues written by world authorities.

Cerilli GJ (ed): Organ Transplantation and Replacement. JB Lippincott, Philadelphia, 1988

A textbook on solid organ transplantation. It devotes chapters to history, immunology, as well as most organs transplanted today.

Starzl TE, Demetris AJ, Van Thiel D: Liver transplantation. Parts 1 and 2. New Engl J Med 321:1014, 1092, 1989

A two-part article written by the surgeon who pioneered liver transplantation.

QUESTIONS

1. Which of the following common technical complications of OLT require reoperation?

    A. HAT.

    B. Intra-abdominal bleeding.

    C. Biliary leakage.

    D. All of the above.

2. The imminent and most devastating postoperative infection is caused by?

    A. *Staphylococcus aureus.*

    B. *E. coli.*

    C. CMV.

    D. Human immunodeficiency virus.

(See p. 604 for answers.)

64 BURNS

MALCOLM LESAVOY

Thermal injuries are a result of the destruction of the skin envelope of the body due to traumatic injury from thermal energy such as heat, chemicals, electricity, radiation, or severe cold. The treatment of these severe and sometimes catastrophic injuries requires knowledge of the management of not only the local burn wound, but also the confounding problems of the hemodynamic, metabolic, nutritional, psychological, and immunologic phenomena that occur. Discussion in this chapter is

predominantly on heat thermal injuries. Chemical and electrical burns are significant problems, but occur less frequently.

CASE 1
A CAR EXPLOSION

A 45-year-old mechanic was cleaning a carburetor when a spark from the lamp he was using ignited the gasoline. His co-workers extinguished his burning clothing rapidly, but he still had charring of his right upper arm, chest, and abdomen. He was quickly undressed on arrival at the hospital and his burn was estimated at 40% TBSA. No evidence of burn about the face or singed nasal hair was noted. He was asked to cough and produced a small amount of clear sputum that had no carbonaceous particles. He was able to breathe without difficulty. Oxygen by nasal cannulae at 4 L/min was begun. An arterial blood gas showed a carboxyhemoglobin concentration of less than 5%. Several intravenous catheters were placed through nonburned skin. The physicians planned to administer 5,600 ml of lactated Ringer's solution to this 70-kg patient over the next 8 hours (700 ml/hr).

On arrival at the burn unit, nasogastric and bladder catheters were placed. Tetanus toxoid was given, and intravenous narcotics were administered. Additional blood samples were sent for CBC, electrolytes, fasting blood sugar, and cross-matching. A chest x-ray and ECG were obtained. His wounds were cleansed and superficial debris removed. The burned areas were dressed with silver sulfadiazine and sterile dressings.

CASE 2
ELECTRICAL WIRING INJURY

A 40-year-old male decided to replace his porch light. The moment his screwdriver touched the wiring he saw a bright flash, felt his muscles contract, and fell to the ground. On arrival at the emergency room he was dazed and sore. He had obviously broken his left arm because of the pain he felt and the visible deformity. An IV catheter infused lactated Ringer's solution at 150 ml/hr. His ECG, head CT, and chest x-ray were all normal. He had a small burn on the dorsum of his right forearm, but otherwise seemed unscathed. He was amazed when the nurse told him that he was being admitted to the ICU for observation.

GENERAL CONSIDERATIONS

Burn injuries cause destruction of the skin. The amount of tissue destruction is related to the intensity of the heat and to the time of exposure. In general, a burn is produced by an agent with a temperature of 40°C or above. Hot baths and showers are common causes of burns around the house, as parents of young children or caretakers of the elderly may not realize how hot the water actually is. Fires and explosions are other common causes (Case 1) when people become careless around flammable liquids. House and office fires are particularly dangerous not only because of the burns they produce, but also because of the toxic fumes that wood and plastics emit when they burn. Victims of closed space fires (cars and unvented rooms) may sustain severe inhalational injuries from these products of combustion. Additionally, inhalation of carbon monoxide produces carboxyhemoglobin in which hemoglobin is unavailable for transport of oxygen. Chemical burn severity depends on the nature of the agent (gasoline, phenol, hydrofluoric acid, white phosphorous, etc.). Electrical injuries depend on the type of circuit (AC or DC), the voltage, the resistance offered by the body, the duration of contact, and the amperage of current flowing through the tissue (Case 2). When there is no direct path through the patient to ground, the injury tends to be less. Use of insulating rather than conductive materials around electric circuits helps increase the resistance and decrease the flow through the patient. Tissue resistance to electrical current increases from nerve (which is the least resistant) to vessel, muscle, skin, tendon, fat, and finally bone (most resistant).

KEY POINTS

- Burn is produced by agent with a temperature of 40°C or above

- Victims of closed space fires (cars and unvented rooms) may sustain severe inhalational injuries from these products of combustion

- Electrical injuries depend on type of circuit, voltage, resistance offered by body, duration of contact, and amperage of current flowing through tissue

DIAGNOSIS

The diagnosis of thermal injuries relates to two major factors: burn size (the percentage of total surface area burned) and depth of the burn (first degree, second degree, third degree, and fourth degree). Other factors related to burns include age of the patient, location of the burn that may cause special problems (e.g., hand, face), inhalational injuries, circumferential burns, and associated injuries such as fractures.

The burn size or percentage of total body surface area (TBSA) that is burned can be estimated by the "rule of nines." This divides the body into multiples of nine. The chest and abdomen are 18% combined, and the back and buttocks are also 18% combined. The anterior portion of the one lower extremity is 9%, the posterior aspect is 9%, each upper extremity is 9%, the head and neck area is 9%, and the genitalia are 1%. In children, the head and neck and the chest and abdomen are relatively larger than the extremities (Fig. 64.1).

The depth of the burn is dependent on the amount of superficial or deep tissue destruction (Fig. 64.2). First-degree burns are limited to the epidermis and are self-limiting and self-healing. Second-degree burns include destruction of the epidermis and portions of the dermis, leaving the mid- to deep dermis intact. Superficial blisters with clear fluid can appear. Because nerve endings are still intact (Fig. 64.3), second-degree burns are extremely

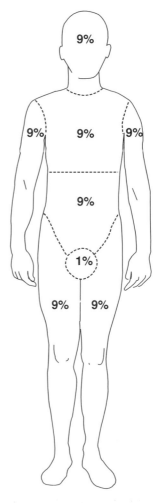

FIGURE 64.1 *The "rule of nines" permits rapid estimation of burned body surface area in adults. It must be adapted for children whose body surface is larger with respect to weight.*

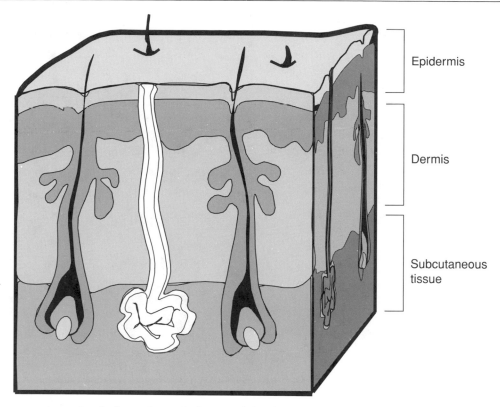

FIGURE 64.2   *Burn depth depends on the layers of the skin involved. This diagram illustrates the normal skin appendages (hair follicles and sweat glands) with respect to their depths.*

painful. These injuries will re-epithelialize without skin grafting within 2 weeks, assuming local infection does not occur. Third-degree burns destroy the epidermis and full thickness layers of the dermis down into the subcutaneous fat and/or muscle and bone (Fig. 64.4). Nerve endings are destroyed, making the affected area anesthetic. Dermal protein is denatured by the heat and becomes a tough, leather-like layer. On palpation, the burn is hard and insensate. Re-epithelialization and self-healing cannot occur because the basal cell layer of the dermis has been destroyed. Skin grafting or flap reconstruction will be necessary.

KEY POINTS

• Diagnosis of thermal injuries relates to burn size (percentage of TBSA) and depth of burn (first degree, second degree, and third degree)

• Other factors related to burns include age of patient, location of burn that may cause special problems (e.g., hand, face), inhalational injuries, circumferential burns, and associated injuries such as fractures

• Burn size or TBSA can be estimated by rule of nines

• First-degree burns limited to epidermis and are self-limiting and self-healing

• Second-degree burns include destruction of epidermis and portions of dermis, leaving mid- to deep dermis intact

• Second-degree burns are extremely painful

• Third-degree burns destroy epidermis and full thickness layers of dermis down into subcutaneous fat and/or muscle and bone; nerve endings destroyed, making affected area anesthetic; dermal protein denatured by heat and becomes tough, leather-like layer; on palpation, burn is hard and insensate

DIFFERENTIAL DIAGNOSIS

It is difficult to differentiate between second- and third-degree burns. Frequently, at the initial injury, they can appear identical; however, it is important to realize that a second-degree burn will "heal by itself" (re-epithelialization) and a third-degree burn will only heal by wound contraction and/or skin grafting. Occasionally, one can differentiate between second- and third-degree burns by testing for sensibility. Feeling in the skin can be present in second-degree burns because the sensory end organs are usually preserved, whereas in third-degree burns, the wound area is totally anesthetic because of the destruction of sensory neural end fibers.

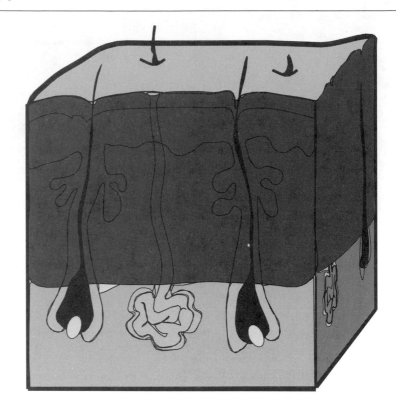

FIGURE 64.3 *A second-degree burn involves a portion of the dermis and the epidermis. Because it is not full thickness, the burn spares the nerves and is extremely painful. Follicles are left intact and will continue to grow hair.*

TREATMENT

Since first-degree burns are self-limited (sunburn) and heal themselves, various topical over-the-counter ointments suffice. There are no sequelae or residual scarring from first-degree burns.

Second- and third-degree burns are treated similarly clinically, with some exceptions. One must understand the differentiation between treating the local wound area and the metabolic effect of second- and third-degree burns. In second-degree burns, the wound can be minimally debrided, topically treated with antibacterials, and allowed time for re-epithelialization. Third-degree burns usually should not be debrided (unless contaminated). They should be topically treated with antibacterial agents until the wound bed is ready for surgical excision, then skin grafted.

When second- or third-degree burns affect more than 20% of the body surface area in any age group (or 10% of the body surface area in patients under 10 or over 60 years of age), these patients should be hospitalized for treatment of not only the local wound, but most importantly, the hemodynamic and metabolic affects of this large and sometimes devastating injury.

The management of a severely burned patient begins with assessment of the airway and breathing. Only rarely is a surgical airway such as a cricothyroidotomy required. When the patient has been in a closed space, they frequently will have singed facial and nasal hair as well as carbonaceous sputum in their oro- or nasopharynx. When

these are present, bronchoscopy is indicated to determine the extent of any inhalational injury.

Plastics and wood emit large amounts of carbon monoxide when they burn. The carbon monoxide binds avidly to hemoglobin and interferes with normal oxygen transport by forming carboxyhemoglobin. At room air oxygen concentration, carboxyhemoglobin has a half-life of 4 hours, while at 100% oxygen, its half-life is reduced to 1 hour. A blood gas sample should be obtained and sent for carboxyhemoglobin saturation shortly after the patient's arrival. Levels less than 5% are normal, while concentrations greater than 30% may be rapidly lethal. Patients who present with singed facial or nasal hairs should be suspect for inhalational injuries. Burning plastics and synthetic fabrics emit a number of compounds that are extremely toxic to the lungs. Fiberoptic bronchoscopy should be performed quickly to determine whether such injury is present in appropriately selected patients. Although a chest x-ray should be obtained in all burn victims to exclude associated trauma, this study is generally not helpful in detecting inhalational injuries (Case 1).

The major physiologic derangement of a second- or third-degree burn comprising more than 20% of the body surface area is hypovolemia. This occurs because of massive edema formation due to loss of the integrity of endothelial cells within capillaries. Fluid is lost from the intravascular space to the interstitial space, causing a "third-space phenomenon." Patients can rapidly develop hypovolemic shock. Massive fluid resuscitation is necessary to replace this volume so that cardiac output can be restored.

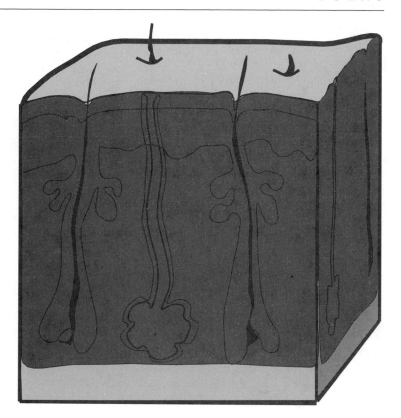

FIGURE 64.4 *A full thickness burn involves all layers down to (and often including) the subcutaneous tissue. Because nerves are destroyed the burn is anesthetic. Coagulation of the skin's proteins produces a white appearance that is "leathery" to the touch. Because hair follicles are destroyed, hair will not regrow. The involved eschar must be excised and replaced with a skin graft.*

Baseline laboratory studies, including hematocrit, urinalysis with specific gravity, electrolytes, chest x-ray, and arterial blood gases, are important before fluid resuscitation.

The treatment of burn hypovolemia requires the intravenous replacement of fluids and electrolytes computed (Baxter or Parkland Hospital formula) as follows: 24 hr requirement (ml) = TBSA burn · 4 · wt (kg). This is provided using lactated Ringer's solution or normal saline. Dextrose should not be used in the initial postburn period. One-half of the amount calculated is given in the first 8 hours following the burn (not the arrival to the emergency room), and the second half is given over the ensuing 16 hours of the 24-hour period (Case 1).

Urine output and specific gravity should be used to monitor the adequacy of resuscitation. As with all formulas, increased or decreased volumes of fluid may be required depending on the patient's response. Following the first day, plasma protein (albumin) can be administered at 0.3–0.5 ml/kg/% burn. Crystalloid can be changed to 5% dextrose in water to maintain urinary output and to keep the serum sodium at a normal level. The monitoring of this resuscitation is extremely important and a urine output of 50 ml/hr or more in adults and 2 ml/kg/hr in children less than 10 years old is paramount. Central venous or pulmonary wedge pressures in these kinds of acute burns are usually unreliable. Routine vital signs should be constantly monitored.

Nutrition is an extremely important part of burn management and should be instituted as quickly as possible. Most patients can tolerate internal feeding through a nasogastric tube. Caloric intake should be at least 40 Kcal/kg/day and protein intake at least 1.2 g/kg/day.

Cure of the burn wound should begin at the time of fluid resuscitation. Burns should be cleansed gently with a surgical soap to remove nonviable epidermis. Bullae should be left in place as they form a biologic dressing. Several topical antimicrobial agents are available that decrease the incidence of invasive burn wound infection and systemic sepsis. All have been associated with improved survival of burn patients. Silver sulfadiazine (Silvadene) is the most commonly used agent. It has limited penetration of the eschar, but is painless on application and has excellent activity against many organisms, with the notable exception of many strains of *Pseudomonas* and virtually all *Enterobacter* species. Its most important undesirable effect is that it can cause a reversible neutropenia. Mafenide acetate (Sulfamylon) has excellent eschar penetration and is particularly useful in patients with heavily contaminated wounds or those known to contain *Pseudomonas*. Its disadvantages are that it causes discomfort when applied to partial thickness burns and it acts as a carbonic anhydrase inhibitor, thereby producing a metabolic acidosis. Both silver sulfadiazine and mafenide acetate are applied every 12 hours, with the excess removed before the next application. Silver nitrate (0.5%) solution and povidone iodine are used occasionally. Silver nitrate is usually reserved for patients with sulfa allergies, since it must be applied every 8 hours and is messy to handle. It causes transeschar leaching of sodium, potassium, chloride, and calcium, which must be replaced as required.

Antibiotic use is not indicated in the initial treatment of burned patients. Studies have shown that such prophylaxis actually increases the rate of several infections (such as pneumonia) in the early postburn period. Clostridial infections and tetanus are not uncommon. Therefore, each patient's tetanus immunization status should be assessed and toxoid administered if required.

Patients should be examined carefully for the presence of circumferential burns, which might restrict blood flow or mobility. This is particularly important on the extremities (including the hands and feet) as well as on the chest where a circumferential eschar may limit ventilatory excursions. When such wounds exist, escharotomy is indicated. Escharotomy involves placing bilateral longitudinal incisions through the length of the eschar to permit blood flow or movement beneath the burn. Escharotomy should be performed quickly since ischemia can occur rapidly. The procedure can be done in the emergency room if required, but is best done at the bedside in the burn unit. Anesthesia is not usually required since the eschar is anesthetic. The incision is carried through the full thickness of the burn until viable (bleeding) tissue is reached beneath. The most commonly used topical antibacterial agent placed as a cream on the burn wound after the removal of necrotic tissue is silver sulfadiazine (Silvadene). Occasionally, biopsies of the burn wound for quantitative and qualitative bacteriology can be helpful. Once the burn wound is cleaned, skin grafts should be applied at periodic operative interventions.

Complications in acute burns can be devastating. Renal failure from hypovolemia can occur and must be diagnosed if not avoided. Gastrointestinal bleeding occurs in over 40% of acute burns and has a correlation with an increased risk of burn wound sepsis. Burn wound sepsis can be diagnosed by tissue biopsies for qualitative and quantitative analysis. The bacterial count should be kept below 10^5 of bacteria per gram of tissue.

KEY POINTS

• At room air oxygen concentration, carboxyhemoglobin has half-life of 4 hours; at 100% oxygen, its half-life is reduced to 1 hour

• Major physiologic derangement of second- or third-degree burn comprising more than 20% of body surface area is hypovolemia

• Treatment of burn hypovolemia requires intravenous replacement of fluids and electrolytes computed (Baxter or Park-Hospital formula) as follows: 24 hr requirement (ml) = TBSA burn · 4 · wt (kg)

• Caloric intake should be at least 40 Kcal/kg/day and protein intake at least 1.2 g/kg/day

• Burns should be cleansed gently with surgical soap to remove nonviable epidermis; bullae should be left in place as they form biologic dressing

• Antibiotic use indicated in initial treatment of burned patients; studies have shown that prophylaxis increases rate of several infections (such as pneumonia) in early postburn period

• Escharotomy involves placing bilateral longitudinal incisions through length of eschar to permit blood flow or movement beneath burn

• Burn wound sepsis can be diagnosed by tissue biopsies for qualitative and quantitative analysis

FOLLOW-UP

Following the successful treatment of the acute thermal injury, further soft tissue reconstruction, splinting, and rehabilitation (physical and psychological) may be necessary. The burn patient can be the sickest patient in any hospital, since all organ systems are often involved. Increased nutritional and metabolic needs must be met during the acute and subacute stage. Various aspects of hyper- or hypothermia, congestive heart failure, pulmonary edema, ileus, mental status changes, azotemia, thrombocytopenia, hypofibrinogenemia, and hyper- or hypoglycemia can all occur. Long-term follow-up, including the prevention of wound contracture and hypertrophic scarring, must be maintained by splinting and compression. Further reconstruction is frequently warranted.

Full thickness burn eschars are nonviable and must be removed. Such tangential excision requires grafting of the underlying bed to allow new skin growth. Most centers now prefer early excision (within several days after injury) of the eschar with skin grafting to aid in mobility and early healing. Studies have shown that early excision and grafting decreases hospital stay and improves subsequent functional outcome.

Electrical injuries present special challenges, including cardiopulmonary difficulties such as ventricular fibrillation. There is also a high risk of renal failure due to hemoglobin and myoglobin deposits in the renal tubules, fractures, spinal cord injuries, intra-abdominal problems, and vascular derangements such as thrombosis of small vessels. Tissue destruction under the eschar of an electrical injury is often worse than might be expected from the appearance of the surface burn (Case 2). Hence, these patients require hospitalization with aggressive management. Fluid requirements are greater than predicted by the formulas, since muscle destruction is more widespread than just the area of the eschar. Injuries due to lightning strikes are particularly hazardous because of the amount of current conducted.

Patients suffering from cold injuries such as frostbite and systemic hypothermia require rapid rewarming in 40°C hydrotherapy tanks as necessary. One must monitor cardiac, vascular, and respiratory function during this rapid rewarming. A urine output of 50 ml/hr should be maintained.

KEY POINTS

• Early excision (within several days after injury) of eschar with skin grafting to aid in mobility and early healing

• Early excision and grafting decreases hospital stay and improves subsequent functional outcome

• Tissue destruction under eschar of an electrical injury is often worse than might be expected from appearance of surface burn

SUGGESTED READINGS

Plastic and Reconstructive Surgery—Essentials for Students. 4th Ed. Plastic Surgery Educational Foundation, Arlington Heights, IL, 1993

A good student manual that has an overview of burn injuries.

Atturson MG: A pathophysiology of severe thermal injury. J Burn Care Rehab 6:129, 1985

A good overview that discusses underlying pathophysiologic mechanisms.

Pruitt BE Jr: The diagnosis and treatment of infection in the burn patient. Burns 11:79, 1984

An outstanding article on burn-related infection, one of the most feared complications. The author is among the best known burn surgeons.

QUESTIONS

1. Clinically, a third-degree burn may be differentiated from a second-degree burn because the former?

   A. Is more superficial.
   B. Is anesthetic.
   C. Has the potential to regenerate normal skin.
   D. Generally has no infection risk.

2. The half-life of carboxyhemoglobin in a patient breathing room air is?

   A. 30 minutes.
   B. 1 hour.
   C. 4 hours.
   D. 1 day.

3. Silver sulfadiazine (Silvadene) is a frequently used topical antimicrobial agent in the treatment of burn wounds. Which of the following items is not one of its characteristics?

   A. Good coverage of *Pseudomonas*.
   B. Incomplete eschar penetration.
   C. Broad spectrum antimicrobial coverage.
   D. Painless on application.

(See p. 604 for answers.)

65

INFECTIONS

AND INJURIES

OF THE HAND

MALCOLM LESAVOY

EDWARD PASSARO, JR.

T he hand is a complex and unique organ that, to a large extent, distinguishes humans from other species. It is highly specialized and anatomically complex, and its function is integrated to a relatively large portion of our brain.

Because the hand is such an active portion of our body it is frequently affected by trauma and infections. Treatment of hand injuries is demanding and highly specialized. The results of improper treatment can be devastating.

This chapter reviews some of the salient features of hand infections and injuries with presentation of two of the most common hand-related problems. Emphasis is placed on prompt recognition of those conditions so that they can be cared for promptly by experts in hand care.

CASE 1
LACERATED TENDONS

A 35-year-old laboratory technician lacerated the palmar surface of her right dominant index finger at the proximal phalanx on a piece of broken laboratory glassware. The laceration was 2 cm in length and bled briskly when pressure was removed. She was unable to flex the fingers at the distal or proximal interphalangeal joints. She also had numbness along the radial aspect of the index fingertips distal to the laceration. A diagnosis of lacerations of the

flexor profundus and flexor superficialis tendons was made. In addition, it was recognized that there was disruption of the radial digital nerve.

In the emergency room, no attempt was made to probe the laceration for pieces of glass. The bleeding was adequately controlled with gauze bandages and manual pressure and subsequently, a pressure dressing. She was given tetanus toxoid and antibiotics and was brought to the operating room. A regional block of the right arm was established by the anesthesiologist, following which the arm was elevated, desanguinated by a tight wrap down the arm with an elastic bandage (Esmark), and then, a blood pressure cuff was inflated on the proximal upper arm to 250 mmHg. This provided a bloodless field for the hand surgeon, who ligated the end of the lacerated digital artery and repaired the severed profundus and sublimis tendons. The ends of the digital nerve were gently reapproximated. At the end of the repair the arm cuff was de-

475

flated and the wound was dry. The hand was placed on a padded forearm splint in the "position of rest" (i.e., with the fingers in slight flexion). The thumb was free. Two weeks later the splint was removed and passive exercises of the fingers made with the help of a physiotherapist. The patient was instructed to carry out a range of passive motion of the fingers several times a day and to reapply the splint at all other times. Two weeks thereafter the splint was discontinued and more active hand and finger exercises instituted by the physiotherapist and surgeon. At the end of 2 months, she had regained full function and strength of her hand, but the radial aspect of the tip of the index finger continued to feel numb.

CASE 2
CELLULITIS

A 30-year-old warehouseman noted slight swelling and tenderness of his right (dominant) hand at the end of a day's work. The following day he was unable to put his gloves on because it produced pain in the right hand, and he reported to the company physician. The hand was now visibly swollen throughout and slightly erythematous. It was uniformly sensitive to pressure, but there was no focal pain. A radial pulse was present. Digital pulses could not be palpated, but the capillary filling time at the fingertips was excellent. He could both partially flex and extend the fingers but was limited by the pain it produced. There were no obvious breaks in the skin. The patient indicated that at work he wore his gloves frequently, but not always, when moving 55-gallon metal drums filled with oil. He did not recall any unusual trauma, strain, or effort, puncture wound, lacerations, or abrasions. In a 4-year period of doing the same type of work he had not had any hand problems. He was not a gardener.

The company physician prescribed oral antibiotics and a tetanus toxoid injection. He sent the patient to a nearby hospital where radiographs of the hand were taken, looking for a sliver of metal from one of the drums that may have penetrated the hand. None was found. No fractures were noted. The hand was immobilized in a sling, and the patient was instructed to return the following morning to the company physician.

On his return, the hand was noted to be more swollen than the day before. The motion of the fingers was now very limited because of the pain. The patient complained of feeling poorly. He had spent a restless night, because moving in bed elicited pain in his hand. His oral temperature was 38°C. The company physician contacted an orthopaedist specializing in hand problems, who arranged to see the patient in the hospital emergency room. His examination confirmed the findings of the company physician. In addition, he now noted edema extending into the wrist and some faint reddish streaks in the volar aspect of the

right forearm. One lymph node was palpable in the right axilla and none in the left axilla. He admitted the patient to the hospital.

Following admission, the right arm was elevated in a suspended sling. An intravenous line was started in the left arm and an infusion of ampicillin started. The following morning the edema was nearly resolved, and 24 hours later it was completely resolved. Full range of motion of the fingers was now possible, although the patient noted that the hand felt tight or stiff. He was discharged and given oral antibiotics for the next 5 days. A week thereafter he was allowed to resume his warehouse duties.

GENERAL CONSIDERATIONS

The human hand is a marvel of construction and function. Its abilities result from an intricate and compact arrangement of bones, nerves, muscles, tendons, and blood vessels. As a consequence, any injury or infection of the hand is liable to affect not one, but several of these important structures, as well as alter the environment of the tendons, bursae, and palmar and dorsal fascial areas. Thus, seemingly inconsequential injuries or infections can have devastating effects on the function of this unique organ (Case 2). Most of us, either directly or indirectly, are dependent on the normal function of the hand for our livelihood. Any disability of the hand has the potential to disable the patient and dependents.

The most important features of the management of the common injuries of the hand, including those caused by trauma (Case 1) and infection (Case 2), are both a history of the trauma or cause of infection and a detailed, carefully documented physical examination or assessment. As in both the cases presented, socioeconomic factors such as hazards in the workplace and workers' compensation become important issues. Thus, a carefully documented assessment of the injury or infection is not only important for the individual patient, but becomes an important issue for both society and the physicians involved in the care of the patient. A thorough and repeated assessment also is the basis for determining conditions that can be managed safely by the primary physician and cases that need the expertise of specialists in the management of these problems (Case 2).

As indicated, the initial assessment is a combination of a detailed history of the injury or infection and an examination of the (1) vascular, (2) neural, (3) mechanical (functional), and (4) infectious causes of the disability. Each of these are examined in a practical and efficient manner, so that a complete assessment can be made by the student or physician without relying on the detailed anatomical and functional knowledge possessed by only a few specialists.

As the hand is richly supplied by communicating arterial arches in both the palmar and dorsal aspects, vascular compromise to the hand seldom results from a single injury localized to the hand. It is more likely to occur from proximal injuries (brachial or axillary artery) or when the hand is involved in multiple extensive injuries that crush or mangle it. Swelling or edema of the hand from such injuries or from an infection can create sufficient pressure to compromise the blood supply to the hand. Often, the extent of the swelling makes examination of the important arterial pulses of the hand (radial, ulnar, digital) impossible. The color and the capillary filling time as observed at the tip of the fingers (Case 2), compared to the uninvolved hand, is a good measure of the arterial circulation to the hand.

Three major nerve trunks—radial, median, and ulnar—supply all the sensory and motor function of the hand. The motor function of each nerve can be tested individually and collectively. For example, if the patient is able to oppose the thumb to each fingertip in succession from 5th to 2nd (index), all motor neural and mechanical systems are intact. Similarly, closing all fingers together in a cone requires intact neural, motor, and mechanical units to all the fingers.

The important ulnar nerve motor function can be tested by spreading the fingers apart (abduction) and approximating them. The thumb and index finger cannot oppose themselves perfectly. The important median nerve motor function can be tested by flexing the finger at the metacarpals and by having the thumb oppose itself to the fingertips of the other fingers. The radial nerve can be tested by extending the fingers and dorsi flexor of the hand. The important sensory components to each of the nerve trunks can be isolated by testing for pinprick sensitivity over the dorsum or back of the hand (radial); the lateral aspects of the thumb, index, and middle fingers (median); and the lateral aspect of the 4th and 5th fingers (ulnar).

Mechanical (functional) impairment occurs when structural components such as tendons are severed (Case 1). Isolated functional impairment can be ascertained at two levels, the wrist and the metacarpophalangeal (MP) joint. Wrist motion, ventroflexion, depends on the integrity of the tendon flexors of the wrist (flexor carpi radialis and flexor carpi ulnaris), while dorsi flexion (extension) of the wrist depends on the extensor carpi radialis.

The flexion of the proximal phalanges at the MP joint depends on the integrity of the flexor sublimis (Case 1), while flexion of the tip of the finger held in extension (Case 1) is dependent on the flexor sublimis.

Lastly, investigation of infectious causes of hand disability involves careful inspection of the compartments that may contain the infection. The compartments are those at the base of the thumb (thenar space), the base of the 5th finger (hypothenar space), and the palm (deep palmar space). Infections can also be confined to the sheaths (tenosynovitis), involving the tendon of the fingers. Infections in these confined spaces are ascertained by gentle palpation in these respective areas, which elicits focal tenderness corresponding to these areas.

KEY POINTS

- Because the hand is such an active portion of the body, it is frequently affected by trauma and infections

- Results of improper treatment can be devastating

- Any injury or infection of the hand is liable to affect not one, but several important structures (bones, nerves, muscles tendons blood vessels), as well as alter the environment of the tendons, bursae, and palmar and dorsal fascial areas

- Most important features of the management of common injuries of the hand, including those caused by trauma and infection, are both a history of trauma or cause of infection and a detailed, carefully documented physical examination or assessment

- Examination includes the vascular, neural, mechanical, and infectious causes of the disability

- As the hand is richly supplied by communicating arterial arches in both palmar and dorsal aspects, vascular compromise to the hand seldom results from single injury localized to hand

- Often, extent of swelling makes examination of important arterial pulses (radial, ulnar, digital) impossible

- Three major nerve trunks—radial, median, and ulnar—supply all sensory and motor function of the hand; motor function of each nerve can be tested individually and collectively

- Important ulnar nerve motor function tested by spreading fingers apart (abduction) and approximating them; thumb and index finger cannot oppose themselves perfectly

- Important median nerve motor functions can be tested by flexing finger at metacarpals and having thumb oppose itself to fingertips of other fingers

- Investigation of infectious causes of hand disability involves careful inspection of compartments that may contain infection

DIAGNOSIS

Hand injuries, whether from trauma or infection, are sufficiently disabling that patients present themselves for treatment earlier than with many other conditions. Establishing that the hand has been impaired and/or infected is often self-evident. The most difficult aspect with either trauma or infection is trying to determine whether the process is uncomplicated and self-limiting so that it can be treated by a primary physician, or whether it should be promptly referred to a specialist. As the patient in Case 2 demonstrates, this can often be a difficult task, even for those with considerable experience in dealing with hand problems.

Several factors can be identified that help distinguish the more complex problems requiring prompt referral to a specialist from those that can be managed by generalists. Extensive trauma as occurs in crush or mangle injuries should be managed by specialists. Similarly, laceration or breaks in the skin that occur with fractures of the bones of the hands (open fractures) require special care. Extensive trauma to several fingers requires sophisticated treatment lest the treatment of the fingers adversely affect the function of the whole hand, for example, by improper splinting for inappropriate lengths of time.

In cases of extensive or multiple trauma, or whenever there is doubt or suspicion that other or occult bones or structural (tendon) injuries are possible, radiographs of the hand should be taken. If the patient has degenerative bone disease (see below), radiographs of the uninvolved hand may be helpful for comparison. Occult fractures, dislocations, or avulsion of tendons with a small spicule of bone can be detected in this way.

The environment in which the injury occurred is also important. The same laceration from a broken but clean piece of laboratory glassware is very much different from that caused by a piece of steel coated with oils or chemicals. The latter will require extensive cleaning and debridement in the operating room, while the former might undergo primary suturing in an emergency room setting. Above all, as emphasized under General Considerations, a carefully done assessment (that is carefully recorded with a drawing or sketch, if possible) of the vascular, neural, structural, and functional aspects of the injured hand must be made.

Infections of the hand are more difficult to diagnose and manage (Case 2). Not only is the assessment mentioned above critical in diagnosing and managing the patient, it is often difficult or limited by the tissue swelling that may be present. A history of the primary event leading to the infection (e.g., stuck by a thorn on a plant) and the time since the initial event are important prognostic factors. Longer durations and obvious gross contamination (e.g., being punctured by a dirty nail) are infections best handled by a specialist. Failures of conservative therapy should be quickly brought to the attention of specialists (Case 2).

KEY POINTS

- Most difficult aspect of diagnosis with either trauma or infection is trying to determine whether process is uncomplicated and self-limiting so that it can be treated by primary physicians, or whether it should be promptly referred to a specialist

- Extensive trauma as occurs in crush or mangle injuries should be managed by specialists

- Similarly, laceration or breaks in skin that occur with fractures of bones of hands (open fractures) require special care; extensive trauma to several fingers requires sophisticated treatment lest the treatment of the fingers adversely affect function of whole hand, for example, by improper splinting for inappropriate lengths of time

- Enviroment in which injury occurred also important

- Carefully done assessment (that is carefully recorded with drawing or sketch, if possible) of vascular, neural, structural, and functional aspects of injured hand must be made

- Infections of hand more difficult to diagnose and manage

- History of primary event leading to infection and time since initial event important prognostic factors

G DIFFERENTIAL DIAGNOSIS

Generally, a good history is sufficient to assist in the differential between trauma and infection and other conditions that can mimic them. The latter are predominately chronic degenerative diseases, which can affect the hand, and chronic forms of trauma or idiopathic changes, which produce limitations of motion.

Chronic systemic degenerative processes that affect the hand include osteoarthritis, rheumatoid arthritis, and vasospastic disorders such as Raynaud's disease. At times, they can be confused with infections of the hand, as they can produce swelling, erythematous changes, and pain on motion. Aids in the differential diagnosis include a previous history of similar attacks, lack of antecedent trauma or cause for infection, and that most of these systemic disorders will involve both hands to some degree, while trauma or infections are usually confined to a single hand. The best strategy is careful documentation of the limitations in vascular, motor, and sensory components and frequent re-examinations to look for progression or resolution of the process.

Mechanical limitations to the hand that can be mistaken for acute trauma include tenosynovitis (i.e., "trigger finger") or early palmar contractures (Dupuytren's contracture) from chronic trauma or idiopathic causes. Again, a thorough history usually allows differentiation from more immediate traumatic causes. Both chronic tenosynovitis and Dupuytren's contracture are marked by a chronic and indolent course. Both may be related in some patients to repetitive forms of hand trauma over long periods. Both tend to involve one hand primarily.

KEY POINTS

- Generally, a good history is sufficient to assist in differential between trauma and infection and other conditions that mimic them

- At times, chronic systemic degenerative processes that affect hand can be confused with infections, as they produce swelling, erythematous changes, and pain on motion

- Both chronic tenosynovitis and Dupuytren's contracture marked by chronic and indolent course

A TREATMENT

Acute trauma to the structural elements of the hand, bones, and tendons requires special care and is best done by experts in this field (Case 1). Note that in Case 1, an attempt was made to repair the injured digital nerve, but the small arterial injury producing the disturbing bleeding was managed by simple ligation.

Minor traumatic injuries occurring in a relatively clean environment, such as a 3-cm laceration of the dorsum of the hand from a clean kitchen knife, can be sutured primarily by a competent physician. Lacerations crossing flexion creases or injuring blood vessels and/or nerves should be dressed with bandages and referred to a hand specialist for repair. Similarly, complex injuries as described above involving more than one finger, extensive tissue injury, or a dirty environment should be referred for the special care they require.

Infections are both more difficult to recognize early and to treat, particularly if no identifiable source is found (Case 2). If the infection is confined to a small area and to a relatively "less risky" area, such as the back of the hand, an initial course of antibiotic therapy, immobilization, and elevation of the hand is warranted. Frequently, because of our dependence on our hands, the degree of immobilization and elevation is suboptimal. Because of this and the difficulty in determining the extent of the infection, frequent repeat examinations carefully noting the changes or lack of improvement are crucial to further management. Whenever a failure to improve promptly is noted, the patient needs to be referred for management (Case 2). Infections of the hand in particular, because of the difficulty in ascertaining their extent and the consequences of improper management, should be seen early by a specialist rather than later.

KEY POINTS

- Minor traumatic injuries occurring in relatively clean environment, such as 3-cm laceration of dorsum of the hand from a clean kitchen knife, can be sutured primarily by competent physician

- If infection confined to small and relatively less risky area, such as back of hand, initial course of antibiotic therapy, immobilization, and elevation of hand is warranted

- Infections of hand in particular, because of difficulty in ascertaining their extent and consequences of improper management, should be seen early by specialist rather than later

FOLLOW-UP

Injury and infections of the hand require careful follow-up to rehabilitate the hand and restore function to normal (Case 1). This involves not only careful evaluation by the surgeon but usually physiotherapists as well. As the hand is complex in both structure and function, any period of immobilization or limitation of motion will produce some decrement in its function. A careful plan to progressively exercise and strengthen, if not retrain, the hand is necessary after any major trauma or infection. In particular, since the use of the hand is often crucial for employment, there is a tendency to reuse the hand fully as

soon as possible rather than wait until complete healing has taken place.

Minor wounds and infections treated by the nonspecialist should be seen at very frequent intervals initially and subsequently at longer intervals, after the patient has resumed normal activities.

KEY POINTS

- Careful plan to progressively exercise and strengthen, if not retrain, hand is necessary after any major trauma or infection

SUGGESTED READINGS

Gaul JS Jr: Management of acute hand injuries. Ann Emerg Med 9:139, 1980

A systemic evaluation of the hand, looking for functional or structural damage to each of its six tissue components, is the first step in managing the acute hand problem.

Phipps AR, Blanshard J: A review of in-patient hand infections. Arch Emerg Med 9:299, 1992

A retrospective review is presented of 64 patients with infections of the hand requiring admission to hospital.

QUESTIONS

1. The major aid in distinguishing between an injury or infection of the hand that can be treated by nonspecialist rather than a specialist is?

   A. CT and MRI scans of the affected hand.

   B. A period of observation.

   C. Consultation with an orthopaedist.

   D. A carefully taken and documented history and physical examination of the hand.

2. Injuries that should be referred promptly to a specialist include?

   A. The multiple injury or mangled hand.

   B. Injuries involving two or more fingers or two or more components (e.g., tendons and bones).

   C. Lacerations across critical areas such as the flexure crease.

   D. All of the above.

3. Infections of the hand?

   A. Are usually promptly detected because of the signs of infection (rubor, calor, dolor).

   B. Can be ascertained because of the history of injury with potentially infected sources.

   C. Invariably respond to immobilization, elevation, and antibiotics.

   D. Can be difficult to detect and treat and have devastating consequences when not managed appropriately.

(See p. 604 for answers.)

66

MANAGEMENT

OF THE

NECK MASS

MARILENE B. WANG

The patient who presents with a new mass in the neck poses a diagnostic challenge because errors in diagnosis and/or therapy may have dire consequences. Such a patient should be approached in a systematic and thorough manner to make appropriate management decisions. In

this chapter, the three broad categories of neck masses will be delineated (congenital, inflammatory, and neoplastic), with emphasis on the workup of the neoplastic neck mass. A complete head and neck history and physical examination will aid in the differential diagnosis of a neck mass. Further laboratory studies, radiographs, and invasive procedures are obtained on an individual case basis where appropriate.

CASE 1
THYROGLOSSAL DUCT CYST

An 8-year-old boy presented to his pediatrician with a history of intermittent swelling in the anterior midline neck region. His mother stated that this mass first appeared 2 years previously and that it got larger and painful when he had a cold. There have been a total of six episodes of swelling in the past 2 years, and recently the mass had persisted. He was otherwise healthy. On physical examination, a 3 × 3-cm firm, nontender nodule was palpable in the midline of the neck, about midway between the chin and the sternal notch. There was no drainage from the mass or erythema of the overlying skin. The mass moved up and down with swallowing. There were no other masses. The remainder of the neck examination was normal.

FNA of the mass yielded straw-colored fluid and cells noted by the cytologist to have features of thyroid follicle epithelium. Based on the presumptive diagnosis of a thyroglossal duct cyst, the boy was scheduled for excision of this mass.

At operation, a 2 × 3-cm cystic nodule was identified at the level of the thyrohyoid membrane. There was a thin stalk that traveled down to the thyroid gland and also a stalk tracking superiorly into the hyoid bone. The entire cyst with its stalk was removed, including the mid-portion of the hyoid bone, and the stalk was followed up to the base of the tongue. He has had no further problems with swelling of the neck.

CASE 2
LUDWIG'S ANGINA

A 31-year-old female presented to her physician with a 4-day history of increasingly painful swelling underneath her chin. She also had had temperatures up to 38°C for 2 days. She was finding it difficult to swallow food and liquids at first, and then was also unable to swallow her saliva.

On examination, the patient appeared lethargic and was more comfortable in an upright position with her head tilted forward. She was breathing rapid, shallow, labored breaths, her mouth was open, and she was holding a basin to spit out saliva. Her temperature was 39°C and her pulse was 115 bpm. The submental area of her neck was swollen, erythematous, and very tender to palpation. In her oral cavity, she had marked swelling of the floor of her mouth, pushing her tongue up to the roof of her mouth. Her dental hygiene was extremely poor.

Because of her impending airway compromise, she was taken emergently to the operating room. A tracheostomy was first performed under local anesthesia, then the submental area was widely opened and drained. Copious, foul-smelling fluid flowed forth from the submental incision. The wound was irrigated with large amounts of saline and antibiotic solution. Large drains were placed and the wound was closed loosely. Cultures from the neck grew out *Streptococcus pneumoniae* and mixed anaerobic flora. Postoperatively, she was maintained on intravenous penicillin and oxacillin for 5 days. Dental consultation was obtained, and radiographs revealed an abscess of her right lower second molar tooth. This tooth was extracted and her clinical course rapidly improved. Her drains, then her tracheostomy, were taken out and she was discharged home on the 8th postoperative day.

CASE 3
SQUAMOUS CELL CARCINOMA, METASTATIC

A 67-year-old male presented with a new finding of a painless lump in the right anterior neck. He first noticed it while shaving and thought that it had enlarged over the 4 weeks prior to presentation. It was poorly mobile and nonfluctuant. He had a history of smoking two packs of cigarettes a day for 50 years, and drank two to three six-packs of beer per week. He had had about a 10-lb weight loss over the past 2 months and attributed that to a general loss of appetite. He had a chronic cough with the production of whitish phlegm in the mornings. His voice had always been "rough." He had an occasional sore throat and right ear pain. He had not noticed any fevers or night sweats. His past medical history was significant for mild hypertension and a "heart condition," for which he took an occasional nitroglycerin tablet.

On examination, he appeared to be a thin, elderly gentleman, alert and oriented. There was a 4-cm, only slightly mobile, nontender, firm mass at the anterior border of his right sternocleidomastoid muscle. There were no changes of the overlying skin. His ears and nose were normal. His oral cavity and oropharynx had changes consistent with a smoker, showing poor dental hygiene, discolored tongue, and erythematous mucosa. There were no discrete ulcerations or exophytic growths. The base of the tongue and floor of the mouth were soft. Examination of his larynx

and nasopharynx was difficult because of his active gag reflex, but no obvious lesions were noted.

The patient was concerned about cancer and requested that the lump in his neck be taken out. A chest x-ray was first obtained, along with a CT scan of his neck from the base of the skull to the clavicles. His chest x-ray showed changes consistent with emphysema, but no other pathology. On CT scan, there was a 4 × 5-cm mass in the right jugulodigastric region, as well as several smaller lymph nodes along the jugular chain.

FNA was obtained of the right neck mass and the cytologist identified malignant epithelial cells consistent with a squamous cell carcinoma.

The patient was then prepared for examination under anesthesia, direct laryngoscopy, and esophagoscopy. During examination, the base of the tongue and floor of the mouth were palpated and found to be soft. The nasopharynx was examined and blind biopsies taken. The larynx was examined with direct laryngoscopy, and a small exophytic lesion was identified at the apex of the pyriform sinus. A biopsy was taken of this lesion. Rigid esophagoscopy was also done. There were no obvious lesions noted.

The biopsy from the pyriform sinus lesion revealed a moderately differentiated squamous cell carcinoma. Because of the location of the cancer adjacent to the larynx, the patient required a total laryngectomy. He underwent operation—total laryngectomy with a right modified radical neck dissection. The specimen had clear margins around the tumor and additional positive lymph nodes were found in the neck. He received postoperative radiotherapy for 6 weeks and was doing well at 1 year follow-up.

GENERAL CONSIDERATIONS

When evaluating a patient with a neck lump, keep in mind three broad categories—congenital, inflammatory, and neoplastic masses. Each of these categories requires a different approach in workup, diagnosis, and treatment. Although treatment of a congenital neck mass is usually excision, inflammatory masses often require antibiotic therapy instead of, or in addition to, open drainage. Neoplastic neck masses are usually metastatic, and mandate a thorough search for a primary site before initiating any further therapy (Fig. 66.1).

Congenital neck masses are generally first discovered in children and young adults but may present at any age. The most frequently encountered congenital neck mass is the thyroglossal duct cyst, which occurs due to faulty migration of the thyroid gland during embryologic development in its descent from the foramen cecum in the tongue. Normally, the gland descends inferiorly, in a path traversing the hyoid bone, to eventually settle anterior to the tracheal rings. The tract of the gland then resorbs; however, failure of resorption at any point along the de-

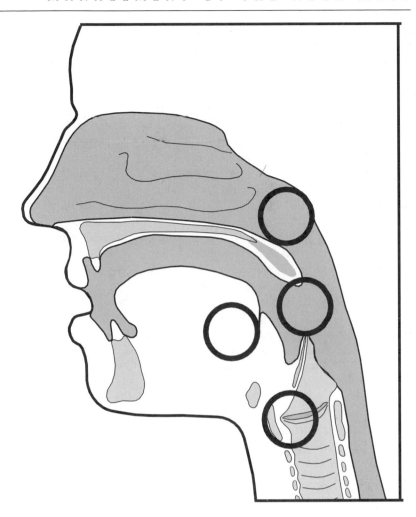

FIGURE 66.1 *Common sites of primary head and neck malignancies.*

scent can result in formation of a thyroglossal duct cyst. Thus, these cysts are located in the midline of the neck, between the base of the tongue and the thyroid gland. They frequently swell and become infected during upper respiratory infections. Because of their attachment to the thyroid gland and hyoid bone, they will move up and down with swallowing. Also, because of the descent pathway, surgical resection requires following the cyst up to the base of the tongue and removing the mid-portion of the hyoid bone with the specimen (Case 1).

Branchial cleft cysts and sinuses are another type of congenital neck mass. The branchial arches and pouches are formed during the fourth to eighth week of gestation, and contain precursors to the vital structures of the head and neck region. Incomplete resorption of these arches will result in a branchial cleft cyst or a draining branchial cleft sinus when there is communication to the skin. The most common of these is a second branchial cleft cyst. Second branchial cleft cysts are usually located anterior to the sternocleidomastoid muscle and may grow to be very large in size, especially following upper respiratory infections. First branchial cleft cysts are usually located in the preauricular area and may be intimately involved with the

facial nerve. Excision usually requires a concomitant superficial parotidectomy with identification and preservation of the facial nerve. Third and forth branchial cleft cysts are exceedingly rare.

Inflammatory masses in the neck are common at any age due to the rich lymphatic network that drains the head and neck region. Ludwig's angina refers to a specific deep neck infection that involves the sublingual and submandibular fascial spaces of the neck. Dental infections are the most common sources of these abscesses. Because of the swelling of the sublingual space, the tongue is elevated up to the roof of the mouth and the airway is severely compromised (Case 2). Early cases of Ludwig's angina may be managed with intravenous antibiotics alone. However, for later cases in which there is impending airway compromise, urgent surgical intervention is mandatory. If there is a great deal of swelling of the floor of the mouth, intubation may not be possible and a tracheostomy is necessary. In all cases, not only is incision and drainage of the abscess mandatory, but the offending tooth needs to be extracted.

Other causes for deep neck infections include peritonsillar abscesses, upper aerodigestive tract trauma, salivary gland infections, and congenital cyst and fistula infections. Cervical adenitis frequently occurs in young children during or following an upper respiratory infection. Treatment consists of appropriate antibiotic therapy. Occasionally, incision and drainage are necessary for fluctuant adenitis or in case of airway compromise or failure to respond to antibiotics.

Less common infectious etiologies for cervical adenitis include tuberculous adenitis, atypical mycobacteria, fungi, and cat-scratch disease. In these cases, the history and pertinent stains of aspirated material will aid in diagnosis. Actual cultures of these organisms may be difficult to obtain due to their fastidious growth requirements.

In the older patient with a history of smoking and alcohol abuse, a new neck mass should be considered a malignancy until proved otherwise. Such a malignancy would represent a metastatic carcinoma in a lymph node from a primary site located elsewhere in the head and neck. A fine needle aspiration (FNA) is the most useful diagnostic examination to determine malignancy (Case 3). A thorough examination of the head and neck is imperative to search for a primary site. Squamous cell carcinoma of the upper aerodigestive tract is by far the most common type of malignancy in the head and neck, and is closely linked to tobacco and alcohol use. Metastatic cancer in a lymph node should not be excised without first performing an exhaustive workup to search for the primary site of malignancy (see below).

KEY POINTS

- Patients who present with new neck mass pose diagnostic challenge because errors in diagnosis and/or therapy may have dire consequences

- When evaluating patient with neck lump, keep in mind three broad categories—congenital, inflammatory, and neoplastic masses

- Congenital masses generally discovered in children and young adults, but may present at any age

- Most frequently encountered congenital neck mass is thyroglossal duct cyst, which occurs due to faulty migration of thyroid gland during embryologic development in descent from foramen cecum in tongue

- Inflammatory masses in neck are common at any age due to rich lymphatic network that drains head and neck region

- Ludwig's angina refers to specific deep neck infection that involves sublingual and submandibular fascial spaces of the neck; dental infections most common source

- In older patient with history of smoking and alcohol abuse, new neck mass should be considered malignant until proved otherwise

- FNA is most useful diagnostic examination to determine malignancy

DIAGNOSIS

In evaluating a patient with a new neck mass, a careful history can give initial clues as to the diagnosis. In younger adults and children, a congenital or inflammatory mass is more likely; however, the possibility of a neoplasm cannot be ignored. In an older adult with a history of tobacco and/or alcohol abuse, weight loss, and cachexia, malignancy needs to be strongly considered.

FNA and appropriate cultures are invaluable in the workup of all three types of neck masses (Fig. 66.2). An experienced cytologist will be able to recognize malignant squamous cells that are aspirated from a lymph node in a patient suspected of harboring a malignancy. In younger patients, identification of branchial or thyroglossal duct cyst epithelium will yield a diagnosis, which only needs to be correlated with the clinical findings. Granulomatous, lymphoid cells and/or actual bacteria may be seen in FNA from inflammatory neck masses.

Computed tomography (CT) or magnetic resonance imaging (MRI) scanning can be very helpful in the evaluation of a neck mass. Clues may be obtained as to the origin and pathway of complex congenital neck masses, and to the extent of deep neck inflammatory masses or abscesses. A CT or MRI may reveal the site of an otherwise hidden primary squamous cell carcinoma in a patient with a neck metastasis, particularly in the hard-to-examine areas of the tongue base, tonsil, and pyriform sinus.

The definitive diagnostic test for a congenital neck mass is an actual histologic examination of the excised specimen. Inflammatory neck masses may not need to be excised if a good response to appropriate therapy is obtained.

If FNA reveals metastatic squamous cell carcinoma, an aggressive workup must be initiated to identify the source (Case 3). An open biopsy of the neck mass should not be undertaken as such a procedure would result in spillage of malignant cells and violation of the tissue planes of the neck. Patients who have had open biopsies of metastatic carcinoma in the neck have poorer survival because of inadvertent spread of tumor cells beyond the capsule of the lymph node.

If a complete examination of the head and neck in the clinic fails to reveal a primary site of the cancer, further studies are warranted. These include a chest x-ray, CT, and/or MRI of the head and neck from the base of the skull to the clavicles, and, if necessary, endoscopy and examination under general anesthesia. At the time of endoscopy, the entire upper aerodigestive tract is thoroughly examined, with special attention placed on areas likely to harbor unknown primary carcinoma. These sites include the nasopharynx, base of tongue, tonsil, and pyriform sinus. Palpation of the base of tongue, floor of mouth, and the nasopharynx is an essential part of the workup. If no obvious primary site is identified at endoscopy, blind biopsies are taken from these areas in case of a possible microscopic primary site. In approximately 90% of patients who present with metastatic neck

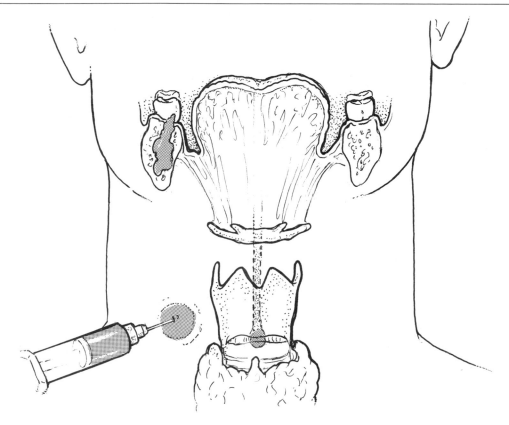

FIGURE 66.2   *Fine needle aspiration of a neck mass.*

disease with an unknown primary, such a thorough workup will result in discovery of a primary site (Case 3). Patients in whom a primary site is never identified may be treated with radiotherapy and/or a radical neck dissection. It may be assumed that these patients have a small, hidden primary cancer that will be effectively eradicated with radiation. Interestingly, such patients have no worse a prognosis than those in whom a primary site is identified and treated.

There may be instances in which FNA cytology is not available or results are equivocal. In these cases, the physician is faced with the dilemma of having a neck mass without a diagnosis of malignancy, yet no recourse exists but to perform an open biopsy to obtain tissue for diagnosis. To avoid violation of tissue planes and possible extracapsular spread of cancer cells from an open biopsy, the patient is taken to the operating room and prepared for endoscopy and biopsy. Prior consent is obtained for an open biopsy, with the possibility of a formal radical neck dissection should the frozen section show malignancy. First, a thorough examination is done of the upper aerodigestive tract, including endoscopy of the larynx and esophagus and palpation and inspection of potential hidden primary sites. If no obvious primary carcinoma is identified, an incision is planned that can be converted into a neck dissection incision. The neck node is biopsied and the tissue is sent for frozen section analysis. If the diagnosis of metastatic carcinoma is made, the incision is extended and a radical neck

dissection is carried out. In this way, a complete operation is performed, removing the gross malignant disease without spillage of tumor cells into the field. In addition, the patient may be treated with radiotherapy postoperatively.

KEY POINTS

- FNA and appropriate cultures invaluable in workup of all three types of neck masses (Fig. 66.2)

- CT or MRI can be helpful in evaluation of neck mass; clues obtained as to origin and pathway of complex congenital neck masses, and to extent of deep neck inflammatory masses or abscesses

- In approximately 90% of patients who present with metastatic neck disease with unknown primary, thorough workup results in discovery of primary site

- To avoid violation of tissue planes and possible extracapsular spread of cancer cells from open biopsy, patient is taken to operating room and prepared for endoscopy and biopsy

DIFFERENTIAL DIAGNOSIS

The list of differential diagnoses for patients who present with a mass in the neck is long; the categories of congenital, inflammatory, and neoplastic are discussed above. Other disease that must also be kept in mind are thyroid nodules (Ch. 40), parotid tumors, lipomas, lymphomas, and rare soft tissue sarcomas.

TREATMENT

The treatment for most congenital neck masses consists of complete surgical excision. This is not always an easy task, especially in cases of recurrent thyroglossal duct or branchial cleft cysts a history of repeated infections. It is of utmost importance, however, to attempt to perform as complete an operation as possible, as reoperation is fraught with danger to nerves and other vital structures in the neck. In the excision of a thyroglossal duct cyst, this necessitates following the cyst up to the hyoid bone, removing the mid-portion of the hyoid bone, and tracking the pathway all the way to the base of the tongue. During excision of branchial cleft cysts, it is necessary to follow the cyst pathway along the embryologic pathway of development to completely remove the specimen.

Inflammatory neck masses generally require antibiotic therapy before or in conjunction with operative drainage. If the mass responds completely to medical therapy alone, operation is not necessary. Occasionally, a residual nodule remains despite a prolonged course of antibiotic therapy, particularly in mycobacterial and atypical mycobacterial infections. In these instances, it may be beneficial to excise the residual nodule for complete eradication of the disease.

Patients with a cancer of the head and neck need to be carefully evaluated for multidisciplinary treatment. Such patients frequently have concurrent medical illnesses such as heart disease, diabetes, and malnutrition. These issues need to be addressed when planning for a major operation. A thorough radiologic assessment also should be done to assess the extent of the primary lesion as well as nodal metastases. Reconstruction efforts may require collaboration with a plastic surgeon. Radiation oncology consultation is also mandatory in planning either pre- or postoperative radiotherapy. In addition, psychosocial support should be arranged before surgery, for many of the ablative cancer operations leave patients with major functional and cosmetic deficits that may prove to be a difficult adjustment dilemma for them and their families.

KEY POINTS

• Treatment for most congenital neck masses consists of complete surgical excision

• Inflammatory neck masses generally require antibiotic therapy before or in conjunction with operative drainage

• Patients with cancer of head and neck need to be carefully evaluated for multidisciplinary treatment

FOLLOW-UP

Patients who have undergone complete resection of a congenital neck mass should experience no further problems with swelling or infection. However, if residual tissue is left behind at the time of the operation, recurrences are common. These recurrent congenital cysts often prove difficult to eradicate completely; the importance of an initial complete resection cannot be overemphasized.

After appropriate treatment, inflammatory neck masses usually do not pose problems with recurrence. It is important to evaluate and treat the underlying cause of the infection, such as a decayed tooth or an unusual granulomatous infection.

Cancer patients require close follow-up for the rest of their lives, even after complete eradication of their disease. During the initial postoperative period and during radiotherapy, they should be examined every few months. As they progress farther out from their treatment period, these intervals may be lengthened. In addition, the patient should be taught to be alert to any changes in the head and neck area and in general health that may indicate recurrence.

KEY POINTS

• Recurrent congenital cysts often prove difficult to eradicate completely; the importance of initial complete resection cannot be overemphasized

• Cancer patients require close follow-up for rest of their lives, even after complete eradication of disease

SUGGESTED READINGS

Canler JR, Mitchell B: Branchial cleft cysts, sinuses and fistulas. Otolaryngol Clin North Am 14:175, 1981

A detailed synopsis of the most common congenital neck masses. Embryologic events, clinical features, and histopathology are described.

McGuirt WF, McCabe BF: Significance of node biopsy before definitive treatment of cervical metastatic carcinoma. Laryngoscope 88:594, 1978

A classic article describing the worsened prognosis for patients who have undergone open biopsy of a neck node before definitive treatment of their head and neck cancer.

Patterson HD, Kelly JH, Strome M: Ludwig's angina: an update. Laryngoscope 92:370, 1982

A summary of the clinical features of Ludwig's angina, along with recommended treatment.

QUESTIONS

1. *The three broad categories of neck masses are?*
    A. Benign, moderately differentiated, anaplastic.
    B. Anterior triangle, posterior triangle, submental.
    C. Congenital, inflammatory, neoplastic.
    D. Fluctuant, moveable, fixed.

2. *Following a careful history and head and neck examin-ation, the initial approach for diagnosis of a firm, immo-bile, nontender mass at the anterior border of the stern-ocleidomastoid muscle should be?*

    A. Chest film and CT scan of neck.
    B. Simple excision and frozen section.
    C. Direct triple endoscopy and biopsy.
    D. FNA of the mass.

3. *The important etiologic factor in deep neck infection and abscess is?*

    A. History of a recent respiratory tract infection or cold.
    B. Poor dental hygiene.
    C. Infected sinuses.
    D. AIDS.

(See p. 604 for answers.)

67

NASAL AND

SINUS DISEASE

MARILENE B. WANG

This chapter discusses common disorders of the nose and paranasal sinuses. A wide range of disease processes affect the nose and paranasal sinuses in both children and adults. Practitioners of almost every specialty in medicine need to be familiar with these diseases, recognize frequently encountered symptoms, and understand when emergency measures are necessary. Epistaxis (nosebleed) in most instances can be managed effectively with simple measures; however, in rare cases, it can be life

threatening and exceedingly difficult to control. The same pertains to sinus infections. The ordinary case of acute sinusitis can be treated on an outpatient basis with oral antibiotics. In cases of preseptal cellulitis, juvenile nasal cellulitis or abscess, or orbital cellulitis or abscess, urgent drainage in the operating room may be necessary. Juvenile nasal angiofibroma is a disease affecting young males that must be recognized and worked up properly. A careless nasal biopsy in this case may prove fatal because of hemorrhage.

CASE 1
EPISTAXIS

A 52-year-old male presented to the emergency room in the evening with rapid bleeding from his nose. The bleeding had started earlier in the day, and after about 4 hours, he had soaked through five washcloths. He had tried ice, pressure, and plugging with tissue paper, all to no avail. He had a history of previous nosebleeds, but they usually stopped with simple measures. His past medical history was significant for recently diagnosed hypertension for which his family doctor had prescribed a diuretic. He was about 30 lb overweight but had no other major medical illnesses.

On examination, he appeared to be a pale, anxious gentleman, sweating and holding a washcloth to his nose. His pulse was 110 bpm; BP, 210/110 mmHg; and temperature, normal. Rapid initial examination of his nose revealed blood pouring out of the left nostril without a visible bleeding vessel. Blood was in the back of his throat and he was spitting blood-tinged saliva. His lungs were clear, abdomen soft, and his heart rate, although rapid, was regular.

The emergency room staff placed two large bore IV catheters in the patient and began to infuse lactated Ringer's solution while also attempting to control his high blood pressure. Meanwhile, the otolaryngology consultant arrived and began to prepare the nose for packing. An initial dose of 10 mg of sublingual nifedipine was given, resulting in a BP of 160/90 mmHg. The otolaryngologist suctioned out the nose and mouth and applied topical cocaine for vasoconstriction and anesthesia. A pumping vessel was identified in the area of Kiesselbach's plexus on the left anterior septum. Silver nitrate was applied to the vessel for cauterization. Most of the bleeding stopped after these measures; however, there was still a slight amount of oozing. An anterior nasal pack, consisting of Vaseline gauze strips coated with Polysporin ointment, was placed to further control the bleeding. An oral antibiotic was prescribed and the patient placed on a new antihypertensive medical regimen. On follow-up 2 days later, the nasal packing was removed without further bleeding. His BP was 150/80 mmHg on the new medication.

CASE 2
JUVENILE NASAL ANGIOFIBROMA

A 14-year-old male presented to his pediatrician with a 2-month history of increasing nasal congestion, particularly on the right side. He reported three episodes of brisk bleeding from his nose, also on the right side. There was no previous history of nasal or allergy problems.

The pediatrician found a reddish, bulging mass in the right nostril. The left nostril was clear. The mass in the right nostril was not bleeding at the time of examination. However, it appeared to be pulsatile and vascular.

The boy was referred to an otolaryngologist, who diagnosed a juvenile mass angiofibroma in the right nostril, on the basis of the history and findings. A CT scan confirmed the presence of a mass in the right nostril and nasopharynx. Surgical resection, preceded by embolization of the feeding vessels, was planned. After an angiogram and embolization of several large vessels from the internal maxillary artery, a transpalatal resection of the angiofibroma was done. At 3 years follow-up, there was no sign of recurrence.

CASE 3
SINUS ABSCESS

A 9-year-old female had an upper respiratory infection for 5 days with symptoms of cough, sore throat, nasal congestion, and headaches. She had a temperature at night of about 38°C. Her mother had given her analgesics and other over-the-counter cold medications, without improvement. By the time she was taken to the pediatrician, her nasal congestion and headaches had worsened, and she had begun to have swelling around her left eye.

On examination, she was lethargic, with a temperature of 38.5°C. Her tympanic membranes were clear, her nose had some thick greenish yellow drainage, and her lips and mouth were dry and cracked. Her left eye was almost swollen shut, and there was redness of the periorbital tissues. Her vision was grossly intact in both eyes, and there was no limitation or pain with extraocular movement. A radiograph of her sinuses revealed near total opacification of the left maxillary and ethmoid sinuses.

Because of the child's acute sinus infection, with involvement of the periorbital tissues, and her dehydration, she was admitted to the hospital for intravenous antibiotics and fluids. She was also monitored closely for worsening of her visual examination. Despite 4 hours of intravenous amoxicillin/sulbactam therapy, her left eye swelling increased. She continued to have fevers, and began to have decreasing vision in the left eye. Since she had poor response to medical therapy, she was operated on and found to have purulent material in her left maxillary and ethmoid sinuses. After drainage of the infected sinuses, she recovered rapidly.

GENERAL CONSIDERATIONS

The nose and paranasal sinuses may be involved in a variety of disease processes. Symptoms or complaints in these areas may signal a more serious systemic disorder (Case 1). Epistaxis is a common problem, which rarely can be life threatening. There are many different etiologies, the most common one being trauma. Nosebleeds are common after trauma to the face, or, more frequently, digital manipulation or nose-picking. The incidence of nosebleeds increases during periods of hot, dry weather when the nasal mucosa may become thin, and crack. Other less common but more serious disorders that can result in epistaxis are uncontrolled hypertension (Case 1) and bleeding diatheses, including platelet abnormalities, clotting factor deficiencies, and prolonged aspirin use. A careful history will generally reveal the underlying process responsible for such bleeding. Treatment of not only the nosebleed but also the more serious disease process is absolutely essential for proper, successful management of these patients.

Juvenile nasal angiofibroma (JNA) (Case 2) is an uncommon but important neoplasm found most frequently in young adolescent males. It is a benign tumor containing numerous dilated vascular channels amid loose connective tissue, and can cause symptoms of nasal congestion and intermittent brisk bleeding. These tumors are hormonally related, and often enlarge during puberty. A patient suspected of having a JNA should never be biopsied in the office. Such a careless biopsy may lead to potentially fatal hemorrhage. Instead, a unilateral vascular nasal mass in a pubertal-aged male must be assumed to be JNA until proved otherwise. The patient should be worked up carefully with radiographic imaging such as a computed tomography (CT) scan or magnetic resonance imaging (MRI), and plans made for treatment (Case 2).

Acute sinus infections are common at all ages, and usually respond to simple supportive measures and oral antibiotics. Children in particular are susceptible to serious sequelae if a sinus infection remains inadequately treated. Because of the delicate tissue planes in children, maxillary and ethmoid sinus infections may spread to the periorbital area (Case 3). Unchecked, there may be subsequent extension to the eye and even the cavernous sinus. Visual acuity and extraocular movements will be affected in these situations; thus, a careful visual examination is imperative when evaluating a child with sinusitis and periorbital cellulitis.

Allergic disease is the most common etiology in patients with chronic sinus infections. In allergic rhinitis, the continual irritation and inflammation of the mucosal lining of the nasal passages and sinuses leads to blockage of the natural ostia that drain the sinuses. This results in fluid buildup and thickening of the mucoperiosteum of the sinuses, with subsequent secondary bacterial infections. Symptoms of chronic sinusitis include nasal congestion, sinus pressure and pain, and postnasal drip. The underlying allergy must be addressed when evaluating and treating a patient with chronic sinusitis.

KEY POINTS

• Treatment of not only the nosebleed but also the more serious disease process absolutely essential for proper, successful management of these patients

• Visual acuity and extraocular events will be affected in patients with acute sinus infections that spread to the periorbital area; thus, a careful visual examination is imperative when evaluating a child with sinusitis and periorbital cellulitis

A DIAGNOSIS

thorough history is essential in a patient with nasal or sinus disease. A patient who presents with a nosebleed needs to be questioned for any history of previous bleeding episodes, family history of bleeding disorders, systemic illness such as hypertension or liver disease, or other etiologies for bleeding diatheses. After control of the nosebleed, a complete medical evaluation is necessary, including laboratory evaluation of coagulation parameters. Stigmata of chronic liver disease or hypertension can give clues as to an underlying disease process in a patient with a nosebleed.

An adolescent male with a history of nasal congestion and intermittent nosebleeds must be carefully examined for the presence of a JNA. The characteristic appearance of a reddish, pulsatile, unilateral nasal mass should alert the physician to the possible diagnosis of JNA. A CT scan or MRI study can confirm the diagnosis, by showing a vascular mass involving the nasal cavity and nasopharynx. A biopsy of the mass should *never* be done in the office, as severe and/or fatal hemorrhage can occur. An angiogram is usually done in patients with JNA, both for diagnostic purposes and for preoperative embolization of the major feeding vessels.

Acute sinusitis usually follows or occurs concomitantly with an upper respiratory infection. Symptoms of thick yellow-greenish nasal drainage, pressure behind the cheeks, eyes, or nose, and postnasal drip are common in acute sinusitis. Severe episodes of acute sinusitis can progress to involve the tissues around the eye, resulting in periorbital cellulitis and/or visual impairment (Case 2). A patient with

acute sinusitis will usually have tenderness over the affected sinus, nasal congestion, and drainage. Patients with involvement of the eye or extraocular muscles should undergo a careful visual acuity examination initially, as well as frequently during the course of their treatment. Sinus x-rays or CT scans are essential in diagnosing acute sinusitis at all stages. Early sinusitis will show fluid levels in one or more sinuses, while later stages will progress to complete opacification of the sinuses with extension into the periorbital tissues (Case 3). The most serious late stage sequelae of unchecked acute sinusitis are orbital abscess and cavernous sinus thrombosis.

Chronic sinusitis is more insidious, both in onset and symptoms, and therefore may be more difficult to diagnose. A history of allergic nasal and/or reactive airway disease is common in patients with chronic sinusitis, and inquiry should be made into patterns of allergic symptoms upon exposure to offending agents such as pollen, dust, or other particulate matter. Patients with chronic sinusitis will have complaints of dull headaches rather than acute sinus tenderness. Examination of the nose will reveal swollen, boggy turbinates, and often there will be a clear or white rhinorrhea. In severe cases of allergic rhinitis with chronic sinusitis, there will often be extensive nasal polyposis as well. As in acute sinusitis, radiographs or CT scans are very useful in the diagnostic process. They will usually reveal mucoperiosteal thickening of the sinus mucosa, patchy opacification of the ethmoid air cells, and/or nasal polyposis (Fig. 67.1).

KEY POINTS

• Biopsy of mass should *never* be done in the office, as severe and/or fatal hemorrhage can occur

P DIFFERENTIAL DIAGNOSIS

atients with recurrent episodes of epistaxis must be carefully evaluated for the presence of a neoplasm in the nasal cavity or paranasal sinuses. After control of the acute bleeding episode, removal of the packing, and recovery, the patient should be carefully examined, with fiberoptic nasopharyngoscopy if necessary. In addition, CT or MRI of the paranasal sinuses may be indicated to rule out neoplastic disease.

A patient with acute sinusitis may present with symptoms very similar to meningitis. In the absence of nasal symptoms, headache, fever, nuchal rigidity, or lethargy should alert the physician to possible meningitis. CT scan or sinus x-rays, along with a diagnostic lumbar puncture, will differentiate between the two.

In diabetic or immunocompromised patients, sinusitis may be a life-threatening emergency, due to infection with fungal or other virulent organisms. Mucormycosis and as-

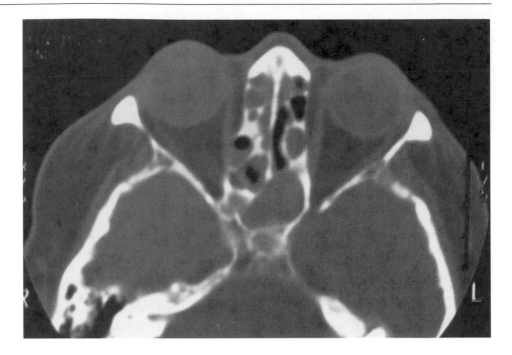

FIGURE 67.1 *CT scan of patient with chronic sinusitis.*

pergillosis are two fungal etiologies for severe sinus infections in immunocompromised patients. The diagnosis is made on biopsy of characteristic black necrotic tissue and examination for hyphae. Prompt debridement of tissue and systemic amphotericin β should be initiated emergently, for the prognosis is grave.

Uncommon granulomatous diseases are occasionally seen in patients with nasal complaints. Sarcoidosis, syphilis, Wegener's granulomatosis, lethal midline granuloma, leprosy, and tuberculosis are examples. Diagnosis is established by biopsy and culture of the lesions. In addition, a thorough search should be made for systemic lesions associated with these disease entities.

KEY POINTS

- In diabetic or immunocompromised patients, sinusitis may be a life-threatening emergency, due to infection with fungal or other virulent organisms

---

TREATMENT

Nosebleeds are common at all ages. Usually, simple measures will suffice to stop the bleeding, such as cold packs, manual pressure, or light packing. When these measures fail, the patient usually seeks aid in a doctor's office or emergency room. A patient with a nosebleed that presents in such a manner may be expected to be quite anxious. Rapid assessment of vital signs should be done, but attention is quickly directed to the actual bleeding nose. The physician should be appropriately equipped with an adequate light source and suction. Protective garb for the eyes, face, and body should be worn, as frequently the patient will be coughing and spraying blood. The patient should be positioned upright in a chair during evaluation and treatment (Case 1). The nose should be suctioned carefully of clots and fresh blood and the bleeding site searched for. If a definite vessel is identified, it can be cauterized with a silver nitrate stick. Usually, however, it is difficult to visualize a specific bleeding source, and therefore, the nose should be prepared for anterior packing. Cocaine or another local anesthetic/vasoconstrictive agent is applied. Packing material may consist of Vaseline gauze coated with Polysporin ointment, or an absorbable material such as Gelfoam and/or a thromboplastic mesh may be used. An oral antibiotic is given for as long as the packing is in the nose (Case 1), to prevent toxic shock syndrome and/or sinusitis from blockage of the sinus ostia. Anterior nasal packing is effective for the vast majority of nosebleeds, but on rare occasions the patient continues to bleed despite these measures.

In severe cases of epistaxis, a posterior nasal pack is necessary. In this type of pack, a Foley catheter is inserted through the nose into the nasopharynx and the balloon is inflated with saline (Fig. 67.2). Gentle forward traction is applied to stop the bleeding. After placement of a posterior nasal pack, the patient needs to be admitted to an intensive care unit for close observation, as there may be hypoxia and vagally mediated adverse cardiac reflexes, even in young, healthy adults. Two to 3 days of a posterior nasal pack is usually sufficient to control even the most severe nosebleeds. Those rare cases that continue to bleed require embolization or surgical ligation of the bleeding vessel.

After initial stabilization with intravenous fluid and an anterior nasal pack, treatment for the underlying cause of the bleeding must be instituted. Immediate control of high

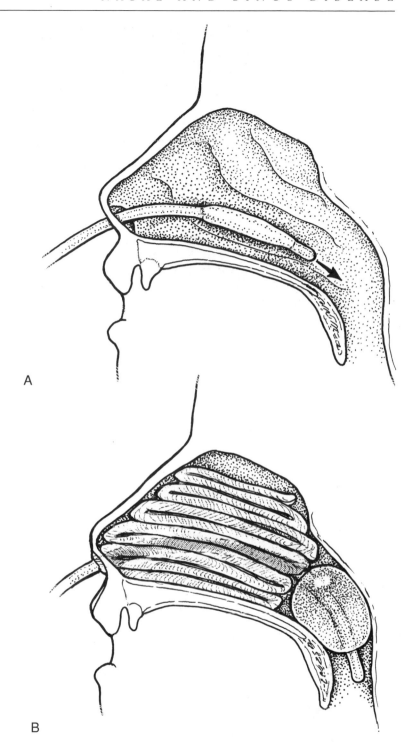

A

B

FIGURE 67.2   *(A & B)*
Foley catheter insertion for
treatment of severe epistaxis
(see text for details).

blood pressure is important, using an appropriate rapid-acting antihypertensive agent (Case 1). Correction of any coagulopathy should be done with appropriate platelet or other blood product transfusions.

Treatment for juvenile nasal angiofibroma is generally surgical, except in cases of intracranial extension or feeding vessels. Surgical resection is usually preceded by embolization of the major vessels feeding the tumor (Case 2). This maneuver greatly decreases the blood loss during the

operation. In patients in whom surgical resection is not feasible because of intracranial involvement, radiotherapy may be given.

Early and mild cases of acute sinusitis respond well to oral antibiotic therapy. In patients with more severe cases (Case 3), more aggressive treatment is needed. Admission to the hospital and intravenous antibiotics are required when there is worsening of symptoms and/or involvement of the eye or extraocular muscles. Topical nasal decongestants may be helpful to decrease the swelling around the sinus ostia and promote better drainage. When there is no improvement, despite maximal medical therapy, surgical drainage is indicated. Cultures taken during the procedure can aid in the choice of antibiotic used postoperatively.

Chronic sinusitis must be treated with the underlying allergic disease in mind. Antibiotics, antihistamines, and nasal steroids are the mainstay of therapy. Surgical drainage of the sinuses may be helpful in cases unresponsive to medical treatment. Consultation with an allergist for skin testing and desensitization shots are also indicated, as combined medical/surgical treatment provides the optimal care for these patients.

KEY POINTS

• After placement of posterior nasal pack, patient needs to be admitted to ICU for close observation, as there may be hypoxia and vagally mediated adverse cardiac reflexes, even in young, healthy adults

FOLLOW-UP

Patients with a history of recurrent nosebleeds must be carefully evaluated for an underlying systemic illness such as hypertension, coagulopathy, or liver disease. In addition, after the acute bleeding episode has resolved, a mass lesion in the nose or nasopharynx should be ruled out by fiberoptic examination and/or radiologic imaging studies.

After complete surgical resection of JNA, recurrence is rare. However, in cases in which surgical resection is not done, treatment with radiotherapy must be followed up closely with periodic MRI or CT scans to determine the extent of regression of the tumor. Instead of complete regression, most often extensive fibrosis is found in the area of the original lesion.

Patients who recover fully from one episode of acute sinusitis generally do not require specific follow-up. A patient with a history of recurrent sinusitis warrants evaluation for structural abnormalities of the sinuses or nose, allergic disease, and immunologic deficiencies. Patients with recurrent or chronic sinusitis with an underlying allergic etiology require long-term therapy.

SUGGESTED READINGS

Economou T, Abemayor E, Ward P: Juvenile nasopharyngeal angiofibroma: an update of the UCLA experience, 1960–1985. Laryngoscope 98:170, 1988

A report of the treatment results for juvenile nasopharyngeal angiofibroma at UCLA over a 25-year period. Surgical resection within 48 hours of embolization is recommended for most lesions, with radiotherapy reserved for those with intracranial feeding vessels.

Grybauskas V, Parker J, Friedman M: Juvenile nasopharyngeal angiofibroma. Otolaryngol Clin North Am 19:647, 1986

An excellent article outlining the etiology, clinical behavior, and recommended therapy for juvenile nasopharyngeal angiofibroma.

Mackay I: Rhinitis, Mechanisms and Management. Royal Society of Medicine Services Limited, London, 1989

A concise text that covers major topics in allergic and nonallergic rhinitis.

QUESTIONS

1. A 58-year-old female is seen because of a persistent nosebleed that has not responded to pressure, cold packs, position changes, and so forth. The best treatment plan is to?

A. Apply an anterior nasal pack soaked in a cocaine solution.

B. Obtain intravenous access, control blood pressure, if necessary, and examine the nostril carefully with adequate illumination and suctioning.

C. Admit patient to hospital, administer vitamin K and fresh frozen plasma, and prepare patient for examination and treatment in an operating room.

D. Insert a posterior nasal pack.

2. In a 10-year-old boy, febrile from infected sinuses, treatment should be?

A. Oral antibiotics with a return visit in 24–48 hours.

B. Prompt surgical drainage of the infected sinuses.

C. An initial course of intravenous antibiotics in hospital followed by operation, if necessary.

D. Irrigation of the sinuses with an antibiotic solution.

(See p. 604 for answers.)

68 OTITIS
MEDIA

PAVEL DULGUEROV

CLAUDINE GYSIN

Otitis media (OM) is an inflammatory process of the mucosa lining the middle ear cavities that occurs in different forms. OM is the most common illness in children and its surgical treatment, namely tympanostomy tube placement, is the most frequent operation performed today. Recurrence is a frequent problem in children, and persistent OM can lead to hearing loss, delays in language acquisition, and chronic middle ear sequelae. This chapter discusses the diagnosis and

treatment of the various forms of OM and its differentiation from other diseases of the ear.

CASE 1
BILATERAL SEROUS OTITIS MEDIA

A 3½-year-old male was referred to an otolaryngologist after failing a school screening for hearing loss. At 3 months of age, the child had had his first episode of acute otitis and by the age of 2 years, he had had seven episodes of acute OM, all treated by antibiotics. Bilateral tympanostomy tubes were placed and remained in place for 6 months. The patient was not seen again until the referral for hearing loss.

The mother believed her son was not paying attention because she frequently had to repeat herself. He snored at night and had a runny nose. The otoscopic examination showed a dull and retracted right tympanic membrane and a middle ear fluid level on the left. Thick nasal secre-

tions were present, and the child was unable to breathe with the mouth closed. Adenoid hypertrophy was noted on examination of the nasopharynx. The audiogram revealed a 25-db conductive hearing loss, and the tympanogram was flat. The diagnosis of bilateral serous otitis media was made. A full course of antibiotics was administered without improvement. Because of the long-lasting history of otitis media, adenoidectomy and placement of tympanostomy tubes were done. No further recurrence of OM was noted in the following 3 years, and the patient had a normal language acquisition.

CASE 2
ACUTE MASTOIDITIS WITH FACIAL NERVE PARALYSIS

A 6-year-old male presented to the clinic with right side otalgia (earache) of 1-week duration and an acute right facial nerve paralysis. He had no other medical problems.

At the age of 3 years, he had a single episode of left acute OM treated with antibiotics.

The right tympanic membrane was dull and hypomobile. The posterior wall of the right external ear canal was swollen and the auricle was pushed forward and downward by a large and tender retroauricular swelling. Complete peripheral facial nerve paralysis was present. The left tympanic membrane was normal. No meningeal signs were noted.

His temperature was 37.8°C, and the WBC count was 14,000 with a left shift. The audiogram showed a 20-db conductive hearing loss. A CT scan demonstrated an opacified right middle ear and an erosion of the mastoid cortex with a large retroauricular soft tissue swelling (Fig. 68.1). The diagnosis of acute mastoiditis with facial nerve paralysis was made.

An emergency right mastoidectomy was performed and a right tympanostomy tube was placed. Mucoid fluid was present in the middle ear and a large purulent collection was found in the mastoid and subcutaneous tissues. The additus ad antrum was blocked by granulation tissue, which was removed. The facial nerve canal was found to be dehiscent at the level of the second genu. Intravenous antibiotics were given. The patient improved quickly, and some facial movements were noted at 10 days. Recovery was complete at 1 month.

GENERAL CONSIDERATIONS

The middle ear cavities consist of (1) the tympanic cavity, (2) the mastoid air cells, and (3) other air cells of the temporal bone. This complex system of cavities is aerated through the eustachian tube, which allows communication with the nasopharynx. The tympanic cavity communicates with the mastoid cells through a narrow opening called the *additus ad antrum.* It is separated from the external ear by the tympanic membrane. The entire cavity system is generally involved during inflammation or infection. Otitis media is an inflammation of the middle ear mucosa without reference to etiology or pathogenesis. The classification shown in Table 68.1 is based on clinical grounds.

Otitis media is the most common infection among infants and children and presents a real public concern.

About two-thirds of children have had one or more episodes of acute OM (AOM) before the age of 3 years. At this age, children can be divided into three groups of equal size: one-third are free of ear infections, one-third have occasional AOM (<3/yr), and the remaining one-third have recurrent episodes (>6/yr). Having the first episode of AOM during the first 6 months of life is a predisposing factor for recurring episodes and is often re-

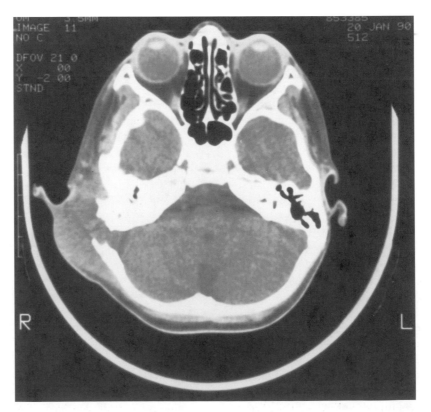

FIGURE 68.1 *CT scan demonstrating opacified right middle ear and erosion of mastoid cortex with large retroauricular soft tissue swelling.*

TABLE 68.1 *Classification of otitis media*

Myringitis	Inflammation localized to the tympanic membrane
Acute otitis media	Otitis media of rapid onset with signs and symptoms of infection
Secretory otitis media	Middle ear effusion behind an intact tympanic membrane without signs of acute infection
Chronic otitis media	A permanent perforation of the tympanic membrane (>3 months). It can be active (purulent drainage) or inactive (no drainage)
Sequelae of otitis media	Chronic inflammatory processes remaining within the mucoperiosteum of the middle ear
Complications of otitis media	Acute inflammatory process extending beyond the mucoperiosteum of the middle ear

ferred to as the "otitis prone" condition. Other predisposing factors are cleft palates and other craniofacial malformations, decreased immunocompetence, abnormalities of the cilia, breast feeding less than 2–3 months, bottle feedings in supine position, and allergies. Infections are more common during colder months.

Bacteria or viruses can gain access to the middle ear through the eustachian tube, and they initiate an inflammatory response followed by the production of an exudate within the middle ear cavities. The tympanic membrane is erythematous, dull, and bulging. When fluid is present in the middle ear, a conductive hearing loss is observed, and the mobility of the tympanic membrane is reduced. This fluid collection may be seen as an empyema, resulting in fever and otalgia.

Without treatment, a spontaneous perforation of the eardrum can occur with marked diminution of pain and other symptoms, or the infection might spread to produce various temporal bone or intracranial complications. Antibiotics tend to relieve the clinical symptons of AOM but fluid often persists in the middle ear for a variable duration.

The epidemiology of secretory OM (SOM) is more controversial, since children rarely complain of hearing loss, the main symptom of SOM. Monthly screenings of asymptomatic children, aged 2 and 6 years, revealed that 20% of children will develop an episode of SOM during a 1-year period. Most of the children have only a single episode of SOM, and most episodes are of short duration (<1 month) and resolve without treatment. Most are associated with an episode of upper respiratory infections.

Dysfunction of the eustachian tube is probably the most important factor in the pathogenesis of SOM in children. The eustachian tube function is less efficient as it is shorter, straighter, and has a lesser vertical slope. Children also present frequently with episodes of upper respiratory

tract infection that result in mucosal congestion and abnormal ciliary motion. These infections are probably caused by a lack of mucosal immunity against common viral pathogens. During acquisition of this immunity, adenoid hypertrophy is common and is an additional factor of eustachian tube obstruction.

KEY POINTS

- Entire cavity system generally involved during inflammation or infection
- Otitis media an inflammation of the middle ear mucosa without reference to etiology or pathogenesis
- Recurring episodes referred to as "otitis-prone" condition
- When fluid present in middle ear, a conductive hearing loss is observed and mobility of tympanic membrane is reduced
- Dysfunction of eustachian tube probably most important factor in pathogenesis of SOM in children; eustachian tube function is less efficient, as it is shorter, straighter, and has less vertical slope

DIAGNOSIS

AOM often occurs after an upper respiratory infection. It is a clinical diagnosis. The patients complain about fever, earache, a sense of fullness, and decreased hearing. With small children, symptoms are not as obvious. They are irritable, tug at their ears, and sometimes present only with diarrhea or vomiting. The most important examination is otoscopy (i.e., the visualization of the tympanic membrane through the external ear canal). In AOM, the tympanic membrane is red, opaque, and sometimes bulging. Landmarks are absent, and the mobility of the tympanic membrane is decreased.

The main symptom of SOM is hearing loss. The parents or teachers note that the child does not hear well or speaks loudly. Otoscopy shows either a yellowish or bluish, dull, and retracted tympanic membrane without light reflex. A fluid level or bubbles can occasionally be seen behind the tympanic membrane.

The presence of a tympanic membrane perforation is easily diagnosed on careful otoscopy. Chronic OM (COM) can be inactive (dry) or active (pus drainage). Conductive hearing loss is often present. The principal concern in evaluating COM is not to miss a cholesteatoma because of its progressively destructive nature. This requires thorough inspection of the tympanic membrane.

KEY POINTS

- AOM is a clinical diagnosis
- Principal concern in evaluating COM is not to miss a cholesteatoma because of its progressively destructive nature

DIFFERENTIAL DIAGNOSIS

Otalgia (earache) can result from ear diseases, or the pain can be referred from other head and neck affections through cranial nerves V, VII, IX, and X. In ear disease, pain can arise from the external or middle ear. In external otitis, the pain is increased when the auricle is displaced. The patients are afebrile and secretions are present in the external canal. Most complications of OM are associated with ear pain, most often located over the mastoid. Frequent causes of referred otalgia include pharyngitis, oropharyngeal tumors, and dysfunction of the temporomandibular joint (pain increases with chewing).

Otorrhea (ear discharge) can originate from external otitis or from the middle ear, through a perforation of the tympanic membrane. In AOM, the otorrhea is sudden and is accompanied by a relief of pain. The eardrum is often injected and the perforation is small. In active COM, the ear discharge could be continuous or intermittent, otalgia is rarely present, and general signs of infection are absent; the eardrum is often sclerotic, retracted, and exhibits a large perforation. Cholesteatoma is generally associated with marginal perforations in the pars flaccida.

Hearing loss can be conductive or sensorineural. Conductive hearing loss is due to diseases of the external or middle ear. All forms of OM generally result in conductive hearing loss. Sensorineural hearing loss can result from lesions of the inner ear or central auditory pathways.

TREATMENT

The most frequent pathogens found in AOM are *Streptococcus pneumoniae, Haemophilus influenzae,* and *Moraxella (Branhamella) catarrhalis.* A recent study demonstrates a similar proportion of pathogens in children and adults, except for *Moraxella catarrhalis,* which is more common in children. An increasing proportion of *H. influenzae* (15–35%) and *Moraxella catarrhalis* (60–80%) strains produce β-lactamase.

Bacteria found in SOM are similar to those found in AOM, in different proportions. In one-third of SOM cases, no pathogen can be cultured. Other bacteria, like staphylococcus or gram-negative rods, are seen in special populations such as neonates in the intensive care unit (ICU).

The recommended antibiotic for empiric therapy for uncomplicated episodes of AOM is amoxicillin, because it is safe, inexpensive, and is active against almost all strains of *S. pneumoniae* and most strains of *H. influenzae.* For a child less than 5 years of age, where the incidence of β-lactamase producing bacteria is higher, β-lactamase resistant drugs such as amoxicillin plus clavulanate, cefaclor, newer third generation cephalosporins, and erythromycin plus sulfafurazole are recommended. If the patient is allergic to penicillin, erythromycin plus sulfafurazole or co-trimoxazole could be prescribed.

In general, symptoms improve after 2–3 days. If not, a paracentesis (a small perforation of the eardrum with either a needle or a specially designed scalpel) is recommended in order to obtain a sample for bacteriology and/or to switch the antibiotic to a β-lactamase resistant drug. Oral decongestant-antihistamine preparations and oral steroids have been shown not to provide additional benefit.

Treatment of SOM is more controversial, since most of the episodes will resolve spontaneously. In persistent cases (>3 months), a full course of antibiotic therapy, similar to the treatment for AOM, should be tried. Resolution mandates a periodic follow-up until 7–8 years of age, after which SOM is less frequent. If it recurs, or in the case of frequently recurrent AOM, a trial of antibiotic prophylaxis has been shown to be effective. The recommended drugs are amoxicillin (2 mg/kg/day) or sulfisoxazole (75 mg/kg/day) in one daily dose.

Failure of medical treatment signals the need for surgical treatment. Tympanostomy tube placement has been shown to improve both SOM and recurrent AOM. Tympanostomy tubes provide drainage of the fluid, correct the associated hearing loss, and permit ventilation of the middle ear, thereby allowing the regression of mucosal inflammation and the development of a normal pneumatization of the temporal bone. The procedure requires general anesthesia in children.

The tubes extrude spontaneously after an average of 6–9 months. Some children tend to resume the cycle of AOM-SOM after the closure of the tympanic membrane. If they fail medical management again, adenoidectomy should be performed along with another placement of tympanostomy tubes.

The final cure of the eustachian dysfunction problem is provided by the growth of the child. The aim of the above treatments is to allow the child to develop normal language by relieving the hearing loss and to have the child reach the age of 8–12 years with a middle ear that is as close to normal as possible.

The microbiology of COM is different from AOM and SOM. Close to 50% of the germs recovered are gram-negative rods, mostly *Pseudomonas aeruginosa* and *Proteus. H. influenzae* and *Branhamella catarrhalis* are present only exceptionally. Medical treatment aims to render the COM inactive and consists mainly of topical ear drops active against gram-negative rods, and frequent debridement by suctioning.

A patient with COM should be evaluated by an otolaryngologist because (1) surgery is necessary in most cases, (2) periodic cleaning, using a microscope, is often necessary, (3) it is often difficult to rule out a cholesteatoma, and (4) COM can result in intratemporal and intracranial complications.

FOLLOW-UP

The need for frequent follow-up (every few months) is evident, since AOM and SOM tend to recur, and because SOM does not generate any complaints from children. Even after a tympanostomy tube placement, children have to be followed after extrusion to rule out recurrence of OM.

COM patients, once the infection is under control, need to be followed for several years to ensure that cholesteatoma does not develop or has not recurred.

SUGGESTED READINGS

Casselbrandt ML, Brostoff LM, Cantekin EI et al: Otitis media with effusion in preschool children. Laryngoscope 95:428, 1985

Casselbrandt ML, Kaleida PH, Rockette HE et al: Efficacy of antimicrobial prophylaxis and or tympanostomy tube insertion for prevention of recurrent otitis media: results of a randomized clinical trial. Pediatr Infect Dis J 11:278, 1991

Gates GA, Avery CA, Prihoda TJ, Cooper JJ: Effectiveness of adenoidectomy and tympanostomy tubes in the treatment of chronic otitis media with effusion. N Engl J Med 317:444, 1987

The above articles are clinical studies on controversial topics.

Goycoolea MV, Jung TTK: Complications of suppurative otitis media p. 1381. In Paparella MM, Shumrick DA, Gluckman JL, Meyerhoff WL (eds): Otolaryngology. 3rd Ed. WB Saunders, Philadelphia, 1991

A good and complete overview of the complications of otitis media.

QUESTIONS

1. *Dysfunction of the eustachian tube is considered the most important factor in the development of SOM. The dysfunction can result from?*
    A. Adenoids.
    B. Upper respiratory tract infection.
    C. Allergies.
    D. All of the above.

2. *The major concern from the presence of cholesteatoma is?*
    A. Infection.
    B. Destruction of the ossicles.
    C. Malignant degeneration.
    D. Tympanosclerosis.

3. *Which of the following is not true? Tympanostomy tube placement in children*
    A. Provides drainage of fluid.
    B. Corrects associated hearing loss.
    C. Permits ventilation of the middle ear.
    D. Can be inserted with local anesthesia.

(See p. 604 for answers.)

69 FACIAL PARALYSIS

JOEL A. SERCARZ

RINALDO CANALIS

Facial nerve paralysis produces a severe cosmetic and functional deformity. The most common cause of facial paralysis is Bell's palsy, a diagnosis that should only be made after treatable conditions such as neoplasms or infections have been excluded. The aims of this chapter are to (1) describe some of the causes of facial paralysis other than Bell's palsy, (2) outline the anatomy and physiology of the facial nerve, and (3) describe the causes of facial paralysis that require medical or surgical therapy.

CASE 1
FACIAL NERVE SCHWANNOMA

A 38-year-old female noted a gradual onset of left facial paralysis over the 3 months before evaluation. She also described a progressive hearing loss of a year's duration. She denied having tinnitus, vertigo, ear pain, or otorrhea.

She had no history of serious illnesses. She had undergone a previous tonsillectomy and appendectomy.

On examination, she appeared healthy. There was incomplete left facial paralysis with sparing of some function in the muscles supplied by the ramus mandibularis branch of the nerve. The patient had incomplete eye closure, but there was no evidence of corneal injury. The tympanic membranes were normal in appearance. On tuning fork examination, the Weber's test, with the tuning fork placed on the forehead, lateralized to the left ear. The Rinne test indicated that bone conduction was better than air conduction for the left ear. The remainder of the head and neck examination was normal.

An audiogram demonstrated a 30-decibel conductive hearing loss in the left ear. An MRI scan with gadolinium showed a contrast enhancing lesion in the middle ear, near the second genu of the facial nerve.

The left middle ear was explored through a combined mastoidectomy and transcanal approach, and the acoustic tumor was excised. Resection of the tumor resulted in a 14-mm facial nerve gap. A greater auricular nerve graft was placed to bridge the defect, with one interrupted 10–0 nylon suture placed at the distal anastomosis.

One year following the procedure, the patient had regained significant tone in the facial musculature and fair to good volitional movement on the operated side. An MRI scan demonstrated no recurrence of the tumor.

CASE 2
HERPES ZOSTER OTICUS

A 35-year-old male presented to the otolaryngology clinic with a 5-day history of a painful rash involving the left auricle. He also described a 1-day history of near total left facial paralysis. He denied previous surgery or trauma involving the ear or temporal bone. His past medical history was noncontributory.

On examination, the left ear demonstrated multiple vesicular skin lesions, approximately 2 mm in size, involving the cartilaginous canal, concha, and antihelix. The tympanic membrane was normal. The Weber's test was midline. The Rinne test revealed air conduction better than bone conduction bilaterally.

There was a complete paralysis of the left face with incomplete eye closure. Bell's phenomenon, in which the globe rotates superiorly with attempted eye closure, was present in the left eye. The nose, oral cavity, oropharynx, and larynx were normal.

An audiogram demonstrated a mild high frequency sensorineural hearing loss in the left ear. Hearing in the right ear was normal. An MRI scan performed with gadolinium contrast was normal.

The patient was treated with oral acyclovir, 200 mg 5 times per day for 10 days. He experienced gradual recovery of facial function over 3 months. The vesicles gradually resolved. His facial function 1 year later was excellent, except for weakness of the forehead musculature. There was also mild postherpetic neuralgia of the left auricle.

GENERAL CONSIDERATIONS

These cases illustrate two possible etiologies for facial paralysis and demonstrate the importance of investigating the cause of facial paralysis. Idiopathic (Bell's) facial paralysis is a diagnosis of exclusion.

After entering the internal auditory canal, the nerve courses within the fallopian canal. The intratemporal portion of the nerve has three branches: (1) the greater superficial petrosal nerve, which supplies the lacrimal gland, (2) the nerve to the stapedius muscle, which contracts and stabilizes the stapes during loud noise exposure, and (3) the chorda tympani nerve, which supplies taste and sensation to the anterior two-thirds of the tongue and parasympathetic supply to the submandibular gland. The function of the greater superficial petrosal nerve can be evaluated by Schirmer's test, which measures lacrimation. The stapedius branch of the nerve is routinely tested when a complete audiologic profile is obtained by an audiologist. The function of the chorda tympani is usually assessed by history only, but electrogustometry and submandibular gland flow may be measured in certain situations.

The main extratemporal branches of the facial nerve are the cervical, mandibular, buccal, zygomatic, and temporal. These branches course within the substance of the parotid gland after the nerve exits at the stylomastoid foramen.

KEY POINTS
• Most common cause of facial paralysis is Bell's palsy; diagnosis should only be made after treatable conditions such as neoplasms or infections excluded, that is, idiopathic (Bell's) facial paralysis is diagnosis of exclusion

DIAGNOSIS

The most important part of the evaluation of a patient with facial paralysis is a thorough history and physical examination focusing on the head and neck region and neurologic system. It is especially important to evaluate the ear canal, eardrum, and mastoid for evidence of infection or neoplasm. The parotid gland should be palpated carefully for evidence of tumor. Mastoid tenderness should be elicited if present. A complete neurologic examination should be performed to exclude associated deficits and localize the site of the lesion.

The interview should be detailed: the history of adenopathy, rash, trauma, ear infection, or tick bite should be elicited, the latter raising the possibility of Lyme disease. The onset, duration, associated symptoms, and rate of progression of the paralysis should be sought.

An audiogram is always performed for patients with facial paralysis. This allows assessment of both hearing and stapedial reflex. Some causes of facial paralysis, including tumors of the cerebellopontine angle, may affect both the 7th and 8th cranial nerves. An MRI scan of the temporal bone is currently an important part of the evaluation of facial paralysis. This is especially true if the history and physical examination do not support the diagnosis of Bell's palsy or when the paralysis is gradual in onset or associated with other neurologic findings. The scan should be performed with gadolinium, which is helpful in detecting small tumors such as acoustic and facial neuromas.

KEY POINTS
• MRI of temporal bone important part of evaluation of facial paralysis, especially if history and physical examination do not support diagnosis of Bell's palsy or when paralysis gradual in onset or associated with other neurologic findings

DIFFERENTIAL DIAGNOSIS

Many illnesses can present with facial paralysis (Table 69.1). A history of a sudden loss of facial function, without evidence for another cause, suggests the diagnosis of Bell's palsy. Some authorities believe that this disorder is caused by a virus of the herpes family, but this hypothesis is yet to be proved. When the nerves of patients with Bell's palsy are surgically explored, erythema and swelling may be observed. The site of lesion remains controversial, although the geniculate ganglion and tympanic portion are believed to be the most frequently affected. Bell's palsy can also involve other cranial nerves, particularly the 5th (30%) and 8th.

Herpes zoster oticus (Case 2) has a worse prognosis than Bell's palsy. It is clinically distinguished by the pres-

TABLE 69.1 *Causes of facial paralysis*

Trauma

    Forceps delivery

    Temporal bone trauma

    Penetrating trauma

    Iatrogenic: parotid/mastoid surgery

Neoplastic

    Parotid malignancies

    Schwannoma

    Parotid tumor

    Carcinoma

    Fibrous dysplasia

    Von Recklinghausen's disease

Inflammatory

    External otitis

    Otitis media

    Mastoiditis

    Herpes zoster oticus

    Coxsackie virus

    Lyme disease

Idiopathic

    Bell's palsy

    Guillain-Barré syndrome

    Myasthenia gravis

    Sarcoidosis

    Amyloidosis

ence of painful vesicles, which often precede the onset of facial paralysis.

Infections of the ear and temporal bone, such as otitis media and mastoiditis are important causes of facial paralysis in which rapid intervention can favorably alter its course. When an acute ear infection is present on the same side as a facial paralysis, immediate treatment, including intravenous antibiotics and drainage of the middle ear, is mandatory. Both chronic and acute infections of the mastoid can be responsible for facial paralysis. A chronic ear infection may be complicated by cholesteatoma, which can destroy the fallopian canal and injure the facial nerve directly.

Neoplasms of the temporal bone, ear canal, and parotid can cause facial paralysis. In the parotid, the facial paralysis associated with a malignant tumor carries a poor prognosis. Facial nerve schwannomas (Case 1) are rare, but may produce paralysis late in the course of their growth. Acoustic neuromas can cause facial paralysis, but usually late in the course of the disease, when they are very large.

Many lesions of the brain can cause facial paralysis. These include infections, tumors, or cerebrovascular lesions of the brain or brain stem. Lesions of the cortex produce contralateral facial paralysis because the upper division has bilateral representation.

Some infants are born with congenital facial paralysis. Birth trauma is an infrequent cause of facial paralysis, sometimes seen in difficult forceps deliveries. Congenital paralysis occurs in many syndromes, including the Möbius syndrome, in which infants present with multiple cranial neuropathies.

KEY POINTS

- Bell's palsy can also involve other cranial nerves, particularly 5th (30%) and 8th

- When acute ear infection present on same side as facial paralysis, immediate treatment, including intravenous antibiotics and drainage of middle ear is mandatory

TREATMENT AND PROGNOSIS

Treatment for patients with facial paralysis varies according to its etiology. Patients with trauma to the facial nerve, especially when the nerve is completely severed, are best treated with immediate exploration and nerve repair. When the nerve is severed, a primary reanastomosis produces the best functional recovery.

Many infections of the temporal bone that produce facial paralysis require surgical treatment. For example, patients with cholesteatoma and concurrent 7th nerve weakness require a mastoidectomy, facial nerve decompression, and control of the cholesteatoma.

The therapy for other causes of facial nerve paralysis is somewhat controversial. There is evidence that short-term steroid therapy is beneficial for patients with Bell's palsy. Most physicians use a rapidly tapering course of oral prednisone over a period of 10 days. In herpes zoster oticus, acyclovir is a rational treatment approach, but proof of its efficacy is lacking. Ideally, it should be initiated during the avascular eruption, before onset of facial paralysis.

Neoplasms that cause facial paralysis are generally treated with surgical excision. In the parotid area, malignant tumors are usually resected in continuity with the facial nerve, which is then repaired with a graft. When grafting is not possible, the nerve can be rehabilitated in selected cases with a hypoglossal to facial transfer. After reinnervation takes place, patients can be trained to move the tongue to produce specific facial movements.

Patients with permanent facial paralysis generally require rehabilitation. For eye closure, gold weights are a popular method of eye protection. The weight is placed in the upper lid just anterior to the tarsus. The weight is light enough so that the eye can be opened by the levator palpebrae superior, which are innervated by the 3rd cranial nerve.

The facial nerve has a significant level of resistance to insult. The prognosis of facial nerve paralysis varies according to its etiology and the general condition and age of the patient. Young, healthy patients tend to recover faster and more completely than older and debilitated individuals.

Bell's palsy has a recovery rate between 85% and 90%. Approximately 10% of patients will have only partial recovery and in 5%, no volitional movement may return, exhibiting significant flaccidity. Prognosis for herpes zoster oticus is less favorable, with some series showing only 50% of patients achieving full recovery. Tics and synkinetic movements are a common occurrence in all patients with incomplete functional recovery, regardless of the original cause of the paralysis.

Patients with facial nerve paralysis secondary to temporal bone infections have an excellent prognosis if treated early and aggressively. When paralysis becomes complete and fails to show recovery in approximately 12 weeks, significant fiber degradation may be assumed. This is also true when the paralysis is secondary to trauma.

Reanastomosis, decompression, and grafting work exceptionally well when they are properly performed. The degree of functional recovery depends upon the patient's age, degree of nerve injury, length of the damaged segment, and the technical ability of the surgeon.

KEY POINTS

• Patients with trauma to facial nerve, especially when nerve completely severed, are best treated with immediate exploration and nerve repair

• There is evidence that short-term steroid therapy is beneficial for patients with Bell's palsy

• Bell's palsy has recovery rate between 85% and 90%; approximately 10% of patients will have only partial recovery and in 5%, no volitional movement may return

---

FOLLOW-UP

Close repeated evaluation of patients with facial paralysis is critical, particularly to detect complications such as ocular exposure keratitis. It is also important to be certain that patients with presumed Bell's palsy do not have an unsuspected neoplasm. Such patients usually will have some other evidence on history or physical examination that suggest the possibility.

SUGGESTED READINGS

Adour KK: The diagnosis and management of facial paralysis. N Engl J Med 307:348, 1982

An excellent review concerning the approach to the patient with facial paralysis.

May M: The Facial Nerve. Thieme-Stratton, New York, 1986

A comprehensive textbook for those interested in a comprehensive description of facial nerve function, anatomy, paralysis, injury, and repair.

QUESTIONS

1. Bell's palsy, the most common cause of facial paralysis?
   A. Is a diagnosis of exclusion of causes of treatable facial paralysis.
   B. Is suggested by a sudden loss of facial function.
   C. May also involve the 5th facial nerve as well.
   D. All of the above.

2. Infectious causes of facial paralysis where rapid intervention can favorably alter its course are?
   A. Otitis media.
   B. Mastoiditis.
   C. Herpes zoster.
   D. All of the above.

(See p. 604 for answers.)

70

HOARSENESS

AND

STRIDOR

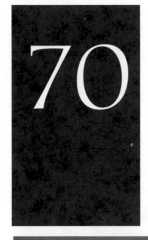

JOEL A. SERCARZ

SINA NASRI

Hoarseness and stridor (noisy breathing) are two important symptoms of laryngeal and airway disease. It is generally possible to identify a tumor or inflammation on physical examination of the upper airway in hoarse or stridorous patients. Fiberoptic instruments have recently made examination of the airway, especially in children, much easier.

The aims of this chapter are to (1) describe the causes of hoarseness and stridor and (2) familiarize the reader with the principals of laryngeal disorders. Some patients with laryngeal symptoms, such as an adolescent with persistent hoarseness after shouting at a football game, do not require urgent evaluation. Other patients, such as an elderly smoker with a change in the voice, or *any* patient with stridor, require immediate attention.

CASE 1
HOARSENESS

A 65-year-old male was referred for evaluation of a change in his voice for the previous 3 months. He reported frequent vocal fatigue and a harsh voice quality, which he described as "raspy." He also complained of a sharp pain that occurred on swallowing, particularly with hot foods. His past history was significant for mild hypertension. He had smoked 2 packs of cigarettes per day for 38 years and was a moderate drinker of alcohol.

There was a 1-cm area of leukoplakia on the floor of mouth. Indirect laryngoscopy was performed with a flexible endoscope. There was a 2-cm exophytic lesion of the left vocal cord with extension. There was no significant vocal cord mobility, and therefore the lesion was staged as T3 (Table 70.1). No subglottic extension was present. On examination of the left neck there was a 2-cm lymph node high in the jugulodigastric chain.

A direct laryngoscopy was performed under general anesthesia. A cancer of the left true vocal cord was identified, which extended to the anterior commissure and posteriorly to a point just anterior to the vocal process of the arytenoid (Fig. 70.1). The tumor appeared to cross the laryngeal ventricle but did not extend significantly to the false vocal cord.

The patient was treated with a partial laryngectomy and a left neck dissection. The larynx was reconstructed with a strap muscle flap. Two nodes in the specimen contained metastatic squamous cell tumor; all of the surgical margins were free of tumor. He underwent postoperative radiotherapy to 5,500 cGy. At his most recent fol-

TABLE 70.1 *Carcinoma of the vocal cord*

Tis: Carcinoma in situ

T1: Tumor confined to the vocal cord with normal mobility

T2: Supraglottic or subglottic extension of tumor with normal or impaired vocal cord mobility

T3: Tumor confined to the larynx with vocal cord fixation

T4: Massive tumor with thyroid cartilage destruction or extension beyond the confines of the larynx, or both

low-up he was free of disease 2 years following treatment.

CASE 2
STRIDOR IN AN INFANT

An 8-day-old male infant was referred because of stridor. Since the time of birth, he has had marked expiratory stridor and intermittent cyanosis. He had remained hospitalized because of the airway distress and was intubated 2 days after birth following a desaturation to 50% PaO₂. Since extubation 5 days after birth, the child continued to have noisy, high-pitched stridor.

He was the product of a normal gestation and delivery. After a careful evaluation by a neonatologist, no other medical problems were identified.

Examination of the larynx performed with a flexible laryngoscope demonstrated no supraglottic or vocal cord lesions. The mobility of the vocal cords was normal bilaterally. There was an apparent circumferential area of stenosis at the immediate subglottic level (this area is difficult to visualize in an awake infant).

The child was taken the next day to the operating room, where a direct laryngoscopy and bronchoscopy were performed under general anesthesia. A firm, circumferential scar band was present in the subglottis; only a 2.5-mm diameter subglottic airway was present, making it impossible to pass the 3-mm rigid bronchoscope past the obstruction.

The pediatric otolaryngologist decided to perform an anterior cricoid split during the same anesthetic in order to avoid the need for tracheostomy. This was performed by dividing the cricoid cartilage and first two tracheal rings in the midline and placing a small cartilage graft into the cartilage defect (Fig. 70.2). A cuffless endotracheal tube was left in the airway as a stent for the first 5 postoperative days. The child remained on the ventilator in the ICU during that time. The endotracheal tube was removed on postoperative day 6 in the operating room. At the time, the subglottic airway was approximately 3.5 mm in diameter (borderline size for infants).

Postoperatively, the patient had mild stridor during the first 2 postoperative days that resolved shortly thereafter. One year following surgery, the child was asymptomatic, and bronchoscopy demonstrated that the subglottic airway was adequate but a mild degree of stenosis was still apparent.

GENERAL CONSIDERATIONS

The normal voice is produced by a regular oscillation of the vocal cords, driven by the air flowing past the glottis. A wave-like motion is produced by the sliding of the mucosa over the underlying muscular portion of the vocal cord, which is visible only with the slow-motion perspective of laryngeal stroboscopic examination (Fig. 70.3).

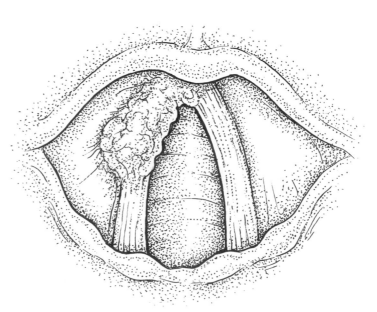

FIGURE 70.1 *A carcinoma of the vocal cord with extension to the anterior commissure and the laryngeal ventricle (Case 1).*

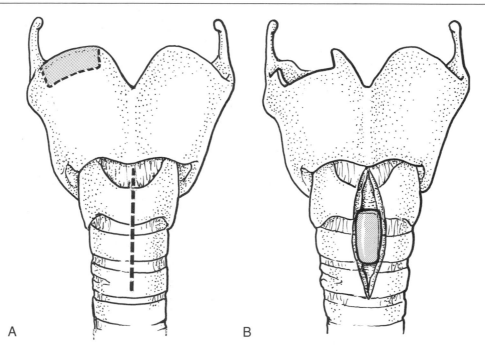

A B

FIGURE 70.2 *(A & B) A cricoid split involves an anterior incision through the cricoid without violation of the mucosa and the placement of a cartilage graft (harvested from the thyroid lamina). If successful, this procedure widens the subglottic airway and avoids the necessity of tracheostomy in patients with subglottic stenosis.*

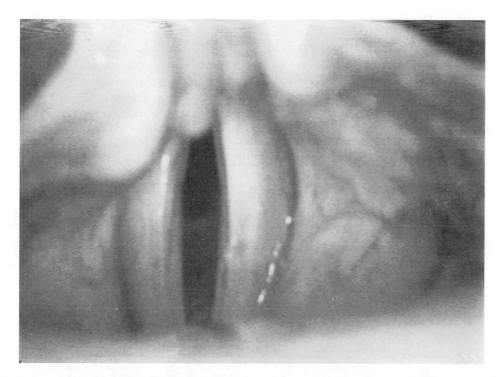

FIGURE 70.3 *When viewed on high speed photography, a wave-like motion of the vocal cord mucosa can be visualized. These waves "crash" along the surface of the cord, approximately 200 times per second.*

Any process that prevents normal vibration of the vocal cords can produce hoarseness. This includes a variety of benign and malignant tumors and many inflammatory causes. When the history suggests acute laryngitis, it is acceptable to make a presumptive diagnosis and treat the patient with oral antibiotics for 1–2 weeks. In an elderly smoker, however, it is unwise to attribute hoarseness to laryngitis. Likewise, persistent hoarseness in any patient should be evaluated with an office examination of the larynx. The goal is to differentiate inflammation of the larynx from potentially lethal neoplasms of the airway, which require immediate biopsy and treatment.

The detection of laryngeal squamous cell carcinoma is critical. Ten thousand new cases of laryngeal carcinoma are diagnosed yearly in the United States, particularly in smokers. Preservation of the larynx (Case 2) depends on early diagnosis of laryngeal cancer. If the tumor arises on the true vocal cord, the diagnosis is usually made early in the course of the disease, because the patient develops hoarseness while the tumor is still small. In early laryngeal carcinomas, radiotherapy or a voice-preserving operation is possible (Case 2). Fortunately, the vocal cord has few lymphatic vessels, and vocal cord tumors therefore rarely spread to regional lymphatics at the time of diagnosis. When the tumor has spread to the laryngeal ventricle, the area between the false and true vocal cords, metastasis is more common (Case 2).

The need for laryngeal examination is especially critical if the patient is an adult with other signs of laryngeal or hypopharyngeal cancer, such as odynophagia (painful swallowing) or dysphagia. Smokers with such symptoms require immediate evaluation. As seen in Case 2, premalignant white patches, or leukoplakia, can occur in multiple areas in the upper airway mucosa of smokers. Therefore, a careful head and neck examination is critical in the workup of such patients.

Tumors of the supraglottic larynx and hypopharynx (a region that includes the pyriform sinus) usually become extensive before symptoms such as hoarseness occur. A patient with such a tumor may complain of referred ear pain (otalgia) mediated through the 9th and 10th cranial nerves. The hypopharynx is richly supplied with lymphatics, and therefore, metastasis to the neck occurs early in the disease process.

Stridor is a sign of significant airway obstruction, because about 70% of the airway must be obstructed before stridor is clinically obvious. Inspiratory stridor is most often due to supraglottic (above the vocal cord) obstruction, while expiratory stridor is usually caused by infraglottic lesions. As one might expect, airway obstruction at the level of the glottis produces both inspiratory and expiratory stridor. Stridor is more common in infants because the cross-sectional area of the newborn larynx is much narrower, particularly at the subglottic level.

KEY POINTS

- Persistent hoarseness in any patient should be evaluated with office examination of larynx

- If tumor arises on true vocal cord, diagnosis is usually made early in course of disease, because patient develops hoarseness while tumor is small

- Tumors of supraglottic larynx and hypopharynx (region that includes pyriform sinus) usually become extensive before symptoms such as hoarseness occur

- Hypopharynx richly supplied with lymphatics, and therefore, metastasis occurs early in disease

- Stridor is sign of significant airway obstruction; about 70% of airway must be obstructed before stridor is clinically obvious

- Stridor more common in infants because cross-sectional area of newborn larynx is much narrower, particularly at subglottic level

DIAGNOSIS

The diagnosis of laryngeal disease begins with an examination of the airway. In the recent past, this was performed with a laryngeal mirror and reflecting headlight. Today, examination with a flexible fiberoptic laryngoscope is the preferred method in both adults and children. The mucosa of the pharynx, pyriform sinuses, epiglottis, and false and true vocal cords can be examined and recorded on videotape. The subglottis and trachea can be examined in adults with the use of the flexible bronchoscope, provided that topical anesthesia is generously applied to the larynx.

In children, the flexible laryngoscope has allowed the relatively easy examination of the larynx, although visualization of the subglottis and trachea are limited. A comprehensive examination of the airway in children is usually performed with a combination of direct laryngoscopy and bronchoscopy under general anesthesia. This approach allows both careful examination of the airway mucosa and biopsy of suspicious lesions.

KEY POINTS

- Diagnosis of laryngeal disease begins with examination of airway

- Today, examination with flexible fiberoptic laryngoscope most preferred method in both adults and children

DIFFERENTIAL DIAGNOSIS

The most common causes of hoarseness are inflammatory. Acute laryngitis can be caused by either bacteria or viruses. On examination, the vocal cords generally appear reddened and mildly edematous. Laryngitis usually will resolve without treatment, although penicillin will hasten the recovery in bacterial laryngitis. Other inflammatory conditions that may lead to hoarseness include tuberculosis, which generally involves the supraglottis, causing a pale inflammation. Fungal infections involving the larynx produce hoarseness if there is vocal cord involvement.

Reflux of stomach acid can cause chronic inflammation of the posterior larynx, and is a common cause of hoarseness. On examination, the area between and adjacent to the arytenoids is inflamed. In addition to hoarseness, the patient may complain of a globus sensation (i.e., feeling) lump in the throat. Reflux laryngitis has recently shown to be a risk factor for carcinoma of the larynx.

Numerous benign and malignant neoplasms of the larynx are capable of producing hoarseness. The identification of squamous cell carcinoma is paramount. Other, less common laryngeal tumors include chondrosarcoma and adenocarcinoma. Benign tumors of the larynx are relatively common. Vocal cord nodules are caused by abuse of the voice, as is often the case with cheerleaders or heavy metal singers. These lesions are often reversible with speech therapy and avoidance of the abusive practices. Operation is reserved for nodules that do not respond to speech therapy. Granulomas of the vocal cord most often occur following an endotracheal intubation. They produce hoarseness by preventing closure of the larynx during speech. Laryngeal papillomas, caused by the human papilloma virus, frequently present with hoarseness; laryngeal examination demonstrates characteristic multiple white lesions.

Finally, trauma, either iatrogenic or accidental, can scar the vocal cord tissue and prevent normal laryngeal vibration, producing hoarseness.

The three most common causes of stridor in infants are vocal cord paralysis, subglottic stenosis, and laryngomalacia. Laryngomalacia is caused by an immaturity of the laryngeal cartilage, often at the supraglottic level, which causes airway instability and stridor. Laryngomalacia has an excellent prognosis, generally resolving with age.

Subglottic stenosis usually occurs in infants following prolonged intubation. There is also a congenital form of the disease (Case 2). The introduction of the cricoid split technique (Fig. 70.2), has allowed resolution of stridor in infants who previously would have required tracheostomy. The cricoid split widens the narrowest portion of the airway, just below the vocal cords.

Inflammatory conditions such as croup or epiglottitis are causes of stridor in older children. Croup is a viral inflammation of the larynx and trachea. Epiglottitis is a rapidly progressive infection of the epiglottis. Due to the recent introduction of a vaccine against *Haemophilus influenzae*, the incidence of epiglottitis in children has dramatically decreased. Meanwhile, in adults, the incidence of epiglottitis has increased in the population with human immunodeficiency virus (HIV) infection. Because the airway obstruction of epiglottitis can progress rapidly, immediate intubation or tracheostomy is usually necessary.

Rarely, stridor is caused by a foreign body at the laryngeal level. In general, a foreign body should be suspected in a young child with an unexplained acute airway problem, especially one marked by shortness of breath, chest retractions, desaturation, or unexplained lobar pneumonia. Other rare causes of stridor in children include hemangiomas, malignant tumors, and vascular abnormalities, such as the presence of a double aortic arch.

Unilateral cord paralysis does not cause stridor in adults because abduction of the single mobile vocal cord produces an adequate airway diameter in most patients. Adults with cord paralysis usually present with a breathiness or weakness of the voice due to inadequate adduction of the paralyzed cord.

Bilateral cord paralysis can occur in either adults or children. In adults, the most common cause is surgical trauma during thyroidectomy. In infants, a central etiology, including severe hydrocephalus or Arnold Chiari malformation can produce bilateral paralysis. In either age group, immediate airway intervention is necessary.

The etiology of stridor is somewhat different in adults because of the larger airway diameter. Obstructive laryngeal tumors cause stridor when the tumor either restricts motion of the vocal cords or becomes so bulky that adequate air passage is impossible. Finally, severe infections of the larynx in adults can occasionally produce stridor if the airway diameter is sharply reduced.

KEY POINTS

- Most common causes of hoarseness are inflammatory

- Reflux of stomach acid can cause chronic inflammation of posterior larynx, and is common cause of hoarseness

- Numerous benign and malignant neoplasms of larynx are capable of producing hoarseness

- Vocal cord paralysis, subglottic stenosis, and laryngomalacia three most common causes of stridor in infants

- Foreign body should be suspected in young child with unexplained acute airway problem, especially one marked by shortness of breath, chest retractions, desaturation, or unexplained lobar pneumonia

- Etiology of stridor somewhat different in adults because of larger airway diameter

TREATMENT

The treatment for patients with hoarseness is individualized based on the diagnosis. Inflammation of the larynx can usually be treated with appropriate medical therapy such as antibiotics; the hoarseness is usually self-limited. Patients with benign neoplasms on the vocal cord can often be treated by excisional biopsy during direct laryngoscopy. Care must be taken to avoid injury to the muscular portion of the vocal cord during the excision of benign tumors, because permanent scarring and a hoarse voice can result. Nodules on the larynx often respond to changes in the use (or abuse) of the voice. Speech therapy is the first line of treatment.

The treatment of laryngeal cancer is somewhat controversial. Early tumors can be treated with either radiotherapy or laser surgery. We favor radiotherapy in most patients with small vocal cord malignancies (T1 or small T2), because the speech quality is better following radiation. In the above example (Case 1), the lesion was staged clinically as T3, and could have been treated with either operation or radiotherapy.

In Case 1, a vertical partial laryngectomy was performed. With this operation, the entire hemilarynx including the arytenoid, is resected. Following this procedure, the intact vocal cord vibrates against a muscle flap, producing a hoarse but serviceable voice. A total laryngectomy is necessary for extensive tumors (T4), such as lesions with extension through the thyroid cartilage. Following a total laryngectomy, esophageal speech or prosthetic speech through a tracheoesophageal puncture is possible in motivated patients.

Laryngeal preservation in patients with large cancers, employing chemotherapy and radiotherapy, is being actively investigated. Currently, combined treatment with operation and radiotherapy results in the highest cure rate.

The stridulous patient requires correction of the underlying problem or rapid establishment of a safe airway. It requires clinical judgment to decide whether a patient requires a tracheostomy to bypass the airway obstruction, or can be safely followed clinically and given medical therapy. When laryngeal or tracheal inflammation is a component of the problem, intravenous steroids can be used to reduce the airway edema. Recent studies have shown, for example, that croup responds favorably to the systemic administration of steroids.

Children with laryngomalacia or unilateral vocal cord paralysis can be observed and do not require immediate airway intervention. By contrast, patients with bilateral vocal cord paralysis at any age usually require tracheostomy, at least temporarily. In infants with severe subglottic stenosis who are not candidates for cricoid split, tracheostomy is usually necessary until definitive surgery can be performed later in life. Unfortunately, tube occlusion in a tracheostomized child can lead to death, so vigilance is necessary for parents and caretakers.

Epiglottitis can be largely prevented by vaccination for *H. influenzae*. Epiglottitis in children is treated by airway support, usually an endotracheal tube, and appropriate antibiotics. Finally, croup is treated with systemic steroids, humidification, and topical racemic epinephrine; intubation is usually not necessary.

KEY POINTS

• Treatment of laryngeal cancer is somewhat controversial; early tumors can be treated with either radiotherapy or laser surgery

• Stridulous patient requires correction of underlying problem or rapid establishment of safe airway

FOLLOW-UP

Patients with hoarseness should be followed regularly, especially smokers, in whom the risk of laryngeal cancer is highest. If there is any doubt about the presence of a malignancy, a biopsy of the larynx under general anesthesia should be performed.

Patients with stridor need to be closely observed until an airway is established or the problem resolves. Acute airway decompensation is always a possibility in the stridulous patient.

Patients with cancer of the larynx need lifetime follow-up, to detect both recurrences and new primaries in the upper aerodigestive tract.

KEY POINTS

• If any doubt about presence of malignancy, biopsy of larynx should be performed under general anesthesia

SUGGESTED READINGS

Cohen SR, Thompson JW, Geller KA et al: Voice change in the pediatric patient: a differential diagnosis. Ann Otol Rhinol Laryngol 92:437, 1983

Fried M (Ed): The Larynx: A Multidisciplinary Approach. Mosby–Year Book, 1995

An excellent textbook for students seeking a more detailed account of laryngeal and tracheal disease.

Sercarz JA, Berke GB, Ming Y et al: Videostroboscopy of human vocal cord paralysis. Ann Otol Rhino Laryngol 101:567, 1992

This article discusses the basics of laryngeal vibration in normal and paralysis states.

QUESTIONS

1. *Stridor?*
   A. Is more common in children, as the tracheal diameter is small.
   B. Is, in adults, a sign of significant obstruction.
   C. Requires prompt correction of underlying problem and rapid establishment of a safe airway.
   D. All of the above.

2. *Tumors of the hypopharynx and supraglottic larynx?*
   A. Present late.
   B. Provide hoarseness commonly.
   C. May have neck metastases when first seen.
   D. All of the above.

(See p. 604 for answers.)

71 TUMORS OF THE PHARYNX

SINA NASRI

JOEL A. SERCARZ

The pharynx is a tubular structure extending from the base of the skull superiorly to the esophageal inlet inferiorly. It is composed of three distinct areas: nasopharynx, oropharynx, and hypopharynx. The pharyngeal walls are composed of the superior, middle, and inferior pharyngeal constrictor muscles.

The aim of this chapter is to give the reader an understanding of the risk factors, treatment, and early diagnosis of tumors in the pharynx. The symptoms of pharyngeal cancer can be subtle, but must be recognized early for effective treatment.

CASE 1
UNDIFFERENTATED NASOPHARYNGEAL CARCINOMA

A 39-year-old Chinese male developed progressive right hearing loss over several months. On examination, he had fluid in the right middle ear and was treated with a 2-week course of oral antibiotics. The fluid in the middle ear persisted for 1 month and he was referred to an otolaryngologist.

There was serous effusion in the right middle ear cavity. Weber's test lateralized to the right ear. The right Rinne test indicated that bone conduction was better than air conduction, consistent with a right conductive hearing loss. Fiberoptic nasopharyngoscopy showed a mass in the right nasopharynx obstructing the eustachian tube orifice. No cervical lymphadenopathy was noted.

An MRI scan showed a mass in the right lateral nasopharynx not extending posterosuperiorly. No extension of the tumor into the nasal cavity, oropharynx, or skull base was present. The neck was free of disease. A biopsy of the mass showed undifferentiated nasopharyngeal carcinoma.

The patient received 7,000 cGy of radiotherapy to the primary site and 5,500 cGy to the neck, and was free of disease 13 months following the completion of the radiotherapy.

CASE 2
SQUAMOUS CELL CARCINOMA

A 63-year-old male presented with right-sided ear pain for over 3 months. He was initially treated with two consecutive courses of antibiotics, without improvement. On indirect laryngoscopy, an ulcerative mass was noted in the right pyriform sinus. There was a 1×2-cm mass in the right midanterior neck. He smoked three packs of cigarettes per day for 45 years and drank a 12-pack of beer each day.

FNA biopsy of the neck mass showed metastatic squamous cell carcinoma. He underwent a rigid laryngoscopy, esophagoscopy, bronchoscopy, and biopsy. The right pyriform sinus mass involved the apex of the pyriform fossa and postcricoid area (the portion of the hypopharynx behind the cricoid and superior to the esophageal inlet). No other lesion was noted. The biopsy of the mass showed a moderately well differentiated squamous cell carcinoma. The lesion is diagrammed in Figure 71.1.

He underwent a total laryngectomy, partial pharyngectomy, and right modified radical neck dissection with preservation of the spinal accessory nerve. Because there was a lack of mucosa available to reconstruct the pharynx, a radial forearm free flap was used. He recovered from the operation without swallowing disability. He was given a full course of radiotherapy (6,800 cGy) to the primary site and 5,500 cGy to the neck after the resection. Unfortunately, he presented with an inoperable recurrence in the right neck 1 year after treatment.

GENERAL CONSIDERATIONS

Tumors of the pharynx may present with nonspecific findings such as otalgia or unilateral otitis media. Frequently, patients are seen after a considerable delay in diagnosis. Patients with otalgia but no apparent ear pathology should have a complete examination of the upper aerodigestive tract, including the larynx. This is especially critical in smokers.

Anatomically, the nasopharynx is connected anteriorly to the nasal cavity through the choanae. Inferiorly, it is bounded by the upper aspect of the soft palate. Superiorly, it is bounded by the base of the skull (occipital bone) and the body of the sphenoid bone. Laterally, each side contains the opening of the eustachian tube posteriorly, and a submucosal cartilaginous structure (torus tubarius), behind which is a depression (fossa of Rosenmueller).

Nasopharyngeal carcinoma arises from the epithelium of the nasopharynx. Nearly all tumors of the nasopharynx are malignant epithelial lesions. The epithelium of the nasopharynx varies from stratified squamous to ciliated columnar. The variety of underlying epithelium results in heterogeneity of nasopharyngeal tumors.

Nasopharyngeal carcinoma is subtyped into three histologic variants: keratinizing (25%), nonkeratinizing (15%), and undifferentiated (about 60%). A prominent non-neoplastic lymphoid component is frequently present, leading to the misnomer "lymphoepithelioma."

The fossa of Rosenmueller is the most common site of occurrence of nasopharyngeal carcinoma. An increased incidence of nasopharyngeal carcinoma is observed in some

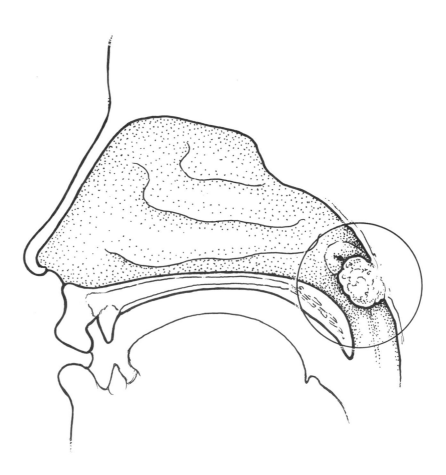

FIGURE 71.1 *A tumor of the nasopharynx involving the lateral wall, including obstruction of the eustachian tube orifice.*

parts of China and Taiwan. The incidence among Chinese people decreases after they migrate outside the country. However, Chinese-Americans still have a higher incidence than other North Americans. Elevated titers of Epstein-Barr virus (EBV) antibodies are associated with the undifferentiated and nonkeratinizing types. The precise role of EBV in the pathogenesis of nasopharyngeal carcinoma is being investigated.

The hypopharynx includes the pyriform fossae and the posterior and lateral pharyngeal walls (Fig. 71.2). The postcricoid area is immediately behind the larynx superior to the esophageal inlet. The hypopharynx extends from the level of the hyoid bone superiorly to the lower border of the cricoid cartilage inferiorly. Anteriorly, it is bounded by the mucosa on the medial aspect of the posterior thyroid cartilage. The lateral walls attach to the hyoid bone and thyroid cartilage. Medially, it is bounded by the larynx. The pyriform fossa (sinus) is the part of the hypopharynx that extends forward around the sides of the larynx and lies between the thyroid cartilage and the larynx.

The most common hypopharyngeal tumor is squamous cell carcinoma (>95%), which is most commonly found in males in the sixth and seventh decades of life. Pyriform sinus lesions are much more common than postcricoid or posterior pharyngeal wall carcinomas.

The most important predisposing factors in hypopharyngeal carcinoma development are tobacco and alcohol use. Alcohol abuse plays a more significant role in hypopharyngeal than endolaryngeal tumors. The Plummer-Vinson syndrome characterized by glossitis, splenomegaly, iron deficiency anemia, esophageal stenosis, and achlorhydria has strong correlation with postcricoid squamous cell carcinomas. This syndrome is seen mainly in Northern European women.

Compared to the larynx, the hypopharynx has fewer natural barriers to the spread of malignancy. The pyriform sinus lesions are characterized by submucous spread of the carcinoma to both the lateral pharyngeal wall and postcricoid area (Fig. 71.2). Needless to say, surgeons attempt wide resection of these tumors.

The hypopharynx has a rich lymphatic drainage. The pyriform sinus has the highest density of lymphatic vessels, followed by the posterior hypopharyngeal wall and the postcricoid area. Overall, more than 75% of hypopha-

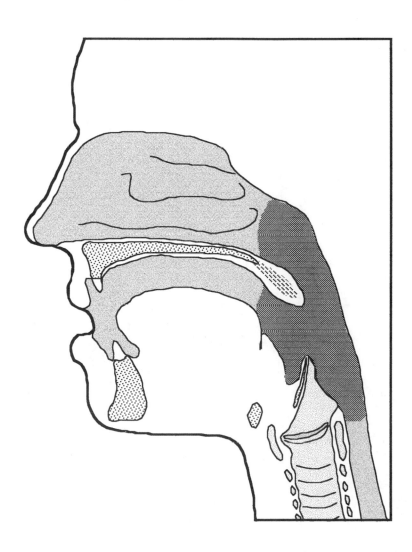

FIGURE 71.2 *Diagram of the larynx and pyriform sinus.*

ryngeal squamous cell carcinomas have cervical lymphatic involvement at the time of diagnosis. Therefore, treatment of the neck is mandatory in these tumors.

Patients with hypopharyngeal tumors develop otalgia because the 9th and 10th nerves supply the pharynx and also the ear, through Jacobson's (9th) and Arnold's (10th) nerves. Patients with pharyngeal tumors may complain of ear pain and not mention sore throat, hoarseness, or other pharyngeal symptoms.

KEY POINTS

• Pharynx is tubular structure extending from base of skull superiorly to esophageal inlet inferiorly

• Pharynx composed of three distinct areas: nasopharynx, oropharynx, and hypopharynx

• Pharyngeal walls composed of superior, middle, and inferior pharyngeal constrictor muscles

• Tumors of pharynx may present with nonspecific findings such as otalgia or unilateral otitis media

• Nasopharyngeal carcinoma arises from epithelium of nasopharynx; nearly all are malignant epithelial lesions

• Nasopharyngeal carcinoma subtyped into three histologic variants: keratinizing (25%), nonkeratinizing (15%), and undifferentiated (about 60%); prominent non-neoplastic lymphoid component frequently present, leading to misnomer "lymphoepithelioma"

• Fossa of Rosenmueller most common site of occurrence of nasopharyngeal carcinoma

• Most common hypopharyngeal tumor is squamous cell carcinoma (>95%); most commonly found in males in sixth and seventh decades of life

• Pyriform sinus lesions much more common than postcricoid or posterior pharyngeal wall carcinomas

• Tobacco and alcohol use most important predisposing factors in hypopharyngeal carcinoma development

• Alcohol abuse plays more significant role in hypopharyngeal than in endolaryngeal tumors

• Patients with hypopharyngeal tumors develop otalgia because 9th and 10th nerves supply pharynx and also the ear, through Jacobson's (9th) and Arnold's (10th) nerves

---

ryngeal carcinoma. Special attention should be paid to the symptoms of unilateral nasal obstruction and/or bleeding. Flexible nasopharyngolaryngoscopy and palpation of the neck should be done if there is any suspicion of nasopharyngeal mass.

Any nasopharyngeal mass or mucosal asymmetry should be biopsied. Before biopsy, however, a magnetic resonance imaging (MRI) scan of the nasopharynx and cervical region may be useful for accurate localization and extent of the mass. A computed tomography (CT) scan is the study of choice for determination of invasion of the bony base of the skull. It is preferable to obtain the radiographic studies before the biopsy in order not to mistake postbiopsy changes with the lesion itself.

Unilateral sore throat is the most common symptom of hypopharyngeal carcinomas. Others include dysphagia, odynophagia, referred otalgia, and hoarseness. Approximately 25% of patients present with otalgia; another 25% present with a neck mass.

Rigid or flexible laryngopharyngoscopy is used to visualize the hypopharynx. The apex of the pyriform sinus and the postcricoid areas, however, cannot be examined in this fashion. Salivary pooling and asymmetry may indicate a hypopharyngeal mass. Lateral manipulation of the thyroid cartilage normally produces crepitance. With the postcricoid lesions, this sound is usually lost.

KEY POINTS

• Persistent unilateral otitis media in adults should raise strong suspicion of nasopharyngeal carcinoma; special attention should be paid to symptoms of unilateral nasal obstruction and/or bleeding

• Flexible nasopharyngolaryngoscopy and palpation of neck should be done if any suspicion of nasopharyngeal mass

• Any nasopharyngeal mass or mucosal asymmetry should be biopsied; before biopsy, an MRI scan of nasopharynx and cervical region useful for accurate localization and extent of mass

• Unilateral sore throat most common symptom of hypopharyngeal carcinomas; other signs include dysphagia, odynophagia, referred otalgia, and hoarseness

---

DIAGNOSIS

Nasopharyngeal carcinoma is uncommon in the United States (0.25% versus 18% in China). More than half of patients have a painless neck mass. Other presenting signs and symptoms include serous otitis media, cranial nerve involvement (the 5th and 6th are the most common), epistaxis, and nasal obstruction.

History and examination are the most important parts of the diagnostic evaluation. Persistent unilateral otitis media in adults, should raise a strong suspicion of naspha-

DIFFERENTIAL DIAGNOSIS

Other malignancies in the differential diagnosis of the nasopharyngeal mass include lymphoma and rhabdomyosarcoma. Biopsies differentiate these tumors.

TREATMENT

The treatment of choice for nasopharyngeal carcinoma is high dose radiotherapy (6,500–7,500 cGy) to the nasopharynx and a lesser dose to the neck. The response varies according to the histology of the tumor. Keratinizing tumors are not radiosensitive; however, they remain localized without dissemination. Their 5-year survival rate is 10–20%. Nonkeratinizing tumors are variably radiosensitive and have a 5-year survival rate of 35–50%. They metastasize to regional lymph nodes. Undifferentiated tumors are radioresponsive with a 5-year survival rate of 55–65%. Radical neck dissection is indicated for persistent neck disease following radiotherapy. Some surgeons have attempted resection of persistent disease in the nasopharynx, which has proved to be successful for small tumors. The role of chemotherapy is currently being studied.

Several factors are important in the prognosis. One is age; younger patients have a better prognosis, partly because the nasopharyngeal carcinoma occurring in younger patients is predominantly of undifferentiated type. Another factor is lymphatic metastasis. Involvement of lymph nodes decreases the overall 5-year survival by 10–20%. Other factors include clinical stage and histologic variant of the disease, as outlined above.

Treatment of hypopharyngeal cancers includes operation and postoperative radiotherapy. Small tumors can be treated with radiation alone, but most patients present with advanced stage tumors. For T2 lesions, if the apex of the pyriform sinus is not involved, a trial of irradiation may be curative and operation is reserved for salvage. If the apex is involved, a total laryngectomy is required to obtain adequate margins, even though the endolarynx may not be involved. More advanced pyriform sinus lesions (T3 and T4) are treated with total laryngectomy, partial pharyngectomy, and postoperative radiation.

Radiotherapy is the primary treatment for the posterior pharyngeal wall tumors. Occasionally, radiation failures can be treated with pharyngectomy. For more advanced lesions, total laryngopharyngectomy and gastric pull-up may be used for ablation and reconstruction. Postcricoid tumors generally require total laryngectomy because of their location. If the tumor is extensive, a free flap may be necessary (Case 2). The radial forearm flap is useful to repair subtotal defects of the hypopharynx.

The treatment of the neck in head and neck cancer remains somewhat controversial. The neck requires treatment if there is adenopathy present or, in the absence of disease, if there is a greater than 20% chance of occult involvement. The neck is treated with irradiation if radiation alone is used for the treatment of the primary lesion. When a combined modality is used for the treatment of the hypopharyngeal disease, a neck dissection and resection of the primary is followed by irradiation.

The 5-year survival rate with all early stage hypopharyngeal squamous cell carcinomas is 35–45% and for more advanced stages, 20–25%. In the advanced stages of the disease, there is considerable risk of distant metastasis. The best results are obtained in patients whose tumors are detected early, particularly before the presence of adenopathy.

KEY POINTS

- Treatment of choice for nasopharyngeal carcinoma is high dose radiotherapy (6,500–7,500 cGy) to nasopharynx and a lesser dose to the neck

- Treatment of hypopharyngeal cancers includes operation and postoperative radiotherapy; small tumors can be treated with radiation alone, but most patients present with advanced stage tumors

- For T2 lesions, if apex of pyriform sinus not involved, a trial of irradiation may be curative and operation reserved for salvage

- If apex involved, a total laryngectomy is required to obtain adequate margins, even though endolarynx may not be involved

FOLLOW-UP

Patients with tumors of the pharynx need close observation for the first 5 years after therapy, when they are at risk of local or regional recurrence. There is also considerable risk of developing a second primary tumor in patients who continue to smoke and drink alcohol.

KEY POINTS

- Patients who continue to smoke and drink alcohol have considerable risk of developing a second primary tumor

SUGGESTED READINGS

Hongzheng S, Haixia J: Combined therapy for carcinoma of nasopharynx: a report of 49 cases. J Laryngol Otol 107:201, 1993

Some new thinking on combined treatment of nasopharyngeal carcinoma.

Thawley SE, Panje WR: Comprehensive Management of Head and Neck Tumors. WB Saunders, Philadelphia,

An excellent introductory chapter on pharyngeal tumors.

Wenig BM: Atlas of Head and Neck Pathology. WB Saunders, Philadelphia,

A brief, to-the-point chapter on nasopharyngeal carcinomas.

QUESTIONS

1. *Which of the following nerves is responsible for referred otalgia in upper aerodigestive tract tumors?*

    A. Vagus nerve.

    B. Arnold's nerve.

    C. Jacobson's nerve.

    D. Glossopharyngeal nerve.

    E. All of the above.

2. *Which of the following statements about nasopharyngeal carcinoma is false?*

    A. Nasopharyngeal cancer is associated with Epstein-Barr virus exposure.

    B. Chinese people who emigrate to the United States have the same rate of nasopharyngeal carcinoma as other Americans.

    C. The most common presenting signs of nasopharyngeal cancer are neck mass and hearing loss.

    D. Unilateral serous otitis media in an adult requires evaluation of the nasopharynx.

3. *The need to treat the neck in head and neck cancer depends on?*

    A. The location of the primary tumor.

    B. The likelihood of subclinical metastasis.

    C. Whether surgery or radiation is the primary modality of treatment.

    D. The experience of the surgeon.

(See p. 604 for answers.)

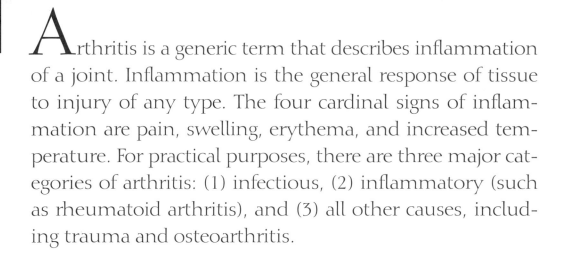

72 ARTHRITIS

THOMAS P. SCHMALZRIED

Arthritis is a generic term that describes inflammation of a joint. Inflammation is the general response of tissue to injury of any type. The four cardinal signs of inflammation are pain, swelling, erythema, and increased temperature. For practical purposes, there are three major categories of arthritis: (1) infectious, (2) inflammatory (such as rheumatoid arthritis), and (3) all other causes, including trauma and osteoarthritis.

The goals of this chapter are to (1) illustrate differences in the clinical presentations of arthritis, (2) describe an approach to the evaluation of joint symptoms, (3) briefly review the pathophysiology of rheumatoid and osteoarthritis, and (4) outline available treatments and associated indications.

CASE 1
ACUTE HIP INFECTION

A previously healthy 4-year-old male had been avoiding motion of his right hip and refusing to walk. For the past 12 hours, he had been feeling sick and had a fever. His temperature was 38.5°C. Movement of the hip was very painful. His other joints were normal. Radiographs of the hips and pelvis showed slight widening of the distance between the proximal femoral metaphysis and the medial wall of the acetabulum on the right side, suggesting a joint effusion. The WBC count was elevated with increased segmented neutrophils. The sedimentation rate was more than double the upper limit of normal. Two sets of blood cultures were drawn.

Empiric intravenous antibiotic therapy was started with oxacillin (for *Staphylococcus aureus*) and a third-generation cephalosporin (for *Haemophilus influenzae*). Six hours later he was taken to the operating room and the hip joint aspirated of slightly cloudy joint fluid. It was sent for cell count, differential, culture, and sensitivity. The clinical presentation, blood studies, and gross appearance of the fluid were all consistent with an acute hip infection, and an open irrigation and drainage of the hip was done. A small drainage tube was left in the hip. The blood and joint fluid cultures subsequently grew *S. aureus* sensitive to oxacillin and the cephalosporin was discontinued. Drainage stopped after 36 hours and the drainage tube was removed. Intravenous antibiotics were given for 1 week and oral antibiotics (dicloxacillin) for an additional 5 weeks.

Five years later hip function and radiographs were normal.

CASE 2
RHEUMATOID ARTHRITIS

A 32-year-old female complained of pain and swelling in the small joints of her hands and feet. She also had some pain in her knees and elbows. Her hips and shoulder were normal, although she did have diffuse joint stiffness for about 1 hour on awaking. She had no malaise, skin lesions, or rashes. There was no known family history of arthritis. Although she appeared well, she had slight swelling of the small joints of her hands, accompanied by slight erythema and warmth. Radiographs of the hands showed soft tissue swelling, some periarticular osteopenia, and slight uniform reduction of the joint spaces. There were small erosions at the margins of several of the joints on both hands. Her WBC count was not elevated; however, the sedimentation rate was more than double the upper limit of normal. Her serum tested positive for rheumatoid factor but negative for ANAs. She was started on an oral NSAID.

Her rheumatoid arthritis progressed, and subsequent medical management included separate trials of several different NSAIDs, oral gold, methotrexate, and prednisone. Years later she complained of persistent, severe bilateral knee pain that was not relieved by the oral medicines. The knees were injected with corticosteroids about every 3 months, but pain relief was not long-lasting. The pain was nearly constant and occasionally awakened her at night. Her ambulation was limited to about one block.

She had moderate effusions, slight erythema, and increased skin temperature of both knees. There was a roughly symmetric amount of valgus and flexion deformity of both knees. There was diffuse tenderness involving the patellofemoral joint as well as the medial and lateral joint lines.

Radiographs showed diffuse osteopenia and roughly symmetric loss of joint space involving all three compartments of the knee—patellofemoral, medial, and lateral—but no significant osteophytes.

She was considered for bilateral total knee replacement. A right total knee replacement was done, followed in 2 weeks by a left total knee replacement. She had an uncomplicated postoperative course. Five years later she had no knee pain, had full active extension, and her ambulation was not limited by her knee function. She was very satisfied with the function of her knees.

CASE 3
DEGENERATIVE MENISCAL TEAR

A 50-year-old male complained of pain on the medial side of his right knee. The pain was associated with prolonged walking and had been slowly increasing in intensity over the past year. He described an occasional "catching" sensation, and there had been intermittent swelling of that knee. He denied any history of acute injury. He had no other joint symptoms. There was a moderate effusion, a slight increase in skin temperature, and tenderness over the right medial joint line. There was pain and a "catching" or "popping" sensation from the posteromedial aspect of the knee when the leg was rotated with the knee in flexion. Weight-bearing radiographs of the knee confirmed the varus alignment noted on physical examination and showed medial joint space narrowing, subchondral sclerosis and small peripheral osteophytes. The lateral joint space was normal. No blood or joint fluid studies were obtained.

The mechanical symptoms of "catching" combined with the ability to reproduce and palpate this event on physical examination suggested a torn meniscus. An MRI was not obtained. Arthroscopy showed a degenerative tear of the posterior horn of the medial meniscus. It was resected. The articular and meniscal cartilage of the medial compartment were diffusely yellow (oxidation) and fibrillated (worn). The articular cartilage was thin in the central portion of the tibial plateau and there was a small area of full-thickness loss of articular cartilage (exposed subchondral bone) in the most medial portion of the plateau. The lateral and patellofemoral compartments were relatively well preserved, having only slight yellowing, softening, and limited fibrillation. Under the same anesthetic, in order to correct the varus alignment of this knee, an HTO was performed. A lateral incision was made over the proximal tibia. A 10 degree wedge of bone was removed from between the joint line and the tibial tubercle. The base of the wedge was lateral and the apex was medial. A valgus stress was applied to the leg that approximated the bone laterally (closed the wedge). Internal fixation was used to stabilize the osteotomy.

Five years later, the patient had slight medial side knee pain, which only occurred occasionally with heavy work or sports. He had no "catching" and no swelling. He was very satisfied with the function of his knee. At age 60, 10 years after surgery, he had diffuse pain in his knee. Oral NSAIDs and intra-articular injections provided partial and temporary relief of pain. He eventually developed pain at rest that disturbed his sleep; he required a cane to walk one block, and had difficulty with stairs. His general health was good. Radiographs at age 62 showed extensive loss of joint space in the medial, lateral, and patellofemoral compartments, with subchondral sclerosis and marginal osteophytes. He elected to have a total knee replacement. He had an uncomplicated postoperative course. Five years after surgery he had no pain in the knee and could walk unlimited distances. He was highly satisfied with the function of the prosthetic knee.

GENERAL CONSIDERATIONS

Arthritis per se is not a disease, but rather a term that describes the inflamed condition of a joint. With this generic definition, arthritis is very common (the inversion ankle sprain is a good example). Inflammation is the general response of tissue to injury of any type and is characterized by pain, swelling, erythema, and increased temperature. The injury can be primarily due to physical forces, which includes both acute and chronic (repetitive) trauma or injury, or it can be due to chemical factors, including acute enzymatic degradation of articular cartilage in suppurative infections and chronic degradation in rheumatoid arthritis.

In the management of any disease process, appropriate therapy is based on making an accurate diagnosis. For practical purposes in making a diagnosis and prescribing treatment, it is useful to consider arthritis in three broad etiologic categories: primary infection (suppurative: staphylococcosis; nonsuppurative: tuberculosis), primary inflammatory (such as rheumatoid arthritis), and all other causes, including acute trauma and osteoarthritis. The case presentations were specifically chosen to illustrate the breadth of pathologic processes that present as inflammation of a joint. Although suppurative infections account for only a small fraction of arthritis cases, it is important to consider sepsis as an etiology of acute arthritis, because accurate diagnosis and prompt treatment are key to obtaining a satisfactory outcome.

Because it is a systemic disease, a team approach is often used in the management of rheumatoid arthritis and includes a rheumatologist and physical or occupational therapist, as well as the primary care provider. Surgery is indicated when nonsurgical modalities are unsuccessful. Most arthritis cases, however, fall into the diagnostic category of osteoarthritis, often referred to as degenerative joint disease (Case 3). Primary osteoarthritis and osteoarthrosis are diseases with a primary abnormality of articular cartilage composition. In secondary osteoarthritis, which is much more common than primary osteoarthritis, the composition of the articular cartilage is normal but the cartilage wears at an accelerated rate due to abnormal stresses.

KEY POINTS

- Arthritis is not a disease per se but rather describes inflammation of a joint

- Cardinal signs are pain, swelling, erythema, and increased temperature

- Useful to consider arthritis in three broad etiologic categories; primary infection; primary inflammatory (such as rheumatoid arthritis) causes; and all other causes, including acute trauma and osteoarthritis

- Although suppurative infections account for only a small fraction of arthritis cases, it is important to consider sepsis as an etiology of acute arthritis, because accurate diagnosis and prompt treatment are key to obtaining satisfactory outcome

- Most arthritis cases fall into diagnostic category of osteoarthritis, often referred to as degenerative joint disease

DIAGNOSIS

The accurate diagnosis of arthritis is dependent on identifying (1) the temporal progression of symptoms, (2) several key associated features in the history, (3) characteristic findings on physical examination, and (4) supportive laboratory and radiographic tests. For example, osteoarthritis frequently presents in middle age, starts insidiously, and is aggravated by use and relieved by rest (Case 3). Symptoms typically follow an intermittent course, and often involve either hip or knee and the interphalangeal joints. Movement is always restricted and may be accompanied by crepitus. Radiographs show nonuniform loss of joint space.

Bacterial arthritis continues to be the most rapidly destructive form of joint disease. The causal organism is *S. aureus* in about 60% of cases (Case 1). The knee joint is the most commonly involved, followed by the hip, shoulder, wrist, ankle, elbow, and hand. The most common source is via hematogenous dissemination of an infection localized in another area of the body. The synovial membrane is extremely vascular, and an organism circulating in the blood may become trapped in the synovial space. Other causes of joint contamination include contiguous spread from soft tissues or periarticular osteomyelitis, direct inoculation secondary to penetrating trauma, and diagnostic or therapeutic joint aspiration. Factors that predispose to joint infection include closed trauma to the joint, intravenous drug abuse, pre-existing joint disease such as rheumatoid arthritis, and impaired host defense mechanisms such as concurrent steroid usage or other immunosuppressive medications, diabetes mellitus, sickle cell anemia, or advanced age. Polymorphonuclear leukocytes and other inflammatory cells migrate to the multiplying bacteria in the joint (a functionally closed space). The white blood cells (WBCs) release various cytokines and the cartilage is ultimately destroyed by enzymes released by the inflammatory cells, bacterial enzymes, and enzymes released from the synovium.

The infected joint usually presents as acutely swollen, red, painful, and warm, with marked tenderness and restricted movement (Case 1). The patient may also show systemic signs, such as malaise, fever, and tachycardia. The patient should be examined for possible sources of the infection and questioned about intravenous drug abuse and exposure to sexually transmitted disease, especially gonorrhea. Radiographs should be obtained, although early in the course of the disease they will be normal. Joint space narrowing and erosions may be detectable within 7–14 days, and the timing of their appearance is dependent on the virulence of the organism. Late changes include osteoporosis, marginal erosions, uniform joint space narrowing, and periostitis.

Blood studies may reveal an elevated WBC count with a left shift. The erythrocyte sedimentation rate (ESR) is often markedly elevated. The diagnosis is usually made, however, by joint aspiration. Synovial fluid analysis shows a WBC count of more than $50,000/mm^3$, with greater than 75% neutrophils (Case 1). Joint fluid should also be sent for Gram stain, culture, and sensitivity. Blood cultures should be sent. On occasion, the joint aspirate may be sterile and bacterial identification is made on blood culture.

Tuberculous arthritis also arises from either direct extension from bone or following hematogenous dissemination of organisms from a pulmonary or other focus of infection. Bones or joints are affected in about 5% of patients with tuberculosis. The most common skeletal site is the spine (Pott's disease) followed by the hip. Eighty percent of cases are monoarticular. The tuberculous bacilli elicit a chronic inflammatory reaction with the characteristic granuloma made up of epithelioid and multinucleated giant cells. Tuberculous arthritis, which may go undiagnosed for months or years, can result in extensive fibrosis and obliteration of the joint space.

Radiographs show periarticular osteopenia, marginal erosions, uniform loss of joint space, and may have subchondral cysts in a paired or "kissing" position on both sides of the joint. The diagnosis is supported by a positive PPD (purified protein derivative) skin test and confirmed by the demonstration of acid-fast bacilli (present in 10–20% of the cases) and "rice bodies" (fibrin globules) in joint fluid. Growth of the bacilli may take weeks, but synovial fluid cultures are positive in 50% of the cases. Synovial biopsy is more reliable, as cultures of the synovium are positive 80% of the time. Treatment includes long-term antituberculous drugs (frequently including rifampin and isoniazid), and operative drainage in cases of more serious joint involvement (loculated fluid, loose bodies, neurologic involvement, or exuberant synovial pannus).

Mycotic infections of joints most often are caused by direct extension from bone infection. Most cases are seen in immunocompromised hosts. The indolent course of most fungal joint infections often leads to delayed diagnosis. Common pathogens include *Candida albicans, Histoplasmosis,* and *Sporotrichosis.* Radiographic changes are variable and nonspecific. Synovial fluid analyses are variable and depend on the stage of the disease. Potassium hydroxide (KOH) preparations are helpful, but culture of the involved tissue or synovial fluid remains the most reliable method of definitive diagnosis. Treatment is directed at the causal organism. Amphotericin B is the drug of choice for *C. albicans* and can be delivered intra-articularly with less side effects. Operative debridement is required in the presence of purulent fluid.

Lyme disease is a multisystem disease caused by the spirochete *Borrelia burgdorferi* that is transmitted by ticks endemic to the United States. Lyme disease mimics classic rheumatic diseases and occurs in three stages: (1) rash (erythema chronicum migrans [ECM]), (2) neurologic symptoms, and (3) arthritis. If musculoskeletal symptoms occur early in the illness, the typical pattern is one of migratory pain in joints, tendons, bursae, muscle, or bone, usually without joint swelling. Later in the course of the disease, about 60% of patients develop monoarticular or oligoarticular arthritis, frequently affecting the knee and shoulder. The attacks are acute, intermittent joint swelling that generally last for months. In about 10% of patients the joint involvement becomes chronic, resulting in erosion of cartilage and bone. If Gram stain and cultures of the joint aspirate show no organisms, diagnosis can be confirmed by enzyme-linked immunosorbent assay (ELISA) testing. Making the correct diagnosis is important, as Lyme disease can be eradicated with tetracycline or penicillin.

Rheumatoid arthritis is an autoimmune disease (or diseases) characterized by joint inflammation due to systemic and/or circulating factors. The typical patient is a woman between 30 and 40 years old who complains of morning stiffness, or stiffness after periods of inactivity, in multiple joints, often including the proximal joints of the fingers, wrists, feet, knees, and shoulders (Case 2).

The disease process in rheumatoid arthritis primarily affects the synovial membrane, not the articular cartilage as in osteoarthritis. Autoantibodies (both IgG and IgM; rheumatoid factor), are produced to the body's own IgG. Rheumatoid factors can be found in 60–80% of patients with rheumatoid arthritis, although a positive test is not diagnostic, since rheumatoid factors are found in 1–5% of subjects without other signs of rheumatoid arthritis. High titers of rheumatoid factor are generally associated with more severe and/or active joint disease, the presence of nodules, greater frequency of systemic complications, and a poorer prognosis. These autoantibodies and the immune complexes they form are concentrated in the synovium. The synovial inflammation is associated with massive T-cell infiltration as well as B-cell reactivity. The joint capsule becomes thickened, the synovium becomes edematous and undergoes villus hyperplasia, and an effusion forms in the affected joints and tendon sheaths. The articular cartilage is eroded by proteolytic enzymes released by the inflammatory cells, by vascular folds in the thickened synovium, and by creeping granulation tissue (pannus). Similar changes occur in the supporting tendons, which can lead to tendon rupture. The combination of the changes and damage to the articular cartilage, capsule, and tendons results in progressive instability and deformity of the joints.

As determined by the American College of Rheumatology, four of the following seven criteria are needed for the diagnosis of rheumatoid arthritis: (1) morning stiffness lasting at least 1 hour, (2) arthritis of three or more regions, (3) arthritis of the hands, (4) symmetric arthritis of the same joint (left and right), (5) rheumatoid nodules, (6) radiographic changes typical of rheumatoid arthritis, and (7) serum positive for rheumatoid factor.

The physical signs often include swelling and tenderness of metacarpophalangeal (MCP) joints, proximal interphalangeal (PIP) joints, and wrists, with ulnar deviation of these small joints. Larger joints may demonstrate warmth, synovial thickening ("boggy synovium"), and effusions. Systemic manifestations may include nodules (pathognomonic for rheumatoid arthritis) in the back of the elbows and in the tendons, pericarditis, and pulmonary disease (pleurisy, nodules, and fibrosis).

Radiographs generally demonstrate periarticular osteopenia and marginal bone erosions with uniform narrowing of the joint space. Blood studies are characterized by an elevated ESR and C-reactive protein. At some point in the course of the disease, rheumatoid factor can be detected in up to 80% of patients. The inflammatory synovial fluid is thin and watery with WBC counts ranging from 5,000–20,000/mm^3 and with 50–70% polyps. Rheumatoid factor can be demonstrated, and complement levels are decreased.

Juvenile rheumatoid arthritis (JRA) is a persistent noninfectious arthritis lasting more than 3 months. The cause is probably similar to that of rheumatoid disease, a response to an autoantigen, although rheumatoid factor is usually absent. The diagnosis is based on arthritis plus one of the following: intermittent fever, rash, presence of rheumatoid factor, iridocyclitis, cervical spine involvement, pericarditis, tenosynovitis, or morning stiffness.

The pathology is similar to that of rheumatoid arthritis with synovial proliferation leading to joint destruction. There are three general presentations. (1) Systemic JRA or Still's disease, where the clinical manifestations include fever, rash, hepatosplenomegaly, and pericardial or pleural effusions. Chronic polyarthritis develops in many individuals, and about 25% progress to develop severe chronic arthritis. (2) Pauciarticular JRA is the most common form of JRA. Only a few joints are involved and frequently they are "medium-sized": knees, ankles, and elbows. A serious manifestation is iridocyclitis, which develops in 10–15%. (3) Polyarticular JRA affects multiple joints, and these children frequently have constitutional symptoms, including low grade fever, adenopathy, mild organomegaly, anemia, and growth retardation. Involvement of the cervical spine (particularly C2 and C3) and temporomandibular joint is also seen. The general prognosis for JRA is good, as 75% of patients have a long remission and show little or no residual. Initial therapy includes salicylates, range of motion exercises, night splinting, and occasionally, synovectomy.

Ankylosing spondylitis is a chronic inflammatory condition that affects mainly the spine and the sacroiliac joints. Ankylosing spondylitis is one of the seronegative spondylarthropathies (rheumatoid factor-negative). There are two general types of lesions: (1) synovitis of sacroiliac and vertebral facet joints, and (2) inflammation of tendon and ligament insertions into bone (enthesopathy) at intervertebral discs, sacroiliac ligaments, symphysis pubis, and manubrium sterni. Peripheral joints (hips, shoulders, knees) are involved in approximately one-third of cases. Radiographs show blurring of the sacroiliac joint initially and sclerosis later in the disease. The vertebral bodies often lose their normal anterior concavity and become "squared" accompanied by syndesmophytes (ossification bridging the intervertebral disks). The ESR is elevated during the active phases of the disease, and more than 75% of the patients have HLA-B27. Patients are encouraged to maintain an active lifestyle. Physical therapy including gentle range of motion exercises and nonsteroidal anti-inflammatory drugs (NSAIDs) are helpful in decreasing the soft tissue inflammation and reducing pain. Lower spinal deformities coupled with hip arthritis and flexion contractures can be helped by total hip arthroplasty.

Reiter syndrome is another seronegative spondylarthropathy and is a reactive arthritis that generally affects the weight-bearing joints. Onset often follows dysentery or venereal infection, with the classic presentation being a triad of arthritis, uveitis/conjunctivitis, and urethritis. Reiter syndrome generally affects young men between the ages of 20 and 40. The acute phase frequently involves asymmetric involvement of lower extremity joints and lasts a few weeks or months. The chronic phase is characterized by recurrent episodes of mild polyarthritis, often involving the upper extremities. Similar to ankylosing spondylitis, Reiter syndrome has a close association with HLA-B27, and there is no specific treatment for it. Initial symptomatic therapy includes physical therapy and NSAIDs.

Psoriatic arthritis is a polyarthritis seen in 7% of patients with psoriasis. Similar to the other seronegative spondylarthropathies, it is associated with the HLA-B27 locus. The patients commonly present with a mild, asymmetric polyarthritis affecting the interphalangeal joints of the fingers and toes, although as many as 30% will eventually suffer from sacroiliitis and spondylitis. Psoriasis of the skin and nails usually precedes the arthritis, but the diagnosis is difficult to distinguish from psoriasis with seronegative rheumatoid arthritis. Physical therapy and NSAIDs are used to reduce the inflammation present in the joints.

Systemic lupus erythematosus (SLE), like rheumatoid arthritis, is a systemic condition of autoimmune etiology. It has a marked predisposition for young females, particularly black females. A number of systemic manifestations may be seen, including fever, butterfly (malar) rash, splenomegaly, pericarditis, nephritis, and polyarthritis. Arthralgias and arthritis are among the most common presenting features of SLE and nearly all patients complain of joint pains at some point during the course of illness. Progressive joint deformity is unusual in SLE. A complication of SLE is avascular necrosis (frequently involving the femoral head) that may occur because the disease predisposes to bone ischemia, or it may be a complication of systemic corticosteroid treatment. Anemia, leukopenia, and an elevated ESR are common. Antinuclear antibodies (ANAs) appear in almost all patients with SLE. The fluorescent ANA test has become the standard screening test for SLE. Treatment of the disease is related to its activity and the target organ. NSAIDs, corticosteroids, and immunosuppressive agents all are used in the treatment of lupus arthritis.

Sjögren syndrome is a chronic inflammatory disorder characterized by diminished lacrimal and salivary gland secretion (sicca complex) that results in keratoconjunctivitis and xerostomia. The most common presentation is in women over 50 years of age. This autoimmune disorder affects many organ systems and the musculoskeletal manifestations include polymyopathy, polymyositis, and polyarthritis. The sicca complex can accompany rheumatoid arthritis, SLE, systemic sclerosis, or it can exist as a primary pathologic entity with no associated disorder. Treatment is aimed at symptomatic relief and limits the damaging effects of chronic xerostomia and keratoconjunctivitis.

Osteoarthritis, often referred to as "degenerative joint disease," is the largest group of joint diseases. Most patients with osteoarthritis are over 50 years of age. There is a higher incidence in Northern European and American whites, lower in black Americans, and infrequent in Asians. Pain is the usual presenting symptom associated with stiffness of the hip, knee, or interphalangeal joints of the fingers. Symptoms start insidiously and progress over months to years. Symptoms are aggravated by exertion and relieved by rest.

The etiology of osteoarthritis is multifactorial and is actually several disorders, which results in a similar clinical picture. Although inflammation is an important component of the disease, the initiating events are not inflammatory, hence the term *osteoarthrosis*. Etiology can be divided into two groups: (1) abnormal cartilage exposed to normal stresses, and (2) normal cartilage exposed to abnormal stresses. Primary osteoarthritis or osteoarthrosis is a clinical diagnosis of exclusion; if there is no evidence of a developmental or other acquired abnormality that has disturbed the joint, it is assumed that the articular cartilage is the primary abnormality. In cases with a primary cartilage abnormality, one would expect multiple joints to be involved.

Secondary osteoarthritis occurs when the articular cartilage is initially healthy but there is a primary congenital or acquired abnormality such as developmental dysplasia, trauma, or infection (Case 3). This primary event results in increased stress or inadequate stress distribution and/or otherwise damages the cartilage, resulting in secondary accelerated deterioration of articular cartilage. Conditions predisposing to secondary osteoarthritis include (1) congenital conditions that affect epiphyseal growth and development (developmental dysplasia of the hip, slipped capital femoral epiphysis, multiple epiphyseal dysplasia; (2) structural disorders arising in childhood (Legg-Calvé-Perthes disease; tibia vara (Blount's disease); (3) trauma and associated mechanical disturbances (growth plate fractures and/or arrest, intra-articular fractures, meniscectomy, ligament disruptions and/or joint instability, malunion of long bones, massive obesity); (4) crystal deposition (uric acid, gout, calcium pyrophosphate, pseudogout); and (5) metabolic abnormalities affecting cartilage (ochronosis).

The physical signs of osteoarthritis include effusion, local tenderness, and reduced range of motion. The four radiographic signs of osteoarthritis are (1) joint space narrowing, (2) subchondral sclerosis, (3) osteophytes at the margins of the joint, and (4) cysts adjacent to the joint surface. The synovial fluid is characterized by moderate viscosity. The WBC count is low (<200 WBCs with <25% polymorphonuclear neutrophils [PMNs]); glucose and protein concentrations are equal to serum. Calcium pyrophosphate dihydrate and/or apatite crystals are seen in many osteoarthritic joint effusions.

Crystal deposition comprises a number of disease entities that result in the formation of crystals in joints, bursae, and tendons. The major crystal deposition diseases are monosodium urate (gout), calcium pyrophosphate dihydrate (pseudogout), and calcium oxalate (seen in chronic renal failure).

Gout is a disorder of nucleic acid metabolism that results in hyperuricemia and deposition of monosodium urate crystals in joints. It is seen more commonly in males, particularly between the ages of 40 and 60. Women are rarely affected before menopause. Two forms are recognized: (1) primary gout (95%) is an inherited disorder with overproduction or underexcretion of uric acid, and (2) secondary gout, which results from acquired conditions that cause uric acid overproduction (e.g., myeloproliferative disorders) or underexcretion (e.g., renal failure). Although the risk of developing gout increases with increasing levels of hyperuricemia, only a fraction of those with hyperuricemia develop gout. Factors, including trauma, intercurrent illness, increased exercise, and alcohol, may be important in triggering crystal formation. Crystal formation is temperature dependent; thus, peripheral joints are more often affected.

The presenting symptom is often pain in the first metatarsophalangeal joint (podagra) or in the ankle or wrist. Radiographs show soft tissue changes (swelling) in acute attacks, and "punched out" periarticular erosions with sclerotic borders and joint space narrowing in the chronic setting. Diagnosis is confirmed by the identification of sodium urate crystals within neutrophils and free-floating in synovial fluid. Under a polarizing microscope, these crystals are needle-shaped and negatively birefringent (appear yellow).

Treatment includes resting the affected joint and the use of NSAIDs. Patients with an established diagnosis of gout should be monitored by a rheumatologist. Acute gouty attacks can be treated with NSAIDs (particularly indomethacin), adrenocorticotropic hormone (ACTH), or colchicine. Long-term treatment of patients with recurrent gouty episodes may prevent recurrent attacks. Between attacks, attention should be given to simple measures such as losing weight, cutting out alcohol, and eliminating diuretics. Patients who are underexcretors of uric acid and have normal renal function can be managed with uricosuric drugs (such as probenecid or sulfinpyrazone) or allopurinol (a xanthine oxidase inhibitor). These drugs should never be started during an acute attack and their administration should be accompanied by an anti-inflammatory medication or colchicine; otherwise they may actually precipitate an acute attack.

Chondrocalcinosis or calcium pyroprosphate deposition disease occurs in certain metabolic disorders (including hyperparathyroidism, hypothyroidism, Wilson's disease, and hemochromatosis) that cause a critical change in ionic calcium and pyrophosphate equilibrium in cartilage. Calcium pyrophosphate crystals are deposited in the synovial fluid and in articular cartilage. The knee and other large joints are most frequently affected. Pseudogout is often confused with infection. Radiographs show fine linear calcification parallel to the joint in hyaline cartilage that is often bilateral and symmetrical. In the fibrocartilaginous menisci and discs, it produces fluffy irregular opacities. Degenerative changes are similar to those of osteoarthritis but involve unusual sites such as non-weight-bearing joints. Diagnosis is confirmed by identification of weakly positively birefringent (green), short, rhomboidal crystals of calcium pyrophosphate dihydrate that are seen in neutrophils. Treatment of pseudogout is like that of gout: rest and anti-inflammatory therapy. Intra-articular injections of steroids or yttrium-90 have been found to be successful in chronic cases.

KEY POINTS

• Rheumatoid arthritis is autoimmune disease characterized by joint inflammation due to systemic and/or circulating factors

• As determined by the American College of Rheumatology, four of seven criteria are needed to diagnose rheumatoid arthritis: (1) morning stiffness lasting at least 1 hour, (2) arthritis of three or more regions, (3) arthritis of the hands, (4) symmetric arthritis of the same joint (left and right), (5) rheumatoid nodules, (6) radiographic changes typical of rheumatoid arthritis, and (7) serum positive for rheumatoid factor

• Osteoarthritis, often referred to as degenerative joint disease, is the largest group of joint diseases

• Secondary osteoarthritis occurs when articular cartilage is initially healthy but there is a primary congenital or acquired abnormality such as development of dysplasia, trauma, or infection

• Physical signs of osteoarthritis include effusion, local tenderness, and reduced range of motion; four radiographic signs are (1) joint space narrowing, (2) subchondral sclerosis, (3) osteophytes at the margins of the joint, and (4) cysts adjacent to the joint surface

DIFFERENTIAL DIAGNOSIS

The key to generating a differential diagnosis is to remember the three major categories: (1) infectious, (2) inflammatory (rheumatoid arthritis), and (3) all other causes (trauma and osteoarthritis). It is very helpful to first try to classify arthritis into one of these three basic categories.

This is practically important because of the dramatic differences in acute treatment, especially for infection. Remember, the presentation of gout may mimic infection and vice versa. The prevalence of tuberculosis is rising, and tuberculosis can present in many ways. Opportunistic infections should be considered in immunocompromised hosts.

If acute trauma, infection, and crystalline deposition are unlikely, the diagnostic dilemma is often between rheumatoid arthritis and osteoarthritis. Table 72.1 outlines the differences between rheumatoid arthritis and osteoarthritis in clinical presentation, radiographic appearance, and laboratory studies.

KEY POINTS

• Key to generating differential diagnosis is to remember the three major categories: (1) infection, (2) inflammatory (rheumatoid arthritis), and (3) all other causes (trauma and osteoarthritis)

TREATMENT

The goals in the management of arthritis are to (1) relieve pain, (2) delay progression of disease, (3) maintain functional level, and (4) improve the functional level. Nonsurgical treatment of arthritis includes rest and/or activity modification, orthotics (splints, braces), walking assists (cane, crutch), physical and occupational therapy, oral medications such as analgesics and NSAIDs, and local injections of corticosteroids. The surgical treatment of arthritis is reserved for cases in which nonsurgical forms of management have failed. The general indication for surgical intervention is pain and subsequent loss of function. Treatment is both diagnosis and patient specific. In each individual case it is important to consider the diagnosis, patient age, patient demands and expectations, systemic health, and the presence or absence of arthritis in other joints.

The broad categories of surgical treatment are (1) debridement (synovectomy), (2) osteotomy, (3) fusion arthrodesis, and (4) arthroplasty (resection or prosthetic). In general, timely diagnosis of septic arthritis allows successful treatment with organism-specific antibiotics. Because the blood supply to the femoral head may be compromised by increased intracapsular pressure resulting from the infection, there is general agreement that septic arthritis of the hip should be treated by immediate open drainage and appropriate antibiotics. There is ongoing controversy concerning the need for surgical treatment of acute pyarthrosis in most other joints, which may be managed by repeated aspirations. Chronic joint infections may require open drainage with debridement, including synovectomy. Although this treatment may be successful in controlling the infection, the long-term prognosis for

TABLE 72.1   *Differences between rheumatoid arthritis and osteoarthritis*

	RHEUMATOID ARTHRITIS	OSTEOARTHRITIS
Symptoms		
	Multiple joints, roughly symmetric	Rarely less than 44 years of age
	Morning stiffness	Insidious onset
	Small joints (hands and feet)	Large joints frequently
	MCP and PIP joints (Bouchard's nodes)	DIP joint (Herberden's nodes)
	Hips infrequently symptomatic	
Radiographs		
	Uniform loss of joint space	Nonuniform loss of joint space
	Juxta-articular osteopenia	Subchondral sclerosis
	Marginal joint erosions	Osteophyte formation
		Subchondral cysts
Laboratory findings		
	RF+	Blood/serum studies within normal limits

Abbreviations: MCP, metacarpophalangeal; DIP, distal interphalangeal; RF, rheumatoid factor.

chronically infected joints is poor, as the articular cartilage has been irreparably damaged.

Joint debridement is indicated in cases of chronic infection and in cases with extensive or chronic noninfectious synovitis, loose bodies, and/or cartilage aberrations with mechanical symptoms (locking, catching, giving way). Arthroscopic techniques are very useful in the knee, shoulder, ankle, wrist, elbow, and, to some degree, in the hip. Open techniques are generally used in smaller joints, and often in the hip because of the anatomy and extent of the soft tissues around the hip. Examples include arthroscopic debridement of degenerated meniscal cartilage in the knee, arthroscopic debridement of rotator cuff tears, and arthroscopic removal of loose bodies in the hip. Rheumatoid synovectomies can be performed arthroscopically, although there has been some success in effecting synovectomy by injection of radioactive materials. Synovectomy at the wrist is more commonly performed with open technique.

Osteotomy is a generic term for those operations that simply cut the bone. The procedure is done to correct angular deformities and/or increase the congruency of a joint in order to improve the distribution of forces in joint loading (Case 3). The deformity or joint abnormality may be congenital (e.g., developmental dysplasia of the hip) or acquired (e.g., malunion of a long bone). Osteotomies are often named by simply using descriptive terms, such as "proximal femoral varus osteotomy." A varus osteotomy corrects a valgus deformity and vice versa.

High tibial osteotomy (HTO) (Case 3) describes an osteotomy through the proximal tibia. Although a valgus HTO (which corrects a varus deformity) is more commonly performed (Case 3), a varus HTO can be performed

to correct a valgus deformity. The basic principles of an osteotomy in the treatment of arthritis treatment are nicely illustrated by the HTO. In tibia vara (bowed leg) the anatomic alignment deformity results in a mechanical axis that passes through the medial compartment of the knee. This results in an increased load being transmitted to the medial compartment structures, including the meniscal and articular cartilage. In youth, the reparative capacity of the cartilage can keep pace with the increased stresses. However, with age, the reparative capacity of the cartilage decreases and consequently, so do the mechanical properties of the cartilage. If the stresses remain high but the repair process fails, the net results is degeneration or wearing out of the cartilage. This is seen radiographically as a narrowing or loss of the medial joint space on weight bearing films. Loss of medial compartment cartilage thickness increases the varus deformity and thus further increases the loads seen by the medial compartment, which further accelerates cartilage loss. This increasingly adverse mechanical situation can be interrupted by an HTO.

Removing a lateral based wedge of bone from the proximal tibia and closing the gap (a valgus HTO) can correct the malalignment and improve the mechanical axis of the limb (Case 3). Following this operation, stress will be shifted from the medial compartment onto the lateral compartment, where the cartilage thickness and general health are much better. It is important to recognize that the operation does not improve the poor condition of the medial cartilage. The operation simply transfers load from the worn cartilage to less worn cartilage. The operation is analogous to balancing a tire to redistribute load to the better tread.

The HTO is durable and allows the patient to perform heavy work and play sports. The 5-year result of a valgus

HTO is generally quite satisfactory. However, the most common cause of pain following an HTO is progression of degenerative arthritis in the other compartments of the knee. It is important to note that a good HTO can defer knee arthroplasty for many years (Case 3).

Fusion or *arthrodesis* is a generic term for those operations that surgically eliminate the joint and unite the adjacent bones. They are simply named for the joint involved, for example, "knee arthrodesis" or "thumb metacarpophalangeal joint arthrodesis." Although simple in concept, these operations can be technically challenging. Fusion is the preferred method of treatment for advanced arthritis if there is active infection or concern about the possibility of latent infection. In almost all circumstances, fusion is the best method of treatment for advanced arthritis of the ankle (tibiotalar joint), the hindfoot (subtalar and talonavicular joints), and the first (great toe) metatarsophalangeal joint of the foot. Fusion of the wrist is more stable and durable than wrist arthroplasty, but less functional due to loss of motion. Fusion is currently the only generally available surgical treatment for advanced arthritis of the spine (spondylarthropathy).

In young patients, preferably less than about 5 ft, 10 in. tall, fusion of the hip or knee is a good durable alternative to joint arthroplasty. Taller patients with hip or knee fusions have difficulty sitting. Many years later, a hip fusion can often be converted to a satisfactory total hip replacement. However, due to functional loss of the extensor mechanism and collateral ligaments as a result of the fusion, a knee arthrodesis generally cannot be converted to total knee replacement. Employed only as a last resort, fusion of the shoulder or elbow does not provide a good functional result.

Arthroplasty is a generic term for those operations that in some way reconstruct joint surfaces. These operations are also simply named for the joint involved, although there are a few commonly used eponyms. Sometimes the arthroplasty simply resects the arthritic joint surfaces (resection arthroplasty). In these cases, only the fibrous tissue (scar) that forms in the space is the interposed material. Primary resection arthroplasty of the hip, a Girdlestone procedure, provides a far less functional result than a hip arthrodesis and is generally done for chronic infection or because bone and/or soft tissue deficiencies do not permit arthrodesis or some other form of reconstruction. Resection arthroplasty is the preferred treatment of advanced arthritis of the small joints of the lesser toes (metatarsophalangeal and interphalangeal joints). Another category, interpositional arthroplasty, interposes some host tissue in the resection space. The choice of resection or interpositional arthroplasty is often made because there is simply no other choice. More commonly performed in the past before the availability of prosthetic joint implants, the interpositional material may be a strip of fascia lata or a tendon. Interpositional arthro-

plasty as treatment for advanced arthritis at the thumb carpometacarpal joint is commonly performed using the palmaris longus tendon as the interpositional material.

One of the most important advances in surgery over the past 50 years is *prosthetic joint arthroplasty* (total joint replacement or reconstruction, or "artificial joints"). Categorically, this technology has dramatically improved the quality of life of millions of patients worldwide. Total hip and total knee replacement surgery are two of the most consistently successful of all surgical procedures. Further, by returning patients to an independent lifestyle, they are also two of the most cost-effective.

The general indications for prosthetic joint arthroplasty are pain and associated loss of function, caused by advanced arthritis with extensive loss of articular cartilage on both sides of the joint (Cases 1 and 2). In addition, nonsurgical treatment will have failed and lesser or nonprosthetic techniques will either have been tried and failed or cannot provide a satisfactory result. Important contraindications include active local or systemic bacterial or fungal infection or a medical condition that makes the patient a poor surgical or postoperative risk.

Mostly because of differences in the applied technology, a distinction is made between small joint arthroplasty (hands and feet) and large joint arthroplasty (hip, knee, shoulder, and elbow). Small joint prostheses are generally made of silastic. Because of higher loads and/or bending forces, current large joint prostheses utilize a combination of titanium- or cobalt-based "super-alloys" and a tough plastic, ultra-high molecular weight polyethylene. These metals are preferred not only because of their strength but also because of outstanding corrosion resistance. The implant material (that which is actually implanted into or attached to the bone) is generally one of the metals, while the bearing surfaces (the actual articulating parts of the joint) have one side made of metal alloy (ceramics are often used in this application) and one side made of polyethelene (i.e., a metallic femoral head articulating against a polyethylene socket).

It is well documented that for absence of pain and long-term clinical success, large joint implants must be firmly anchored to bone with practically no relative motion between the implant and the adjacent bone. Techniques for attaching the implant to bone are generally divided into two categories: with bone cement and without bone cement. Bone cement is a self-curing acrylic (polymer), polymethylmethacrylate. At the time of surgery, a powder containing acrylic polymer granules is mixed with liquid acrylic monomer (methylmethacrylate). The resultant paste subsequently takes on a doughy consistency and, through an exothermic reaction (a chemical initiator and an accelerator are included in the mix), becomes completely solid in about 15 minutes. During this time, the cement is applied to and pressurized into the bone, and the prosthesis is inserted. The three-dimensional mechanical interlock that the cement forms with the interstices of cancellous bone anchors the implant. There is no inherent adhesive property to the cement; it functions more like a grout.

Fixation to bone can also be obtained without using cement. Two general categories describe this technology: porous ingrowth and press-fit. Bone will grow into the interstices of a metallic surface if they are of a certain size and shape. Thus, appropriate porous surfaces allow "biologic" fixation to bone. Porous ingrowth technology has been successfully developed and applied using both titanium- and cobalt-based alloys. In addition to having an appropriate surface, the prerequisites for obtaining bone ingrowth are intimate apposition of the porous surface with bone (bone does not cross gaps very well) and absence of relative motion (bone cannot hit a moving target very well). Titanium-based alloys are extremely biocompatible. Consequently, bone will grow in intimate apposition with no intervening material along a smooth titanium alloy surface (not so with cobalt-based alloys). This type of fixation is the basis of smooth or press-fit implants. It has been shown that the addition of a thin layer of hydroxyapatite improves both the rate and extent of bone apposition. Thus, many smooth titanium press-fit implants now have a hydroxyapatite coating.

Regardless of the type of fixation technology, in the case of large joint implants, initial stability (absence of relative motion) must be achieved at the time of surgery. Motion begets more motion; a loose implant will never become firmly attached to bone. A loose large joint implant is likely to be painful. Further, relative motion can mechanically remove bone and can also induce cellular processes, which resorb bone. Regardless of the type of fixation technology, maintenance of long-term implant fixation to bone is highly dependent on exacting surgical technique.

For all practical purposes, the implant materials are biocompatible when in bulk form. However, when of a small enough size to be phagocytized by a macrophage (generally on the order of $\leq 10\ \mu m$), these same materials evoke a foreign body response. The intensity of the response is a function of material composition, and the plastics appear to be more inflammatory than the metals. The intensity of the response is also a function of the number of particles (a dose-response effect) and their shape. When a macrophage has been exposed to a sufficient number of particulates, the cell enters into a heightened state of metabolism referred to as *activation*. A complex series of biochemical events ensues that includes the production and release of factors (including prostaglandins, interleukins, and matrix metalloproteinases) that are capable of either directly or indirectly effecting periprosthetic bone resorption.

Although highly successful, prosthetic joints do fail on occasion for a variety of reasons. The largest general category of failure is loosening, which can be subdivided into septic and aseptic categories. The inert prosthetic implants have no blood supply and are therefore at increased risk of infection, as is any devitalized material. Bacteria will grow on the joint implants in an adherent mode encased in a glycocalyx, which can impede detection and response by the immune system. The avascularity of the implants and the adherent mode of growth of the bacteria make eradication of infection difficult and often necessitate removal of the implants followed by a minimum of 6 weeks of organism-specific intravenous antibiotic therapy. At a later time, another prosthetic joint can be inserted in most cases. Prophylactic perioperative antibiotics have greatly reduced the incidence of deep sepsis resulting from the surgical implantation procedure to less than 1% in most series. The real risk of infection is from hematogenous spread of bacteria from another site, including the urinary tract, or cutaneous, dental, and pulmonary sources. The risk is present for the life of the patient and the implant. This presents a case for prophylactic antibiotics whenever diagnostic or therapeutic instrumentation or manipulation (i.e., dental work, bronchoscopy, colonoscopy) can create transient bacteremia.

Aspectic loosening can broadly be considered in two categories, mechanical and biologic. There is some controversy over the relative role of mechanical factors (e.g., the repetitive forces of joint loading) versus biologic factors (e.g., inflammatory cellular reactions to the particulates) in the initiation and progression of aseptic loosening. In reality, an interplay of multiple factors occurs in such complex prosthetic-biologic systems and for this reason it is difficult to separate loosening that occurs primarily as a result of mechanical forces from that which occurs primarily as a result of inflammatory response. Mechanical factors, which include stress shielding and relative motion at the implant-bone interface, as well as biologic factors (the inflammatory reaction to particulates), can cause periprosthetic bone loss. It is important to recognize that periprosthetic bone loss is a cause of loosening as well as a result.

The current limitations of prosthetic joint arthroplasty are related to the generation and release of wear particles. Wear is the removal of material, with the generation of wear particles, that occurs because of relative motions between two opposed surfaces under load. The greatest number of small particles (<1 μm in length) are composed of polyethylene and are generated from the intended motion of the articulation (i.e., the metallic femoral head moving against the polyethylene socket). Although the bulk polyethylene is essentially inert, as described above, the small polyethylene wear particles incite a foreign body inflammatory response, which can result in periprosthetic bone resorption. The rate and degree of bone resorption are related to that rate of wear of the polyethylene, which is a function of the number of loading cycles—or use of the prosthesis. Thus, similar to a set of automobile tires, the longevity of a prosthetic joint is a function of use, not time. For this reason, it is generally expected that a prosthetic joint will last 15–20 years, and possibly the rest of the patient's life, in an older and relatively inactive person. By contrast, due to the greatly increased amount of use, young and active patients have accelerated wear rates, release more polyethylene particles to the periprosthetic tissues, and have greater degrees of periprosthetic bone loss and earlier failure of the arthroplasty. For this reason, it is generally desirable to seek alternatives to arthroplasty in younger and/or more active patients and defer total joint arthroplasty as long as possible.

Materials with better wear characteristics are desirable, and this is an area of intense investigation. Regeneration or replacement with living articular cartilage is theoretically an excellent alternative to prosthetic joint replacement. There are, unfortunately, a number of practical problems, and this is also an area of intense research (Case 3).

KEY POINTS

• Surgical treatment of arthritis reserved for cases in which nonsurgical forms of management have failed; general indication for surgical intervention is pain and subsequent loss of function

• *Osteotomy* is generic term for those operations that simply cut the bone; the procedure is done to correct angular deformities and/or increase the congruency of a joint in order to improve the distribution of forces in joint loading

• *Fusion* or *arthrodesis* is generic term for those operations that surgically eliminate the joint and unite the adjacent bones

• *Arthroplastly* is generic term for those operations that in some way reconstruct joint surfaces; prosthetic joint arthroplasty (total joint replacement or reconstruction) is one of the most important advances in surgery over the past 50 years

E FOLLOW-UP

ffective follow-up of arthritis patients is based on the fact that there are currently no cures for rheumatoid arthritis and osteoarthritis. The course of these diseases is highly variable. In general, the patient's level of pain and loss of function will determine the frequency of follow-up. This principle is also applied to patients treated with nonprosthetic surgery (arthrodesis, osteotomy, resection, or interpositional arthroplasty). It is recommended that patients with prosthetic joints have annual clinical and radiographic assessments. This can allow early detection of problems such as accelerated wear, and bone resorption and/or loosening, thus allowing intervention before extensive loss of bone stock.

KEY POINTS

• Currently no cures available for rheumatoid arthritis and osteoarthritis

• Course of these diseases is highly variable

• Patient's level of pain and loss of function will determine frequency of follow-up

SUGGESTED READINGS

Goldenberg DL: Infectious arthritis: bacterial. p. 192. In Schumacher HR (ed): Primer on Rheumatic Diseases. 10th Ed. Arthritis Foundation, Atlanta, 1993

An excellent overview of infectious etiologies, presentations, and treatment.

Moskowitz RW, Howell DS, Goldberg VM: Osteoarthritis. WB Saunders, Philadelphia, 1992

For the student interested in comprehensive information on the most common type of arthritis.

Sledge DB, Harris ED, Ruddy S et al: Arthritis Surgery. WB Saunders, Philadelphia, 1994

Good overview of the spectrum of procedures useful in the surgical treatment of arthritis.

QUESTIONS

1. Plain radiographs that exhibit osteophytes, joint space narrowing, subchondral sclerosis, and cysts would best characterize which of the following?

    A. Rheumatoid arthritis.
    B. Gout.
    C. Pseudogout.
    D. Reiter syndrome.
    E. Osteoarthritis.

2. Synovial fluid analysis can yield clinically useful information. A fluid aspirate that is turbid, of low viscosity, contains more than 100,000 WBCs, 75% of which are neutrophils is most consistent with?

    A. Osteoarthritis.
    B. Gout.
    C. Rheumatoid arthritis.
    D. Bacterial arthritis.
    E. Ankylosing spondylitis.

3. Gout and pseudogout can be differentiated by the use of polarized light. Match the type of inflammatory arthritis with its characteristic crystal.

    A. Gout   1. Yellow, negatively birefringent.
    B. Pseudogout   2. Blue, positively birefringent.

(See p. 604 for answers.)

73

BONE

TUMORS

CYNTHIA M. KELLY

Bone tumors, both benign and malignant, are relatively uncommon and therefore often receive little attention. Either type may have a startling appearance on radiographs, and the patient's presentation may be relatively dramatic with pathologic fractures and/or other physical limitations or deformities.

The goals of this chapter are to (1) aid in the identification of classic signs and symptoms of bone cancer, (2) differentiate between benign and malignant tumors, (3) determine which diagnostic tests are most helpful, (4) understand the methods of treatment, and (5) identify the most common patterns of tumor spread and treatment failure.

CASE 1
KNEE PAIN (OSTEOGENIC SARCOMA)

An 18-year-old male presented to his family physician with a chief complaint of vague knee pain for approximately 4 months. He related the beginning of his complaints to an episode of minor trauma when he fell from a skateboard. Since then, he noticed a slight progression in the intensity of his complaints with the recent onset of night pain, some minor swelling, and a feeling of warmth about the knee. Initially his pain was relieved by rest and anti-inflammatory medications; however, more recently, these measures had become less effective. The right knee had increased tactile temperature without erythema or joint irritability, diffuse swelling about the medial aspect of the distal thigh that was slightly tender to palpation, and 15 degrees less flexion than the contralateral knee. The neurovascular examination of the extremity was normal. His Hct was 41%; WBC count, 5,600/mm³; and ESR, 21 mm/hr.

Orthogonal radiographs of the knee were obtained. A lesion of the medial femoral condyle that had destroyed the cortex and had a "sunburst" pattern to the matrix and the presence of a "Codman's triangle" were noted. The surrounding soft tissues appeared to be distorted and more "full" than normal. An MRI scan demonstrated an abnormal signal in the intramedullary canal of the bone, extending 14 cm proximal to the distal femoral articular surface and a large soft tissue mass that extended medially and posteriorly. The tumor did not involve the neurovascular bundle. A CT-guided biopsy showed a high grade osteosarcoma. A chest x-ray showed a possible right lower lobe peripheral nodule and subsequently, a chest CT scan failed to reveal evidence of metastatic disease in the pulmonary parenchyma.

The patient received preoperative chemotherapy and at operation the tumor and affected bone were resected en bloc. Intraoperative frozen section analysis of the margins of resection were negative for the presence of tumor and a reconstruction of the distal femur was performed. The patient's postoperative recovery was uneventful and he began early physical therapy on the second postoperative day, with knee range of motion maneuvers and muscle strengthening exercises. Histologic analysis of the tumor revealed 95% necrosis of the tumor parenchyma, and margins of resection were negative for tumor. After the wound had healed, he completed the chemotherapy protocol for the treatment of osteosarcoma.

CASE 2
KNEE PAIN
(OSTEOCHONDROMA)

A 15-year-old female presented to her basketball team trainer with a chief complaint of knee pain and a burning sensation over the lateral aspect of the knee, particularly after repetitive jumping. She also complained of the presence of a mass over the lateral aspect of her distal thigh that was mildly tender to palpation. She stated that this mass had increased in size over the previous 6 months; however, she denied any night pain or other constitutional symptoms. Her symptoms were responsive to rest, ice, and anti-inflammatory medications. A thorough family history was notable for a brother with a mass about his proximal arm and a father with a mass over the medial aspect of his proximal tibia that had been resected at 18 years of age. On examination there was a firm, mildly tender mass over the lateral aspect of the distal femur. Knee range of motion was symmetric with the contralateral side, and no ligamentous laxity was noted. A snapping sensation was noted over the lateral aspect of the knee with flexion and extension that was painful and associated with a burning sensation. There was no increased tactile temperature or joint effusion. Orthogonal radiographs were obtained as well as oblique radiographs that demonstrated a pedunculated mass intimately associated with the lateral aspect of the femur. The mass was not associated with cortical destruction or erosions. The bony trabeculae of the mass were noted to be in continuity with the trabeculae of the distal femur and the apex of the mass was at the level of the distal femoral metaphysis. In addition, a pelvic x-ray that had been obtained for minor trauma 8 months prior was available for review and demonstrated a 3-cm pedunculated lesion at the proximal portion of the femur.

Because of the location of the tumor, its steady increase in size over the prior 6 months, and its associated symptoms, resection was recommended. Resection was done and histologic analysis noted a 1-cm cartilage cap covering the end of a pedunculated mass of benign lamellar bone. Postoperatively, she had restoration of normal knee function and returned to playing basketball with no residual pain.

GENERAL CONSIDERATIONS

The basic approach to a patient with a musculoskeletal neoplasm begins with the history and physical examination. The goal is to determine a differential diagnosis, whether a biopsy is indicated, and what further treatment should be rendered. The age of the patient should be noted, as certain tumors are characteristic in certain age groups.

Bone tumors can be either benign or malignant. Many benign tumors are asymptomatic and are often discovered as an incidental finding when a diagnostic test is performed for other reasons. As a result, the true incidence of benign bone tumors is not known. Overall, primary malignant bone tumors constitute approximately 1% of all malignant lesions. The most common malignant tumor in bone is a metastatic lesion from another primary tumor. Except for multiple myeloma, osteosarcoma is the most common primary neoplasm of bone. It is estimated that there are approximately 700–800 newly diagnosed cases of osteosarcoma in the United States annually. Tumor spread of sarcomas is almost exclusively hematogenous and therefore, thorough evaluation of the pulmonary parenchyma is indicated (Case 1). Most patients who develop a malignant tumor of bone have no known risk factors. There are a few identified etiologic factors for the development of malignant tumors of bone, such as chromosomal transpositions, prior radiation exposure, and a few hereditary diseases.

Before the advent of modern chemotherapy regimens, the 5-year survival rate of patients with osteosarcoma was approximately 20% and the mainstay of surgical treatment was amputation, except for patients with lesions in expendable bones. With virtually all metastases occurring within 2 years of the surgical resection it was surmised that nearly 80% of the patients must have had circulating micrometastases at the time of surgery. Based on these observations, a trial of adjuvant chemotherapy was initiated, and a significant increase in 5-year survival was noted. Subsequently, neoadjuvant (chemotherapy given before surgery) protocols have been implemented that allow for early tumor kill and less morbid operative procedures to be performed with improved limb function postoperatively (Case 1).

KEY POINTS

- Basic approach to musculoskeletal neoplasm begins with history and physical examination

- Most common malignant tumor in bone is metastatic lesion from another primary tumor; except for multiple myeloma, osteosarcoma most common primary neoplasm of bone

- Tumor spread of sarcomas is hematogenous; thorough evaluation of pulmonary parenchyma indicated

DIAGNOSIS

Nearly 90% of patients with tumors relate the onset of their symptoms to a traumatic event (Case 1). Night pain is a traditionally classic complaint for patients with a malignancy. It is important to note whether the lesion was discovered incidently or because the patient had symptoms such as pain, a mass, or pathologic fracture. During the physical examination, attention should be given to the characteristics of the lesion, particularly size, consistency, depth, and involvement of surrounding structures (Cases 1 and 2). Tumors that are deep, more than 5 cm in diameter, firm, and fixed to surrounding tissues are more likely to be malignant.

Diagnostic tests may include routine radiographs, computed tomography (CT) scan, magnetic resonance imaging (MRI), and radionuclide scans. Laboratory studies, including complete blood count (CBC), erythrocyte sedimentation rate (ESR), calcium, phosphorus, alkaline phosphatase, and serum protein electrophoresis (SPEP) should be judiciously ordered. High quality plain radiographs should be obtained on the initial evaluation as they can provide a significant amount of pertinent information. It is important to note the location of the lesion in the bone (epiphyseal, metaphyseal, diaphyseal, proximal, or distal), which bone is involved, and whether it is eccentric, or centrally located in the bone or on the surface. The response of the bone to the tumor is also essential to note, such as periosteal reaction, cortical erosion, sclerotic borders, and fractures. It is also essential to examine the matrix of the tumor for the presence of calcifications.

If the identity of the lesion remains in question, further diagnostic studies should be obtained. A CT scan is excellent for evaluating the extent of bony involvement, particularly endosteal erosion, and for detecting the presence of calcifications. A CT scan of the chest is necessary for completion of the metastatic workup of sarcomas. MRI is useful for determining the extent of soft tissue involvement, proximity of neurovascular structures (Case 1), and the intramedullary involvement of the bone, including the presence of skip lesions. Malignant tumors "light up" on T_2-weighted images. Bone scan may be useful for identifying the presence of other distant lesions and assessing the activity of the lesion. Several processes lead to a false-negative or "cold" bone scan—multiple myeloma, lymphoma, eosinophilic granuloma, some metastatic tumors, overwhelming sepsis, and very rapidly growing lesions.

A carefully performed biopsy by a surgeon experienced in tumor surgery is the mainstay of obtaining adequate tissue for diagnosis. Alternate methods of obtaining tissue are available; however, they are more likely to be subject to sampling error. Preferably, a small incision is made in a carefully planned location and is used to obtain samples from several areas of the tumor, since many bony tumors are heterogenous, and accurate diagnosis depends on adequate sampling of the tumor. Biopsy incisions are preferably made in a location that permits subsequent wide excision at the time of definitive surgery without adding to the morbidity of the procedure or precluding a limb salvage procedure. Inappropriately performed biopsies cause or contribute to 5% of unnecessary amputations.

KEY POINTS

- Night pain classic complaint of patients with malignancy
- During physical examination, attention should be given to lesion characteristics such as size, consistency, depth, and involvement of surrounding structures

- Tumors that are deep, more than 5 cm in diameter, firm, and fixed to surrounding tissues are more likely to be malignant
- Location of lesion in the bone (epiphyseal, metaphyseal, diaphyseal, proximal, or distal) is noted, which bone involved, whether eccentric or centrally located in bone or on surface, and response of bone to tumor
- Chest CT scan necessary for completion of metastatic workup of sarcomas
- Malignant tumors "light up" on T2-weighted images
- Several processes lead to false-negative bone scan—multiple myeloma, lymphoma, eosinophilic granuloma, some metastatic tumors, overwhelming sepsis, and very rapidly growing lesions
- Carefully performed biopsy by surgeon experienced in tumor surgery is mainstay of obtaining adequate tissue for diagnosis

DIFFERENTIAL DIAGNOSIS

Combined clinical and radiologic information determines the differential diagnosis. From the history, physical examination, and interpretation of the radiographs, the physician should be able to formulate a reasonable differential diagnosis. There are conditions that can mimic musculoskeletal tumors and should be included in the differential diagnosis of these lesions. These pseudotumors include infection, hematoma, hyperparathyroidism, and myositis ossificans. Infection can radiographically appear to be an aggressive process with bony destruction and periosteal reaction and can be diagnosed based on laboratory values and culture of the affected tissues. Hematomas occur after trauma and can later organize to simulate a tumor. Myositis ossificans is an extraosseous bone formation that occurs in muscle or other soft tissues. It is usually associated with decreasing pain in time, an intact bony cortex, and radiographically, a zonal pattern. Histologic analysis reveals a central area of immature fibrous tissue that transitions to a peripheral zone of more mature bone. In osteosarcoma the opposite scenario is present, with the central bone being more mature than that in the periphery.

The following is a list of some of the more common tumors of bone, both benign and malignant (Table 73.1).

1. Osteogenic tumors (bone forming)

A. Osteoid osteoma: a benign osteoblastic lesion with a small oval or round nidus and surrounding zone of dramatically sclerotic bone in the cortex of any bone. The lesions are usually less than 1.5 cm in diameter and are classically associated with pain that is worse at night, relieved by salicylates, and exacerbated by alcohol. Patients are usually in their second or third decade. Bone scan reveals marked uptake by the lesion, and histologic analysis reveals interlacing osteoid arranged in a "meaningless tangle of numerous anastomoses." Treatment can be medical

TABLE 73.1 *Differential diagnosis of bone tumors*

Tumor	Sex	Decade	Location	Common Site	Radiograph	Treatment	Prognosis
Osteogenic (making bone)							
Osteoid osteoma	M>F	2–3	Me/D	Femur Tibia Vertebrae	<1.5-cm nidus with sclerotic rim	Excision; acetylsalicylic acid (aspirin)	Recurrence rare
Osteoblastoma	M>F	3	V	Vertebrae	>2 cm with sclerotic rim	Excision	Recurrence rare
Osteosarcoma	M>F	2–3	Me	Knee Proximal humerus	Lytic and sclerotic Codman's triangle	Radical excision	Fair
Chondrogenic (making cartilage)							
Enchondroma	M=F	2–5	D	Hands Feet	Stippled calcification; expanded cortex	Curettage and bone graft	Rare occurrence
Osteochondroma	M=F	2	Me	About the knee and humerus	Pedunculated or sessile; cartilage cap	Excision	Rare recurrence
Chondrosarcoma	M=F	3–7	Me/D	Pelvis Shoulder girdle Femur	Lytic lesion with mottled calcification; fusiform expansion	Wide excision	Fair to good
Fibrogenic							
Simple cyst	M=F	1–2	Me	Proximal humerus Femur Tibia	Lytic lesion; fallen leaf sign	Steroid injection	50% recurrence
ABC	M=F	2	Me	Femur Tibia Vertebrae	Cystic expansion; zone of rarefaction	Curettage and bone graft	15% recurrence
Fibrous cortical defect	M=F	2	Me	Distal femur Tibia	Eccentric oval lytic lesion with sclerotic margin	Observation	Good
MFH	M>F	2–7	Me/D	All bones	Lytic lesion with poor margins	Radical excision	Poor

Hematopoietic

Tumor	Sex	Age	Location	Bones	Radiographic findings	Treatment	Prognosis
Eosinophilic granuloma	M=F	1–2	D	Pelvis, Femur, Spine	Discrete lytic lesion with sharp margins, vertebrae plana	Observation, radiotherapy	Good
Myeloma	M>>F	5–7	D	Vertebrae, Bones with hematopoietic tissue	Punched out lesions, diffuse osteopenia	Chemotherapy, radiotherapy	Fair to good

Vascular

Tumor	Sex	Age	Location	Bones	Radiographic findings	Treatment	Prognosis
Hemangioma	M=F	3–7	V	Cranium, Vertebrae	Jailhouse vertebrae	Observation, radiotherapy	Good

Neurogenic

Tumor	Sex	Age	Location	Bones	Radiographic findings	Treatment	Prognosis
Chordoma	M>F	5–7	V	Sacrum, Skull	Irregular destruction with soft tissue mass	Excision	High recurrence

Other

Tumor	Sex	Age	Location	Bones	Radiographic findings	Treatment	Prognosis
Ewing's sarcoma	M>>F	1–2	D	Fibula, Femur, Pelvis	Onion skinning; lytic lesion	Excision, chemotherapy, radiotherapy	Fair
Metastasis	M=F	4–7	D/Me	Proximal bones	Lytic or blastic	Based on patient's primary tumor	Poor to fair

Abbreviations: M, male; F, female; ABC, aneurysmal bone cyst; MFH, malignant fibrous histiocytoma. D, diaphysis; Me, metaphysis; and V, vertebra.

with the use of high dose salicylates, or surgical with resection of the tumor. Incomplete removal can lead to recurrence of the lesion.

B. Osteoblastoma: a benign lesion similar in histologic appearance and clinical presentation to osteoid osteoma but usually more than 2.0 cm in diameter. These tumors have a distinct predilection for the vertebral column, particularly the posterior elements and the mandible (cementoblastoma). Patients complain of pain at the site of the tumor and may also have nerve root compression depending on the tumor location. Treatment involves curettage and bone grafting with or without cryosurgery.

C. Osteosarcoma: the most common primary bone malignancy in children and young adults; it affects males more often (Case 1). A painless mass is a frequent presentation; however, pain may be the chief complaint (Case 1). Several subtypes of osteosarcoma exist and the most common is the central osteosarcoma. Radiographically, one sees a "sunburst" appearance with radiodense areas, lucent areas, areas of permeative destruction, and soft tissue extension (Case 1). Codman's triangle, which is an area of periosteal elevation and reaction, indicates the presence of an aggressive (but not necessarily malignant) lesion. Skip lesions may be present in 20% of cases, and either bone scan or MRI is helpful in identifying these. Histologically, the hallmark of osteosarcoma is the presence of osteoid produced directly by the malignant stromal cells. Juxtacortical osteosarcomas do not communicate with the intramedual canal (in contrast to the benign osteochondroma), and usually occur in patients between 30 and 40 years old, and have a better prognosis. These include paraosteal, periosteal, and high grade surface osteosarcomas. Adjuvant chemotherapy has profoundly improved 5-year survival rates, and current operative procedures have improved limb salvage rates. In spite of amputation or limb salvage, the local recurrence rate still remains at approximately 10%.

2. Chondrogenic tumors (cartilage forming)

A. Enchondroma: a benign tumor of mature hyaline cartilage, usually located within bone. These tumors may be solitary, multiple, or associated with hemangiomas (Maffucci syndrome). Enchondromas are usually asymptomatic and can be seen in any bone but are especially seen in the tubular bones of the hands and feet. Histologically, nodules of normal hyaline cartilage with small uniform chondrocytes are seen. Malignant transformation is more likely in older patients with larger lesions (>4.5 cm) and in bones outside the hands and feet. Radiographically, the diaphyseal lesion may contain stippled calcifications, central rarefaction, and expansion of the overlying cortex. Endosteal scalloping is indicative of possible malignant transformation.

B. Osteochondroma: a benign tumor resulting from normal enchondral growth arising from the cortex of a long bone adjacent to the epiphyseal plate. The lesions may be either pedunculated or sessile. Radiographically, these prominent bony lesions lie adjacent to the epiphysis with intramedullary trabeculae of the normal bone being contiguous with those of the tumor (Case 2). A cartilage cap is present over the end of the tumor and measures 1–2 cm in thickness. Histologically, the cap resembles a disorganized epiphyseal plate consisting of hyaline cartilage. Malignant transformation to chondrosarcoma is possible and more likely in patients with multiple lesions (hereditary) and a cartilage cap more than 3 cm. Additionally, patients may complain of tumor growth. A CT scan is the most helpful diagnostic study to assess the status of the cartilage cap. Malignant and benign lesions that are problematic due to impingement or angular deformity should be excised, with care being taken not to enter the growth plate.

C. Chondrosarcoma: ranks second to osteosarcoma in prevalence of bony sarcomas, and is usually associated with dull, deep pain. Radiographs demonstrate a lytic lesion with or without a sclerotic border, endosteal scalloping, and calcifications. Histologically, increased cellularity, cellular atypia, mitotic figures, and multiple nuclei within cells are characteristic of malignant lesions. Low grade tumors can be difficult to differentiate from a benign enchondroma and careful examination by an experienced pathologist is essential. Treatment is wide local resection. Recurrence is notorious by implantation of cells at the time of resection.

3. Fibrogenic tumors

A. Simple cyst: this is also referred to as unicameral bone cyst. This occurs during growth, is located adjacent to the epiphyseal plate, and is usually asymptomatic until a pathologic fracture occurs. Radiographically, it appears as a lucent lesion with sclerotic margins and a "fallen leaf" sign if pathologic fracture is present. Histologically, numerous cell types are seen including a cuboidal cell lining, loose mesenchymal cells, giant cells, chronic inflammatory cells, macrophages, and hemosiderin. Treatment includes conservative treatment of any pathologic fracture, aspiration of the cyst, and injection with methylprednisolone after fracture healing. Curettage and bone grafting may also be performed; however, this is a procedure of larger magnitude than aspiration and steroid injection.

B. Aneurysmal bone cyst: these may occur in any bone. Radiographs reveal an expansile, eccentrically located lesion with thin septae and a thin sclerotic margin. These are blood-filled cavities and CT scan may demonstrate a fluid level within the cyst. Histologically, these tumors are characterized by giant and endothelial cells lining cystic cavities filled with red blood cells. Treatment is curettage and bone grafting.

C. Fibrous cortical defect (non-ossifying fibroma): it is the most common skeletal lesion (most are incidental findings on radiographs). This lesion is a localized defect in the cortex of long bones, usually metaphyseal, and often around the knee. These lytic lesions with sclerotic margins represent an area where bone failed to form. Microscopically, whirling fibrous tissue and smaller giant cells are present in a thin shell of reactive bone. Most lesions will ossify by 25–30 years of age and therefore management is observation alone.

D. Malignant fibrous histiocytoma: this high grade malignant tumor is often found in the metaphyses of the distal femur and proximal tibia. Radiographs reveal a lytic lesion with minimal periosteal reaction, no bone formation, and cortical disruption (histologically, spindle cells in a storiform pattern intermingle with bizarre, giant, foamy histiocytes). This tumor may be associated with Paget's disease or occur in previously irradiated tissue. The prognosis is poor, and adjuvant chemotherapy along with surgical resection is recommended.

4. Hematopoeitic tumors

A. Eosinophilic granuloma: one of the reticuloendothelioses with an unknown etiology. Radiographs are notable for a lytic "punched out" lesion in long bones and vertebrae plana in spine. Histologically, sheets of Langerhans cells and eosinophils dominate the field. Treatment consists of observation initially, and if the lesion does not spontaneously resolve, it may be treated with low dose radiation, curettage, or excision.

B. Myeloma: this is the most common primary malignant tumor of bone. This lesion represents an uncontrolled proliferation of plasma cells (B lymphocytes). Patients present with pain, anemia, a monoclonal spike on SPEP (serum protein electrophoresis), and UPEP (urine protein electrophoresis) with an elevated M spike. Radiographs reveal multiple punched out lesions (if solitary = plasmacytoma). Histologically, sheets of plasma cells are seen. A peripheral blood smear may demonstrate "roleaux" formation. Aggressive systemic therapy and radiotherapy with surgical stabilization of pathologic lesions is the treatment of choice.

5. Vascular tumors

A. Hemangioma: the most common vascular lesion of bone, it usually involves the vertebral body or skull. Radiographs reveal a typical "corduroy" or "jailhouse" pattern in the vertebrae. Histologic examination is notable for large vascular lakes lined by flattened endothelial cells. Treatment is usually observation since it is often asymptomatic; however, these tumors are radiosensitive.

6. Neurogenic tumors

A. Chordoma: this lesion arises from remnants of the notochord and is most commonly found at opposite ends of the spinal column, at the base of the skull, and in the sacrococcygeal region. Radiographic destruction of vertebrae is seen on plain radiograph and soft tissue extension is noted on additional imaging studies. Microscopically, physaliferous cells are the histologic hallmark of this tumor and are combined with vascular fibrous septae. Patients usually present late and resection is difficult because of the tumor location, therefore recurrence is common. This tumor is relatively insensitive to both chemotherapy and radiotherapy. Radiation is often used but is of limited usefulness.

7. Other tumors

A. Ewing's sarcoma: a malignancy of childhood often associated with systemic signs such as fever, weight loss, local tenderness, palpable mass, and erythema, and is therefore often confused with osteomyelitis. Radiographs reveal a radiolucency without bone formation. Often a periosteal reaction resembling onion skin is seen. Histologically, uniform sheets of small round cells are present and may at times form pseudorosettes. Special stains reveal periodic acid-Schiff (PAS) positivity as well as positive reticulum staining. Treatment with newer chemotherapeutic agents has improved survival dramatically and surgical resection is also recommended.

B. Metastatic tumors: are the most common malignancies of bone. Spread to the bone is via a hematogenous route, and therefore multiple lesions are often present. Lesions in bone occur commonly in the metaphyseal region and may progress to the point of impending or actual pathologic fracture. These should be stabilized in addition to treatment of the primary tumor. The most common primary tumors that metastasize to bone are breast, lung, kidney, prostate, and thyroid cancer. Prophylactic fixation and stabilization of impending pathologic fractures is indicated for lesions more than 2.5 cm in diameter, involving more than 50% of the cortex, or in patients having pain.

KEY POINTS

- Conditions that mimic musculoskeletal tumors should be included in differential diagnosis of these lesions; these pseudotumors include infection, hematoma, hyperparathyroidism, and myositis ossificans

- Osteoid osteoma lesions are less than 1.5 cm in diameter and classically associated with pain that is worse at night, relieved by salicylates, and exacerbated by alcohol

- Osteoblastoma is benign lesion usually more than 2.0 cm in diameter

- Osteosarcoma is most common primary bone malignancy in children and young adults, affects males more often; radiographically one sees "sunburst" appearance with radiodense areas; osteoid produced directly by malignant stromal cells; in spite of amputation or limb salvage, local recurrence rate still remains approximately 10%

- Osteochondroma is pedunculated or sessile, with intramedullary trabeculae of normal bone being contiguous with those of tumor

- Chondrosarcoma ranks second to osteosarcoma in prevalence of bony sarcomas; low grade tumors can be difficult to differentiate from benign enchondroma and careful examination by experienced pathologist is essential

- Fibrous cortical defect (nonossifying fibroma) is most common skeletal lesion, mostly incidental findings on radiograph; most lesions ossify by 25–30 years, and therefore managed by observation alone

- Malignant fibrous histiocytoma may be associated with Paget's disease or occur in previously irradiated tissue

- Myeloma is most common primary malignant tumor of bone; patients present with pain, anemia, and monoclonal spike on SPEP, and histologically, sheets of plasma cells and possibly "roleaux" formation on peripheral blood smear

- Chordoma found at base of skull and sacrococcygeal region; physaliferous cells are histologic hallmark

- In Ewing's sarcoma, periosteal reaction resembling onion skin is seen

- Metastatic tumors most common bone malignancy; most common primary tumors that metastasize to bone are breast, lung, kidney, prostate, and thyroid; prophylactic fixation and stabilization of impending pathologic fractures is indicated for lesions greater than 2.5 cm in diameter, involving over 50% of the cortex, or in patients in pain

TREATMENT

Both chemotherapy and radiotherapy have become increasingly more important in the treatment of tumors of the musculoskeletal system. Neoadjuvant (Case 1) and adjuvant (postoperative) chemotherapy have had a significant effect on the survival rate of patients with bony malignancies. Survival rates and the ability to perform limb salvage surgery have improved dramatically in the last 20 years. Five-year survival rates have increased from rates near 20% in the early 1970s to a current rate near 70%. Survival is site dependent, with certain locations having a more favorable prognosis than others. Secondary malignancies induced (rarely) by chemotherapy include leukemias and bladder and skin cancer.

Preoperative radiotherapy may be combined with operation to create a firm rind around the reactive zone and allow for less tissue resection at the time of operation. Radiotherapy is especially useful in treating round cell tumors and soft tissue tumors, but is not particularly useful in primary malignancies of bone. Postirradiation sarcoma is a recognized factor in the development of secondary malignancies and is associated with a poor prognosis.

With current surgical techniques, nearly all bones in the body can be considered "expendable" and limb salvage procedures have become more usual in recent years. There are two parallel goals in the treatment of extremity sarcomas. First and foremost is the intent to save the pa-

tient's life, and the second consideration is to save the limb. Limb preservation efforts are predicated on the ability to completely resect the tumor and preserve a limb that will function better than a prosthesis on an amputated limb.

Staging of bony tumors is based on the surgical grade, surgical site of the tumor, and the presence or absence of metastases. Enneking introduced the surgical staging system adopted by the musculoskeletal tumor society (Table 73.2).

Intracompartmental tumors are surrounded in all dimensions by natural barriers to extension. Extracompartmental tumors extend beyond natural barriers because of tumor growth or iatrogenic spread, or they may arise primarily in extracompartmental locations.

Classification of the surgical procedure is based on the plane of dissection in relation to the tumor. In intracapsular resections the incision is made through the capsule or pseudocapsule directly into the tumor. Gross tumor is left behind and the entire operative field is potentially contaminated. Marginal resections remove the entire tumor with the plane of dissection passing through the capsule or pseudocapsule and therefore, 50% of the time leave microscopic disease in the field. Wide or en bloc resection includes the tumor, the reactive zone, and a cuff of normal tissue. Radical resections are extracompartmental and remove all tissue components that contain tumor. Previously, radical resection meant an amputation; however, limb salvage surgery is now possible in most cases. If limb salvage is performed, the oncologic result must be similar to amputation and the limb function should be useful and acceptable.

Several methods are available for reconstruction of skeletal defects after tumor resection. The basis of these procedures is to replace the defect with metallic prostheses, allografts, a combination of materials, or bone transport.

TABLE 73.2   *Enneking's surgical staging system*

STAGE	GRADE	SITE
IA	Low	Intracompartmental
IB	Low	Extracompartmental
IIA	High	Intracompartmental
IIB	High	Extracompartmental
III	Metastases	

KEY POINTS

- Neoadjuvant and adjuvant chemotherapy significantly affect survival rate of patients with bony malignancies; 5-year survival rates increased from 20% in early 1970s to 70% currently

- Two parallel goals in treating extremity sarcomas: first, to save the life; second, to save the limb

- Limb preservation efforts predicated on ability to completely resect the tumor and preserve a limb that will function better than prosthesis on an amputated limb

- Classification of the surgical procedure based on plane of dissection in relation to tumor

FOLLOW-UP

Follow-up treatment for patients after having completed their entire regimen of adjuvant therapies includes physical therapy to restore limb function and evaluation of areas at risk of disease recurrence. These measures focus primarily on the pulmonary system and the area of tumor resection to rule out pulmonary metastases and local recurrence respectively. CT scans are particularly sensitive for assessment of the pulmonary parenchyma and are ordered at regular intervals (every 6 months for 5 years). Physical examination of the area of tumor resection and plain radiographs are usually sufficient for evaluation of local recurrence. In the case of abnormal findings an MRI is often indicated for further diagnostic evaluation. Screening laboratory tests generally prove not to be particularly informative, even in patients with recurrence of disease. Local recurrence rate of tumor is approximmately 10% when performed by a skilled, knowledgeable surgeon. Rates of metastatic spread to the lungs varies with the grade of the tumor, with higher grade tumors having higher rates of spread (≤30% in grade III tumors).

KEY POINTS

- CT scans sensitive for assessment of pulmonary parenchyma; ordered at 6-month intervals for 5 years

- Physical examination of tumor resection and plain radiographs usually suffice for evaluation of local recurrence

- In cases of abnormal findings, MRI indicated for further diagnostic evaluation

SUGGESTED READINGS

Miller MD: Orthopaedic Pathology, Review of Orthopaedics. WB Saunders, Philadelphia, 1992

Basic review of orthopaedic oncology.

American Academy of Orthopaedic Surgeons: Orthopaedic Knowledge Update 4, 1993

A current overview of orthopaedic oncology.

Simon MA, Biermann JS: Biopsy of bone and soft tissue lesions. J Bone Joint Surg Am 75: 611, 1993

A review of biopsy techniques and histologic examination.

Simon MA, Finn HA: Diagnostic strategy for bone and soft-tissue tumors. J Bone Joint Surg Am 75:622, 1993

A pertinent article discussing diagnostic strategies for musculoskeletal tumors.

QUESTIONS

1. *The most common bone tumor is?*
    A. Multiple myeloma.
    B. Osteosarcoma.
    C. Chondrosarcoma.
    D. Fibrous cortical defect.
    E. Metastatic.

2. *Appropriate evaluation of a suspected malignant bone tumor may include?*
    A. MRI scan of the area.
    B. CT scan of the chest.
    C. Excisional biopsy.
    D. Angiography.
    E. All of the above.

(See p. 604 for answers.)

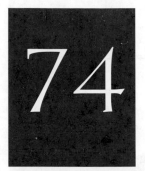

74

ORTHOPAEDIC

TRAUMA

DANIEL ZINAR

Musculoskeletal trauma can be divided into two main groups. First is the patient with an isolated musculoskeletal injury such as a fracture of the tibia. The second type is the musculoskeletal injury that presents as part of a polytraumatized patient, such as the patient who suffers a pelvic fracture and femur fracture in a motor vehicle accident. These two types of patients must be treated differently. The rationale and explanation for the specific treatment of each of these types of orthopaedic trauma are

often poorly understood. The aims of this chapter are to elucidate (1) the correct method of evaluating the patient with a musculoskeletal injury, either monotrauma or polytrauma, (2) the difference between initial and definitive management of the orthopaedic trauma patient, (3) the complications associated with both types of patients with orthopaedic injuries, (4) available treatment options for patients with orthopaedic trauma, and (5) the basic principles in the management of open fractures.

CASE 1
LOWER LEG PAIN, SWELLING, AND DEFORMITY

A 22-year-old Hispanic female presented to the emergency room with complaints of left leg pain, swelling, and deformity following a twisting injury during a collision in a soccer game. The injury occurred 2 hours before her arrival in the emergency room. She was brought to the hospital by her friends, who had placed her leg in a homemade cardboard splint. She denied any other injuries suffered in this accident. There was no history of prior trauma to this leg. Physical examination was significant for

diffuse swelling of the leg, with a circumferential measurement of the leg demonstrating 3 cm of increased size as compared to the opposite leg. A moderate amount of ecchymosis was present about the anteromedial aspect of the tibia. There was an obvious deformity of the leg, with the lower portion externally rotated. The injured leg was about 1 cm shorter than the uninjured leg. The pulses and motor and sensory neurologic evaluation were normal.

Radiographs of the lower leg revealed a comminuted fracture of the tibia and fibula at the middle one-third of the bones. Significant displacement was noted at the fracture site, with about 1 cm of shortening. Radiographs of the knee and ankle revealed no other injuries.

The patient was counseled regarding options, and a treatment plan was discussed. Initially, after intravenous sedation as well as a local anesthetic block, a closed manipulation and reduction was performed. A long leg cast was applied, and repeat radiographs demonstrated satisfactory angular alignment, correction of prior rotational deformity, and only 5 mm of limb shortening. The patient was admitted to the hospital for observation because of the significant swelling that had been present. After 24 hours, she was discharged home with crutches, having maintained a normal neurovascular examination. The patient returned for a follow-up visit 3 days and again 1 week after her injury. Repeat radiographs at each visit revealed preservation of her alignment. She was seen at weekly intervals during the next month until the 4-week mark, when she was placed into a below knee tibial fracture brace. Radiographs were taken every 3–4 weeks as an outpatient. The patient began partial weight bearing at the 6-week mark, and progressed to full weight bearing over the next 2–3 months. Radiographs demonstrated healing of the fracture with bridging callus after 4 months. Clinical examination revealed no tenderness of motion at the fracture site.

CASE 2
MULTIPLE ORTHOPAEDIC INJURIES

A 59-year-old white male was driving under the influence of alcohol when he lost control of his car and was thrown over an embankment. He was brought into the hospital by paramedics, who found him conscious at the scene with stable vital signs. On arrival in the emergency room, he complained of pain in the right leg, lower abdomen, and left wrist. He had no other complaints, other than slight numbness in the left index finger and thumb. After evaluation by the trauma service, he was cleared of any other systemic injuries. Physical examination showed tenderness and swelling over the suprapubic area; pain, swelling, and deformity of the right thigh; and obvious deformity with localized tenderness at the left wrist. The neurovascular examination was normal except for decreased sensation to pinprick in the region of the median nerve of the left hand.

Laboratory studies revealed an Hct of 39.5%, which, when repeated 1 hour later, was 35.0%. Radiographs revealed a pelvic fracture with diastasis of 5 cm at the pubic symphysis. In addition, a midshaft femur fracture was seen with about 3 cm of shortening, and a displaced fracture of the distal radius was identified. A cystourethrogram was performed and no urologic injury was noted. A CT scan of the pelvis showed no evidence of posterior pelvic instability.

The patient had placement of a sugar tong splint on the left upper extremity fracture and was counseled regarding treatment options. He was brought to the operating room within 24 hours and underwent uneventful intramedullary rodding of the right femur fracture, open reduction/internal fixation of the pubic symphysis diastasis, and closed reduction and percutaneous pinning of the left distal radial fracture. The patient remained hemodynamically stable both intraoperatively and postoperatively. The patient was sitting upright in bed on postoperative day 1 and was seen by physical therapy for gait training with crutches on postoperative day 3. Resolution of his paresthesias in the left hand had occurred by the time of his discharge home on day 7.

GENERAL CONSIDERATIONS

Musculoskeletal trauma is the number one cause of lost work time in the United States. It is also the leading cause of death in the 20–40 year age range. Most musculoskeletal injuries are isolated and do not involve polytraumatized patients. The wide spectrum of possible orthopaedic injuries can involve any age range from infant to geriatric patient. The mechanism of injury is vital to the assessment of the patient. Injuries are often separated into low energy versus high energy injuries. Athletic injuries are for the most part considered to be of the low energy variety, but still may be quite severe. High speed motor vehicle, motorcycle, or pedestrian-versus-auto accidents make up most high energy orthopaedic injuries. Equally important is that over 70% of orthopaedic trauma patients in the emergency room have either alcohol or drugs as a contributing etiologic factor to their accident (Case 2). Despite advances in preventative measures such as motorcycle helmets, more attention is still given to methods of treating orthopaedic injuries after they occur than to preventative measures. Use of protective athletic equipment, seatbelts, and airbags are examples of some progress that has been made.

Long bone fractures (i.e., femur, tibia, and humerus) usually occur as a result of direct trauma. A bending, twisting, or axial loading force is usually responsible for creating the fracture. The amount of energy imparted to the traumatized area is responsible for the magnitude of the injury. A highly comminuted (>2 fracture fragments) fracture or open fracture usually implies a higher level of energy responsible for the trauma. A fracture is just part of a severe soft tissue injury that involves the bone. The significant swelling and ecchymosis in the limb of both cases presented is just as significant as is the bony injury. The amount of deformity present after a fracture is directly related to the amount of soft tissue injury (i.e., muscle and ligamentous damage, periosteal stripping, neurovascular injury). The degree of soft tissue injury may be significant, leading to the development of a compartment syndrome. The higher the energy of injury, the higher the likelihood of significant bleeding that can lead to a compartment syndrome.

The amount of soft tissue damage present in an orthopaedic injury greatly influences the type of treatment and management. Low energy injuries such as the tibial fracture (Case 1) with less soft tissue damage are more likely to be treated nonoperatively, with a splint or casts. Higher energy injuries such as the motor vehicle accident (Case 2) with more severe soft tissue damage are more often unstable and require operative stabilization with either internal or external fixation.

The presence of fractures in the multiply injured patient requires a more aggressive approach in the management of pelvic, spine, and femur fractures. All of these injuries, if not stabilized early, can result in mandatory bed rest for the patient, with a concomitant increase in mortality and morbidity secondary to pulmonary complications. Extremity injuries, such as a distal radius fracture in a polytrauma patient, do not require the same level of aggressiveness because a delay in stabilization does not affect the patient systemically. The patient can still be mobilized in a splint or cast with any fracture other than the spine, pelvis, or femur.

DIAGNOSIS

The diagnosis of most musculoskeletal trauma requires a careful history with regards to the mechanism of injury, a detailed physical examination focusing on the injured area, and appropriate radiographs. The history will alert the physician as to the seriousness of the injury, as well as to the need to focus or generalize the musculoskeletal examination. The diagnoses of the orthopaedic injuries in both cases is fairly apparent. As a general rule in any extremity injury, the physician must rule out the presence of an injury to the joint above as well as the joint below the injury by both clinical and radiographic examination. When the diagnosis of tibia fracture (Case 1) is made, radiographs and clinical examination must include the knee and ankle joint.

The diagnosis of the spectrum of injuries suffered in a multiply traumatized patient presents a more complex problem. After a routine musculoskeletal examination is done, the patient should be carefully re-examined 24–48 hours after the initial injury, to rule out the presence of a more subtle or minor injury. More trivial but ultimately functionally significant injuries may be overlooked initially, especially closed upper extremity injuries of the hand, forearm, and shoulder, as well as ligamentous injuries to the knee.

The diagnosis of a displaced, partially unstable pelvic fracture should alert the physician to perform other diagnostic tests, including a computed tomography (CT) scan to examine the posterior integrity of the pelvis as well as inlet and outlet oblique radiographs. Diastasis of the public symphysis greater than 5 cm is often associated with disruption of posterior pelvic anatomy. With significant anterior pelvic disruption, routine urologic evaluation with a cystourethrogram is recommended before Foley catheter insertion.

KEY POINTS

• As a general rule in any extremity injury, the physician must rule out the presence of an injury to the joint above, as well as the joint below the injury, by both clinical and radiographic examination

DIFFERENTIAL DIAGNOSIS

Severe swelling due to bleeding within an enclosed fascial space may occur after any significant trauma to an extremity. Although the tibia fracture (Case 1) occurred with a low energy mechanism of injury, the comminution and significant displacement of the fracture, along with the clinical findings of ecchymosis and swelling, should be viewed with a high level of suspicion for development of a compartment syndrome. This is a clinical diagnosis that is made in the presence of unremitting pain and tense swelling, despite adequate fracture immobilization. Since a compartment syndrome is an easily treated entity by means of a fasciotomy, its presence or absence should always be in the differential diagnosis of major extremity trauma. Compartment syndromes can exist even in the presence of open fractures, because not all fascial spaces are decompressed with open fractures.

The presence of a fracture must alert the examiner to ensure that the fracture is closed as opposed to open. Open fractures require immediate attention because of the significant risk of infection. The treatment protocol for open fractures includes (1) intravenous antibiotics, (2) operative debridement of devitalized bone and soft tissue, with irrigation to reduce contamination, (3) skeletal stabilization with internal or external fixation, (4) aggressive soft tissue coverage, and (5) early limb rehabilitation. Open fractures are classified according to the system of Gustilo. Grade I is considered a lower energy injury with a soft tissue wound usually less than 1 cm; grade II involves a higher energy with either further fracture comminution or a wound greater than 1 cm; grade III injuries are subdivided into IIIA, IIIB, and IIIC. All grade III injuries are high energy injuries, with type A involving large soft tissue flaps with periosteal stripping; type B requiring soft tissue coverage with a local or free muscle flap; and type C requiring arterial vascular reconstruction.

Abdominal, urologic, and neurologic sequelae of displaced pelvic fractures should always be included in the differential diagnosis. In the hemodynamically unstable patient, a supraumbilical diagnostic peritoneal lavage should be performed to rule out significant intra-abdominal bleeding. Careful neurologic examination must be done to document any lumbosacral plexus injury that may occur with displaced posterior pelvic structures. A multidisciplinary approach is necessary in these patients. In addition, complete examination of the perineal area must be done to evaluate for the possibility of an open pelvic fracture. Rectal and vaginal examination is mandatory in order to exclude a tear or perforation.

TREATMENT

The goal of fracture treatment is restoration of function. Having diagnosed a fracture of the midshaft of the tibia and fibula (Case 1), what information is needed to make a decision regarding management? The initial displacement of the fracture, the condition of the soft tissue, and the functional demands of the patient should all be considered in treating any long bone fracture. The decision to use cast treatment rather than internal or external fixation operative treatment in Case 1 was made based on the results of the closed reduction. Acceptable alignment of a fractured long bone is individualized depending on the particular fracture being treated. For the tibia, less than 1 cm of shortening, less than 5 degrees of angulation, and less than 10 degrees of malrotation is acceptable. If the fracture had not maintained alignment within these limits, surgical stabilization with an internal plate or rod versus external fixation would have been necessary. Many patients are unable to tolerate cast treatment because of the length of time needed for limb immobilization. Joint stiffness can occur in any area after prolonged immobilization. The decision of what type of definitive treatment to be used should be made within the first 7–10 days after the injury in order to expedite return to full function. Operative treatment has the advantage of earlier restoration of function with the added (minimal) risk of infection. All risks and benefits of each treatment should be discussed with the patient before deciding the management course.

Femoral fracture treatment in the adult is noncontroversial. Intramedullary nailing is the preferred method in both the isolated and polytrauma patient (Case 2). This is a low risk, safe, and effective procedure that allows the patient to be mobilized early and return to normal function. Traction treatment or cast immobilization are not recommended for adult femoral fractures because of the long healing time of 3–4 months, and the limitation of the patient's return to normal function. Prompt treatment of all fractures whenever possible is preferred, especially in the multiply injured patient whose fractures of the spine, pelvis, or femur would otherwise confine them to bed rest. The combination of the supine, bedridden patient whose chest is horizontal has been shown to lead to an increase in pulmonary complications in the polytrauma setting, including pulmonary emboli.

Pelvic fracture treatment is based on stability. Fractures that are stable to both vertical and rotation forces (type A) can be treated without surgery. Partially stable fractures (type B) (Case 2) may do better after surgical stabilization because they decrease pain by limiting fracture motion, decrease bleeding, and restore the normal anatomy. Completely unstable fractures (type C) (i.e., with both rotation and vertical instability) require stabilization in order to restore fracture stability and normal function. The timing of surgery depends on the condition of the patient. The concern with most unstable pelvic fractures is the risk of hemorrhage due to venous injury in the posterior pelvis. Surgical skeletal stabilization can be done emergently to assist in the resuscitation of the patient by closing the pelvic volume and reducing the hemorrhage. In the hypotensive trauma patient this is best done with external fixation. The patient in Case 2 was hemodynamically stable at the time of arrival so internal fixation could be performed as *definitive* pelvic stabilization. Polytrauma

patients should have the majority of their musculoskeletal injuries stabilized within the first 24 hours. A well-resuscitated trauma patient is usually in the best state of health at the time of admission. Isolated musculoskeletal injuries do not require the same degree of aggressiveness.

The distal radius fracture (Case 2) differs from the other injuries in that it represents an intra-articular fracture. These fractures require exact alignment of the articular portion of the fracture within 1–2 mm. The same treatment options exist: casting, external fixation, and internal fixation. This decision depends on the fracture stability, the condition of the soft tissue of the limb, and individual surgeon experience. The particular fracture in Case 2 was treated with closed reduction and percutaneous internal fixation.

KEY POINTS

- Initial displacement of the fracture, condition of the soft tissue, and functional demands of the patient should all be considered in treating any long bone fracture

- Concern with most unstable pelvic fractures is risk of hemorrhage due to venous injury in the posterior pelvis; surgical skeletal stabilization can be done emergently to assist in the resuscitation of the patient by closing the pelvic volume and reducing the hemorrhage

- Polytrauma patients should have the majority of their musculoskeletal injuries stabilized within the first 24 hours; a well-resuscitated trauma patient is usually in the best state of health at the time of admission

---

E FOLLOW-UP

Effective postoperative follow-up requires an understanding of the average healing time of most fractures. Although most fractures may be healed in 3–5 months, it may take up to 1 year for full functional recovery. Intra-articular fractures require at least 2 years' minimum follow-up to see whether any post-traumatic arthritis will develop. Patients can expect functional improvement for up to 2 years following most fractures. Radiographs should be taken at monthly intervals for the first 3 months and then every 6–12 months for 2 years. At each visit an assessment of functional recovery should be measured by recording the range of motion of adjacent joints, muscle strength, and the level of function—both work and recreational. Despite appropriate management of fractures, some patients may never regain full function because of irreversible damage to soft tissues (muscle, tendon, ligament, and cartilage).

KEY POINTS

- Intra-articular fractures require at least 2 years' minimum follow-up to see whether any post-traumatic arthritis will develop

- At each visit an assessment of functional recovery should be measured by recording range of motion of adjacent joints, muscle strength, and level of function—both work and recreational; despite appropriate management of fractures, some patients may never regain full function because of irreversible damage to soft tissues (muscle, tendon, ligament, and cartilage)

SUGGESTED READINGS

Bone L, Johnson K, Weigelt J et al: Early versus delayed femoral fracture stabilization: a prospective randomized study. J Bone Joint Surg Am 71:336, 1989

Multiply injured patients with femoral shaft fractures have a lower mortality and morbidity if their fractures are stabilized within the first 24 hours of injury.

Ghanayem A, Wilber J, Lieberman J, Matta A: The effect of laparatomy and external fixation stabilization on pelvic volume in an unstable pelvic injury. J Trauma 38:3, 1995

Demonstrates the effect of reducing the pelvic volume by placement of an external fixation device, which in turn can reduce hemorrhage.

Gustilo RB, Anderson JT: Prevention of infection in the treatment of 1,025 open fractures of long bones: retrospective and prospective analysis. J Bone Joint Surg Am 58:453, 1976

Outlines the classification system of open fractures, and a protocol of management to reduce complications.

QUESTIONS

1. *Early repair of fractures may?*
   A. Improve pulmonary function.
   B. Be dictated by the patients' hemodynamic status.
   C. Allow improved functional outcome.
   D. Be performed by external or internal fixation.
   E. All of the above.

2. *Pelvic fractures?*
   A. Usually require urgent operation.
   B. Require body casting and prolonged bed rest.
   C. May be associated with significant hemorrhage.
   D. Make evaluation of the abdomen with open peritoneal lavage mandatory.
   E. All of the above.

(See p. 604 for answers.)

75 PROSTATE DISEASE

MARK S. LITWIN

GERHARD J. FUCHS

JACOB RAJFER

The prostate is a doughnut-shaped, walnut-sized gland situated on the male pelvic floor just below the bladder (Fig. 75.1). The urethra passes through the center of the prostate, as it conducts urine down into the penis for elimination. In the postpubertal male, the prostate and nearby seminal vesicles are responsible for generating and expressing semen, the carrier fluid that bathes and nourishes spermatozoa after ejaculation. After the fertility years are over, the prostate continues to secrete semen, but its physiologic usefulness diminishes. As the male ages, the prostate grows and may become a source of morbidity or mortality. This chapter discusses the basic elements of diagnosis and treatment for the two most common pathologic conditions of the prostate: prostate cancer and benign prostatic hyperplasia.

CASE 1
PROSTATIC CARCINOMA

An asymptomatic 66-year-old black male was found on digital rectal examination to have a 1-cm firm nodule in the left lobe of his prostate. He had stable mild essential hypertension. He took one baby aspirin per day as prophylaxis against heart attacks. His father and a maternal uncle had died of prostate cancer in their early 70s. The patient claimed normal erections and had full urinary continence. His serum PSA was 9.2 ng/dl and Hct was 43%.

A transrectal ultrasound-guided prostate needle biopsy was performed after discontinuation of aspirin for 10 days, 24 hours of prophylactic antibiotics, and a cleansing enema. The biopsy revealed a Gleason 3 + 2 adenocarcinoma confined to the left lobe. Chest x-ray and nuclear bone scan were normal.

The patient elected to undergo nerve-sparing radical retropubic prostatectomy with bilateral pelvic lymph node dissection. He tolerated the operation without incident and recovered uneventfully. Pathology examination showed that the entire left lobe of the prostate was replaced by a Gleason 3 + 2 adenocarcinoma with 2 small foci of tumor in the right lobe as well. The lymph nodes and seminal vesicles were free of tumor. Although he suffered from temporary stress urinary incontinence, within 6 months he was completely dry and had experienced return of his erectile function.

CASE 2
BENIGN PROSTATIC HYPERPLASIA

A 73-year-old male was seen for a 1-year history of progressive obstructive voiding symptoms. He complained of hesitancy in initiating his stream, decreased flow, intermit-

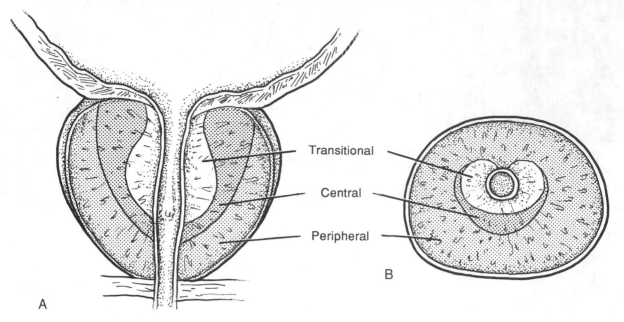

FIGURE 75.1   *Normal prostate. (**A**) Coronal section. (**B**) Transverse section.*

tency of his stream, a sensation of incomplete emptying, and nocturia three times per night. Digital rectal examination revealed an enlarged prostate.

The serum PSA was 2.8 ng/dl. Uroflowmetry revealed a maximum flow rate of 6.6 ml/sec, with an average flow of 4.5 ml/sec and a total voided volume of 230 ml. Postvoid residual measured by bladder ultrasound was 70 ml. His AUA symptom score was 24/35.

The patient chose to try an oral 5_α-reductase inhibitor; however, after 7 months he had experienced only minimal improvement in his symptoms. He therefore elected to undergo TURP under spinal anesthesia. He tolerated the procedure well and experienced a dramatic improvement in urinary symptoms. At a follow-up visit 12 weeks after surgery, his symptom score was 6/35, and he was pleased with the results.

GENERAL CONSIDERATIONS

Prostate cancer is the most common malignancy and the second most common cause of cancer death in American males. Its incidence increases with advancing age. In autopsy studies, up to 60% of men over 60 years old have been shown to have prostate cancer, although it was often subclinical during life. Prostate cancer is two to three times more common and more lethal in black men than in white men. There also appears to be a hereditary component. Although its cause is unknown, its incidence may be enhanced by a high fat, low fiber diet. Most prostate cancers are asymptomatic (Case 1). Almost all prostate malignancies are adenocarcinomas arising from the glandular lining of the prostatic ducts. At the time of initial diagno-

sis, 60% are organ-confined and 40% have evidence of regional or distant spread. In the past, most prostate cancers were identified on routine rectal examinations; however, the popularity in recent years of prostate-specific antigen (PSA) as a screening tool has led to an increase in the diagnosis of prostate cancer based on elevated PSA alone. The value of population-based screening for prostate cancer is highly controversial; however, the American Cancer Society currently recommends annual digital rectal examinations beginning at age 50 for most men and at age 40 in blacks, or if there is a paternal or maternal family history of prostate cancer.

Prostate cancer is often indolent, with many men living for years after the diagnosis. Some prostate cancers are more aggressive and, if left untreated, will lead to early death. The challenge in treating this malignancy is to discern which patients need therapy and which do not.

Benign prostatic hyperplasia (BPH) is a nonmalignant condition in which progressive enlargement of the prostate can cause bothersome urinary symptoms (Fig. 75.2). Although BPH also affects older men and may occur simultaneously with prostate cancer, there is no known causal relationship between the two. BPH leads to obstructive voiding symptoms (Case 2) simply by blocking urine flow from the bladder to the outer urethra. As the prostate grows larger, the bladder works harder, and the obstructive symptoms worsen. In some cases the prostatic urethra may become completely obstructed, causing acute urinary retention. Prostate enlargement is very common in older men. It may or may not cause functional impairment, and this impairment may or may not be bothersome to each individual. Both function and bother must be considered when evaluating patients and recommending therapy.

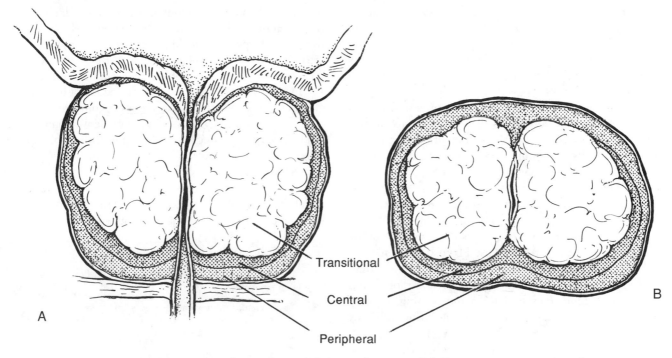

Transitional

Central

Peripheral

A

B

FIGURE 75.2 *Benign prostatic hyperplasia. (**A**) Coronal section. (**B**) Transverse section. Note the greatly hypertrophied central or periurethral component, and the corresponding decrease in urethral cross-sectional area.*

KEY POINTS

• Prostate cancer is two to three times more common and more lethal in black men than in white men

• Most prostate cancers are asymptomatic

• Prostate cancer is often indolent, with many men living for years after the diagnosis

• Both function and bother must be considered when evaluating patients and recommending therapy

DIAGNOSIS

Prostate cancer can only be definitively diagnosed by tissue biopsy. Usual indications for prostate biopsy are palpation of a suspicious firm nodule on rectal examination (Case 1), or elevation of the PSA. Typically, biopsy is performed as an outpatient procedure with transrectal ultrasound guidance. A spring-loaded, Tru-cut needle is passed through the ultrasound probe into the prostate gland and several cores of tissue are removed. If there is no obvious palpable or ultrasonographic lesion, then several random tissue samples are taken. Prostate biopsy carries a minimal risk of morbidity and is very well tolerated without anesthesia. Occasionally, patients require small intravenous doses of a tranquilizer. The primary risks are bleeding and infection; patients are asked to avoid aspirin-containing

products or anticoagulants for several days before the biopsy. Many urologists also prescribe prophylactic antibiotics and a cleansing rectal enema (Case 1).

The pathologist measures the volume of cancer present in the biopsy specimen and determines the grade of the tumor. The Gleason grade ranges from 1 (well differentiated) to 5 (anaplastic). Each tumor is given two scores, one for its most common and one for its second most common area of cytologic appearance. Hence, the total Gleason score ranges from 2–10 and is usually presented as both individual scores separated by a plus sign (Case 1).

Before therapy can begin, tumors must be stratified as organ confined or metastatic. Staging workup begins with a digital examination to determine whether the tumor extends outside the prostate. It also includes a chest x-ray and whole body nuclear scintigraphy bone scan, since bone is the most common site of spread. A PSA level of 4–8 is mildly elevated, above 8 is clearly abnormal, and above 50 is strongly suggestive of metastasis. Serum acid phosphatase measurement is also used to identify metastatic cases. Cancers are clinically staged as A (incidental without palpable abnormality), B (palpable but confined to the prostate), C (extending locally outside the prostate), and D (metastatic to lymph nodes, bone, or other organs). BPH is diagnosed with a combination of subjective and objective measures. The American Urologic Association (AUA) symptom scale comprises seven questions that are answered by the patient and each is scored from 0–5.

They are then summed into a total AUA symptom score that ranges from 0–35 (Case 2). The higher the score, the more severe are the symptoms. Patients must also be asked how bothered they are by their symptoms, since this may vary tremendously from patient to patient. Objective measures include uroflowmetry, in which the patient urinates into a computerized funnel that records volume and flow rate. An average flow of less than 15 ml/sec usually indicates obstruction (Case 2). Measurement of the postvoid residual urine by ultrasound or catheterization provides objective evidence of how well the patient empties his bladder. The prostate size is estimated by digital rectal examination but can be more accurately measured with transrectal ultrasound. Intravenous pyelography (IVP) is sometimes used to demonstrate upper tract dilatation or deviation of the distal ureters caused by prostatic enlargement. Cystourethroscopy can also be helpful by providing direct visualization of the obstructing prostate lobes and the strained bladder muscle. Urodynamic testing, a highly technical set of pressure measurements at different places in the bladder, prostate, urethra, and rectum, is sometimes required to quantify the degree of obstruction (Case 2). Objective findings must be correlated with subjective complaints, since the latter drives therapy decisions.

KEY POINTS

- BPH is diagnosed with a combination of subjective and objective measures
- Objective findings must be correlated with subjective complaints, since the latter drives therapy decisions

DIFFERENTIAL DIAGNOSIS

Suspicion of prostate cancer is raised when there is a prostate nodule or a PSA elevation. Hence, differential diagnosis includes other conditions that cause these findings. Prostatitis can cause significant elevations in the PSA, despite the absence of malignancy. Chronic prostatitis can also lead to calcifications that are palpated rectally and may be confused with malignant nodules. BPH can cause PSA elevations or asymmetric hyperplastic nodules in the prostate that may feel suspicious to the novice finger. Severe BPH can also cause acute prostatic infarctions that produce pain and elevation in the PSA or acid phosphatase. Rectal masses are usually not confused with prostate masses. Since prostate cancer usually causes no symptoms, other diagnoses must be suspected when the patient presents with specific complaints. Nevertheless, malignancy must be considered and addressed when any older man seeks urologic evaluation. Ultimately, prostate biopsy is the definitive test in correctly diagnosing prostate cancer.

BPH must be differentiated from other causes of obstructive bladder symptoms. The most common nonprosta-

tic cause is hypotonic bladder, a condition in which the detrusor muscle fails to contract and adequately express all the urine. Hypotonic bladder can cause symptoms of decreased flow that are similar to those of BPH. Another common cause of urinary symptoms that can be confused with BPH is prostatitis. Inflammation or infection of the prostate gland can lead to irritative voiding symptoms that must be carefully differentiated from their obstructive counterparts before therapy is undertaken. Other causes of voiding symptoms include urethral strictures, obstructing bladder calculi, posterior urethral valves in young boys, and rare benign urethral polyps. Age is an important clue in the differential diagnosis of BPH. The younger the patient, the less likely he is to have significant prostatic enlargement.

KEY POINTS

- Prostatitis can cause significant elevations in PSA, despite absence of malignancy
- Prostate cancer usually causes no symptoms

TREATMENT

Currently, prostate cancer treatment is highly controversial. Many physicians fervently believe that because of its usual indolence, prostate cancer requires no direct intervention. Others believe with equal conviction that these tumors must be treated. Therapy is directed at the gland itself in organ-confined disease, and systemically in metastatic disease. In clinically localized tumors, the three options are radical prostatectomy, external beam irradiation, or observation. In younger men or those who have a greater than 10-year life expectancy, operation is indicated. In older men or those who are not good surgical candidates, radiation is most appropriate. Observational follow-up, although controversial in the United States, has been used successfully in Europe, especially in cases in which the tumor grade is not very threatening or when life expectancy is less than the projected survival due to the cancer. Carefully considered treatment decisions must include attention to quality of life as well as survival, and must ultimately be made by the patient.

Radical prostatectomy is usually carried out through a midline suprapubic incision (or occasionally via a perineal approach). The external iliac lymph nodes are sampled to exclude regional spread. If these pelvic nodes are free of tumor, prostatectomy is performed. Otherwise, it is aborted and the patient is treated systemically for metastatic disease. Since the gland is precariously situated between the bladder and the urethra, care must be taken to identify and preserve the anatomic structures that are adjacent to the prostate. These include the neurovascular bundles (lateral) that control penile erection, the urethral sphincter (caudal) that provides the continence mechanism, and the rectum (posterior). The prostatic urethra and seminal vesicles are excised with the gland, and a direct sutured anastomosis reconnects the bladder with the urethra (Fig. 75.3). A closed suction drain protects the anastomosis for several postoperative days, and a urethral catheter is left indwelling for 3 weeks. Most patients experience temporary stress urinary incontinence for several months following surgery (Case 1). Some patients may have persistent problems with urine leakage; others may develop anastamotic strictures that require dilatation. Although ejaculation is not possible after radical prostatectomy, erection and orgasm may be maintained following a nerve-sparing operation. Depending on age and level of preoperative sexual function, patients may experience erectile impotence due to nerve damage during operation. Rectal injury is uncommon and usually repaired primarily at the time of surgery.

Pelvic irradiation may be administered by external beam over the course of several weeks, or with radioactive seeds that are surgically implanted in the prostate gland. Either method is effective at delivering a dose adequate to kill cancer cells. Side effects of radiation are similar to those of surgery, although they are less frequent. Radiation proctitis, cystitis, or dermatitis may cause annoying symptoms; however, they are usually temporary.

Observational follow-up includes regular checkups, measurement of PSA and acid phosphatase levels, and bone scans to identify local or metastatic extension. Symptoms are treated as they arise.

The mainstay of therapy for metastatic prostate cancer is testosterone ablation. Huggins won the Nobel Prize in Medicine for identifying the hormonal dependency of prostate cancer cells (a finding he published in 1941). Testosterone ablation may be accomplished by bilateral orchiectomy, injectable agents that interrupt the hypothalamic-pituitary-gonadal axis, or oral antiandrogens. These are often used in combination.

BPH may be treated with operation, medications, or watchful waiting, depending primarily on the patient's wishes. The historic gold standard therapy for BPH is transurethral resection of the prostate (TURP) (Case 2), an endoscopic procedure in which the central core of the gland is chipped away with an electrocautery loop (Fig. 75.4). Care must be taken not to damage the urethral sphincter, which is located just caudal to the prostate. The prostatic urethra, removed during TURP, spontaneously regenerates within 2 weeks. Since the bladder neck is also resected during TURP, patients generally experience permanent retrograde ejaculation following the procedure. Erection and orgasm are not affected. When the prostate is not large enough to warrant TURP, symptomatic improvement may be obtained by endoscopically incising the prostate (TUIP). If the gland is too large to be adequately resected transurethrally, a simple open prostatectomy may be performed. In this operation, the prostatic capsule is left intact and the adenomatous central portion shelled out. Results from this approach are usually dramatic.

Nonsurgical therapies have recently become the initial treatment of choice for many men with BPH. Oral α-blockers, usually terazosin or prazosin, may be used to relax the smooth muscle found inside the prostate and bladder neck. These drugs may cause dizziness in some men. Alternatively, the 5_α-reductase inhibitor, finasteride, can be used to shrink the size of the prostate gland by blocking the stimulatory effects of androgens (Case 2). It usually takes several months to work and must be continued for life. The only significant side effects of finasteride are decreases in libido, ejaculatory volume, and PSA level. For some patients, these agents provide adequate symptomatic relief and have the advantage of avoiding the risks of operation and anesthesia.

Watchful waiting is appropriate in men who are not terribly bothered by their symptoms, not good surgical candidates, or unable to take any of the oral medications. Patients in chronic urinary retention, for whom surgical and medical therapies are unsuccessful or inappropriate, may be managed with bladder catheterization (intermittent or indwelling).

> ### KEY POINTS
>
> - Prostate cancer treatment is highly controversial
> - In clinically localized tumors, the three options are radical prostatectomy, external beam irradiation, or observation
> - Mainstay of therapy for metastatic prostate cancer is testosterone ablation
> - BPH may be treated with operation, medications, or watchful waiting, depending primarily on the patient's wishes

FOLLOW-UP

Prostate cancer patients are seen every several months following treatment. PSA levels are invaluable in detecting recurrence or progression of disease. PSA should be undetectable following prostatectomy and very low following irradiation. Postsurgical and postirradiation patients must also be evaluated for urinary incontinence and erectile dysfunction. If the patient desires, he can receive effective treatment for either complication. If metastatic disease is detected at any point, the patient is offered hormonal therapy (surgical or medical), continued observation, or in certain cases, irradiation to the prostate fossa. Focal irradiation is also used to treat bone pain arising from metastatic lesions.

BPH patients are followed with careful attention to their symptoms and the degree of bother they experience. Regardless of whether patients opt for operation, medications, or watchful waiting, the AUA symptom score is a useful way to quantify the subjective phenomena associated with BPH. Interval uroflowmetry and measurement

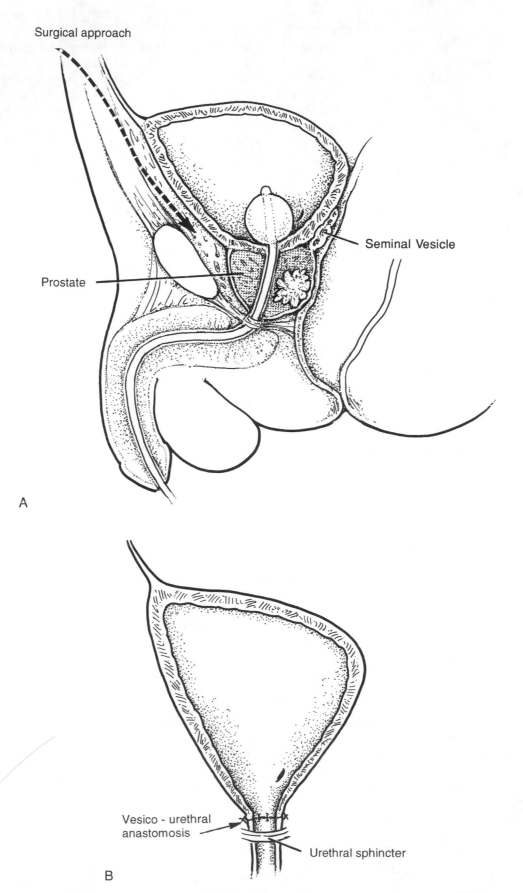

Surgical approach

Seminal Vesicle

Prostate

A

Vesico - urethral
anastomosis

Urethral sphincter

B

FIGURE 75.3 *(A) Prostate cancer is preferably diagnosed at an asymptomatic stage. (B) Open prosta-tectomy restabilizes genitourinary continuity and function.*

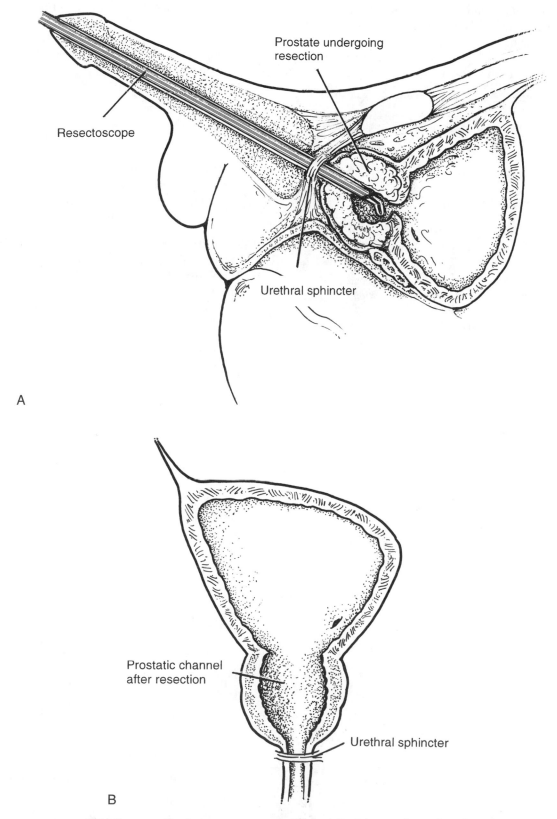

FIGURE 75.4 *(A) Transurethral resection prostatectomy (TURP) is performed with cystoscopic guidance. (B) Following succesful TURP, the obstruction to flow is eliminated.*

of the postvoid bladder residual may also be used (Case 2). Digital rectal examination and PSA screening are also performed at regular intervals to increase the likelihood of diagnosing early stage prostate cancer.

> **KEY POINTS**
>
> • PSA levels are invaluable in detecting recurrence or progression of prostate cancer
>
> • PSA should be undetectable following prostatectomy and very low following irradiation

SUGGESTED READINGS

Chute C, Panser L, Girman C et al: The prevalence of prostatism: a population-based survey of urinary symptoms. J Urol 150;85, 1993

An easy to read documentation of the epidemiology of prostatic obstructive symptoms in the adult population.

Gittes R: Carcinoma of the prostate. N Engl J Med 324:236, 1991

This thorough review succinctly summarizes the current state of basic science and clinical knowledge in the field of prostate cancer.

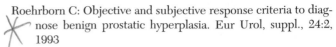

Roehrborn C: Objective and subjective response criteria to diagnose benign prostatic hyperplasia. Eur Urol, suppl., 24:2, 1993

This article concisely summarizes the diagnostic evaluation and therapeutic interventions for men with obstructive voiding symptoms.

QUESTIONS

1. *BPH?*
   A. Is a precursor of prostate cancer.
   B. Requires surgical treatment.
   C. May be treated with radiotherapy.
   D. May be effectively treated with an α-blocker.

2. *Prostate cancer?*
   A. May spread to bone.
   B. May spread to iliac lymph nodes.
   C. May be asymptomatic.
   D. Can be treated with hormonal therapy.
   E. All of the above.

(See p. 604 for answers.)

76

NEPHROLITHIASIS AND OBSTRUCTION

GERHARD J. FUCHS

MARK S. LITWIN

JACOB RAJFER

Urolithiasis accounts for approximately 30% of all urologic emergency room admissions and clinic visits in the United States. Due to the disabling, acute onset of severe abdominal colicky pain with nausea and vomiting, the diagnosis of urolithiasis is often made in the emergency room setting.

Nephrolithiasis usually occurs in the third to fifth decade of life and is a common cause of time lost from work. Prior to the advent of minimally invasive treatment techniques in the early 1980s, including extracorporeal shock wave lithotripsy (ESWL) and endoscopic stone surgery, open surgery of kidney and ureteral stones or "blind" (i.e., under fluoroscopic control, not observed through an endoscope) basketing of ureteral stones were the only treatment options. Since the mid-1980s, most patients are treated without resorting to open surgery, thereby greatly reducing stone-related morbidity, time lost from work, and overall stone-related costs to society.

CASE 1
URETERAL STONE WITH HYDRONEPHROSIS

A 24-year-old white male was admitted to the emergency room with acute onset of severe right-sided colicky flank pain and nausea. He vomited once at home 1 hour after dinner and took two over-the-counter painkillers that did not bring any relief. He had no fever or chills. He had regular bowel movements until the afternoon of his admission and reported no voiding symptoms. There was no history of prior operations, his medical history was unremarkable, and there was no familial history of stone disease. Physical examination showed an otherwise healthy 24-year-old with right flank tenderness, no rebound tenderness, and hypoactive bowel sounds. His vital signs were normal. His urinalysis had 5 RBC/HPF and pH of 6.5. A plain abdominal x-ray showed a 7-mm calcification adjacent to the lateral process of L3 on the right side. A significant amount of abdominal gas overlay the renal shadows. He was presumed to have a right ureteral stone. A right renal ultrasound showed a normal sized kidney with normal parenchyma. Hydronephrosis grade III (out of IV) was seen and no stones were identified in the kidney or proximal ureter. An IV catheter was started and he was then given 75 mg of Demerol and 25 mg IM of Vistaril, which relieved his pain within the next 30 minutes. In the pain-free interval, an IVP confirmed the presence of a partially obstructing right ureteral stone with gross hydronephrosis. He remained asymptomatic after the IVP study and was discharged taking oral pain medications and advised to report to the urology clinic the following morning.

The following day, after discussion of the treatment options of conservative management versus interventional therapy, the patient opted for a trial with conservative management of fluid challenge and oral pain medication as needed. He was instructed to return to the clinic in case of unremitting pain and/or a fever of greater than 38.6°C. Otherwise, he was to return in 2 weeks time to review his progress and the degree of ureteral obstruction. Over the ensuing 2 weeks, he had three more severe pain attacks that responded to the oral pain medication, and he was seen once at an outside emergency room where he received intramuscular pain medication. At his 2-week follow-up, the KUB x-ray showed the stone in the same position at the level of L3 and ultrasound again showed hydronephrosis grade III. Since there was no progress in his status despite the repeated pain attacks, interventional therapy was begun. The patient underwent cystoscopic manipulation of the stone with repositioning of the stone into the kidney pelvis followed by ESWL under the same epidural anesthesia. Due to the amount of ureteral edema, an indwelling ureteral stent was placed. At posttreatment follow-up 2 weeks after the procedure, the patient appeared to be stone-free by KUB and ultrasound, and the hydronephrosis had resolved. The ureteral stent was removed in the office under topical anesthesia. Analysis of the patient's stone showed pure calcium oxalate monohydrate. Since this was his first stone incident with no obvious risk factors, no metabolic workup was performed. He was advised to modify his fluid intake (6 oz/hr) and avoid dehydration.

CASE 2
PYELONEPHRITIS SECONDARY TO STAGHORN STONE

A 46-year-old female with a temperature of 39.7°C, and general malaise was seen by her internist. She had a history of 1 year of intermitent dull left-sided flank discomfort, and three episodes of bladder infections that were treated with oral antibiotics. She related that she had dull flank pain for the past 2 weeks and a low grade temperature of 38°C. She had regular gynecologic examinations, the last of which was 3 weeks previous and normal. Her urinalysis revealed 80 WBC/HPF, 10 RBC/HPF, and pH 7.0; her Hct was 36%; WBC count, 16,000/mm³; creatinine level, 1.5 g/dl; BUN, 20 mg/dl. A KUB x-ray showed a complete staghorn stone of the left kidney filling all renal calyces. Urine and blood cultures were obtained and the patient was admitted to the hospital with a diagnosis of pyelonephritis secondary to left renal staghorn stone. An

intravenous line was started and antibiotics given. She defervesced and an IVP study showed equal excretion of contrast bilaterally and no obstruction. The urine culture grew *Pseudomonas*, sensitive to ciprofloxacin, and she was discharged the following morning taking the antibiotic. Three weeks later, she underwent percutaneous endoscopic stone removal of 80% of her stone burden, including all stone parts from the lower calyceal group, the renal pelvis, and parts of the upper calyceal group. A nephrostomy tube was left in place. The patient was discharged from the hospital on postoperative day 2 with oral antibiotics. She returned 1 week later as an outpatient and the remainder of the stone was fragmented using ESWL under intravenous sedation and analgesia. The patient was discharged the same day. Ten days later, a nephrostogram was obtained confirming patency of the ureter and unimpaired drainage of contrast into the bladder. The nephrostomy tube was clamped and removed 2 days later. Four weeks later, a KUB x-ray and renal ultrasound did not show any residual fragments and there was no evidence of infection.

GENERAL CONSIDERATIONS

Most patients with stones present with unilateral severe flank pain of sudden onset (Case 1). Macro- or microhematuria is present in the majority of cases (Cases 1 and 2). There is a 3:1 predominance of male patients, with female patients being more prone to infection-induced stones; females have a higher incidence of urinary tract infections (UTIs) because of a shorter urethra. The etiology of stone formation in the urinary tract is not completely understood. The most common explanation for stone formation is the concomitant presence of three major parameters, namely, urine supersaturation with stone forming crystals (e.g., calcium oxalate, uric acid, cystine), deficiency of urinary inhibitors such as citrate, and formation of matrix, a mucoprotein that binds calcium. Genetic factors such as certain enzyme defects (in cystinuria, renal tubular acidosis, uric acid) are rare causes of stone formation. However, in these patients, onset of stone disease is usually at a relatively young age and often leads to renal insufficiency.

The most commonly found stones are of calcium oxalate composition (70%) caused by supersaturation of the urine with calcium (Case 1). This is secondary to increased calcium absorption from the bowel (such as seen with high doses of vitamin D, sarcoidosis, and hyperparathyroidism), increased calcium resorption from bone (such as in immobilization and hyperparathyroidism), or high urine calcium concentrations due to a renal "leak" (such as in renal tubular acidosis and congenitally). Another common cause of the formation of calcium stones is a high concentration of oxalate in the urine (hyperoxaluria) from dietary sources (vegetarian diet) or hyperabsorption from the colon and terminal ileum in patients whose status is postintestinal bypass for management of obesity or patients suffering from Crohn's disease. Uric stones are found in 15% of patients and are caused by high urine concentration of uric acid in the presence of acidic urine and low urine volumes. Contributing factors are a diet high in purine, myeloproliferative disorders, and gout. Infection-induced struvite stones are found in approximately 15% of patients, mostly in females (Case 2). These are found concomitant with UTIs caused by urea-splitting bacteria (proteus). Urea-splitting bacteria produce urease, which in turn splits urea into ammonia, thus raising the urinary pH value. This causes lower solubility of ammonium, magnesium, and phosphate in the urine, thus precipitating ammonium-magnesium-phosphate to form stones (struvite). Less frequent are cystine stones (1%) and matrix stones (<1%).

KEY POINTS

- Urolithiasis accounts for 30% of all urologic emergency room admissions and clinic visits

- Because of acute onset of severe abdominal colicky pain with nausea and vomiting, diagnosis made in emergency room

- Common cause of time lost from work

- Patients with stones present with unilateral severe flank pain of sudden onset, and macro- or microhematuria present in majoriy of cases

- Stones form from urine supersaturation with stone forming crystals, deficiency of urinary inhibitors such as citrate, and formation of matrix (mucoprotein that binds calcium); most commonly found stones are of calcium oxalate composition (70%), caused by supersaturation of urine with calcium, secondary to increased calcium absorption from the bowel, increased calcium resorption from bone, or high urine calcium concentrations due to renal "leak"

- Calcium stones also caused by high concentration of oxalate in urine (hyperoxaluria) from dietary sources or hyperabsorption from colon and terminal ileum

- Uric stones found in 15% of patients and caused by high urine concentration of uric acid in presence of acidic urine and low urine volumes

- Infection-induced struvite stones found in 15% of patients, mostly females, caused by urea-splitting bacteria (proteus)

DIAGNOSIS

The examination of the acutely symptomatic patient includes a history and physical examination (vital signs, temperature, abdominal examination), plain abdominal x-ray (kidney-ureter-bladder [KUB]) and ultrasound, blood work (complete blood count, creatinine, blood urea nitrogen, uric acid, urinalysis, and urine culture and sensitivity.

These basic tests will allow the diagnosis or exclusion of urinary stones in the majority of cases. The KUB x-ray will show radiopaque stones in approximately 80–90% of cases (Cases 1 and 2). The renal ultrasound will give important information on renal anatomy showing renal stones (including radiolucent stones) and/or hydronephrosis as an indication of ureteral obstruction. If a stone is identified with KUB and/or ultrasound, an intravenous pyelogram (IVP) study is not required immediately. With the patient in acute ureteral colic, the added diuretic fluid load of the IVP medium may cause forniceal renal rupture and extravasation of urine. Secondly, the quality of an IVP study obtained during an acute renal colic is usually poor because of abdominal gas (paralytic ileus) overlying the shadows of the urinary tract. It is prudent to postpone the IVP study until the pain-free interval, and after appropriate bowel preparation. Also, before an IVP study, one should rule out renal failure and ask whether the patient is allergic to the contrast medium.

Urinalysis will reveal hematuria in almost all cases of symptomatic stones. Pyuria and presence of bacteria suggest UTI, and urine should then be sent for culture and sensitivity testing. The urine pH will give further clues as to the chemical composition of the stone. An acid pH of 5 is found with uric acid stones and cystine stones. An alkali pH of 7.5 and higher suggests an infection-induced struvite stone.

Flank pain, an elevated temperature (>38.6°C), leukocytosis, and a urine specimen containing white blood cells and bacteria hold the possibility of pyelonephritis. If ureteral obstruction is present in this setting, this represents a urologic emergency since urosepsis or pyonephrosis are immediate risks.

When the patient is oliguric/anuric or allergic to contrast media, a cystoscopy and retrograde pyelogram should be performed to assess the course of the ureter, identify the cause of obstruction, and establish ureteral drainage by cystoscopic insertion of an indwelling ureteral stent. If the patient is allergic to the IVP contrast medium, non-ionic contrast can also be used. There is no established role in the diagnosis of suspected urinary stone disease for computed tomography (CT) scans or magnetic resonance imaging (MRI) studies. These imaging modalities are costly and do not add significantly to the information necessary to establish a diagnosis.

KEY POINTS

- Examination includes history, physical examination, plain abdominal x-ray and ultrasound, blood work, urinalysis, and urine culture and sensitivity; basic tests allow diagnosis or exclusion of urinary stones in most cases

- KUB x-ray shows radiopaque stones in 80–90% of cases

- Renal ultrasound shows renal stones (including radiolucent stones) and/or hydronephrosis as indication of ureteral obstruction

- Urinalysis reveals hematuria in cases of symptomatic stones; pyuria and presence of bacteria suggest UTI, and urine should be sent for culture and sensitivity testing

- Flank pain, temperature above 38.6°C, leukocytosis, urine specimen with clumps of white blood cells indicate pyelonephritis; if ureteral obstruction present, is urologic emergency, since urosepsis or pyonephrosis are risks

- In patient who is oliguric/anuric or allergic to contrast media, cystoscopy and retrograde pyelogram should be performed to assess course of ureter, identify obstruction, and establish drainage by cystoscopic insertion of indwelling ureteral stent

DIFFERENTIAL DIAGNOSIS

Any other cause of acute severe abdominal pain, especially unilaterally severe pain with or without nausea and vomiting, needs to be considered when evaluating the patient with presumed stone disease. It is imperative to rule out potentially life-threatening acute abdominal disease (viscus perforation, peritonitis, aortic aneurysm) before labeling a patient as having "only stone disease" and administering pain medication. Using the above-described diagnostic workup, stone disease as the cause of abdominal pain should be readily diagnosed or ruled out within the first 20–30 minutes of a patient's presentation. If this basic examination does not reveal any pathology of the urinary tract, other causes for the patient's pain need to be evaluated. This includes the gamut of differential diagnoses of the acute abdomen. When the pain is predominantly in the right upper quadrant, the more common differential diagnoses are biliary colic, acute cholecystitis, hepatic abscess, pleurisy or pneumonia, peptic ulcer disease, subphrenic or subhepatic abscess, obstructive and inflammatory disease of the ascending and transverse colon, appendicitis of a retrocecal appendix, pancreatitis, myocardial infarction, pulmonary embolism, and dissecting thoracic aneurysm.

In the right lower quadrant, the main differential diagnoses are appendicitis, endometriosis, ectopic pregnancy (ruptured), pelvic inflammatory disease, mittelschmerz, salpingitis, torsion of an ovarian cyst, obstructive and inflammatory disease of the ascending colon, aortic aneurysm, and hip pain (referred).

In the left upper quadrant, the main differential diagnoses include gastritis, pancreatitis, peptic ulcer disease, pericarditis and pleurisy, splenic rupture or infarct, and dissecting aneurysm of the thoracic aorta.

In the left lower quadrant, diverticulitis, obstructive colon disease, aortic aneurysm, referred hip pain, and female organ pathology need to be considered.

TREATMENT

Therapy of stone disease depends on the presenting symptoms as well as the stone characteristics. Stones associated with ureteral obstruction and infection are urologic emergencies and need immediate treatment with removal of the obstruction and broad spectrum antibiotic therapy. All other stones can be treated according to specific stone characteristics such as location, burden, composition, anatomic and functional status of the urinary tract, and concomitant disease.

Ureteral obstruction by a stone (or other cause, see Ch. 21) associated with UTI is an indication for immediate urologic intervention to prevent urosepsis (Case 2). Antibiotic treatment alone will not suffice in treating this condition, since the obstructed kidney may not excrete the antibiotic into the obstructed "dead space" urine. Even if the antibiotic is excreted into the dead space, the patient is at risk of succumbing to toxic shock syndrome secondary to production of toxins. Therefore, it is imperative to remove the obstruction from the kidney by means of bypassing the obstacle (stone) with a ureteral catheter of sufficient caliber or placement of a percutaneous renal drainage tube. An indwelling ureteral drainage stent may be placed via the cystoscope (under fluoroscopy control) with the patient under intravenous sedation and local anesthesia. A percutaneous renal drainage tube is usually placed by the uroradiologist in the radiology suite under intravenous sedation and local anesthesia. Once the patient has defervesced and the infection is appropriately treated, the underlying stone can be addressed following the principles of elective stone treatment. The major determinants of the treatment choice for elective stone treatment are location, burden, composition, and anatomy and physiology of the upper urinary tract.

Stones located in the course of the ureter measuring 5 mm or less have a 90% chance of passing spontaneously. Stones larger than 9 mm have a less than 10% chance of passing spontaneously. Therefore, if the symptoms of pain are intermittent and not disabling, stones smaller than 5 mm are treated conservatively with fluid challenge, pain management, and observation. Stones between 5 mm and 9 mm in size are also managed with expectant waiting (Case 1) if consecutive pain episodes are productive (i.e., stone migrating toward the bladder is documented on serial plain abdominal x-rays). Stones causing disabling pain, progressive obstruction, or those that show no migration despite recurrent pain episodes are treated with minimally invasive therapy (i.e., either ureteroscopic fragmentation and removal or with ESWL [Case 1]). Ureteroscopy utilizes small caliber endoscopes that can be advanced into the ureteric orifice and up the ureter to the level of the stone under direct vision (the endoscope is usually connected to a video camera). The stone can then be removed using a small grasping device or, if the stone is lodged in the ureteral wall, it is fragmented using electrohydraulic, ultrasonic, laser, or pneumatic energy. In experienced hands, success rates with ureteroscopy vary from 100% in the distal ureter below the pelvic brim to 90% in the proximal ureter.

ESWL utilizes shockwave energy to noninvasively fragment stones in the kidney (or ureter). The device consists of a shockwave source, focusing device, and x-ray and/or ultrasound localization. The shockwave is generated outside the body in a semiellipsoid brass cylinder and focused onto the stone inside the body using x-ray (fluoroscopy) or ultrasound equipment. The stone is then broken by repeated shockwave exposures (500–3,000) and the resulting stone fragments are excreted with the urine. Most patients with renal stones can be treated with ESWL (Cases 1 and 2). The current range of indications include approximately 70% of nonselected urinary stone patients. An additional 25% of patients with more complex stones in the upper urinary tract can receive treatment with the lithotriptor when combining the method with endourologic procedures (Case 2).

Approximately 70% of nonselected stone patients are eligible for ESWL monotherapy (Table 76.1). This group includes patients with single and multiple stones (added stone mass of <2.5 cm) in the kidney, selected ureteral stones above the iliac crest (after successful repositioning into the kidney); and staghorn stones that are filling a nondilated collecting system (in the absence of internal

TABLE 76.1 *Treatment of urinary calculi*

SIZE OF STONE	MODALITY OF CHOICE
Nonstaghorn stone	
<1.5 cm	ESWL
1.5–2.5 cm	ESWL (± double-J stent)
>2.5 cm	PCN
Staghorn stone	PCN (± ESWL)
	Open surgery
Ureteral stone	
Proximal ureter	In situ ESWL
	Push back + ESWL
	(bypass stenting + ESWL)
	Ureteroscopy
Distal ureter	Ureteroscopy (ESWL)

Abbreviations: ESWL, extracorporeal shockwave lithotripsy; PCN, percutaneous nephrostomy.

stenosis or dilatation). The remainder of patients present with more complex stone disease (larger stone burdens or anatomic abnormalities that may preclude proper passage of stone debris), or with stones that need auxiliary procedures to maximize the advantage of ESWL). The latter group includes radiolucent and small semiopaque stones that need to be made visible by use of contrast medium, as they cannot be primarily identified on standard fluoroscopy (with the exception of ultrasound-based localization lithotripsy). Success rates with ESWL in the ureter are between 60% and 90%. Therefore, the treatment of choice at dedicated stone centers with experience in all treatment modalities is ureteroscopic removal of ureteral stones rather than ESWL treatment.

For staghorn stones, different treatment strategies are used depending on user bias (monotherapy with ESWL versus the combined treatment of endourologic procedures and subsequent ESWL). Success with ESWL of kidney stones is dependent on (1) the overall stone burden in the kidney, (2) the shape of the renal collecting system, (3) the architecture of the dependent calyces, and (4) stone composition.

Based on these criteria, the following guidelines for the treatment of staghorn stones have been established at our institution. In partial and complete staghorn stones, monotherapy with ESWL (in conjunction with the use of indwelling ureteral catheters) is only preferable to percutaneous surgery in cases where the stone is filling a nondilated collecting system. A planned, staged ESWL procedure is a treatment option in staghorn stones that are filling a slightly dilated collecting system. It must be pointed out, however, that with increasing stone burden, the complication rates of second sessions and follow-up complications are considerably higher than those encountered with smaller stones. Also, the period of stone passage is significantly prolonged compared with percutaneous stone surgery or combination therapy. Auxiliary procedures, namely percutaneous nephrostomy tube placement and ureteroscopic ureteral manipulations, are required in approximately 70% of patients after the ESWL treatment of large branched stones (Case 2). Thus, in staghorn stones with (1) a large stone mass filling a dilated renal collecting system, and (2) with intrarenal anatomic alterations, a percutaneous procedure is performed first for debulking the stone. In a second session, ESWL is employed for the disintegration of the remaining calyceal stone parts, and under the same anesthesia, the patient undergoes a second percutaneous procedure for removal of the stone gravel. Although inherently more invasive than monotherapy with ESWL, this approach is of great benefit for the patient with regard to stone-free rates, hospitalizations, and time lost from work.

Open surgery is rarely indicated (1–2%) in the state-of-the-art management of urinary stones. Severe anatomic abnormalities that cannot be corrected endoscopically or laparoscopically, such as multiple intrarenal or long ureteral strictures, are the only remaining indications for open surgery at experienced centers.

Most procedures for treatment of urinary stones are performed in an outpatient setting. Patients undergo procedures under epidural anesthesia (60%), general anesthesia (30%), or intravenous sedation and analgesia (10%). Perioperative antibiotics (e.g., ampicillin and gentamicin) are administered on-call to the operating theater in all patients undergoing endoscopic instrumentation and in those patients undergoing an ESWL procedure who have a history of previous UTI. After surgery, patients recover in the surgical recovery room and are discharged from the outpatient surgical unit after they have voided spontaneously. Admission to the hospital is routine in patients undergoing percutaneous renal surgery (average hospital stay is less than 2 days) or for the management of concomitant medical disease as preoperatively determined. Unplanned admissions from the recovery room or the outpatient surgical unit are rare exceptions (<2%). Pain management is the usual reason for unplanned hospital admission.

KEY POINTS

• Stones associated with ureteral obstruction and infection are urologic emergencies and require immmediate relief of obstruction and broad spectrum antibiotic therapy

• Other stones treated according to stone characteristics such as location, burden, composition, anatomic and functional status of urinary tract, and concomitant disease

• Antibiotic treatment not enough to treat ureteral obstruction, because kidney may not excrete antibiotic into dead space urine; imperative to remove obstruction by means of bypassing stone with ureteral catheter or placement of percutaneous renal drainage tube

• Major determinants of elective stone treatment are location, burden, composition, and anatomy and physiology of upper urinary tract

• Stones smaller than 5 mm treated conservatively with fluid challenge, pain management, and observation

• Stones causing disabling pain, progressive obstruction, or those that show no migration despite recurrent pain episodes are treated with minimally invasive therapy

• Current range of indications for ESWL include approximately 70% of nonselected urinary stone patients; additional 25% of patients with more complex stones in upper urinary tract can receive treatment with lithotriptor, in combination with endourologic procedures

• Open surgery rarely indicated (1–2%) in state-of-the-art management of urinary stones

• Most procedures for urinary stones done in outpatient setting

• Unplanned admissions from recovery room or outpatient surgical unit rare exceptions (<2%), usually for pain management

FOLLOW-UP

Patients undergoing endoscopic surgery are discharged with oral antibiotics for 5 days (e.g. Bactrim DS by mouth twice a day) and pain medications (e.g., Tylenol 3, 1–2 tablets by mouth, as needed for pain). Patients undergoing ESWL treatment without ureteral manipulation and without a history of UTI do not require routine postoperative antibiotic coverage. Patients are usually seen 1 week postoperatively after uncomplicated ureteroscopy for a KUB and possible stent removal, or after 2 weeks following either ESWL treatment or percutaneous surgery for the assessment of the status of residual stone debris and the possible removal of ureteral/renal drainage stents. Patients with residual stone debris are seen at individualized intervals until either all stone debris has passed or only a small and clinically insignificant amount is present (usually residing in a lower pole renal calyx). Routine stone metaphylaxis in a first-time stone former stresses the importance of avoiding dehydration by increasing fluid intake to 6 oz per waking hour. The rate of stone recurrence in a nonselected group of patients having had a first stone incident is approximately 10%/yr for a maximum of 70% over a 10-year observation period. A metabolic stone evaluation is performed for all patients with recurrent stone disease.

KEY POINTS

• Patients with residual stone debris are seen at individualized intervals until either all stone debris has passed or only clinically insignificant amount is present

SUGGESTED READINGS

Eisenberger F, Miller K, Rassweiler J (ed): Stone Therapy in Urology. Thieme Medical Publishers, New York, 1991
Hanno P, Wein A (ed): A Clinical Manual of Urology. Appleton-Century-Crofts, E. Norwalk, CT, 1986

QUESTIONS

1. *Nephrolithiasis?*
    A. Is most commonly due to calcium oxalate supersaturation.
    B. In females is usually due to infection.
    C. Requires an IVP for diagnosis.
    D. Is often due to uric acid stones when the urine pH is more than 7.5.

2. *Options for removing ureteral stones include?*
    A. Ureteroscopic retrieval.
    B. ESWL
    C. Combined endoscopic and lithotripsy management.
    D. Open surgical treatment.
    E. All of the above.

(See p. 604 for answers.)

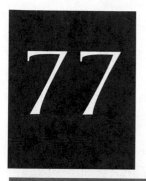

77

UROLOGIC

NEOPLASMS

MARK S. LITWIN

GERHARD J. FUCHS

JACOB RAJFER

Urologic malignancies are most amenable to treatment if they are identified early. Diagnosis and treatment is based on the organ of origin. This chapter focuses on three common forms of genitourinary cancer: bladder, kidney, and testis.

Primary bladder malignancies are usually papillary transitional cell carcinomas (TCCs) that arise from the urothelial lining. They are associated with cigarette smoking and certain occupational chemical exposures. They are easily diagnosed and are almost always endoscopically accessible.

Primary renal cell carcinomas are adenocarcinomas that arise from the proximal tubule cells of the kidney and replace renal parenchyma as they grow. TCCs of the renal pelvis and ureter are not covered in this chapter but follow the same general principles as those of the bladder.

Testis cancer, although relatively rare, is the most common solid tumor in men between the ages of 18 and 35. It is one of the most curable malignancies. A high degree of clinical suspicion is warranted in young men with testis masses. A testis mass in a young man is considered cancer until proved otherwise. Early diagnosis is facilitated by testicular self-examination.

Prostate cancer, the most frequent urologic malignancy, indeed the most frequent malignancy in American males, is discussed in Chapter 75.

CASE 1
BLADDER CANCER

A 64-year-old male smoker, who worked in the dry cleaning industry, was seen by his primary care physician for a single episode of gross painless hematuria lasting less than 24 hours. He denied irritative or obstructive voiding symptoms or any change in his urinary habits. He had symptomatic emphysema treated with twice-a-day bronchodilators, and coronary artery disease for which he underwent coronary artery bypass surgery 3 years ago. Physical examination was remarkable only for prostate enlargement, hypertension, and mild obesity. The primary care physician ordered a urine culture, an IVP, and a urine cytology. The urine culture grew no organisms. IVP revealed normal kidneys and ureters, but suggested a filling defect in the bladder. Urine cytology showed cells that were suspicious for malignancy.

The patient was referred to a urologist, who performed cystoscopy under local anesthesia. This revealed the presence of a 5-cm broad-based polypoid lesion on the left wall of the bladder. Subsequent cystoscopic resection and biopsy under spinal anesthesia revealed a grade III/stage III TCC with invasion deep into the muscular wall of the bladder. Random biopsies of normal appearing urothelium revealed no CIS. Abdominal-pelvic CT scan showed no evidence of nodal metastasis or extension outside the bladder. Chest x-ray was normal.

The patient elected to undergo a radical cystoprostatectomy with bilateral pelvic lymphadenectomy and creation of an ileal conduit urinary diversion. Final pathology revealed a 6-cm grade III/stage III TCC with deep muscle invasion but no extension of the cancer into the perivesical fat. All pelvic lymph nodes were negative for metastasis. The patient stopped smoking and learned to manage his urinary stoma appliance. He was later treated successfully for impotence.

CASE 2
RENAL CANCER

A healthy 50-year-old female had a 3-day history of gross hematuria associated with right flank pain. She denied prior kidney stones or UTIs. An IVP was performed and was suggestive of a mass in her right kidney. Serum creatinine was 1.1 mg/dl. Urine culture and cytology were negative, however, renal ultrasound revealed a 10-cm parenchymal mass in the upper pole of the right kidney and a right renal vein that was free of tumor. Cystoscopy excluded bladder pathology. Abdominal CT scan confirmed the presence of a 10-cm solid right renal mass with a normal contralateral kidney and no obvious lymphadenopathy. Chest x-ray was negative for metastasis.

She underwent right radical nephrectomy through a flank incision. She was well without evidence of recurrence on follow-up CT scan and chest x-ray 24 months after surgery.

CASE 3
TESTIS CANCER

A 23-year-old white male medical student was seen in the student health clinic 1 week after finding a painless lump in his left testicle during self-examination while showering. Past medical history was significant for surgical repair of an undescended left testicle at age 14 months. Physical examination revealed a mass in the left testicle, which was not tender to deep palpation. The patient was seen later that afternoon by a urologist, who confirmed the physical examination and ordered a scrotal ultrasound. It showed a 2-cm heterogenous mass in the parenchyma of the left testis and a normal right testis. Serum tumor markers included AFP 96 ng/ml and BHCG 110 µIU/ml. Chest x-ray was normal. After a thorough discussion, the patient was scheduled for left radical inguinal orchiectomy in the outpatient surgery center the following morning. Final pathology revealed a 1.5-cm nonseminomatous germ cell carcinoma with microvascular invasion, but with no invasion of the spermatic cord or rete testis. Abdominal-pelvic CT scan 3 days later appeared negative for retroperitoneal lymphadenopathy. Serum tumor markers returned to normal within 2 weeks.

After thoroughly considering and rejecting an observational protocol and storing several semen specimens at a local sperm bank, the patient underwent RPLND through a thoracoabdominal incision later that month. At the time of surgery, all nodes felt benign. He did well and was discharged on the fifth postoperative day. Final pathology showed microscopic metastasis of nonseminomatous germ cell carcinoma in 2 of 35 lymph nodes removed. Both positive nodes were less than 2 cm in size. The patient returned regularly for follow-up CT scans, chest x-rays, and serum tumor marker levels. Six years later he remained free of recurrence.

GENERAL CONSIDERATIONS

TCC of the bladder often presents with painless gross hematuria (Case 1). It is more common in males, whites, and individuals exposed to urothelial carcinogens, such as the metabolites of aniline dyes. Bladder cancer is strongly associated with cigarette smoking. Most tumors are superficial and do not invade the bladder muscle. Typically, they appear as narrow-stalked, frondular "mulberries" that are easily identified and excised cystoscopically. Superficial tumors tend to recur over time, but invasion and metastasis are uncommon. Other bladder tumors appear as broad-based, sessile lesions and are more likely to invade the bladder muscle and metastasize to regional lymph nodes or distant sites (Case 1).

Renal cell carcinomas were historically reported to present with a triad of hematuria, pain, and flank mass; however, a minority of renal tumors today are associated with all three symptoms (Case 2). The advent of routine abdominal ultrasound has made renal tumors much easier to diagnose. Since surgical removal of the primary tumor is the most effective treatment, diagnosis at early stages is of paramount importance in this malignancy.

Testis cancer is one of the most curable solid malignancies. Therapy is based on tumor histology: seminomas versus nonseminomas. Seminomas carry a somewhat better prognosis. Cryptorchidism increases the risk of developing testis cancer in both the affected and nonaffected testes, even after surgical orchiopexy (Case 3). One fundamental reason for surgically repairing undescended testes is to facilitate subsequent physical examination to identify tumors early.

When metastasizing, testis cancer typically skips the pelvic lymphatics and spreads directly up the spermatic cord to the retroperitoneal nodes adjacent to the aorta and inferior vena cava, before continuing on to the lung or other distant sites.

KEY POINTS

- A testis mass in a young man is considered cancer until proved otherwise
- Bladder cancer strongly associated with cigarette smoking; most tumors superficial, do not invade bladder muscle; superficial tumors tend to recur

- Routine abdominal ultrasound has made renal tumor easier to diagnose; surgical removal of primary tumor is most effective treatment
- Testis cancer therapy is based on tumor hisotology: seminomas versus nonseminomas
- Cryptorchidism increases risk of developing testis cancer in both affected and nonaffected testes, even after surgical orchiopexy

DIAGNOSIS

TCC of the bladder is easily diagnosed with cystoscopic evaluation and biopsy. The entire tumor can usually be removed through this approach. Deep biopsies must be taken at the tumor site to identify invasion into bladder muscle. In addition, all new bladder cancer patients undergo random bladder biopsies to look for carcinoma in situ (CIS) (Case 1), which carries prognostic significance and requires more aggressive treatment. Prostatic urethral biopsies may also be taken. Care must be taken not to perforate the bladder during biopsy, since this can spread tumor into the perivesical space.

The pathologist determines two important histologic features of the tumor: grade (usually on a scale of 1–4 with 4 being the most anaplastic and thus unfavorable) and stage (level of invasion). The hallmark of tumor aggressiveness is invasion into or through the muscular wall of the bladder (Case 1). An intravenous pyelogram (IVP) is performed to rule out upper tract TCCs, which occur in about 20% of patients with bladder TCCs. Metastatic workup includes chest x-ray and abdominal-pelvic computed tomography (CT) scan. Tumors are clinically staged as A (superficial), B (muscle-invasive), C (extending into adjacent structures), and D (metastatic).

Renal cell carcinoma is diagnosed with great accuracy by radiographic studies alone. Percutaneous biopsy is rarely required and has been reported to cause tumor seeding of the biopsy tract. Preoperative metastatic workup includes chest x-ray to identify pulmonary lesions, and abdominal CT scan to look for involvement of the regional nodes (Case 2). Definitive histologic examination is usually performed on the radical nephrectomy specimen. Pathologic staging is based on tumor size, penetration of the kidney's fascial layers, and extension to regional nodes or distant sites. The tumor is often multicentric within the kidney. Renal cell carcinoma can invade the lumen of the renal vein and extend into the IVC or, rarely, into the right atrium. Renal vein or inferior venus cava extension carries a better prognosis than nodal involvement. Long-term survival is low for patients with nodal or distant metastasis.

Because testis cancer in young males is so curable if found early, urologists tend to be very aggressive in diagnosing these patients. Males older than 50 with testis tumors are more likely to have lymphoma or spermatocytic seminoma, a low grade tumor. Ultimately, testis cancer is a histologic diagnosis made on a radical orchiectomy specimen. Nonseminomas are subclassified as embryonal cell carcinoma, choriocarcinoma, yolk sac tumor, or teratoma. Testis tumors may be a pure cell type (60%) or mixed (40%). In addition to determining the cell type of the tumor, the pathologist looks for several histologic signs in the orchiectomy specimen that are risk factors for metastasis. These include vascular or lymphatic invasion (Case 3), extension into the rete testis, presence of embryonal cell histology, and absence of necrosis, teratoma, or yolk sac elements. Pure choriocarcinoma also carries a worse overall prognosis.

Clinical staging is accomplished with abdominal CT scan, chest x-ray, and serum tumor markers (α-fetoprotein [AFP] and β-human chorionic gonadotropin [β-hCG]) (Case 3). Serum half-lives are 4–6 days for AFP and 24 hours for β-hCG. Tumors are classified as stage I (organ-confined), stage II (metastatic to the retroperitoneal lymph nodes), or stage III (metastatic to distant sites, such as lung or brain).

KEY POINTS

- Hallmark of tumor agressiveness is invasion into or through muscular wall of bladder
- Renal vein or inferior vena cava extension carries better prognosis than nodal involvement

DIFFERENTIAL DIAGNOSIS

TCC of the bladder must be differentiated from other causes of hematuria, such as infection, prostate enlargement, and bladder or kidney stones. Irritative voiding symptoms are usually caused by benign conditions, but may occasionally result from tumors on the trigone. Less than 1% of bladder cancers are adenocarcinomas, and metastatic tumors to the bladder are even rarer. Chronic cystitis can produce lesions that are cystoscopically similar in appearance to superficial TCC.

Renal cell carcinoma must be differentiated from TCC of the renal pelvis, since the approach is different. Oncocytoma, a low grade malignancy without metastatic potential, may mimic renal cell carcinoma radiographically. Xanthogranulomatous pyelonephritis, a benign infectious condition often seen in diabetic patients, may also be confused with malignant renal tumors. Angiomyolipoma, a highly vascular benign renal tumor, sometimes requires removal to avoid rupture and hemorrhage. Kidney stones may grow quite large and cause flank pain with hematuria, but they are usually easy to differentiate from renal malignancy. Occasionally, tumors may metastasize to the kidney from the lung or other organs.

Testis cancer must be distinguished from benign scrotal masses such as inguinal hernias, hydroceles, spermatoceles, varicoceles, tunica albuginea cysts, and rare benign epididymal tumors. Scrotal ultrasound is very sensitive in distinguishing cystic from solid masses (Case 3). Benign testis tumors are rare.

S TREATMENT

uperficial TCC of the bladder is treated with cystoscopic transurethral resection. Intravesical chemotherapy with bacillus Calmette-Guérin (BCG) or antineoplastic drugs may be used against tumors that are multiple, recurrent, high grade, superficially invasive into the lamina propria, or associated with CIS. These agents are given as a series of 6 or 8 weekly bladder installations and are followed with repeat biopsies to measure success.

Muscle-invasive tumors or those with refractory CIS are treated aggressively with surgical excision (Case 1). Because of anatomic considerations, radical cystectomy (also called anterior pelvic exenteration) includes removal of the prostate in the male and the uterus and urethra in the female. Sometimes urethrectomy is also performed in the male.

Numerous surgical techniques have been devised for urinary drainage after bladder removal. The most popular and time-honored is the ileal conduit, in which the distal ureters are connected to a defunctionalized segment of small intestine that is then connected to the skin as a stoma. Urine then drains through the ileal conduit into a plastic bag that is attached to the patient's skin (Case 1).

Chemotherapy may be used as an adjunct to surgery for extensive tumors, or as the sole therapy in metastatic tumors. Radiotherapy can be effective in controlling aggressive local disease in patients too ill to undergo radical surgery.

Renal cell carcinoma is treated with radical nephrectomy, which involves removal of the kidney, its surrounding Gerota's fascia, and the ipsilateral adrenal gland (Case 2). The remaining ureter is left as a nonfunctional remnant (unlike treatment for TCCs of the renal pelvis, which requires removal of the entire ureter). In most patients, the contralateral kidney is sufficient for normal renal function. In cases of renal insufficiency of a solitary kidney, partial nephrectomy is useful. The adrenal is included in the resection since it is a frequent site for metachronous tumor. Regional lymph nodes are biopsied for pathologic staging. Chemotherapy and radiotherapy are not effective in renal cell cancer. Immunotherapy has recently gained attention as a promising treatment for recurrent or metastatic renal cell carcinomas.

Testis cancer is initially treated with radical inguinal orchiectomy (Case 3). This allows removal of the testis, its tunica, and a substantial segment of spermatic cord, the primary route of spread. The scrotum is not violated, to avoid seeding the scrotal lymphatics. Subsequent therapy depends on the histology of the primary tumor. Since abdominal CT scans understage nodal metastases in about 30% of cases, the retroperitoneum must be treated in males with clinically organ-confined tumors: nonseminomas are treated with retroperitoneal lymph node dissection (RPLND) (Case 3), and seminomas are treated with prophylactic irradiation. Those undergoing RPLND for clinical stage I nonseminomas undergo a modified dissection that preserves some lumbar sympathetic nerves and decreases the incidence of postoperative infertility.

Patients with bulky retroperitoneal nodes at diagnosis are treated with highly effective platinum-based chemotherapy. The 10–15% of patients who are partial responders with persistent postchemotherapy retroperitoneal masses are treated with RPLND in nonseminomas or salvage chemotherapy protocols in seminomas. Chemotherapy-resistant nonseminomas also require salvage chemotherapy. Persistent solitary lung nodules may be treated with surgical excision.

KEY POINTS

- Superficial TCC of bladder treated with cystoscopic transurethral resection

- Muscle-invasive tumors or those with refractory CIS are treated aggressively with surgical excision

- Renal cell carcinoma is treated with radical nephrectomy, which involves removal of the kidney, its surrounding Gerota's fascia, and the ipsilateral adrenal gland

- In treatment for testis cancer the scrotum is not violated, to avoid seeding the scrotal lymphatics

- Since abdominal CT scans understage nodal metastases in about 30% of cases, the retroperitoneum must be treated in males with clinically organ-confined testis cancer; nonseminomas treated with RPLND and seminomas treated with prophylactic irradiation

S FOLLOW-UP

uperficial TCC of the bladder requires long-term interval cystoscopy. During the first 2–3 years, cystoscopic examinations are performed every 3 months. In the absence of recurrence, the interval may be increased to 6 or 12 months. Superficial recurrences are treated with repeat transurethral resections or intravesical chemotherapy. Close monitoring is critical since recurrence is common and a small but significant percentage of superficial tumors will progress to invasive disease.

Follow-up after radical cystectomy includes regular pelvic examinations, CT scans, and chest x-rays to rule out recurrence. Long-term complications of urinary diversion include stoma problems and hydronephrosis that can result from scarring of the ureteroenteric anastomoses. Stomas are followed visually and manually, while the upper urinary tracts are followed with IVP or ultrasound.

Patients who have undergone radical nephrectomy for renal cell carcinoma must be monitored closely with chest x-ray and CT scan of the renal fossa. Metastasis may become evident many years after initial therapy even if the patient was thought to be cured.

Testis cancer patients are followed with serum tumor markers, chest x-rays, and abdominal CT scans every 2–4 months for the first 2–3 years, then at greater intervals for the next 2–3 years. Most recurrences occur within the first 24–36 months of treatment.

RPLND can cause infertility if the lumbar sympathetic fibers are damaged during surgery. These patients may be treated later with sympathomimetic drugs for failure of seminal emission or retrograde ejaculation. Chemotherapy can cause temporary or permanent infertility by sterilizing the germinal epithelium of the remaining testis.

SUGGESTED READINGS

Giuliani L, Giberti C, Martorana G, Rovida S: Radical extensive surgery for renal cell carcinoma: long-term results and prognostic factors. J Urol 143:468, 1990

This is a complete review of the surgical management of localized kidney cancer.

Heney N, Ahmed S, Flanagan J et al: Superficial bladder cancer: progression and recurrence. J Urol 130:1083, 1983

This longitudinal study extensively details the long-term follow-up of progression and recurrence in patients treated for superficial bladder cancer.

Richie J: Detection and treatment of testicular cancer. CA Cancer J Clin 43:151 1993

This article provides a state-of-the-art review of the histology, diagnosis, epidemiology, clinical and pathologic staging, and treatment of testicular cancer.

QUESTIONS

1. *Bladder cancer?*
   A. Is usually incurable due to metastases.
   B. Usually requires radical cystectomy.
   C. Is most commonly treated endoscopically.
   D. Is usually of squamous cell origin.
   E. Is usually found in familial syndromes.

2. *Testicular cancer?*
   A. Is more common with an undescended testicle.
   B. May be cured in a majority of cases.
   C. May be diagnosed by orchiectomy.
   D. Can usually be distinguished from benign scrotal tumors by scrotal ultrasound.
   E. All of the above.

(See p. 605 for answers.)

78

UROLOGIC

TRAUMA

MARK S. LITWIN

GERHARD J. FUCHS

JACOB RAJFER

Injuries to the genitourinary tract can involve the kidneys, ureters, bladder, urethra, and external genitalia. Besides the obvious recognition of injuries to the external genitalia, injuries to the urinary tract may be insidious, and often the only suggestion that one of these organs may be involved in trauma is either the proximity of a penetrating wound and/or the presentation of hematuria following the injury. When these wounds are treated, the major caveat is preservation of organ function without compromising the health or life of the individual. Depending on the situation, this may require conservative (nonoperative) management or aggressive surgical therapy.

CASE 1
RENAL TRAUMA

A 21-year-old male was admitted to the emergency room 4 hours after he fell off of a 22-ft cliff. In the emergency room, he was alert and oriented, and on physical examination was found to have a closed fracture of his right femur. A catheter was passed into his bladder and the urine appeared grossly bloody. Following a normal hematologic and chemical profile, an abdominal CT scan was performed with intravenous contrast material, and this revealed a fracture of the upper pole of the right kidney and absence of contrast material within his left kidney. Since no hypotension existed, a renal angiogram was done that showed an occluded left renal artery and minimal extravasation of the right upper pole artery. Because he was 8 hours postinjury after the angiogram was performed, it was elected to follow the patient conservatively. His femur fracture was reduced and aligned under anesthesia by the orthopaedists. His hematuria resolved and his Hct remained unchanged for the next 4 weeks. A follow-up CT scan at 6 weeks postinjury revealed a nonfunctioning left kidney, with almost complete resolution of the injury to the right upper pole.

CASE 2
BLADDER TRAUMA

A 25-year-old male was thrown off his motorcycle following a collision with an automobile. He was stabilized at the accident site and was taken to the emergency room. His examination on admission revealed a BP of 90/50 mmHg, a pulse of 110 bpm, blood on the tip of his penis, and pain in his pelvis. After he was resuscitated with fluids, a radiograph of his pelvis demonstrated a fracture of the pubic symphysis. A retrograde urethrogram was normal, and a catheter was then passed into his bladder. A gravity cystogram was performed with contrast material, and on the drainage film extravasation was seen in the retroperitoneum. The patient was taken to surgery for fixation of his pelvis. On exploration of the bladder, a large lateral laceration of the bladder was identified. The bladder was opened, the bladder laceration was debrided and sutured, and a suprapubic tube was inserted into the dome of the bladder. The catheter was left in place for 2 weeks, at which time another cystogram was performed and no extravasation was visible. The suprapubic catheter was removed after the patient voided successfully.

GENERAL CONSIDERATIONS

Blunt trauma to the genitourinary organs may result from an automobile or motorcycle accident, a blow to the abdomen or flank, or a sudden deceleration of the body. Since the ribs and lumbar vertebrae are in proximity to the kidneys, fractures of these bones should increase suspicion of an upper tract injury. Sometimes, the history of a sudden deceleration injury (e.g., hitting the steering wheel, falling off a cliff) in which the kidneys are thrust against the ribs/vertebral bodies by the steering wheel/dashboard is sufficient in itself to warrant an investigation into the integrity of the kidneys. It is not surprising that there is an approximately 40–50% incidence of associated intra-abdominal injuries (spleen, liver, pancreas, intestine, etc.) when the kidneys are bluntly traumatized.

In a deceleration injury, both the intima of the renal artery and the ureteropelvic junction are susceptible to tearing, resulting in either thrombosis of the artery (Case 1) or extravasation of urine, respectively. It is rare to save a kidney with a thrombosis of the renal artery following a deceleration injury, because after 2–3 hours of ischemia, irreversible injury occurs. Since the surgical reconstruction of a thrombosed renal vessel is a major undertaking in light of the bodily injuries associated with such a trauma, the current thought is to observe these patients unless diagnosis is made within 3 hours of the injury (Case 1).

Penetrating trauma is being seen more and more frequently in urban hospitals, mainly because of the increase in gun-related violence. Since the kidneys are somewhat protected by other intra-abdominal organs, the ribs, and the lumbar vertebrae, only 10% of all penetrating trauma to the abdomen involves the kidneys. Conversely, when the kidneys are involved in penetrating trauma, approximately 80% of these patients have associated abdominal injuries.

Trauma to the bladder is usually the result of a blunt injury to a distended bladder, a pelvic fracture, or a penetrating wound to the bladder. The bladder is attached to the body at its base at the pelvic floor. The dome of the bladder is covered by peritoneum and is the part of the bladder that distends when the bladder fills with urine.

The most common finding in patients with bladder trauma is hematuria. Occasionally, some patients with bladder trauma have a concomitant urethral injury. The finding of blood at the urethral meatus is one of the major clinical signs of a ruptured urethra. When this is found, a urethral catheter should not be passed into the bladder (Case 2). This is important because most patients who enter the emergency room for trauma get a catheter inserted into the bladder for the monitoring of urinary output.

KEY POINTS

- Often, the only suggestion that kidney, ureters, bladder, urethra, or external genitalia may be involved in trauma is proximity of penetrating wound and/or presentation of hematuria following injury

- Since the ribs and lumbar veterbrae are in proximity to kidneys, fractures of these bones should increase suspicion of upper tract injury

- It is not surprising that there is an approximately 40–50% incidence of associated intra-abdominal injuries (spleen, liver, pancreas, intestine, etc.) when the kidneys are bluntly traumatized

- The finding of blood at the urethral meatus is a major clinical sign of a ruptured urethra

DIAGNOSIS

Most patients with renal trauma will have gross or microscopic hematuria, and this finding is usually the sign that prompts urologic investigation. Although an intravenous pyelogram (IVP) is still considered by some to be the test of choice in the evaluation of the upper tracts, most centers utilize the contrast computed tomography (CT) scan as the definitive test (Case 1). With this test, almost all aspects of renal trauma, including perirenal hematomas, intrarenal pathology, and urinary extravasation, in addition to occlusion of the renal artery, are discernible. If the patient presents to the emergency department in an unstable condition and has to be taken to the operating room immediately, evaluation of the kidneys may be accomplished by injecting intravenous contrast when the patient is under anesthesia and taking an abdominal x-ray 5–10 minutes later on the operating room table (one-shot IVP).

A renal angiogram is performed only if embolization of a renal vessel is being considered (such as with the formation of a pseudoaneurysm in the renal arterial system). Otherwise the decision to operate or observe the renal injury is based on the clinical presentation of the patient and the results of the CT scan. The location of the renal injury, whether it is in the upper, lower, or middle part of the organ, is not a major factor in the decision to operate.

Ureteral injuries are extremely rare yet occur with either a penetrating wound or if the ureter is stretched during an acceleration/deceleration injury. A ureteral injury in this latter setting is very difficult to diagnose, since the patient may not present with symptomatic features. If a CT scan is performed, extravasation of contrast material on the side of the ureteral injury suggests such a lesion. A retrograde pyelogram may be performed at the time surgical repair is undertaken.

If blood is seen at the tip of the meatus, the patient should have a retrograde urethrogram performed. If it demonstrates no urethral disruption, a catheter may be safely passed (Case 2). If a disruption is seen, monitoring of the urinary output and bladder drainage should be accomplished via the placement of a suprapubic tube. This can be done percutaneously if the bladder is distended with urine; alternatively, an open surgical procedure is necessary. Attempts at catheterization in the presence of a urethral injury may produce permanent morbidity by extending an injury and/or creating false passages within the penis.

If there is no urethral disruption and a catheter is placed into the bladder, a cystogram is performed. This involves placement of contrast material through the catheter into the bladder under gravity drainage. It is important that a postdrainage film be taken, since extravasation posteriorly may not be discerned radiographically unless the bladder is emptied (Case 2). The radiographic finding of extravasation into the peritoneum usually means that the dome of the bladder has been ruptured, since the dome of the bladder is the weakest and most distensible part of the bladder.

A urethral injury is typically identified by a retrograde urethrogram. The most common site for traumatic urethral injuries is the prostatic-membranous urethra, since the prostate is held rigid against the pubic bones by the paired puboprostatic ligaments. When the pubic bone shears, the prostate with its rigid attachment moves along with the pubic bone, leaving the urethra behind. Most urethral injuries should be initially managed by a suprapubic tube placement as described above. Some trauma centers attempt to place a urethral catheter under direct vision via an open surgical procedure. A series of interlocking catheters is used in this setting both from inside the bladder and the urethral meatus. Most centers do not attempt this immediate repair of the injury because of the possibility of injuring the cavernosal nerve that runs along each posterolateral side of the prostate. This nerve regulates penile erection, and its injury can lead to impotence.

KEY POINTS

- Most patients with renal trauma will have gross or microscopic hematuria

- When performing a cystogram, important that postdrainage film be taken, since extravasation posteriorly may not be discerned radiographically unless the bladder is emptied

DIFFERENTIAL DIAGNOSIS

Hematuria following any traumatic insult to the body indicates the possibility of an injury somewhere along the urinary tract. A malformed kidney or a renal tumor are very susceptible to bleeding from even a minimal traumatic insult. The most common pathologic entities that bleed following trauma are a hydronephrotic kidney secondary to a ureteropelvic junction obstruction and a kidney harboring an unsuspected Wilms' tumor. In fact, any renal mass may bleed from trauma, and this is why all hematuria, particularly gross hematuria, following an injury requires at least an IVP or a CT scan of the kidneys.

KEY POINTS

- All hematuria, particularly gross hematuria, following an injury requires at least an IVP or CT scan of the kidneys

TREATMENT

When surgery is performed, an abdominal incision is made in the midline. Before the kidneys are exposed, vascular control of the renal vessels is obtained. This allows the surgeon to control the amount of blood loss from the kidneys once the retroperitoneum is opened. The first structure that the surgeon encounters in dissecting out the renal hilum for the vascular pedicle is the renal vein, since this is the most anterior structure. The renal artery is usually directly underneath the vein. If the kidneys are exposed in this manner, the goal of surgery is preservation of renal tissue whenever possible. In most cases, if renal tissue is to be excised, a partial rather than a total nephrectomy should be performed. The peripheral renal vessels should be adequately tamponaded to prevent delayed hemorrhage, and the collecting system should be closed tightly to obviate any urinary fistula formation. All injured tissue should be adequately debrided. Sometimes an internal ureteral stent running from the renal pelvis to the bladder is inserted to prevent any urinary extravasation during the healing process. Drains should be used liberally.

Ureteral injuries may be repaired primarily by anastomosing the proximal end of the injured ureter to the bladder (neoureterovesicostomy) or by uretero-ureteral anastomosis. Internal stenting and external drains are used.

Treatment of bladder ruptures is easily performed by a surgical procedure that includes debridement and approximation of the incised ends of the bladder with placement of a suprapubic tube (Case 2). Alternatively, if the bladder rupture is minor and extraperitoneal, bladder drainage alone via a catheter may be sufficient until bladder healing occurs. If surgery is performed for associated intra-abdominal injuries, if it is determined that urethral catheter drainage is inadequate, or if it is impossible to get a suprapubic tube into the bladder percutaneously, an open procedure will be necessary to place a suprapubic tube. Before the suprapubic tube is removed following healing of the injury, a cystogram should be performed to confirm absence of extravasation (Case 2).

P FOLLOW-UP

Postoperatively, attention is directed to the urinary output, renal function, and hematocrit level, in order to determine whether proper healing has occurred. A postoperative CT scan is obtained to confirm completion of the healing process and to identify any potential postoperative complications. A possible long-term sequela of renal trauma is partial ischemia of retained renal tissue, which may lead to renin-mediated hypertension. The ultimate morbidity and mortality of most patients with renal trauma is dependent on the extent of the associated abdominal injuries, in particular, the liver and spleen. Internal ureteral stents may be removed following confirmation of healing by contrast studies, usually in the office and/or cystoscopy suite.

Most bladder injuries heal without long-term sequela. In some patients who have been on long-term catheter drainage for their bladder injury, bacteriuria with pyelonephritis may occur. If there is a urethral disruption along with a bladder injury, urethral strictures and/or impotence (which results from an injury to the cavernosal nerve) may occur.

KEY POINTS

- A possible long-term sequela of renal trauma is partial ischemia of retained renal tissue, which may lead to renin-mediated hypertension

---

SUGGESTED READINGS

Fournier GR Jr, McAninch JW: Complications of genitourinary trauma. p. 218. In Smith RB, Ehrlich RM (eds): Complications of Urologic Surgery. 2nd Ed. WB Saunders, Philadelphia, 1990

A comprehensive overview of complications.

McAninch JW, Carrol PR: Renal trauma: Kidney preservation through improved vascular control—a refined approach. J Urol 22:265, 1982

Advocates vascular control to minimize blood loss and for renal preservation.

Peters PC, Bright TC III: Blunt renal injuries. Urol Clin North Am 4:17, 1977

An extensive overview of the most common form of genitourinary trauma.

QUESTIONS

1. Although hematuria is the most common indicator of GU trauma, other "warning signs" include?

    A. Lower rib fractures.
    B. Pelvic fractures.
    C. A deceleration injury (e.g., a fall).
    D. Lumbar vertebral fractures.
    E. All of the above.

2. Urethral injuries?

    A. Are frequently due to penetrating trauma.
    B. Are best treated by primary repair.
    C. Commonly involve the prostatic urethra.
    D. Are best diagnosed by an IVP and cystogram.
    E. All of the above.

(See p. 605 for answers.)

79

BRAIN

TUMORS

DUNCAN Q. MCBRIDE

Intracranial tumors are highly variable lesions with respect to presentation, clinical course, surgical resectability, and prognosis. The principle determinant of outcome for patients with intracranial tumors is the histologic tumor type. Second in importance is the location of the lesion in the intracranial cavity.

CASE 1
GLIOBLASTOMA MULTIFORME

A 63-year-old male complained of 6 weeks of headaches. For 2 weeks he was aware of speech that was slightly slurred, with difficulty finding words. The day before admission, he began to limp and dropped his coffee cup. On presentation to a neurologist's office, the general physical examination was unremarkable. The mental status examination revealed slurred speech with anomia, but normal orientation to person, place, time, and circumstance. The cranial nerves were found to be normal, except for a subtle right facial droop. The fundi were normal. On power testing, he was found to have a 4+/5 right hemiparesis with a drift and circumduction of the right leg when walking. The deep tendon reflexes were increased on the right, and there was a right-sided Babinski reflex.

He was sent immediately for an MRI scan with and without contrast, which revealed an irregular left frontotemporal enhancing mass that extended deep to the internal capsule (Fig. 79.1). He was started on steroids and was given a loading dose of phenytoin. A craniotomy and resection of the infiltrating lesion was performed. Frozen section identified the tumor as a malignant glioma. The resection cavity was carried to the visible edge of the lesion. Postoperatively, his speech and hemiparesis improved. Final histology was glioblastoma multiforme. After wound healing, the patient was given a 5,000-cGy dose of fractionated radiotherapy with a subsequent regimen of chemotherapy. In follow-up he was found to have gradual regrowth of tumor and recurrence of his previous symptoms, combined with a gradual deterioration of his mental function. Despite these therapies, the patient expired from tumor recurrence 1 year after the diagnosis.

CASE 2
MENINGIOMA

A 48-year-old female had a long history of headaches. She was noted by her family to have had subtle personality changes for about 6 months with poor attention to details, including shopping, meals, and personal hygiene. She began to exhibit memory loss and disorientation. Her behavior became inappropriate and her conduct was occasionally belligerent. She refused to seek medical attention despite occasional episodes of vomiting. On the day of admission, she suffered a grand mal seizure and was brought to the emergency room where she was disheveled and lethargic. Her speech was clear, but she was disoriented to time and place and demonstrated poor short-term memory and attention span. Her cranial nerves were normal, but fundoscopic examination revealed optic pallor on the right with papilledema on the left. She had normal power on individual muscle testing but demonstrated a left pronator drift. The left-sided deep tendon reflexes were slightly increased. The remaining neurologic and physical examinations were normal.

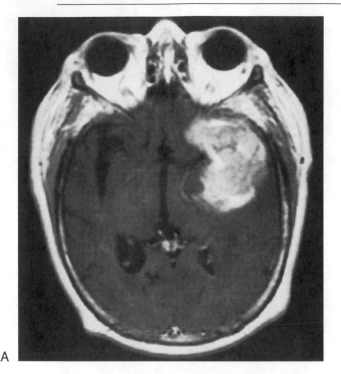

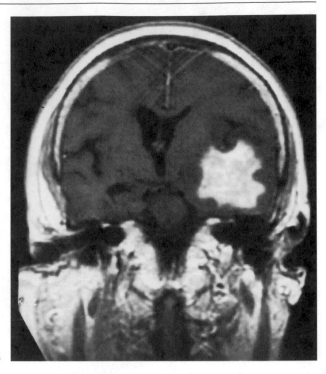

FIGURE 79.1   *(A) Frontal reconstruction of an enhancing mass in the left frontotemporal region that extends deep to the internal capsule (MRI scan). (B) Same mass is seen in a transverse view.*

She was started on phenytoin. CT and MRI studies revealed a large right frontal uniformly enhancing, smooth edged mass with considerable cerebral edema (Fig. 79.2). She was treated with high dose decadron (20 mg IV and then 10 mg IV every 6 hours), which improved her headache and pronator drift. The following week, she underwent gross total removal of a meningioma that was arising from the dura. The dural edge was excised, the dura patched, and the frontal sinus exonerated and sealed. Postoperatively, her cognitive function gradually improved. In long-term follow-up there was no recurrence of tumor and she ultimately returned to her normal premorbid state.

GENERAL CONSIDERATIONS

Brain tumors are second only to stroke as a cause of death from neurologic disease. The overall incidence of these lesions increases with age. Although geographic, racial, and ethnic differences are reported, the general incidence of primary brain tumors averages about 10 cases per 100,000 people per year. About one-half of these are gliomas, about one-quarter are meningiomas, and the remainder are a mixture of lesions.

The etiology of intracranial tumors is unclear. Although association with historic events (such as head injury) and environmental factors (such as exposure to electromagnetic energy, certain chemicals, and radioactive substances) has been implicated, no clear factor has been identified. Considerable research has been directed toward identification of oncogenes as causative factors in brain tumor genesis. Clear genetic relationships have been established for the phakomatoses or neurocutaneous syndromes, including neurofibromatosis II, in which gliomas, neuromas, and meningiomas develop; or tuberous sclerosis, in which subependymal giant cell astrocytomas grow; or von Hippel-Lindau syndrome, in which hemangioblastomas arise.

Oncogenes and their byproducts—such as growth factors, receptors, and kinases—as well as tumor suppressor genes (especially p53) have been clearly related to the growth of malignant brain tumors. Specific genetic chromosomal abnormalities have been identified in malignant gliomas that include monosomy of chromosome 10 and deletions in various other chromosomes, most notably 17. Interestingly, low grade gliomas have been shown to have no deletions in chromosome 10, suggesting that such a chromosomal change might be involved in the degeneration of such tumors to more malignant cell types.

The pathophysiology of brain tumors stems from their growth. Symptoms form from expansion of the mass in the intracranial space: either by direct pressure on neurons, infiltration and damage of neurons, irritation of the cortical surface and resultant seizures, or obstruction of cerebrospinal fluid (CSF) pathways and hydrocephalus. Generally, infiltrating lesions of the glioma cell types spread through the parenchyma of the brain, while benign lesions

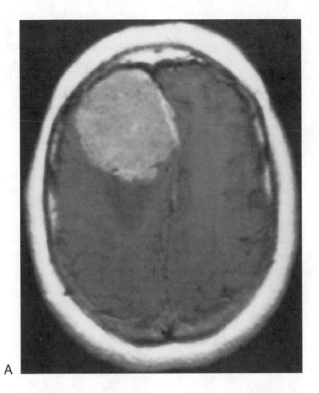

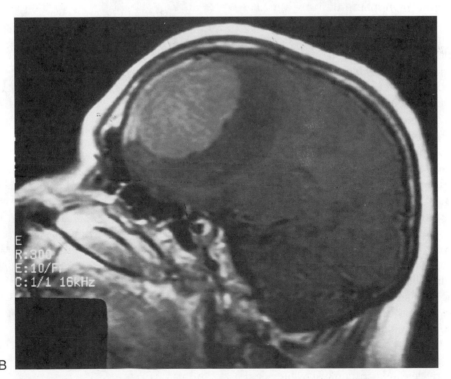

FIGURE 79.2 *(A & B) Two views of the patient in Case 2. The mass is a right frontal lesion that enhances with contrast, indicating breakdown of the blood-brain barrier.*

expand in the extra-axial space and press on brain structures or cranial nerves. In either case, neuronal function is disturbed and neurologic symptoms develop, and eventually, intracranial pressure is elevated. Unchecked, brain tumors of all types have the potential to grow to such size that they cause severe neurologic damage, cerebral herniation, and death.

Development of seizures is a common occurrence with intracranial tumors. About 15% of patients who present with late onset seizures will be found to have an intracranial tumor. Both the type of tumor and its location are determinants in the development of epilepsy. Two-thirds of patients with parietal tumors and one-half of patients with frontal or temporal tumors will develop seizures. Seizures in other locations have a significantly lower rate of epilepsy. Slow growing tumors have a higher incidence of seizures. Two-thirds of meningioma patients and 90% of patients with oligodendrogliomas present with seizures, as opposed to about one-third of patients with gliomas and only 10% of those with metastasis.

The location of a tumor in the intracranial cavity is a major consideration in its presentation, resectability, and prognosis. While adult patients present predominantly with supratentorial tumors, posterior fossa tumors are more frequently observed in the pediatric population. In general, lesions in various locations in the brain have characteristic neurologic deficits. Left hemisphere lesions can cause speech and language deficits. The classic left frontal speech deficit, Broca's aphasia, is a motor problem with delivery of language being impaired (Case 1). A left temporoparietal lesion causes Wernicke's aphasia, which is a fluent aphasia in which both perception of language and delivery of appropriate words is abnormal. Frontal lobe lesions can grow relatively large before symptoms present. Personality changes can be noted (Case 2). Low frontal lesions can cause anosmia or pressure on the optic nerve. Unilateral optic nerve compression with raised intracranial pressure comprises the Foster-Kennedy syndrome, in which optic pallor on one side is associated with papilledema on the other. High frontal lesions close to the central sulcus affect the motor strip and cause contralateral hemiparesis. Lesions in the motor cortex, if discrete, can follow the anatomic distribution of the homunculus, with the lower extremity functions more medial and high, followed by the arm and hand over the convexity and the face and tongue more laterally. Parietal lesions can cause sensory deficits, which are associated with unilateral neglect. Occipital lesions produce hemianopsia. Temporal lobe lesions can cause a quodrantanopsia and are frequently associated with epileptic seizure formation. Deep hemispheric lesions can damage white matter tracts in the internal capsule and have a combination of the above effects. Brain stem lesions affect cranial nerve and long tract functions. Cerebellar tumors present with ataxia, dysmetria, and imbalance, with a wide-based gait if the nuclei are involved. Posterior fossa tumors, as well as pineal and various ventricular tumors are frequently associated with obstructive hydrocephalus, which gives signs and symptoms of raised intracranial pressure. Pituitary tumors will frequently present with hormonal changes, and if large enough, will grow upward out of the sella turcica and compress the optic chiasm, resulting in a bitemporal hemianopsia. Tumors of the skull base or cranial floor will principally affect cranial nerves.

Systemic diseases, such as the phakomatoses, are associated with intracranial tumors. These are congenital disorders in which nervous system tumors are associated with cutaneous lesions. Neurofibromatosis or von Recklinghausen syndrome has multiple subtypes and is associated with café au lait spots on the skin and axial freckling. This syndrome typically harbors only peripheral nerve neuromas. Type II neurofibromatosis, however, is associated with intracranial meningiomas, optic nerve gliomas, and bilateral acoustic neuromas. Tuberous sclerosis, with its sebaceous malar lesions, is associated with subependymal giant cell astrocytoma. Sturge-Weber syndrome, with its facial hemangioma in a trigeminal branch distribution, is associated with subpial calcification and a seizure disorder. Von Hippel-Lindau syndrome is an autosomal dominant disorder in which hemangioma formation may include the brain.

KEY POINTS

- Brain tumors are second only to strokes as a cause of death from neurologic disease; the overall incidence of lesions increases with age

- Oncogenes and their byproducts—such as growth factors, receptors, and kinases—as well as tumor suppressor genes (especially p53) have been clearly related to growth of malignant brain tumors

- Genetic chromosomal abnormalities identified in malignant gliomas include monosomy of chromosome 10 and deletions in various other chromosomes, most notably, 17; low grade gliomas have no deletions in chromosome 10, suggesting that such chromosomal change might be involved in degeneration of such tumors to more malignant cell types

- Development of seizures is a common occurrence with intracranial tumors; about 15% of patients who present with late onset seizures will be found to have intracranial tumor

- Location of tumor in intracranial cavity is a major consideration in its presentation, resectability, and prognosis; while adult patients present predominantly with supratentorial tumors, posterior fossa tumors are more frequently observed in the pediatric population

DIAGNOSIS

As with most neoplastic disorders, diagnosis of intracranial tumors is based on careful history, physical examination, and imaging. Since growth of the intracranial tumor and resultant neurologic dysfunction is the hallmark of these lesions, a history of progressive neurologic deficit is paramount in making this diagnosis. Complaints of headache, vomiting, visual changes, other neurologic deficits, and seizures are all extremely important. A chronic unremitting headache that awakens the patient from sleep, especially in a previously stoic individual, is very suggestive of an intracranial lesion. Yet, surprisingly, only about 50% of patients with documented intracranial tumors will present with headache as a chief complaint.

On physical examination, the neurologic findings, such as speech deficit, mental status changes, motor, coordination, gait, sensory, or pathologic reflexes should all be elicited. Fundoscopic examination is essential to look for papilledema. Examination of the neck for signs of meningeal irritation should be performed. A general physical examination looking for any signs of systemic disease is equally important.

On neurologic testing, there can be false localizing signs that might lead one to misinterpret the anatomic location of a lesion. The classic false localizing sign is a 6th nerve palsy, which results in a lateral deviation of the eye. This can result from any aberration in intracranial pressure and does not localize a lesion to the skull base or the brain stem. Hydrocephalus can result in visual changes and global neurologic signs and symptoms.

Computed tomography (CT) scanning is the primary diagnostic tool for intracranial mass lesions. A CT scan with and without contrast will demonstrate tumors of the brain and intracranial cavity whose uptake of contrast dye is related to the degree of blood-brain barrier breakdown associated with the lesion. Mass effect on the brain is demonstrated by effacement of CSF-containing structures such as ventricles, interhemispheric fissure, sulci, and the basal cisterns. Currently, however, magnetic resonance imaging (MRI) scanning has taken the forefront in localization, surgical planning and execution, and focusing radiotherapy in brain tumors. The availability of sagittal views on MRI scan and the multiple imaging modalities (e.g., MR angiography) have made the MRI scanner essential for the diagnosis of complicated intracranial lesions. Angiography remains important for certain lesions. It identifies their blood supply as well as anomalies of the supply to the brain. Embolization via angiographic techniques is available to treat certain tumors. Other radiographic imaging modalities are of lesser importance in the current management of brain tumors. Although skull x-rays might reveal calcifications or shift of the pineal gland from the midline, they have no current practical usage. Other essentially outdated imaging modalities include nuclear medicine brain scan, pneumoencephalography, and electroencephalogram (EEG). Some imaging techniques are useful in assessing the aggressiveness of various tumors, including thallium scanning for gliomas and bromodeoxyuridine labeling and flow cytometry for

meningiomas. Despite the high quality of modern diagnostic techniques, many intracranial tumors and other mass lesions are indistinguishable from each other. Invasive diagnostic testing in the form of stereotactic needle biopsy is frequently required.

KEY POINTS

- As with most neoplastic disorders, diagnosis of intracranial tumors is based on careful history, physical examination, and imaging

- Since growth of intracranial tumor and resultant neurologic dysfunction is the hallmark of these lesions, a history of progressive neurologic deficit is paramount in making this diagnosis

- Complaints of headache, vomiting, visual changes, other neurologic deficits, and seizures all extremely important; chronic unremitting headache that awakens patient from sleep, especially in previously stoic individual, is very suggestive

- On neurologic testing, false localizing signs can lead one to misinterpret anatomic location of lesion; classic false sign is 6th nerve palsy, which results in lateral deviation of eye

- CT scanning primary diagnostic tool for intracranial mass lesions

- Availability of sagittal views on MRI scan and multiple imaging modalities (e.g., MR angiography) have made MRI scanner essential for diagnosis of complicated intracranial lesions

DIFFERENTIAL DIAGNOSIS

When a patient presents with appropriate signs and symptoms, the differential diagnosis includes intracranial tumors of various types and locations, and other neurologic conditions. Intrinsic brain tumors such as astrocytomas must be distinguished from other tumors of brain tissue. These include ependymomas, medulloblastomas, and oligodendrogliomas. These can usually be distinguished from each other using MRI imaging. Other extraaxial tumors include neuromas, pituitary tumors, craniopharyngiomas, and less frequently, chordomas, keratomas, and cholesteatomas. Acoustic neuromas are schwannomas of the vestibular nerve and can be confused with cerebellopontine angle meningiomas. Metastatic lesions, particularly those that originate in the lung and breast, are frequently seen in the brain and mimic malignant gliomas. Melanomas and renal and gastrointestinal tumors may also metastasize to the brain. Prostate cancer is only known to metastasize to the dura or skull.

Pituitary tumors frequently present with endocrine abnormalities, and if large enough, compress the optic chiasm, resulting in classic bitemporal hemianopsia (Fig. 79.3). Occasionally, apoplexy is the initial event due to hemorrhage, which affects the cranial nerves in the cavernous sinus, causing ophthalmoplegia. Prolactinomas are the most common pituitary tumors. These lesions secrete

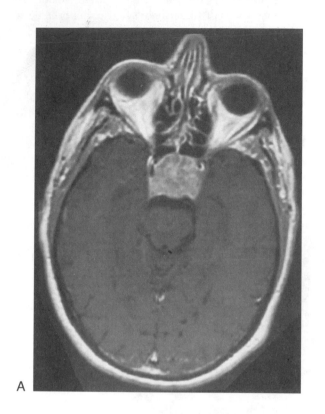

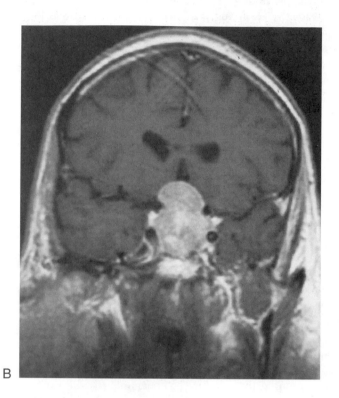

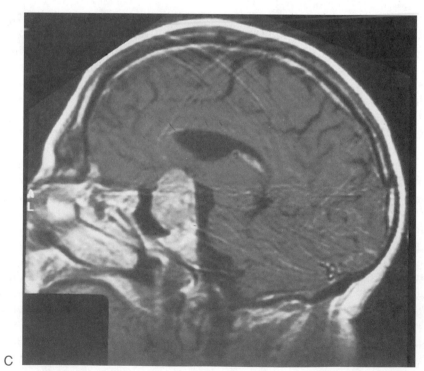

FIGURE 79.3   *(A–C) Three views (MRI) of a large pituitary tumor.*

prolactin, which causes amenorrhea and galactorrhea in females, and gynecomastia and impotence in males. Adrenocorticotropic hormone (ACTH)-producing tumors produce Cushing's disease, with its classic physical findings of moon facies, bloated torso, and abdominal striae. Acromegaly or gigantism results from growth hormone-producing tumors. Frequently, pituitary tumors are non-secreting, and cause global suppression of pituitary hormones with the exception of prolactin, which is normally inhibited. Thus, when the pituitary stock is compressed, the prolactin level is mildly elevated.

Pineal region tumors originate from germ cells and are histologically similar to testicular tumors. Most frequently encountered is the germinoma, which presents in young males and is similar histologically and biologically to the seminoma. Malignant tumors of the pineal region include choriocarcinoma, embryonal cell carcinoma, and pineoblastoma and pineocytoma.

Non-neoplastic, infectious intracranial mass lesions on CT scan occur frequently. These include bacterial abscesses, which appear as ring-enhancing lesions similar to malignant gliomas. The wall of the abscess is typically somewhat smoother and thinner than that of a malignant tumor. Patients with acquired immunodeficiency syndrome (AIDS) present with ring-enhancing mass lesions that are most commonly toxoplasmomas; however, lymphomas, tuberculomas, and other opportunistic lesions arise in the brains of these patients. Cysticercosis is a commonly found parasite that frequently invades the brain of patients who live in areas where personal hygiene is less than fastidious.

Other cerebral conditions can mimic an intracranial tumor. Communicating or obstructive hydrocephalus can arise from other conditions. Cerebral vascular accidents, such as infarct or subarachnoid hemorrhage from an aneurysm, typically have a sudden onset. An arteriovenous malformation can create neurologic symptoms, including seizures and neurologic deficits due to a steal phenomenon. Chronic subdural hematoma and meningitis both can cause symptoms and findings similar to brain tumor. Any adult with new onset of epileptic seizures is a brain tumor suspect; however, such a lesion is not always found. Pseudotumor cerebri is a condition most frequently found in young females who are somewhat overweight and often taking oral contraceptives. This condition causes increased intracranial pressure due to global brain swelling. Other degenerative and demyelinating disorders such as multiple sclerosis can also be confused with intracranial tumors. These conditions typically have a progressive course of increasing neurologic problems similar to tumors; however, the hallmark feature of multiple sclerosis is a waxing and waning of findings. Virtually all neurologic conditions mentioned in the differential diagnoses are easily distinguishable from intracranial tumors using modern diagnostic imaging.

KEY POINTS

- Intrinsic brain tumors such as astrocytomas must be distinguished from other tumors of brain tissue; these include ependymomas, medulloblastomas, and ogliodendrogliomas

- Other extra-axial tumors include neuromas, pituitary tumors, craniopharyngiomas, and less frequently, chordomas, keratomas, and cholesteatomas

- Metastatic lesions, particularly those that originate in the lung and breast, frequently seen in the brain and mimic malignant gliomas

- Pituitary tumors frequently present with endocrine abnormalities, and if large enough, compress the optic chiasm, resulting in classic bitemporal hemianopsia (Fig. 79.3)

- Non-neoplastic, infectious intracranial mass lesions on CT scan occur frequently, including bacterial abscesses, which appear as ring-enhancing lesions similar to malignant gliomas

- Patients with AIDS present with ring-enhancing mass lesions that are most commonly toxoplasmomas; however, lymphomas, tuberculomas, and other opportunistic lesions arise in the brains of these patients

- Cysticercosis commonly found parasite that frequently invades the brain of patients who live in areas where personal hygiene is less than fastidious

TREATMENT

Treatment of brain tumors is as varied as the list of tumors themselves. In general, benign tumors such as meningiomas and acoustic neuromas are surgically excised. Surgical resection of malignant tumors and intrinsic brain tumors is performed to debulk the tumor burden, and such surgery is performed within the boundaries of the tumor to preserve function of the brain surrounding the lesion. Deep lesions are frequently inaccessible to direct surgical approach and thus are treated with stereotactic needle biopsy and subsequent nonsurgical therapies. Pituitary lesions are normally approached through a transseptal transsphenoidal approach. Many newer skull base approaches are used, frequently in concert with head and neck surgeons, to excise lesions along the cranial floor.

Virtually all patients with intracranial tumors receive some benefit from corticosteroids, which reduce the cerebral edema and irritative effects of the tumor. Most hemispheric tumors require anticonvulsant therapy either as a precaution or as a treatment for seizure. The preoperative use of mannitol (an osmotic diuretic) to lower intracranial pressure is often indicated. Obstructive hydrocephalus is treated acutely with ventriculostomy, and chronically with a ventriculoperitoneal shunt.

To prevent recurrence of meningiomas, a margin of dura around the lesion should be excised, and hyperostotic bone removed where possible. The dura then is repaired, typically with a patch, to prevent leakage of CSF. Subtotally resected meningiomas can be treated with postoperative radiotherapy. Preoperatively, angiography with embolization of meningiomas to reduce their blood supply helps to limit intraoperative hemorrhage.

Treatment of malignant brain tumors has been shown to prolong survival; however, a curative therapy has not been developed. Therefore, optional treatment such as radiotherapy has been used to combat these lesions. This may include whole brain radiation of fractionated low dosages. Newer techniques include brachytherapy with ^{125}I implants. Focused beam radiotherapy or "radiosurgery" is more effective in treating smaller lesions by aiming many sublethal radiation beams onto a point to achieve an effective dose at the point of focus. The entire radiation dose can be given at one sitting.

Chemotherapeutic agents are also effective in delaying the recurrence of malignant brain tumors. Nitrosureas and other alkylating agents have been used most commonly. Vinca alkaloids, platinum compounds, and other agents are also in use. Attempts have been made to enhance the delivery of the chemotherapeutic agents to the tumors. These include disruption of the blood-brain barrier, and intra-arterial, intrathecal, and intratumoral injections. Treatments include photodynamic therapy using light-sensitive, free radical-producing agents. Recently, immunotherapy has been utilized against malignant tumors. Interferon, interleukin-2, and lymphokine activated killer leukocytes have all shown some beneficial effect. Attempts to alter the genetic defects are also now feasible. These include retroviral mediated gene transfer therapies.

KEY POINTS

- Benign tumors such as meningiomas and acoustic neuromas are surgically excised

- Surgical resection of malignant tumors and intrinsic brain tumors performed to debulk the tumor burden; such surgery performed within the boundaries of the tumor to preserve function of the brain surrounding the lesion

- Deep lesions are frequently inaccessible to direct surgical approach and thus are treated with stereotactic needle biopsy and subsequent nonsurgical therapies

- Pituitary lesions normally approached through transseptal transsphenoidal approach

- Virtually all patients with intracranial tumors receive some benefit from corticosteroids, which reduce cerebral edema and irritative effects of the tumor

- Newer techniques include brachytherapy with ^{125}I implants

- Focused beam radiotherapy or "radiosurgery" is more effective in treating smaller lesions

- Chemotherapeutic agents also effective in delaying recurrence of malignant brain tumors; nitrosureas and other alkylating agents have been used most commonly, with vinca alkaloids, platinum compounds, and other agents

FOLLOW-UP

The outcome in a patient with an intracranial tumor depends mainly on the tumor type. Location of the lesion, surgical and therapeutic approach, preoperative performance, age, and pre- and postoperative treatment success are also major factors in determining patient outcome. Clearly, completely excised benign extra-axial tumors have the best long-term outcome. Nevertheless, there is an approximately 15–20% long-term recurrence rate after meningioma excision.

Brain tumor patients are typically followed with serial MRI or CT scans to assess completeness of tumor excision and growth of any residual or recurrent tumor. Typically, a gadolinium-enhanced MRI scan is performed on the 3rd postoperative day to assess the initial surgical results. The exception to this general rule is in pituitary tumors, in which early postoperative scans do not appear dissimilar to the preoperative images.

Patients whose tumors require chemotherapy and/or radiotherapy are typically followed by radiation oncologists and neuro-oncologists. Certain intracranial tumors will have spread within the central nervous system and subarachnoid space, but in general, intracranial tumors do not metastasize to the body.

Treatment modalities such as chemotherapy have major systemic side effects. These include fatigue, weight loss, hair loss, and gastrointestinal symptoms. Radiotherapy also has short-term and long-term cerebral side effects. The short-term effects include brain swelling in the acute phase and demyelination in the early delayed phase. Late consequences of radiotherapy include leukoencephalopathy, cerebral necrosis, cerebral vascular injury, and development of other intracranial tumors. In children, there is a decrease in intelligence quotient after brain radiation. For this reason, cranial radiation is typically withheld in patients less than 3 years of age.

Survival after treatment in patients with glioblastoma multiforme averages about 1 year from diagnosis. Patients with less malignant lesions, such as lower grade astrocytomas, oligodendrogliomas, and medulloblastomas can survive in the 5–10 year range. Ependymomas without subarachnoid seeding can be cured with complete surgical extirpation.

Follow-up for patients with brain tumors, particularly intrinsic incurable types, should also include psychological support for patient and family. Survival in malignant tumors is improved by various factors. These include lobar lesions in which repeated surgery is available, young age, tumor grade, and Karnofsky score, which measures the degree of independence in activities of daily living. Interestingly, infection of the operative site has been associated with improved survival in malignant astrocytomas, possibly due to enhanced local immune response.

KEY POINTS

• Brain tumor patients typically followed with serial MRI or CT scans to assess completeness of tumor excision and growth or residual or recurrent tumor

• Typically, gadolinium-enhanced MRI scan performed on 3rd postoperative day to assess initial surgical results

SUGGESTED READINGS

Morantz RA, Walsh JW (eds): Brain Tumors: A Comprehensive Text. Marcel Dekker, New York, 1994

Twijnstra A, Keyser A, De Visser BW: Neuro-oncology: Primary Tumors and Neurological Complications of Cancer. Elsevier, New York, 1993

QUESTIONS

1. *What percentage of patients with late-onset seizures will ultimately be shown to have an intracranial tumor?*

    A. 15%.
    B. 30%.
    C. 50%.
    D. 75%.

2. *The primary diagnostic tool for locating an intracerebral mass lesion is?*

    A. MRI scan.
    B. CT scan.
    C. Angiography.
    D. Skull x-ray.

3. *Outcome in a brain tumor patient depends primarily on?*

    A. Tumor location.
    B. Presenting symptoms.
    C. Tumor stage.
    D. Tumor type.

(See p. 605 for answers.)

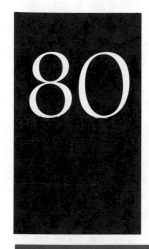

80 ANEURYSMS AND INTRACRANIAL HEMORRHAGE

MARVIN BERGSNEIDER

Intracranial hemorrhage is a common neurologic problem. It occurs in patients of all ages, and may arise secondary to trauma or be a nontraumatic "spontaneous" event. Some type of vascular abnormality, either microscopic or macroscopic, nearly always underlies a spontaneous hemorrhage. The range of presentation varies from the asymptomatic patient to coma. Many patients are found dead. Spontaneous intracranial hemorrhage is a common and important cause of neurologic morbidity,

and therefore, every physician should have a basic knowledge of it. The aims of this chapter are to (1) describe the most common etiologies of spontaneous intracranial hemorrhage, (2) review the diagnostic approach to determining the etiology of the hemorrhage, and (3) outline the treatment rationale for its management.

CASE 1
SUDDEN HEADACHE AND DOUBLE VISION

A 56-year-old female presented to the emergency room complaining of "the worst headache of her life," neck stiffness, and double vision. She stated that the headache began suddenly while she was attempting a bowel movement. She was found on the floor in a confused state by her husband. He brought her immediately to the hospital. Since that time, she reported increased sensitivity to light, and mild nausea. She denied recent fever or trauma, but

did have a history of hypertension, and was poorly complaint with her antihypertensive medications. Her father died of a "brain hemorrhage." General physical examination revealed nuchal rigidity. Neurologic examination was significant for a left 3rd nerve palsy, manifested by a dilated nonreactive pupil, ptosis, and outward deviation of the left eye. There was evidence of mild papilledema on fundoscopic examination. The remainder of the neurologic examination was normal.

A CT scan was ordered immediately and demonstrated diffuse subarachnoid hemorrhage in the left sylvian fissure, suprasellar, and perimesencephalic cisterns (in the area of the left half of the circle of Willis). Mild hydrocephalus was suspected because the temporal horns of the lateral ventricle were mildly enlarged (Fig. 80.1). After reviewing the CT scan, the suspicion of an aneurysm was so great that a confirmatory lumbar puncture was not performed. The patient was given a loading dose of phenytoin for seizure prophylaxis and taken for an urgent four-vessel cerebral angiogram. The angiogram revealed a 9-mm sac-

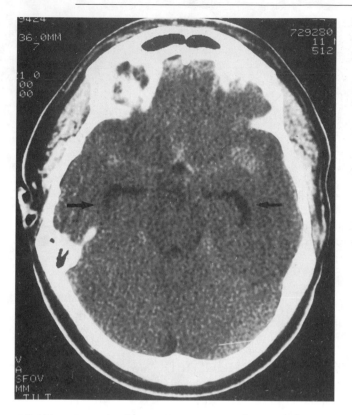

FIGURE 80.1 Axial noncontrast CT scan demonstrating diffuse subarachnoid hemorrhage, seen most clearly in the star-shaped suprasellar cistern. Note the slightly dilated temporal horns (arrows) of the lateral ventricles that indicated hydrocephalus.

cular aneurysm at the origin of the left posterior communicating artery from the internal carotid artery (Fig. 80.2).

She was taken immediately for a right frontotemporal ("pterional") craniotomy, where an aneurysm clip was successfully placed across the neck of the aneurysm (Fig. 80.3). Immediately postoperatively, she remained unchanged neurologically and was managed in the intensive care unit, where the central venous pressure was maintained between 6 and 10 mmHg by intravenous hydration and administration of intravenous 5% albumin. Her blood pressure was kept at or slightly above her normal value. On the fifth postoperative day, she became progressively more lethargic and demonstrated a left pronator drift.

An emergent CT scan was unremarkable. The diagnosis of postsubarachnoid hemorrhage cerebral vasospasm was suspected because the left middle cerebral artery blood velocity was markedly increased on transcranial Doppler ultrasonography (increases in arterial blood flow velocity can indicate a decrease in vessel lumen diameter). The patient was begun on hypertensive and hypervolemic therapy. A pulmonary artery catheter was placed to optimize cardiac filling pressures. The systolic blood pressure was elevated to 180 mmHg by the administration of intravenous phenylephrine. The Hct was at 32%, which was considered opti-

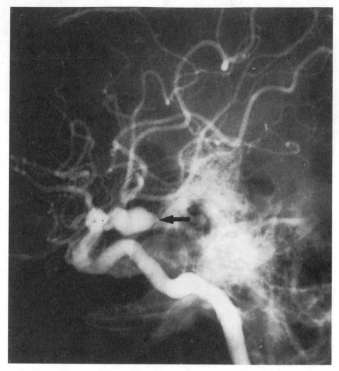

FIGURE 80.2 Lateral cerebral angiogram of a left internal carotid artery injection. A 9-mm elongated saccular aneurysm is seen arising from the region of the takeoff of the posterior communicating artery.

mal. These measures resulted in near complete resolution of her new symptoms. Four days later, the middle cerebral artery velocities began decreasing. A repeat cerebral angiogram confirmed obliteration of the aneurysm by the clip, and resolving vasospasm of the middle cerebral artery. She remained in the hospital 4 more days, and was neurologically intact except for the (resolving) 3rd nerve palsy.

GENERAL CONSIDERATIONS

Aneurysmal subarachnoid hemorrhage most commonly occurs in adulthood, and is often temporally related to a Valsalva maneuver (e.g., physical exertion, sex, bowel movement). Aneurysms most commonly arise at arterial bifurcations involving or in close proximity to the circle of Willis. When an aneurysm ruptures, the hemorrhage occurs at arterial pressures and continues until the subarachnoid pressure tamponades the aneurysmal tear. The extent of the rupture is therefore determined by many factors, including the local subarachnoid space anatomy. Following some aneurysmal subarachnoid hemorrhages, the intracranial pressure momentarily rises to a level near systolic blood pressure, thereby causing a brief loss of consciousness. If the hemorrhage is extensive, the intracranial pressure will remain high—an indication of inadequate cere-

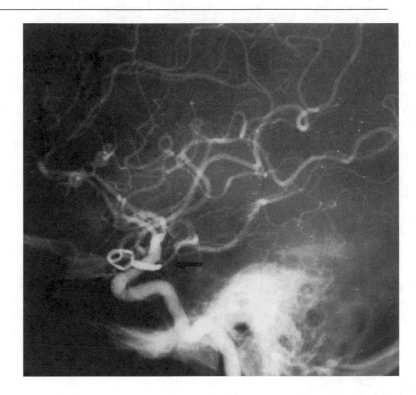

FIGURE 80.3 Postoperative lateral cerebral angiogram of a left internal carotid artery injection. The aneurysm clip is well placed, evidenced by the lack of a residual aneurysm neck and no filling of the aneurysm dome. The posterior communicating artery vessel is now clearly visible (arrow). There is no evidence of vasopasm.

bral blood flow. Because many aneurysmal hemorrhages are extensive, approximately 45% of patients expire before receiving medical attention. Survivors present along a spectrum ranging from mild headache to deep coma. Neck stiffness (nuchal rigidity), nausea, and photophobia are nonspecific findings of meningeal irritation by blood. Meningeal signs can also occur secondary to infection or inflammation involving the meninges.

Cerebral aneurysms are commonly referred to by many names, including berry, saccular, or congenital. Saccular aneurysms appear berry-shaped, and therefore these two terms are used interchangeably. Fusiform dilatations of cerebral arteries (akin to aortic aneurysms) occur as well, but much less commonly. The term *congenital* refers to the theory that patients are born with a congenital weakness of the arterial wall, even though the aneurysm develops in adult life. Hypertension and artherosclerosis are believed to be aggravating conditions. There is a familial tendency for cerebral aneurysms.

The sudden onset of a severe headache is suggestive of an intracranial hemorrhage, specifically aneurysmal subarachnoid hemorrhage. Double vision is caused by a 3rd nerve palsy, which may arise from a variety of etiologies. Most commonly it represents a compression of the nerve as it runs in the basal cistern from the midbrain to the cavernous sinus. A sudden onset of a 3rd nerve palsy in association with severe headache strongly suggests the enlargement or rupture of an aneurysm arising from the internal carotid artery at the posterior communicating artery takeoff (referred to as a "P-comm aneurysm"). Either the expanding aneurysm or the adjacent hematoma

directly compresses the 3rd nerve just before entering the cavernous sinus. An aneurysm arising from the takeoff of the superior cerebellar artery can also compress the 3rd nerve, but aneurysms at this location are relatively rare. Another etiology of 3rd nerve palsy is compression by the medial temporal lobe (uncal herniation). This is most commonly due to temporal lobe swelling or a mass in the temporal lobe. Uncal herniation typically occurs in the context of a comatose patient following severe head injury. Direct trauma to the orbit can also cause "traumatic" mydriasis. A lesion of the midbrain would cause a 3rd nerve palsy in association with a contralateral hemiparesis (Weber syndrome). A dilated pupil without headache may be due to ciliary ganglion disease (Adie's pupil). A 3rd nerve palsy without pupillary dilatation ("pupil-spring") is suggestive of diabetic or other microvascular neuropathy.

An arteriovenous malformation (AVM) should be considered as the possible etiology following the sudden onset of a headache with associated neurologic findings. AVMs most commonly present in young adulthood, and typically occur within the brain parenchyma, causing intracerebral hematomas (also known as intraparenchymal hematomas). Occasionally these lesions hemorrhage into the ventricular or subarachnoid space, and produce meningeal signs. AVMs most commonly present with seizures and/or chronic headache.

Spontaneous hypertensive hemorrhages most commonly occur in the basal ganglia, cerebellar hemisphere, or the brain stem. Similar to strokes, these patients typically present with the sudden onset of neurologic symptoms without significant headache or meningeal signs. A cerebellar hemorrhage large enough to cause obstructive hydrocephalus could cause significant headache, but would likely be associated with ataxia. Hypertensive hemorrhages may occur in conjunction with amphetamine or cocaine abuse. The term "hypertensive hemorrhage" is considered a misnomer by many, since these hemorrhages occur not infrequently in patients without prior history of hypertension.

Spontaneous intracranial hemorrhage can occur secondary to an underlying neoplasm. Brain tumors that are prone to hemorrhage include glioblastoma multiforme and certain metastases (melanoma, renal cell carcinoma, choriocarcinoma). Intracranial infections rarely hemorrhage, with the exception of herpes encephalitis and toxoplasmosis.

In elderly patients, spontaneous intracranial hemorrhages can occur secondary to cerebral amyloid angiopathy. These hemorrhages are most commonly located near the gray-white junction of the cerebral hemispheres. There is no relation to systemic amyloidopathy.

An infectious aneurysm (also known as a mycotic aneurysm) should be considered if fever is present, especially in conjunction with valvular heart disease. Infectious aneurysms arise secondary to an embolic mechanism and are typically found in the distal cerebral vasculature.

KEY POINTS

- Aneurysmal subarachnoid hemorrhage most commonly occurs in adulthood; often temporally related to Valsalva maneuver (e.g., physical exertion, sex, bowel movement)

- Aneurysms most commonly arise at arterial bifurcations involving or in close proximity to circle of Willis

- Because many aneurysmal hemorrhages are extensive, approximately 45% of patients expire before receiving medical attention

- Sudden onset of severe headache is suggestive of intracranial hemorrhage, specifically aneurysmal subarachnoid hemorrhage

- Sudden onset of 3rd nerve palsy in association with severe headache strongly suggests enlargement or rupture of aneurysm arising from internal carotid artery at posterior communicating artery takeoff (P-comm aneurysm)

- Uncal herniation typically occurs in context of comatose patient following severe head injury

- AVM should be considered as possible etiology following sudden onset of headache with associated neurologic findings

- AVMs most commonly present with seizures and/or chronic headache

- Spontaneous hypertensive hemorrhages most commonly occur in basal ganglia, cerebellar hemisphere, or brain stem

- Similar to strokes, these patients typically present with sudden onset of neurologic symptoms without significant headache or meningeal signs

- Spontaneous intracranial hemorrhage can occur secondary to underlying neoplasm

- In elderly patients, spontaneous intracranial hemorrhages occur secondary to cerebral amyloid angiopathy

DIAGNOSIS

The first test that should be ordered is a noncontrast computed tomography (CT) scan (Case 1). This test is much more sensitive to subarachnoid hemorrhage than magnetic resonance imaging (MRI). Still, in about 10% of cases, the CT scan will not demonstrate a subarachnoid hemorrhage. In these cases, a lumbar puncture should be performed to look for blood in the cerebrospinal fluid (or xanthochromia if the hemorrhage occurred several days previously). If neurologic deficits are present, or if there is any indication of raised intracranial pressure, a CT scan should be performed before lumbar puncture to assess the risk of causing tonsillar herniation. A contrast-enhanced CT is not necessary because it is relatively insensitive for the detection of aneurysms. Subarachnoid hemorrhage identified on CT is not necessarily indicative of aneurysmal hemorrhage (trauma is the most frequent cause of subarachnoid hemorrhage). A CT scan is an excellent test to identify an intracerebral hematoma.

If an AVM is suspected, the noncontrast CT scan may not show it unless the AVM is large. A contrast-enhanced CT should be considered, although an MRI scan is the preferred screening test because it shows both the lesion and its relative location to important structures.

For either an aneurysm or AVM, an angiogram is the definitive diagnostic method of choice, since it provides the neurosurgeon with the maximum anatomic information. The most common locations of congenital cerebral aneurysms are in association with the circle of Willis. Approximately 10% of aneurysms occur within the posterior fossa circulation, and therefore, angiography must include visualization of the vertebrobasilar arteries (four-vessel angiogram). In a small percentage of cases, an aneurysm will not be demonstrated on the first angiogram, possibly due to obliteration of the aneurysm by blood clot or lack of filling due to vasospasm. In these cases, a repeat angiogram is sometimes performed approximately 1 week later. Magnetic imaging angiography is not routinely utilized because of marginal sensitivity and poor anatomic detail.

KEY POINTS

- Noncontrast CT scan first test that should be ordered

- If neurologic deficits present, or any indication of raised intracranial pressure, CT should be performed before lumbar puncture to assess risk of causing tonsillar herniation

- Angiogram definitive diagnostic method of choice for aneursym as AVM

DIFFERENTIAL DIAGNOSIS

Several points in a patient's presentation are important. As with most illnesses of the nervous system, the history typically provides the information from which to generate a differential diagnosis of the type of disease process, whereas the neurologic examination is most useful in disease localization. The suddenness of the onset of symptoms strongly suggests a vascular incident, which could be either a hemorrhage or stroke (the term *stroke* is often used in reference to any vascular event, although neurologists and neurosurgeons generally limit its use to infarction). Strokes generally present with a sudden onset of neurologic deficit without headache or altered consciousness. Spontaneous intracranial hemorrhages may present in a wide variety of manners depending on the type and location of hemorrhage. The complaint of the sudden onset of the "worst headache of my life" is highly suggestive of aneurysmal subarachnoid hemorrhage.

KEY POINTS

- Suddenness of onset of symptoms strongly suggests vascular incident

- Complaint of sudden onset of "worst headache of my life" highly suggestive of aneurysmal subarachnoid hemorrhage

---

TREATMENT

Prompt medical attention is required following the diagnosis of a ruptured cerebral aneurysm. The most immediate risk to the patient is rerupture of the aneurysm, since this is associated with a 50% mortality. This risk is highest in the first 48 hours following the initial hemorrhage (20–30%), then declines over the following 2 weeks. The risk of hemorrhage thereafter is cumulative, at 1–2% per year (this is the same risk of an unruptured aneurysm of 1 cm or greater).

The treatment algorithm of ruptured intracranial aneurysms involves many variables, including the neurologic condition of the patient, anesthesia risks, number of days following rupture, and location and size of the aneurysm. In general, surgical exploration is considered as the primary treatment modality in most patients. In order to prevent rerupture, a craniotomy is ideally performed immediately following the angiogram, and a metal clip placed across the neck of the aneurysm (Case 1). In comatose patients, who typically have an edematous brain, some neurosurgeons prefer to delay the surgery 10–14 days because retraction of the swollen brain during surgery may cause further morbidity.

An open craniotomy for clipping of an aneurysm carries a 5–20% combined morbidity and mortality risk, depending on the aneurysm size, location, and condition of the patient. Patients who are at higher operative risk include those with complex or giant aneurysms, previously attempted but failed surgical exploration for clipping, or those who are poor anesthetic risks (due to age or medical condition). In these patients, another therapeutic option is treating the aneurysm by an endovascular approach. Using a transfemoral chatheterization, the aneurysm is filled with detachable metallic coils. This treatment is relatively new, and long term outcome is not presently known.

If the diagnosis is an AVM, the treatment protocol will differ somewhat. Because ruptured AVMs most frequently cause intracerebral hematomas, occasionally a craniotomy must be performed emergently to remove the mass effect caused by the hematoma. AVMs are typically complex lesions, and cerebral angiography is required to determine the arterial supply and venous drainage before treatment. As with aneurysms, most AVMs are managed surgically by excising the AVM nidus. When the AVM is within or immediately adjacent to eloquent brain tissue, focused-beam radiation ("radiosurgery") is considered. It is quite effective (80%) for lesions smaller than 2.5 cm in diameter, and only requires one treatment as an outpatient. The drawback to radiation treatment is that it takes 1–3 years to thrombose the AVM, during which time the patient is still at risk of rupture. AVMs that have not ruptured but are causing neurologic symptoms (most commonly seizures) are treated with either surgery or radiation.

Intracerebral hemorrhages due to hypertensive or amyloid angiopathy are treated expectantly: the hematomas are removed only if they cause life threatening mass effect. Mycotic aneurysms are treated with either antibiotics and/or surgical excision.

The second important cause of morbidity and mortality following aneurysmal subarachnoid hemorrhage is cerebral vasospasm. This typically takes place 4–10 days following the hemorrhage, but may occur as late as 21 days (Case 1). The cause of vasospasm is not known, but is apparently related to hemoglobin breakdown in the periadventitial space surrounding the cerebral arteries. Patients who have the greatest amount of subarachnoid hemorrhage seen on CT scans are at highest risk of vasospasm. Vasospasm typically involves the larger cerebral arteries, and causes morbidity due to ischemia of the brain perfused distal to the constricted vessel. Approximately 30% of aneurysmal subarachnoid hemorrhage patients develop clinically detectable vasospasm.

The primary treatment of cerebral vasospasm is nonoperative—"Triple-H" therapy, consists of hypertension, hypervolemia, and hemodilution (Case 1). The goal is to maintain optimal cerebral perfusion by increasing the systemic blood pressure (occasionally to systolic blood pressures well over 200 mmHg). This is best achieved with adequate cardiac preload, and therefore, either central venous or pulmonary capillary wedge pressure monitoring is required (Case 1). Intravenous colloid is given to optimize the atrial filling pressures. Hemodilution refers to a practice of repeated phlebotomy to achieve an hematocrit (Hct) of 30%. Normally the hypervolemia therapy drops the Hct sufficiently. The rationale for maintaining the Hct in the 23–35% range is that ischemic brain will be more sensitive to a change in oxygen carrying capacity secondary to a low Hct or reduced cerebral blood flow due to high Hct induced sludging of blood in the capillary bed. If triple-H therapy fails to reverse the ischemic conditions, the patient is treated emergently via an endovascular approach with either an arterial vasodilatator (papaverine), or mechanical angioplasty.

Other considerations that cause delayed deterioration are postoperative hematoma formation (intracerebral, subdural, or epidural), or less commonly, a surgical infection. A CT scan or lumbar puncture is obtained emergently to exclude these etiologies (Case 1). Systemic causes such as fever, hypoxia, hypoglycemia, hyponatremia, and endocrine abnormalities should be considered, although they typically cause global neurologic deterioration (as opposed to the focal hemiparesis in Case 1).

KEY POINTS

• Prompt medical attention required following diagnosis of ruptured cerebral aneurysm

• Most immediate risk to patient is rerupture of aneurysm, since associated with 50% mortality

• Surgical exploration considered primary treatment modality in most patients

• Second important cause of morbidity and mortality following aneurysmal subarachnoid hemorrhage is cerebral vasospasm; typically takes place 4–10 days following hemorrhage but may occur as late as 21 days

• Vasospasm typically involves larger cerebral arteries, and causes morbidity due to ischemia of brain perfused distal to constricted vessel

• Primary treatment of cerebral vasospasm is nonoperative

• Systemic causes such as fever, hypoxia, hypoglycemia, hyponatremia, and endocrine abnormalities should be considered, although they typically cause global neurologic deterioration

T FOLLOW-UP

There is no routine follow-up for these patients, since their posthemorrhage course can be quite varied. During the initial weeks following the hemorrhage, the insidious onset of hydrocephalus must be kept in mind. This normally presents several weeks afterward. It is a communicating hydrocephalus, and is presumably due to damage to the arachnoid granulations (which absorb cerebrospinal fluid [CSF] into the venous system) by the blood breakdown products. The treatment is diversion of the cerebrospinal fluid from the ventricles to an alternative site, most commonly the peritoneum (hence, a ventriculoperitoneal shunt).

Aneurysms that are clipped surgically can be considered cured, and do not require angiographic follow-up once the patient is discharged from the hospital. Some neurosurgeons maintain patients on an anticonvulsant for a period of 6–12 months, while others stop prophylaxis within 1 week. Patients who develop seizures require routine follow-up.

Of all patients with aneurysmal subarachnoid hemorrhage, approximately 60% die secondary to the hemorrhage. Of the survivors, many are significantly neurologically impaired and require extensive rehabilitation or prolonged skilled nursing assistance. A significant portion return to normal lives.

KEY POINTS

• During initial weeks following hemorrhage, insidious onset of hydrocephalus must be kept in mind; normally presents several weeks afterward

SUGGESTED READINGS

Greenburg MS: Handbook of Neurosurgery. 3rd Ed. Greenburg Graphics, Lakewood, FL, 1994

This pocketbook is recommended for students rotating on the neurosurgery service. These 41 pages are easily readable in less than an hour.

Ruptured cerebral aneurysms: perioperative management. p. 59. In Ratcheson RA, Wirth FP (eds): Concepts in Neurosurgery. Vol. 6. Williams & Wilkins, Baltimore, 1994

This is a short specialty text that is dedicated to this subject. For the student who wants a more thorough review of the subject that is very up-to-date.

Ojemann RG, Heros RC, Crowell RM (eds): Surgical Management of Cerebrovascular Disease. Williams & Wilkins, Baltimore, 1988

This is a larger textbook that covers neurovascular disorders in an easily readable manner. It is an excellent text for students wishing more in-depth information on aneurysms, AVMs, and other vascular lesions.

QUESTIONS

1. Which cranial nerve is most commonly affected by an expanding intracranial aneurysm?

    A. 3rd.

    B. 4th.

    C. 6th.

    D. 9th.

2. The initial screening test in the diagnosis of a suspected spontaneous intracranial hemorrhage is?

    A. A contrast-enhanced CT scan.

    B. A noncontrast-enhanced CT scan.

    C. A contrast-enhanced MRI scan.

    D. A four-vessel cerebral angiogram.

3. *Unlike strokes, the neurologic deficit associated with a cerebral hemorrhage is?*

    A. Rapid in onset.

    B. Global.

    C. Associated with a severe headache.

    D. More commonly accompanied by visual changes.

4. *The main purpose of craniotomy in patients with intracranial hemorrhage is to?*

    A. Evaluate the hematoma.

    B. Prevent rerupture.

    C. Reduce intracranial pressure.

    D. Reduce brain swelling.

(See p. 605 for answers.)

81 SPINAL DEGENERATIVE DISORDERS

DUNCAN Q. MCBRIDE

Weight bearing, flexion, extension, and rotatory movements all can cause gradual degeneration of intervertebral discs and spinal facet joints. Dehydration, degeneration, collapse, and herniation of intervertebral discs can occur. This causes failure of the spine to bear its normal axial load and can also cause compression and irritation of neural elements. The result is pain and neurologic dysfunction. The specific neurologic deficits are related to the exact location and function of the affected nerves. This chapter introduces the spectrum of degenerative disorders that involve the human spinal column.

CASE 1
CERVICAL SPONDYLITIC MYELOPATHY

A 66-year-old female complained of the insidious onset of neck pain radiating to her shoulders and arms, right greater than left.

She was experiencing tingling, burning, and numbness in her right thumb and index finger. She also noted progressive upper and lower extremity weakness to the extent that she was unable to open a jar or turn a doorknob with her hands. She complained that her gait had become stiff and she was unable to run or to climb stairs without assistance. She denied difficulties with urination or anal sphincter control.

She had mild atrophy of the thenar and hypothenar eminences, right greater than left. Her gait was slightly spastic in nature. Her mental status, cranial nerves, and cerebellar examinations were normal. She had 4+/5 weakness of the right biceps and brachioradialis muscles, and 5–/5 weakness of the wrist extensor on the right and the triceps bilaterally. She also had 5–/5 weakness of the lower extremities diffusely. There was hyperesthesia with tingling sensation on palpation in the index finger and thumb on the right side and into the radial aspect of the forearm. Pin/dull discrimination revealed error in the same distributions bilaterally, with diffuse errors in the trunk and the lower extremities. Joint position sense was intact. Deep tendon reflexes were absent at the biceps and brachioradialis. She had 2+ triceps reflexes and 3+ patellar and Achilles reflexes. The plantar reflexes were extensor bilaterally, and there was mild clonus at the ankles.

Cervical spine radiographs showed the normal lordotic curve with osteophytic spurs at C4-C5 and C5-C6 with evidence of foraminal stenosis. An MRI scan demonstrated circumferential stenotic levels at C4-C5 and C5-C6 due to disc herniation and osteophytes ventrally and ligamentous hypertrophy dorsally (Fig. 81.1). The stenosis at C5-C6 was quite severe with compression of the cervical spinal cord and lack of CSF signal at that level. There was marked stenosis of the neural foramina bilaterally, with greater narrowing on the right side. She was placed in a cervical collar and given dexamethasone acetate. An anterior cervical spinal decompression with discectomies at C4-C5 and C5-C6 was done urgently. The C5 vertebral body underwent corpectomy. The osteophyte and herniated disc segments were carefully elevated and removed. The posterior longitudinal ligament was opened and the dura allowed to relax forward into the defect created in the bone. Foraminotomies were performed at C5-C6 with careful excision of bony material from the neuroforamina. The spine was fused using autologous iliac crest.

Postoperatively, she noted immediate improvement in her pain syndrome in the upper extremities and neck. She had residual numbness in the C5-C6 distribution, which gradually resolved. Her abnormal gait and lower extremity symptoms had begun to improve while on dexamethasone and continued to improve over the course of several months, such that she had a normal gait on long-term follow-up. At 6 weeks postoperatvely, she was able to discontinue the cervical collar orthosis. Cervical spine flexion/extension views demonstrated a good fusion of the bone graft with C4, C5, and C6 moving as one solid unit.

CASE 2
LUMBAR DISC HERNIATION

A 31-year-old male was lifting a couch when he felt a "pop" in his back. He suffered immediate severe lower back pain and could not straighten up properly. Within an hour, he began to note burning of the left leg from his buttock down to the dorsum of his foot. This pain was a shooting, electrical sensation that was quite severe. Whenever he tried to stand, walk, or sit or whenever he coughed or sneezed, he noted increased pain in the lower extremity. He spent 1 or 2 days in bed, which gave some relief; however, he sought medical attention when pain relievers and bed rest did not completely resolve his pain syndrome. He had not had difficulty urinating.

On physical examination, he was in marked distress and unable to straighten, preferring to lie on the examination table. He had decreased light touch in the posterolateral aspect of his left thigh down into his calf and onto the dorsum of his foot, including the lateral aspect onto the plantar surface. He had normal power in his lower extremities except for his left extensor hallucis longus, which was 4/5. He was unable to stand on his toes on the left, and had difficulty with heel standing. The deep tendon reflexes were 2+ at the knees and the right ankle and absent at the

left ankle. The straight leg raising test produced severe pain in the left leg at 30 degrees. The back was nontender to palpation, and there was no paraspinous muscle spasm.

An MRI of the lumbar spine showed a large disc herniation with probable extrusion of disc fragment into the spinal canal on the left side at L5–S1 (Fig. 81.2). The disk caused entrapment of the L5 nerve root exiting at that level as well as the traversing S1 root.

He underwent an L4-L5 hemilaminotomy on the left with microscopic discectomy. A large free disc fragment was found to be compressing the L5 and S1 nerve roots and it was removed.

Postoperatively, he had immediate resolution of his severe pain. He rapidly recovered power in his toe and ankle, although he had persistent absence of the deep tendon reflex at the left ankle on long-term follow-up.

GENERAL CONSIDERATIONS

Degenerative disorders of the spine are quite common. Approximately 50% of individuals over 50 years of age who are studied with lumbar or cervical magnetic resonance imaging (MRI) scans show degenerative changes. Disc herniations can occur acutely with trauma, or insidiously with dehydration and degeneration of the disc and gradual inability of the disc to carry its normal weight and motion load. This causes the disc to lose its height and results in bony osteophyte formation, where bone edges touch that previously did not. This abnormal friction causes overgrowth of bony end-plates and results in bone spur formation (spondylosis). Furthermore, abnormal motion and chronic degenerative changes in posterior facet joints results in hypertrophy of the joint and the adjacent ligamentum flavum. This commonly occurs in the lumbar spine, resulting in progressive circumferential stenosis of the spinal canal with advanced age. In the cervical spine, this can be further aggravated by degeneration and hypertrophy of the uncovertebral joints that lie at the posterolateral aspects of the disc space bilaterally.

The principal manifestations of spinal degenerative disease are pain and neurologic deficit. Patients with cervical spine disc herniation present with a syndrome of neck, arm, and head pain, typically in the dermatomal pattern of the exiting nerve root. Frequently this pain is a severe burning, tingling numbness that awakens the patient at night due to repeated minor trauma to the cervical nerve root. Pain often is felt in the paraspinous muscle area and at trigger points in the interscapular region and occipital areas.

Cervical disc herniation or cervical spondylosis can also cause neurologic deficit in the spinal cord (Case 1). In these circumstances, patients will have long tract upper motor neuron findings manifested below the level of cervical compression, as well as lower motor neuron periph-

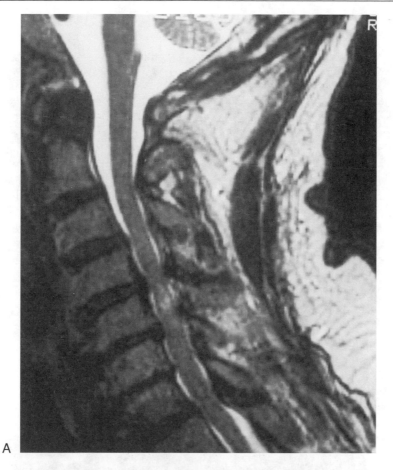

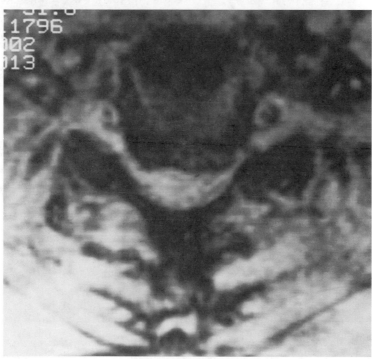

FIGURE 81.1 *(A) Saggital T$_2$-weighted MRI of the cervical spine demonstrating degenerative discs with spinal cord compression maximum at C4-C5 and C5-C6. Note increased signal intensity between these discs indicative of cord edema. (B) Axial CT image through the C5-C6 disc illustrates spinal canal stenosis and spinal cord compression.*

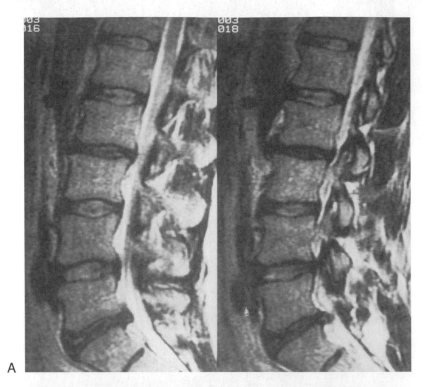

A

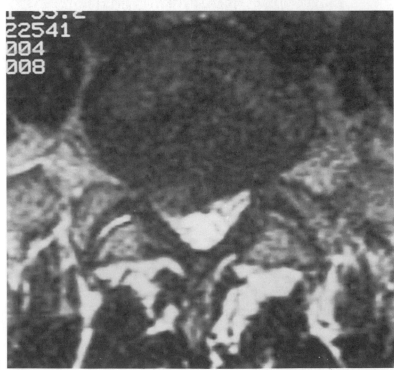

B

FIGURE 81.2 (**A**) *Saggital T$_2$-weighted MRI of the lumbar spine demonstrating degenerated herniated disc at L5–S1 with nerve root entrapment.* (**B**) *Axial view through L5–S1 disc illustrates neural foraminal and nerve root compression on the right from the disc extrusion.*

eral findings in the distribution of the nerve root at the level of compression.

Lumbar spinal degeneration occurs by similar mechanisms. The highest percentage of cases occur below L4, and neurologic signs are virtually always peripheral nerve in nature. Patients with lumbar degenerative disease typically present with varying degrees of a combination of low back pain and leg pain. Radiating leg pain in the distribution of affected nerve roots is often called sciatica. Because low back pain is so common (60–80% incidence) the judicious use of conservative management, diagnostic testing, and surgery is extremely important. Thus, operation is limited to those patients who fail conservative management.

The importance of psychosocial issues in the treatment of spinal degenerative disease cannot be overemphasized. All studies that have examined surgical outcome have demonstrated the effect of litigation. Other forms of secondary gain should also be considered, including familial sympathy, drug seeking, and other psychosocial motivators.

KEY POINTS

• Disc herniations can occur acutely with trauma, or insidiously with dehydration and degeneration of the disc and gradual inability of the disc to carry its normal weight and motion load; this causes the disc to lose height and results in bony osteophyte formation, where bone edges touch that previously did not

• Principal manifestations of spinal degenerative disease are pain and neurologic deficit

• Patients with cervical spine disc herniation present with neck, arm, and head pain, typically in the dermatomal pattern of the exiting nerve root; frequently pain is severe burning, tingling numbness that awakens patient at night due to repeated minor trauma to cervical nerve root

• In circumstances of neurologic deficit of spinal cord, patients will have long tract upper motor neuron findings manifested below the level of cervical compression, as well as lower motor neuron peripheral findings in the distribution of the nerve root at the level of compression

• Highest percentage of cases occur below L4, and neurologic signs are virtually always peripheral nerve in nature

• Radiating leg pain in the distribution of affected nerve roots often called sciatica

DIAGNOSIS

The chief complaint of a patient with cervical degenerative disease is likely to be neck, shoulder, arm, and possibly hand pain. The pain is frequently described as an electrical shooting, pins-and-needles sensation in the more distal regions of the nerve root and more of an ache or stabbing pain in the neck. The pain is exacerbated by

head movements, and often the patient will feel more comfortable with the head tilted away from the side of maximum root compression. The patient may also complain of weakness and numbness in the hand or arm. Specific complaints depend on the level of compression and the degree of neurologic compromise. In those with spinal cord symptoms, the complaints include weakness or abnormal sensation in the legs as well as, potentially, bowel and bladder sphincter disturbance. As in lumbar disease, maneuvers that increase the degree of neural compression cause increased symptoms. These include extreme flexion, extension, or lateral rotation of the spine or Valsalva maneuvers that increase the intrathecal pressure. Thus, the patient's complaints might include increased pain on coughing, sneezing, laughing, or defecation.

Symptoms from lumbar disc disease are similar. Those with disease producing nerve root entrapment have leg symptoms that far outweigh the low back complaints. The patients have abnormal posture, tilting away from the side of disc herniation. The pain can be so severe that they cannot straighten completely or stand upright (Case 2).

Symptoms of lumbar stenosis, without acute disc herniation, differ considerably from those of the acute herniated disc with stenosis. Patients typically have an insidious onset of pain rather than acute pain. The pain is exclusively in the legs and is often bilateral. If back pain does exist, it is typically a low-level dull ache in the uncomplicated stenosis patient. The hallmark feature of lumbar stenosis is onset of leg pain on walking some distance that is relieved by rest. Usually the patient will say they can walk a block or two and then they have to sit down to relieve the burning pain in the posterolateral aspects of their thighs and calves.

In cervical degenerative disease, a wide variety of physical findings may be present. These include pain and tenderness in the paracervical musculature and at trigger points in the interscapular area. Limited range of motion in the neck may also be present. A thorough motor examination of the upper and lower extremities is essential. Motor testing results are given on a five-point scale (Table 81.1). Because the motor power scale is weighted toward the weaker end, clinicians often will include the subcategories of 4+ and 5– power to indicate various degrees of opposition to applied resistance (Case 2). As individual muscle groups are tested, their bulk and tone should also

TABLE 81.1 *Motor power scale*

0	No contraction
1	Palpable or visible contraction with no joint movement
2	Movement of joint only when gravity eliminated
3	Can overcome gravity but not added resistance
4	Can push against added resistance, but weakly
5	Normal strength

be documented. The presence of atrophy should be clearly defined. Sensory testing, including light touch, pin/dull discrimination and joint position sense, aid significantly in the localization of both radicular and spinal cord problems. The testing of deep tendon reflexes, Babinski response, Hoffmann response, and clonus of the ankles is essential in the diagnosis of upper and lower motor neuron problems. Analysis of the patient's gait and ability to stand on heels and toes, and the Romberg test, further define the neurologic deficit that may be present (Table 81.2).

Lumbar degenerative disease examination of the low back for scoliosis, percussion for deep tenderness, and palpation of paraspinous musculature, sacroiliac joint, and the sciatic notch for tenderness is done. Range of motion of the back, and examination of the hip, knee, and ankle should be noted. The typical syndromes for the lumbar and sacral roots are listed in Table 81.3. In herniation, a tension test should be done by straight leg raising. The patient is placed on the back and the leg is elevated by holding the ankle. This puts significant stretch on the nerve root that is compressed by the herniated disc. Absence of straight leg raising or other tension test findings should place significant doubt on the diagnosis of lumbar disc disease that is correctable by operative decompression. In patients with lumbar stenosis, all of the above mentioned root syndromes and tension test findings, are likely to be completely absent. In these patients, careful examination of the hip joint as well as the peripheral vascular pulses in the legs are extremely important to differentiate other commonly occurring sources of similar pain. Additionally, abdominal and rectal examinations are indicated since there are significant abdominal and retroperitoneal conditions (abdominal aortic aneurysm) that may produce leg pain.

A large percentage of plain radiographs of the lumbar spine fail to diagnose the pathology completely, and further imaging is required. At present, MRI scanning is the imaging test of choice for initial evaluation of spinal disorders. Neuronal elements are clearly seen on MRI, and often, disc and bone pathology is adequately imaged by this technique. Computed tomography (CT) scan is superior to MRI in

TABLE 81.3 *Lumbar sacral spine levels*

LEVEL	MOTOR	SENSORY	REFLEX
L1	Iliopsoas	Upper anterior thigh	Cremasteric
L2	Hip flexion, leg adduction	Mid-anterior thigh	None
L3	Hip extension	Anterior thigh, medial knee	None
L4	Quadriceps femoris	Knee, medial calf	Patellar
L5	Ankle dorsiflexors, toe dorsiflexors (EHL)	Lateral thigh and calf, dorsum foot to great toe	None
S1	Ankle, toe plantar flexors	Lateral calf, ankle and foot, sole	Achilles
S2	Hamstrings	Posterior thigh	None
S3–4	Anal sphincter	Perianal	Anal wink

Abbreviation: EHL, extensor hallucis longus.

imaging of bony foramina and for disc versus osteophyte differentiation. On occasion, patients require both MRI and CT scanning to complement each other. The best preoperative test remains the myelogram with postmyelogram CT scan. The myelogram, with intrathecal injection of water soluble contrast material, clearly delineates individual nerve roots as well as spinal cord anatomy. The cross-sectional CT scan with the contrast dye in the thecal sac, gives a superior image of the relationship of disc, bone, ligament, and nerve. In patients with multilevel problems, those with both cervical and lumbar degenerative problems, and those with difficult-to-diagnosis pathology, the myelogram remains the ultimate preoperative imaging test.

KEY POINTS

- Pain exacerbated by head movements; often patient will feel more comfortable with head tilted away from side of maximum root compression

- Patient may also complain of weakness and numbness in hand or arm

- Patients typically have insidious onset of pain rather than acute pain, exclusively in legs and often bilateral

- If back pain exists, typically low-level dull ache in uncomplicated stenosis patient; hallmark feature of lumbar stenosis is onset of leg pain upon walking some distance that is relieved by rest

TABLE 81.2 *Cervical spine levels*

LEVEL	MOTOR	SENSORY	REFLEX
C1–3	Neck muscles	Posterior head and neck	None
C4	Diaphragm	Shoulder	Pectoral
C5	Deltoid	Lateral upper arm	(Biceps)
C6	Biceps, wrist extensors	Radial forearm, thumb, and index finger	Biceps, brachioradialis
C7	Triceps, wrist flexors	Long finger and dorsal web of hand	Triceps
C8	Finger flexors	Ring, little fingers, and ulnar forearm	None

DIFFERENTIAL DIAGNOSIS

Degenerative disorders can present in a similar fashion to cervical spondylitic disease. These include acute disc herniation, gradual disc collapse, osteophyte formation, circumferential spinal stenosis, hypertrophied ligamentum flavum, ossification of the posterior longitudinal ligament (OPLL), and segmental instability. Rheumatoid arthritis and ankylosing spondylitis must also be considered. Tumors of the cervical spine, both intramedullary and extramedullary, can cause nerve root symptoms and long track findings.

Central nervous system disorders such as multiple sclerosis and peripheral nerve entrapment syndromes commonly mimic cervical spine degenerative complaints. Peripheral nerve compression syndromes include carpal tunnel syndrome with entrapment of the median nerve in the wrist, and cubital tunnel syndrome with entrapment of the ulnar nerve at the elbow. The former is distinguished from a C6 or C7 radiculopathy by the presence of normal sensation in the radial nerve innervated portion of the dermatomes (volar aspect of the thumb, index, and long fingers). Tinel's sign (electric shock sensation produced by tapping over the nerve) may be found at the point of entrapment. Often, however, one must perform EMG (electromyograph)/NCV (nerve conduction velocity) testing to distinguish between peripheral entrapment and cervical radiculopathy.

Lumbar disc herniation or degenerative collapse, progressive lumbar stenosis with hypertrophy of the nerve roots in the lateral gutters, and spondylosis with osteophyte formation are all degenerative spinal disorders. Additionally, spondylolisthesis, when a vertebra is out of anteroposterior alignment with its neighbor (subluxation), can be degenerative, congenital, or traumatic. All these disorders can cause nerve root entrapment with varying degrees of associated low back pain. Retroperitoneal and pelvic pathologies including renal stones and neoplasms, can also mimic the lumbar pain syndrome. Back pain and neurologic symptoms and signs in the legs are occasionally caused by thoracic disc herniation.

Claudication is pain in the calf on exertion due to poor arterial inflow. It can be distinguished from lumbar neurogenic claudication by the quality of the pain, which is usually a cramp or a tight sensation that progresses from distal to proximal in vascular disease. This is unlike the burning proximal to distal pain experienced by the patient with lumbar stenosis. In addition, those with vascular claudication will obtain some relief when standing up, whereas the patient with neurogenic claudication usually needs to sit or lie down to get relief from pain in the legs. Physical examination is very helpful in distinguishing these two disorders.

TREATMENT

All patients with cervical radicular signs and symptoms, without myelopathy, are given a course of conservative management in an attempt to relieve their pain. Those with profound motor weakness due to peripheral nerve entrapment who do not have myelopathy may be the exception to this rule. Conservative management of cervical spine disorders is immobilization with a cervical collar. Cervical traction is another option for pain due to a degenerative cervical spine. Application of axial traction in the neutral to slightly flexed position may open the interspace at the disc level and allow the neural foramen some relief of compression from either disc or osteophyte. Traction is applied intermittently during the day for as long as the patient can tolerate. It is used in addition to a soft cervical collar, which should be worn at all other times, especially at night.

Anti-inflammatory agents, particularly nonsteroidal drugs, are most often prescribed. Analgesics can be helpful, but prolonged narcotic use should be avoided. Muscle relaxants are only indicated in patients with severe intermittent muscle spasm. Tricyclic antidepressants, particularly amitriptyline, are often used with considerable success in the nerve root entrapment syndromes. Immobilization and traction may address the cause of the patient's pain, while other approaches merely treat the symptoms. With these modalities, a significant percentage will obtain relief of their symptoms. If significant neurologic findings are absent, the patient should be treated in this manner for at least 6 weeks.

A conservative approach is indicated initially for all patients who present with the low back pain syndrome, with or without pain radiating into the leg. The exceptions to this rule are patients with acute cauda equina syndrome and those with documented progressive motor loss. Similar to cervical pathology, the mainstay of treatment is immobilization. This is best achieved in the lumbar spine by bed rest for at least 7–10 days.

Patients with cervical stenosis and myelopathy, or patients with traumatic soft disc herniations with myelopathy, should be operated on without a prolonged attempt at conservative treatment. High dose steroids, either intravenous or oral, are indicated as a perioperative adjunct. Additionally, those with radicular symptoms who do not significantly improve with conservative management are in need of operation. In those cases, the degree of the patient's pain and neurologic deficit determines the urgency of the elective operation.

There are varying surgical approaches for relief of cervical degenerative radiculopathy and myelopathy. All patients with cervical spine pathology require extremely careful intubation, using an awake fiberoptic nasal technique with minimal head manipulation. In addition, they must be positioned very carefully to ensure that there is no exacerbation of cervical compression while anesthetized. Those with myelopathy should be monitored with intraoperative electrophysiologic evoked potentials.

The typical approach in the presence of ventral cervical compression from a disc or osteophyte is an anterior cervical discectomy. This is done through a small incision in the anterior aspect of the neck, with removal of the intervertebral disc in a piecemeal fashion.

Posterior cervical procedures include a focal laminectomy and foraminotomy for relief of unilateral radiculopathy due to a laterally placed disc or osteophyte. This small operation is often highly effective in relieving compressive symptoms of the root. Occasionally the ventral disc material can be removed as well. The major advantage of this approach is that it does not require cervical fusion. A more extensive bilateral laminectomy is indicated in patients with myelopathy who have greater than two levels of compression, especially those with circumferential compression that includes narrowing of the canal posteriorly. Operation for a lumbar disc should be performed acutely in those with cauda equina syndrome (loss of urinary control, weakness, sensory loss) or progressive motor loss. In addition, when degenerative lumbar stenosis is present, a significant response to conservative management is unlikely. Lumbar disc decompression should be performed only on those with pain syndromes predominantly in the leg. In addition, these patients must have failed a course of conservative management and be free of severe psychosocial problems. For some, litigation revolving around the disc herniation and its consequences is a relative contraindication to operation.

A new, less invasive approach is currently being advocated. This is known as endoscopic discectomy and is performed through a similar posterolateral approach; however, this instrumentation is placed into the neuroforamen. With direct visualization of the disc and root through a microendoscope, the surgeon is able to remove disc material both from the spinal canal and from the intervertebral disc space. As this promising technique is quite new, determination of its safety and efficacy is yet to be made.

P FOLLOW-UP

Patients who are motivated and unencumbered by secondary gain issues, who have clear-cut pathology and whose operation is successful, should have a very high percentage of cure from their pain syndrome. In those with myelopathy, the patient's age and the duration and severity of the myelopathy will determine the outcome. Peripheral nerve injury generally has a favorable long term recovery rate due to wallerian regeneration.

After anterior cervical approach and alignment of the cervical spine, the position of the bone graft and the ultimate fusion of the graft must be assessed. These patients are kept in a cervical collar until the graft is fused. When this occurs at 6 weeks to 2 months postoperatively, the patient is taken out of the collar and flexion/extension lateral cervical spine views are taken to ensure that the fused segment moves as one block. Those who have myelopathy or a significant motor loss from radiculopathy are treated postoperatively with physical and occupational therapy to maximize their recovery.

Patients who have undergone simple lumbar laminectomy are generally mobilized to their feet on either the first or the second postoperative day and go directly into a physical therapy program to exercise their back and abdominal musculature, and assist them in ambulation. Postlaminectomy lumbar instability and recurrent disc herniations are both potential postoperative problems.

SUGGESTED READINGS

Chevrot A, Vallee C: Imaging of degenerative disk diseases. Curr Opin Radiol 4:103, 1992

A very useful reference on current modalities of diagnostic imaging.

Hardin JG, Halla JT: Cervical spine and radicular pain syndromes. Curr Opin Rheumatol 7:136, 1995

A good general review of radicular pain syndromes.

QUESTIONS

1. Lumbar degenerative disease most commonly presents with?

    A. Altered control of voiding.
    B. Sciatica.
    C. Neurogenic impotence.
    D. Lower extremity spasticity.

2. Lumbar stenosis, in contradistinction to acute disc herniation?

    A. Primarily has lower extremity complaints.
    B. Has pain with ambulation not relieved by rest.
    C. Has slower onset of symptoms.
    D. Is associated with severe and constant back pain.

3. The imaging test of choice for the initial diagnosis of spinal disorders is?

    A. Myelography.
    B. CT.
    C. MRI.
    D. Plain films of the spine.

(See p. 605 for answers.)

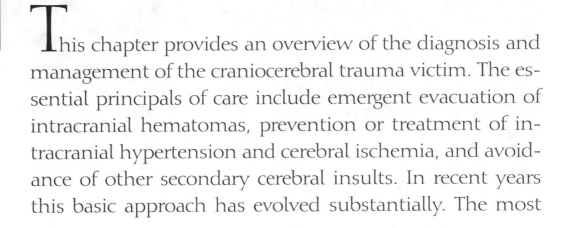

82

HEAD

INJURY

DANIEL F. KELLY

This chapter provides an overview of the diagnosis and management of the craniocerebral trauma victim. The essential principals of care include emergent evacuation of intracranial hematomas, prevention or treatment of intracranial hypertension and cerebral ischemia, and avoidance of other secondary cerebral insults. In recent years this basic approach has evolved substantially. The most

important steps include maintaining adequate cerebral perfusion pressure (CPP) as a means of averting cerebral ischemia and the recognition that excessive hyperventilation to control intracranial hypertension may actually promote ischemia.

CASE 1
EPIDURAL HEMATOMA

A 17-year-old student fell from his bicycle striking his head on the curb. Friends witnessed a brief period of unconsciousness lasting approximately 30 seconds. He gradually regained consciousness over the next several minutes but was confused and somewhat combative on awakening. When paramedics arrived on the scene 15 minutes later, he remained disoriented but was moving all extremities on command and had normally reactive pupils. A right frontotemporal scalp hematoma was noted. He was placed on a spine board and in a stiff cervical collar and transported to the hospital.

On arrival to the emergency room, he was confused, with an initial GCS of 14, a nonfocal neurologic examination, and normal vital signs (BP, 126/78 mmHg; HR, 82 bpm). No other injuries were noted. A three-view cervical spine x-ray series demonstrated no evidence of fracture or subluxation. He was taken urgently for CT of the head,

which demonstrated a right temporal epidural hematoma with effacement of the right lateral ventricle and a slight right-to-left midline shift (Fig. 82.1).

After the CT scan, the patient was noted to be more lethargic, opening his eyes only to painful stimuli, following commands intermittently, exhibiting a left pronator drift and verbalizing inappropriately (GCS, 11). He was taken emergently to the operating room where he was intubated, given a loading dose of phenytoin (18 mg/kg) and a 75-g IV bolus of mannitol. A craniotomy was performed and the epidural hematoma evacuated. A temporal bone fracture and an avulsed bleeding branch of the right middle meningeal artery were found. He was extubated 4 hours after surgery and within 24 hours was fully alert and oriented. A follow-up CT scan demonstrated no reaccumulation of the hematoma. He was discharged home on postoperative day 5 with a nonfocal neurologic examination and mild intermittent headaches.

CASE 2
SUBDURAL HEMATOMA

A 39-year-old male was the unbelted driver in a single car motor vehicle accident in which the car struck a telephone pole. He was found unconscious with shallow respirations and smelling of alcohol. He was extricated, placed on a

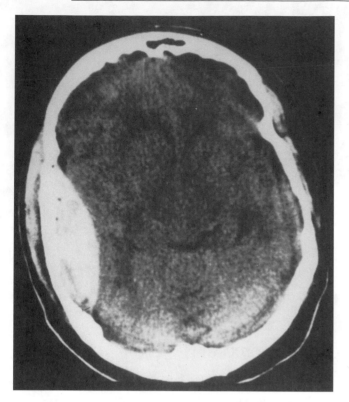

FIGURE 82.1   *Axial noncontrast CT of right middle fossa (temporal) epidural hematoma causing midline shift (Case 1).*

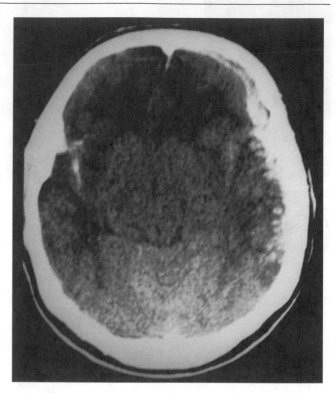

FIGURE 82.2   *Axial noncontrast CT of left convexity acute subdural hematoma with midline shift, early underlying cortical contusions, and thick subarachnoid hemorrhage in the right sylvian fissure (Case 2).*

spine board, and in a cervical collar. On arrival to the emergency room, his BP was 100/65 mmHg; pulse, 88 bpm; and respiration, 8 breaths/min. Initial GCS was 6 with no verbalization or eye opening to painful stimulation, although he withdrew to pain on the right side but extensor postured on the left. The right pupil was 4 mm and briskly reactive, the left was 6 mm and sluggish. Because of the patient's comatose state and focal neurologic deficit suggestive of an intracranial mass lesion with raised intracranial pressure, he was emergently intubated, mildly hyperventilated (PaCO$_2$ 30–35 mmHg), given a 75-g mannitol bolus and treated with phenytoin (18 mg/kg). His mild hypotension was also aggressively treated with a rapid infusion of normal saline. He had a small right temporoparietal cephalohematoma. The chest, abdomen, and extremity examinations were unremarkable. Chest x-ray demonstrated two nondisplaced rib fractures on the right without a pneumothorax. Pelvic films and cervical spine x-rays were normal. He was taken for a head CT, which demonstrated a left frontotemporal subdural hematoma with underlying cortical contusions, diffuse subarachnoid hemorrhage, and a left-to-right shift (Fig. 82.2).

Craniotomy and evacuation of an acute subdural hematoma were performed. A small area of severely contused left frontal lobe was also removed. The brain re-

mained moderately tense but pulsatile after hematoma and contusion removal. A right frontal ventriculostomy was placed for CSF drainage and monitoring of ICP. A central venous pressure line was placed and he was started on dopamine to improve CPP.

On arrival in the ICU, he had a BP of 135/72 mmHg; ICP of 17 mmHg; and CPP of 76 mmHg. Both pupils were now 4 mm, the right briskly reactive and the left sluggish. Over the next 24 hours, his ICP was well controlled (<20 mmHg) with ventricular CSF drainage, narcotic sedation, and mannitol boluses (0.25–0.50 g/kg every 4–6 hours). CPP was maintained over 70 mmHg with volume expansion (CVP 5–10 mmHg) and dopamine. By postinjury day 2, however, the ICP increased from 20 to 35 mmHg and CPP fell to 60 mmHg. He appeared more agitated and was resisting the ventilator. A repeat CT scan showed diffuse swelling, and progression of the frontal and temporal lobe contusions. Therapy was increased accordingly with the addition of a neuromuscular blocking agent and a benzodiazepine for presumed alcohol withdrawal. A pulmonary artery catheter was placed, and after assessing cardiac function, dopamine was maximized and dobutamine added. The patient required aggressive management for the next 4 days, after which his intracranial hypertension began to abate. He was weaned from vasopressor treatment by postinjury day 8 and was extubated on day 10. Over the next several days he began to verbalize but had an obvious expressive dysphasia and a mild right hemiparesis. He was transferred to a rehabilitation facility. At 6 months postinjury, he remained moderately disabled as defined by the Glasgow Outcome Scale.

GENERAL CONSIDERATIONS

Traumatic brain injury continues to pose a serious health care challenge throughout the world. In the United States, trauma is the leading cause of death in individuals under 45 years of age and is a major cause of death and disability in older age groups as well. Brain injury results in more trauma deaths than do injuries to any other specific body region. Approximately half of the 150,000 injury-related deaths that occur annually in the United States involve a serious brain injury that is primarily responsible for the patient's demise. Overall, approximately 500,000 head injuries requiring admission to a hospital occur annually in the United States. Extracranial trauma, including thoracic, abdominal, facial, and extremity injuries, complicate 30–70% of head injuries; approximately 5% of head injury victims also sustain a cervical spine injury. Alcohol intoxication is a compounding factor in at least 25–50% of head injuries (Case 2) and is a contributing factor in almost one-half of all fatal motor vehicle crashes.

A critical factor in early treatment decisions and in long term outcome after head injury is the patient's initial level of consciousness. Although many methods of defining level of consciousness exist, the most widely used is the Glasgow Coma Scale (GCS), first presented by Teasdale and Jennett in 1974 (Table 82.1). The patient's best motor, verbal, and eye-opening responses determine the GCS. A patient who is able to follow commands, is oriented, and has spontaneous eye opening, scores a GCS of 15; a score of less than 15 denotes a diminished level of consciousness (Cases 1 and 2). A patient with no motor response, eye opening, or verbal response to deep pain scores a GCS of 3. The utility of this scaling system is its objectivity, reproducibility, and relative simplicity. It provides paramedics, nurses, and physicians with a rapid measure of a patient's level of consciousness, obviating ambiguous terminology such as lethargic, stuporous, and obtunded. When properly performed, the degree of interobserver difference is negligible. Hence, a change in the GCS from one assessment to the next is indicative of a significant change in the level of consciousness.

Head injury severity is generally categorized into three levels based on the postresuscitation GCS. Minor or mild head injury includes those patients with an initial GCS of 14 or 15 (Case 1), moderate injury includes patients with a GCS of 9–13, and severe injury refers to a postresuscita-

TABLE 82.1 *Glasgow Coma Scale*[a]

Eye opening
   4 = Spontaneously
   3 = To voice
   2 = To pain
   1 – None

Verbal response
   5 = Oriented
   4 = Confused
   3 = Inappropriate words
   2 = Incomprehensible sounds
   1 = None

Motor response
   6 = Follows commands
   5 = Localizes to pain
   4 = Withdrawal to pain
   3 = Abnormal flexion
   2 = Abnormal extension
   1 = None

[a]The postresuscitation GCS is one of the strongest predictors in the head injured patient. Systemic complications of head injuries include coagulopathy, hyperthermia, hyperglycemia, pneumonia, and sepsis.

tion GCS of 3–8 (Case 2) or a subsequent deterioration to a GCS of 8 or less. Approximately one-third to one-half of patients who sustain a severe closed head injury will require craniotomy for evacuation of a traumatic hematoma. Up to three-quarters of cranial gunshot wound victims develop intracranial hematomas, although many are too neurologically devastated to undergo hematoma evacuation.

Meaningful recovery of function after head injury is possible if patients are rapidly and effectively resuscitated, surgical mass lesions are emergently evacuated, and secondary insults are prevented or minimized. A key factor in recovery is reduction of the heightened state of vulnerability in which the brain exists following injury. After such insults, many neuronal, glial, and endothelial cells are functionally impaired. If conditions are favorable, these cells will recover with time. However, if events such as hypotension, hypoxia, or intracranial hypertension go unchecked, injury increases. Optimizing conditions for cellular recovery by maintaining adequate CPP, normalizing intracranial pressure (ICP), and averting additional secondary insults is essential in the overall treatment strategy of the head injured patient.

Several factors have consistently been shown to be strong predictors of poor outcome following head injury. These include older age, a low postresuscitation GCS, an abnormal motor response, pupillary dilatation or asymmetry, and the presence of hypotension, hypoxia, or intracranial hypertension. Computed tomography (CT) findings predictive of poor outcome include mass lesions, particularly acute subdural hematomas, intracerebral hematomas, or multiple contusions, the presence of compressed or absent mesencephalic cisterns, significant midline shift (≥3 mm), or the presence of subarachnoid hemorrhage (Table 82.2). Importantly, these variables have an additive effect on morbidity and mortality; when multiple factors are present in a given patient—such as older age, low GCS, pupillary asymmetry, hypotension and midline shift on CT—the chances for a good recovery are markedly diminished. In recent reports of patients sustaining severe closed head injury, a favorable outcome, defined as a good recovery or moderate disability by Glasgow Outcome Scale, was achieved in approximately 50% of patients, with a mortality rate of approximately 25%. Despite intensive intervention, long-term disability occurs in a large portion of the survivors of severe head injury (Case 2). Significant neuropsychologic sequelae and physical disabilities are also common in patients sustaining milder injuries.

TABLE 82.2 *Major predictors of poor outcome after closed head injury*

Clinical Findings	CT Findings
Older age	Mass lesions (subdural, intracerebral hematoma, multiple contusions)
Lower GCS	
Abnormal motor response	
Abnormal pupillary response	Compressed or absent mesencephalic cisterns
Sustained ICP >20 mmHg	
Hypotension (SBP <90 mmHg)	Midline shift >3 mm
Hypoxia (PaO$_2$ <60 mmHg)	Subarachnoid hemorrhage
Systemic complications	

Abbreviations: CT, computed tomography; GCS, Glasgow Coma Scale; ICP, intracranial pressure; SBP, systolic blood pressure; PaO$_2$, arterial partial pressure of oxygen.

KEY POINTS

• Most important steps include maintaining adequate CPP as a means of averting cerebral ischemia, and recognizing that excessive hyperventilation to control intracranial hypertension may promote ischemia

• Most widely used method of defining level of consciousness is GCS (Table 82.1)

• Meaningful recovery of function after head injury is possible if patients rapidly and effectively resuscitated, surgical mass lesions emergently evaluated, and secondary insults prevented or minimized

• Optimizing conditions for cellular recovery by maintaining adequate CPP, normalizing ICP, and averting additional secondary insults essential in overall treatment of head injured patients

• Strong predictors of poor outcome following head injury are older age, low postresuscitation GCS, abnormal motor response, pupillary dilatation or asymmetry, hypotension, hypoxia, intracranial hypertension

• CT findings predictive of poor outcome include mass lesions (particularly acute subdural hematomas, intracerebral hematomas, or multiple contusions), compressed or absent mesencephalic cisterns, significant midline shift (≥3 mm), or presence of subarachnoid hemorrhage

DIAGNOSIS

Once in the hospital, care of the head injury victim should progress in a rapid yet systematic manner with diagnostic and therapeutic maneuvers proceeding simultaneously. The most immediate concerns are establishing a secure airway, providing adequate ventilation, and correcting or preventing hypoxia and hypotension. Simultaneously, a general survey is performed to determine whether major extracranial injuries are present that may take priority. Initial radiologic studies in the trauma patient include cervical spine, chest, and pelvic films. It is critical that the cervical spine series include a lateral view x-ray, which visualizes the cervicothoracic junction. If the C7-T1 junction is not seen on the lateral view, despite arm traction or a swimmer's view, a CT scan through the level of concern will suffice. An indwelling catheter to monitor urine output and an orogastric or nasogastric tube should be placed. Nasogastric tube insertion is contraindicated when there is a suspected anterior cranial base or midface fracture, given the risk of producing an intracranial injury. Initial laboratory studies should include a type and cross-match for possible blood transfusion, complete blood count, serum electrolytes, an arterial blood gas, clotting studies (including prothrombin time and partial thromboplastin time), and a urinalysis. A blood alcohol level and a urine toxicology screen for amphetamines, cocaine, and phencyclidine (PCP) are also useful.

The depth and pace of the initial neurologic survey in the head injured patient depends largely on the patient's level of consciousness and the extent of associated injuries. In the moderate or severely injured patient (GCS ≤13), the examination is necessarily abbreviated and should focus on the level of consciousness (GCS), the pupillary light reflexes, extraocular eye movements, lower brain stem reflexes for patients in deep coma, and the motor examination (Case 2). An exhaustive neurologic evaluation is not indicated; the primary aim is to assess rapidly the level of consciousness and detect focal neurologic deficits.

As part of the neurologic assessment, the head should be carefully palpated to detect bony step-offs and all scalp lacerations gently probed to assess for depressed fractures and foreign bodies. Signs of a basal skull fracture are also sought, including hemotympanum, cerebrospinal fluid (CSF) otorrhea, or rhinorrhea, and retromastoid or periorbital ecchymosis and tenderness. This initial neurologic survey, along with inspection of the neck and thoracolumbar spine, should take no longer than 5 minutes.

> **KEY POINTS**
>
> • Once in hospital, care of head injury victim should progress in rapid, systematic manner with diagnostic and therapeutic maneuvers proceeding simultaneously
>
> • Most immediate concerns are establishing secure airway, providing adequate ventilation, and correcting or preventing hypoxia and hypotension
>
> • Critical that the cervical spine series include a lateral view x-ray, which visualizes the cervicothoracic junction
>
> • Exhaustive neurologic evaluation not indicated; primary aim is to assess rapidly the level of consciousness and detect focal neurologic deficits

DIFFERENTIAL DIAGNOSIS

The triad of a deteriorating level of consciousness, pupillary dilatation, and an associated hemiparesis is highly suggestive of a hemispheric mass lesion causing transtentorial herniation. However, any one of these findings in a patient after head injury may be a manifestation of a traumatic hematoma and when noted should heighten the urgency of evaluation. The mass lesion is typically located ipsilateral to the side of a dilated pupil and contralateral to the motor deficit, with the pupillary finding being slightly more reliable than the motor examination. The patient with the epidural hematoma (Case 1) demonstrated two components of the triad, namely, a deterioration in consciousness and onset of a mild hemiparesis manifested by a pronator drift. Case 2 is an example of the Kernohan's notch phenomenon in which the motor deficit (extensor posturing) occurs ipsilateral to the side of the lesion. This finding is observed when a mass produces a brain stem shift, resulting in compression of the contralateral cerebral peduncle. Thus, the signs of herniation may be falsely localizing (Case 2), may occur relatively late in the course of injury or not at all, or may be observed in patients with diffuse brain injuries (i.e., in those without mass lesions). Additionally, there are no characteristic neurologic findings that reliably distinguish epidural, subdural, or intracerebral hematomas from each other.

Because the neurologic examination is frequently unreliable in accurately predicting intracranial pathology, radiologic evaluation (preferably with CT) is always indicated in the acutely head injured patient. An axial CT scan without contrast that extends from the skull base to the vertex rapidly and unequivocally defines intracranial lesions and determines whether urgent neurosurgical intervention is required. Obtaining both brain and bone "windows" will help determine the etiology and significance of focal neurologic findings and whether a skull fracture is present, thus obviating the need for skull x-rays. CT is indicated in all head injured patients with a depressed level of consciousness, especially in those who appear to be heavily intoxicated with alcohol. A timely CT scan is also indicated in all patients with a GCS of 15 who sustain a loss of consciousness, are amnestic for the injury, have a focal neurologic deficit, or have signs of a basilar or calvarial skull fracture (Table 82.3).

Other etiologies of a diminished level of consciousness must also be considered in the patient who appears to have sustained a head injury. Such causes include generalized seizures and the postictal state, alcohol intoxication, drug overdose, and severe hypoglycemia. Pharmacologically induced pupillary abnormalities are also common in head injured patients. Opiates such as heroin, morphine, and fentanyl will typically result in miotic but reactive pupils. Atropine, especially when given in large doses during acute resuscitation, may cause poorly reactive mydriatic pupils. Significant hypothermia can also result in nonreactive pupils.

> **KEY POINTS**
>
> • Triad of a deteriorating level of consciousness, pupillary dilatation, and an associated hemiparesis highly suggestive of a hemispheric mass lesion causing transtentorial herniation
>
> • Because the neurologic examination is frequently unreliable in predicting intracranial pathology, radiologic evaluation (preferably with CT) always indicated in acutely head injured patients
>
> • CT indicated in all head injured patients with depressed level of consciousness, especially in those heavily intoxicated with alcohol

TABLE 82.3 *CT scanning criteria following craniocerebral trauma*[a]

GCS of ≤14
GCS of 15 with documented loss of consciousness, amnesia for injury, focal neurologic deficit, and/or signs of basal or calvarial skull fracture

[a]Given the significant risk of rapid deterioration in the mildly head injured patient, the threshold for obtaining a timely CT scan should be low.

TREATMENT

Measures to control intracranial hypertension should begin before obtaining a CT scan in individuals who arrive in coma (GCS ≤8), have a precipitous decline in level of consciousness, or who develop pupillary asymmetry or hemiparesis, given the likelihood that a traumatic mass lesion is responsible for the patient's deterioration (Case 2). Such interventions include airway intubation and assisted ventilation, sedation, bolus mannitol therapy, and administration of prophylactic antiseizure medications (phenytoin). Prevention of hypotension with adequate volume resuscitation and in some cases, vasopressor therapy, is also critical to maintain adequate CPP and to help control ICP (Table 82.4).

Specific indications for endotracheal intubation in the head injured patient include inability to maintain adequate ventilation, impending airway loss from neck or pharyngeal injury, poor airway protection associated with depressed level of consciousness, or the potential for neurologic deterioration when the patient leaves the emergency room. Those who are not verbalizing and cannot follow commands should be promptly intubated. In general, this means that all patients with GCS of 8 or less require intubation and assisted ventilation. Additionally, the great majority of severe head injury patients require ICP monitoring. A ventriculostomy is the preferred method, which allows for both monitoring and treatment of ICP through CSF drainage.

The most critical factors in deciding whether to proceed with surgical evacuation of an intracranial hematoma are the patient's neurologic status and the CT findings. Surgical intervention is indicated in all deteriorating patients harboring an intracranial hematoma causing significant mass effect and brain shift (Case 1). Preemptive measures against intracranial hypertension begun in the emergency department should continue, including narcotic sedation, neuromuscular blocking agents as needed,

hyperventilation to maintain the $PaCO_2$ in the range of 30–35 mmHg, and the administration of mannitol and phenytoin. Over one-half of traumatic intracranial hematomas requiring evacuation are subdural in location; intracerebral and epidural hematomas comprise the remainder. Acute intracranial hematomas cannot be adequately removed through burr holes and a craniotomy is required for their evacuation.

Cerebral perfusion pressure is the difference between the mean arterial pressure (MAP) and the ICP. In normal subjects, mean arterial pressure ranges from 80–100 mmHg and ICP is 5–10 mmHg, resulting in a normal CPP range of 70–95 mmHg. Cerebral autoregulation is the occurrence of vasodilatation in response to a decrease in CPP or the occurrence of vasoconstriction in response to an increase in CPP. Cerebral pressure autoregulation normally has a lower perfusion pressure limit of approximately 40–50 mmHg and an upper limit of approximately 140 mmHg. Below a perfusion pressure of 40 mmHg, compensatory cerebral arteriolar vasodilatation is exhausted and cerebral ischemia results. Above a perfusion pressure of 140 mmHg, cerebral vasoconstriction is overcome, cerebral blood flow increases parallel to CPP, resulting in blood-brain barrier damage and brain edema. After severe head injury, pressure autoregulation is disturbed in up to one-half of individuals. Probably the most important aspect of this derangement is that the lower limit of perfusion pressure at which autoregulation will function is elevated. Consequently, such patients require a CPP of at least 60–70 mmHg to achieve autoregulatory function and optimization of cerebral blood flow. A drop in blood pressure of CPP below this critical level will result in a passive fall in cerebral blood flow, which may lead to ischemia. In individuals with predominantly intact pressure autoregulation, an increase in cerebral blood volume exacerbates intracranial hypertension. Therefore, in either situation (intact or impaired autoregulation), hypotension (low CPP) is deleterious to the already injured brain and must be aggressively corrected or avoided. By maintaining CPP at or above 70 mmHg after severe head injury, the risk of cerebral ischemia is reduced, ICP control is facilitated through enhanced autoregulatory function, and long term outcome is improved.

The first step in establishing adequate CPP is vascular volume expansion. If perfusion pressure remains insufficient after volume therapy and after treatment to reduce ICP, the use of induced hypertension or inotropic support is indicated (Case 2). In patients with precipitous drops in blood pressure or perfusion pressure, urgent and simultaneous use of volume expansion and vasopressors should be instituted. A search for the underlying cause of hemodynamic instability should also be undertaken.

Treatment of intracranial hypertension is performed in a stepwise manner. Routine preemptive measures exercised in all severe head injury patients include mainte-

TABLE 82.4 *Emergent management of intracranial hypertension*[a]

Intubation

Controlled ventilation to $PaCO_2$ of 35 mmHg

Volume resuscitation

Establishment of normotension

Narcotic sedation/neuromuscular blockade

Bolus mannitol 1 g/kg

Phenytoin 18 mg/kg

[a]When head injured patients arrive in coma (GCS of ≤8), precipitously deteriorate in level of consciousness, or have pupillary dilatation or obvious hemiparesis, such interventions are typically implemented even before obtaining a head CT scan.

nance of normothermia, head elevation to 30 degrees with neutral cervical alignment, and mild hyperventilation. When acute and sustained rises in ICP occur, additional therapies to control ICP are utilized as needed, often in a simultaneous fashion. These include ventricular drainage, narcotic sedation and neuromuscular blockade, followed by bolus mannitol administration, and finally, in some select individuals, metabolic suppression therapy with administration of high dose pentobarbital (Case 2) (Table 82.5). Given the risk of acute increases in ICP with generalized seizure activity, prophylactic anticonvulsants should also be administered for at least the first week postinjury; phenytoin with serum levels maintained in the high therapeutic range (15–20 µg/L) is efficacious.

Additional concerns in the moderate or severe head injury patient include nutritional support and management of systemic or extracranial derangement. Traumatic brain injury results in a generalized hypermetabolic and hypercatabolic state. Ideally, full nutritional support is begun within 24–48 hours of injury, preferably through the enteral route. Delivery of jejunal feedings is preferred given that ileus, which typically occurs for several days after head injury, is predominantly restricted to the stomach. Comatose head injured patients are also at high risk of developing electrolyte disturbances, pneumonia, thromboembolic complications, and gastrointestinal hemorrhage. Careful monitoring of these problems is warranted, as are appropriate prophylactic interventions such as subcutaneous heparin for prevention of deep vein thrombosis and pulmonary embolus, and sucralfate therapy for peptic ulcer prevention.

TABLE 82.5 *Medical management of intracranial hypertension*

Preemptive measures

    Head elevation to 30 degrees, neutral alignment

    Mild hyperventilation (PaCO$_2$ 30–35 mmHg)

    Maintenance of euvolemia

    Maintenance of CPP at ≥70 mmHg

    Maintenance of normothermia (<37.5°C)

    Seizure prophylaxis (phenytoin)

Primary therapy

    Ventricular CSF drainage

    Sedation (narcotics, benzodiazepines)

    Neuromuscular blockade

Secondary therapy

    Bolus mannitol administration

    Elevation of cerebral perfusion pressure

Tertiary therapy

    Metabolic suppressive therapy with high dose barbiturates or propofol

KEY POINTS

• Measures to control intracranial hypertension should begin before obtaining a CT in those who arrive in coma (GCS ≤8), have precipitous decline in consciousness level, or who develop pupillary asymmetry or hemiparesis, given likelihood that traumatic mass lesion is responsible for patient's deterioration

• Such interventions include airway intubation and assisted ventilation, sedation, bolus mannitol therapy, and administration of prophylactic antiseizure medication

• Prevention of hypotension with adequate volume resuscitation and vasopressor therapy is critical to maintain adequate CPP and to help control ICP (Table 82.4)

• All patients with GCS of 8 or less require intubation and assisted ventilation, and most require ICP monitoring

• Acute intracranial hematomas cannot be adequately removed through burr holes, because of solid nature; craniotomy required

• CPP is difference between MAP and ICP; in normal subjects, MAP ranges from 80–100 mmHg and ICP is 5–10 mmHg, resulting in CPP of 70–95 mmHg

• Cerebral autoregulation is occurrence of vasodilatation in response to decrease in CPP or occurrence of vasoconstriction in response to increase in CPP; cerebral pressure autoregulation normally has lower perfusion pressure limit of 40–50 mmHg and upper limit of approximately 140 mmHg

• By maintaining CPP at or above 70 mmHg after severe head injury, risk of cerebral ischemia is reduced, ICP control facilitated through enhanced autoregulatory function, and long-term outcome is improved

• First step in establishing adequate CPP is vascular volume expansion

• Treatment of intracranial hypertension is performed in stepwise manner

FOLLOW-UP

In the early weeks after discharge following traumatic brain injury, complaints of persistent headache, confusion, or gait disturbance should prompt a repeat CT to evaluate the development of post-traumatic hydrocephalus. Long-term follow-up is dictated largely by the degree of neurologic and physical disability. For patients who are discharged fully conscious and independent (Case 1), the most common complaints are neuropsychologic in nature, with memory and behavioral disturbances occurring most frequently. Referral to a psychologist for evaluation and counseling may be indicated in some individuals. Patients with significant residual mental and physical deficits (Case 2) are best managed at a comprehensive rehabilitation unit for several months. Recovery of function from the time of discharge to 6 months postinjury can be dramatic, even in severely impaired or vegetative individuals. Improvement generally begins to plateau at 6 months after injury and is typically maximal by 1 year. Individuals sustaining a traumatic intracranial hematoma have an approximate 25% risk of developing late epilepsy. Prophylactic anticonvulsant therapy for late epilepsy is commonly practiced in these patients but its effectiveness remains unproved.

KEY POINTS

• Recovery of function from time of discharge to 6 months postinjury can be dramatic, even in severely impaired or vegetative individuals

• Improvement generally begins to plateau at 6 months postinjury and is maximal by 1 year

SUGGESTED READINGS

Kelly DF, Nikas DL, Becker DP: Diagnosis and treatment of moderate and severe head injuries in adults. p. 1678. In Youmans J (ed): Neurological Surgery. 4th Ed. WB Saunders, Philadelphia, 1995

This chapter provides a relatively comprehensive and current review of the epidemiology, diagnosis, and management of moderate and severe head injury in adults, with attention to emergency resuscitation and initial management decisions.

Marshall LF, Gautille T, Klauber MR et al: The outcome of severe closed head injury. J Neurosurg, suppl., 75:s28, 1991

Summarizes the outcome of over 700 severe closed head injury patients studied in the multicenter, National Institutes of Health-funded Traumatic Coma Data Bank project.

Rosner MJ: Pathophysiology and management of increased intracranial pressure. p. 57. In Andrews BT (ed): Neurosurgical Intensive Care. McGraw-Hill, New York, 1993.

A useful discussion of the pathophysiology and current management of intracranial hypertension. The importance of cerebral perfusion pressure in relation to ICP is stressed.

QUESTIONS

1. Optimized conditions for recovery after head injury include all but one of the following?

    A. Decreased ICP.

    B. Increased CCP.

    C. Decreased MAP.

    D. Averting secondary insults.

2. Transtentorial herniation is suggested by all except one of the following?

    A. Deteriorating level of consciousness.

    B. Pupillary dilatation.

    C. Hemiparesis.

    D. Babinski's reflex.

3. The most critical factors in deciding whether to proceed with evaluation of an intracranial hematoma are?

    A. Neurologic examination and CT scan.

    B. Change in ICP and CCP.

    C. Depressed respiration and exterior posturing.

    D. An epidural location and increased ICP.

4. The first step in establishing adequate CPP in a head injured patient is?

    A. Use of a pressor such as dobutamine.

    B. Vascular volume expansion.

    C. Hyperventilation.

    D. Use of mannitol and phenytoin.

(See p. 605 for answers.)

A N S W E R S

Chapter 2
1. D
2. D
3. C
4. C

Chapter 3
1. D
2. C
3. A
4. D

Chapter 4
1. B
2. C
3. B
4. D

Chapter 5
1. D
2. B
3. A
4. D

Chapter 6
1. B
2. D
3. B

Chapter 7
1. D
2. B
3. C
4. C

Chapter 8
1. B
2. C
3. A
4. C

Chapter 9
1. C
2. D
3. C

Chapter 10
1. A
2. C
3. B
4. C

Chapter 11
1. E
2. B

Chapter 12
1. C
2. D
3. A
4. B

Chapter 13
1. D
2. B
3. D

Chapter 14
1. A
2. B
3. C
4. C

Chapter 15
1. D
2. D

Chapter 16
1. D
2. D

Chapter 17
1. A
2. D

Chapter 18
1. D
2. D
3. D
4. B

Chapter 19
1. D
2. B
3. D

Chapter 20
1. C
2. C
3. C

Chapter 21
1. D
2. C

Chapter 22
1. B
2. B
3. A

Chapter 23
1. D
2. B
3. D

Chapter 24
1. C
2. B
3. D
4. A
5. D

Chapter 25
1. B
2. D
3. C

Chapter 26
1. E
2. D
3. D
4. C

Chapter 27
1. D
2. A
3. D

Chapter 28
1. C
2. A and B
3. B

Chapter 29
1. D
2. E

Chapter 30
1. E
2. C

Chapter 31
1. C
2. E
3. D

Chapter 32
1. C
2. E

Chapter 33
1. C
2. A

Chapter 34
1. B
2. E

Chapter 35
1. D
2. D
3. C

Chapter 36
1. E
2. A

Chapter 37
1. D
2. B

Chapter 38
1. A
2. E

Chapter 39
1. E
2. A

Chapter 40
1. A
2. B
3. E
4. E
5. D

Chapter 41
1. B
2. E
3. E
4. C

Chapter 42
1. E
2. D
3. B
4. F

Chapter 43
1. A
2. D
3. A
4. D

Chapter 44
1. B
2. C
3. D
4. A

Chapter 45
1. C
2. A
3. D
4. A

Chapter 46
1. C
2. D
3. C
4. A

Chapter 47
1. B
2. C
3. D

Chapter 48
1. D
2. A
3. B
4. A

Chapter 49
1. C
2. D
3. A
4. B

Chapter 50
1. A
2. B
3. B
4. B

Chapter 51.
1. D
2. C
3. A

Chapter 52
1. B
2. D
3. B
4. D

Chapter 53
1. A
2. D
3. B
4. A

Chapter 54
1. B
2. D
3. C
4. D

Chapter 55
1. D
2. B
3. A
4. A

Chapter 56
1. C
2. C
3. B

Chapter 57
1. B
2. B

Chapter 58
1. D
2. D
3. A

Chapter 59
1. D
2. E

Chapter 60
1. B
2. A
3. D

Chapter 61.
1. B
2. D
3. C
4. B

Chapter 62
1. B
2. B

Chapter 63
1. D
2. C

Chapter 64
1. B
2. C
3. A

Chapter 65
1. D
2. D
3. D

Chapter 66
1. C
2. D
3. B

Chapter 67
1. B
2. C

Chapter 68
1. B
2. D
3. D

Chapter 69
1. D
2. D

Chapter 70
1. D
2. D

Chapter 71
1. E
2. B
3. B

Chapter 72
1. E
2. D
3. A = 1
   B = 2

Chapter 73
1. D
2. A

Chapter 74
1. E
2. C

Chapter 75
1. D
2. E

Chapter 76
1. A
2. E

Chapter 77
1. C
2. E

Chapter 78
1. E
2. C

Chapter 79
1. A
2. B
3. D

Chapter 80
1. A
2. B
3. C
4. C

Chapter 81
1. B
2. C
3. C

Chapter 82
1. C
2. D
3. A
4. B

INDEX

Page numbers followed by f *indicate figures; those followed by* t *indicate tables.*